Current Anesthesia Practice and Certification Review

Second Edition

Current Anesthesia Practice *and* Certification Review

Sass Elisha
EdD, CRNA, FAANA, FAAN
Assistant Director
Kaiser Permanente School of Anesthesia

Jeremy S. Heiner
EdD, CRNA, FAANA
Academic and Clinical Educator
Kaiser Permanente School of Anesthesia

ELSEVIER

Elsevier
3251 Riverport Lane
St. Louis, Missouri 63043

Current Anesthesia Practice and Certification Review, Second Edition **ISBN: 978-0-443-38100-3**

Previous editions copyrighted 2021.

Executive Content Strategist: Sonya Seigafuse
Senior Content Development Manager: Lisa Newton
Senior Content Development Specialist: Laura Selkirk
Publishing Services Manager: Deepthi Unni
Project Manager: Erragounta Saibabu Rao Erragounta
Senior Book Designer: Amy Buxton

Printed in India at Replika Press Pvt. Ltd.
Plot No. 310-311, EPIP, HSIIDC, Kundli Industrial Park,
Sonipat, Haryana – 131028.

Last digit is the print number: 9 8 7 6 5 4 3 2 1

We dedicate the second edition of *Current Anesthesia Practice and Certification Review* to our dear friend and mentor, Dr. John Nagelhout, who recently passed away. Through his brilliance as an educator, scientist, and practitioner, he has inspired the next generation of leaders to continue his legacy of excellence in anesthesia practice. It is impossible to quantify all of the lives that John touched during his 35-year career as a certified registered nurse anesthetist (CRNA). His teachings will positively affect our nurse anesthesia community for eternity.

PREFACE

To certified registered nurse anesthetists (CRNAs) who provide the highest quality of care to our patients every day, the value that you bring to the lives of so many people is immeasurable. The main objective of *Current Anesthesia Practice and Certification Review* is to serve as a review of the scientific underpinnings that are foundational for competent anesthesia practice. As the pace and critical nature of the operating room continue to become more demanding, and with the increased incidence and complexity of comorbid diseases, nurse anesthetists need a comprehensive resource that will help them improve their recognition, clinical decision making, and treatment of perioperative complications.

As a result of the rigors of modern anesthesia practice, it is difficult to remain proficient in every possible clinical scenario. This book provides a concise synopsis of the principles related to current practice and the elements of crisis management.

At the end of each content area, there are questions, with answers in Appendix A, to help you assess your knowledge and comprehension of key concepts. We sincerely hope that you find yourself frequently reviewing the information contained within this book as you continue to enhance and refine your anesthesia practice throughout your career.

Sass Elisha
Jeremy S. Heiner

CONTENTS

1 **Airway Management,** 1
- Anatomy, 1
- Physiologic Concepts, 17
- Pathophysiologic Concepts, 25
- Airway Blocks, 39
- Airway Assessment, 43
- Airway Equipment, Management of Devices, and Procedures, 47
- Airway Management Concepts, 62

2 **Pharmacology,** 80
- General Principles of Pharmacodynamics and Pharmacokinetics, 80
- Inhalation Anesthetics, 86
- Anesthesia Induction Medications, 94
- Induction Agents, 97
- Opiates, 99
- Neuromuscular Blocking Agents, 106
- Anticholinesterase Agents, 112
- Selective Muscle Relaxant Binding Agent, 115
- Anticholinergics, 118
- Autonomic Nervous System—Sympathomimetic Amines, 120
- α-Adrenergic Blocking Agents, 125
- β-Adrenergic Blocking Agents, 128
- Bronchodilators, 130
- Calcium Channel Blockers, 130
- Antihypertensive Agents, 132
- Vasodilators, 135
- Antiarrhythmics, 137
- Digitalis, 138
- Diuretics, 140
- Nonsteroidal Antiinflammatory Agents, 141
- Miscellaneous Analgesics, 145
- Local Anesthetics, 147
- Oral Antacids, 154
- Antiparkinsonian Drugs, 155
- Antibiotics, 155
- Anticoagulants, 163
- Antiemetics, 168
- Histamine Receptor Antagonists, 174
- Antiepileptic Drugs, 176
- Dantrolene, 177
- Herbal Supplements, 178
- Insulin, 181
- Oral Hypoglycemics, 183
- Intravenous Dyes, 186
- Lipid-Lowering Agents, 187
- Phosphodiesterase Inhibitors, 188
- Psychopharmacology, 189
- Corticosteroids, 193
- Uterotonics, 194

3 **Human Physiology, Pathophysiology, and Anesthesia Case Management,** 196
- Cardiovascular System, 196
- Respiratory System, 236
- Neurologic System, 270
- Endocrine System, 292
- Adrenocortical Insufficiency, 303
- Adrenal Medulla (Inner Layer), 304
- Hepatic System, 314
- Renal System, 339
- Thermoregulation, 368

4 **Anesthesia Equipment and Technology,** 372
- Infection Control: Disinfection, 372
- Monitoring Modalities, 375
- Anesthesia Gas Machine, 411
- Standards for Preanesthesia Evaluation and Informed Consent, 422

Appendix A: Knowledge Check Answers, 425
Index, 431

1

Airway Management

Airway management is a critical aspect of anesthesia practice. A thorough knowledge of airway anatomy, physiology, and pathophysiologic conditions helps providers develop safe and effective airway management plans, and an understanding of the various airway assessments, equipment, procedures, and decision-making strategies assists with the development of a comprehensive airway plan. An awareness of the complications that can occur before, during, or after airway management, as well as an understanding of the different airway management techniques, will help the anesthesia provider keep patients safe as they manage the airway.

ANATOMY

Upper Airway (Above Cricoid Cartilage)

Nose and Nasal Cavity

- The nasal cavity has four functions: (1) to filter pathogens and particulates from inhaled air, (2) to heat and humidify inhaled air, (3) to assist with the sense of smell, and (4) to facilitate the drainage of the paranasal sinuses and lacrimal ducts.
- The nasal cavity extends from the vestibule (area surrounding the anterior opening to the nasal cavity) to the nasopharynx and contains a respiratory conduction region and an olfactory region.
- The *respiratory conduction region* contains ciliated, pseudostriated epithelium with interspersed mucus-secreting goblet cells. This type of cellular structure continues into the lower airway. In addition, the nasal turbinates are located in the respiratory conduction area to facilitate the filtering, heating, and direction of airflow.
- The *olfactory region* is located at the apex of the nasal cavity, and it is lined with olfactory cells, nerves, and receptors.

Turbinates

- The superior, middle, and inferior turbinates (nasal concha) are curved protrusions of spongy bone lined with thick mucosa (mucoperiosteum) that are arranged one above the other on the lateral wall of the nasal cavity. Each contains extensive vascular beds. The turbinates project their free borders downward and inward, curling over themselves similar to how a scroll is rolled. They cover the openings to the paranasal sinuses, which are contained within the superior, middle, and inferior meatus.
- The *superior* and *middle nasal turbinates* arise from the skull and are thus considered part of the cranial bones. Both the superior and middle nasal turbinates project from the inner wall of the ethmoidal labyrinth. The superior nasal turbinate is the smallest turbinate and forms the upper boundary of the superior meatus of the nose. The middle nasal turbinate separates the superior meatus from the middle meatus and extends over the opening of the maxillary and ethmoid sinuses (anterior and middle), protecting these sinuses from pressurized airflow.
- The *inferior nasal turbinates* are the largest turbinates in the nasal cavity. The inferior nasal turbinates are positioned on the right and left lateral walls and extend horizontally within each cavity. They direct the majority of airflow within the nasal cavity and provide the greatest degree of humidification, filtering, and warming of inhaled air. These are the only turbinates that are considered facial bones.
    - Because of their size and position within the nasal cavity, the inferior nasal turbinates are more likely to be traumatized during nasal instrumentation (i.e., endotracheal tube [ETT], nasal airway, nasal gastric tube, and/or endoscopic videoscope insertion and placement).

- Functionally, the turbinates disrupt rapid laminar airflow, causing the flow to become more turbulent. The turbinate configuration within the nasal cavity allows air to contact the large surface area of the turbinates for a prolonged period, promoting better filtration, heating, and humidification. The vasculature contained within the turbinates can dilate or constrict, causing nasal congestion or decongestion, in response to temperature fluctuations. Finally, the turbinates provide humidity to the olfactory epithelium, which helps preserve the sense of smell.
- To avoid trauma to the turbinates during nasal instrumentation (e.g., ETT, gastric tube, or nasal airway placement), devices should be lubricated and directed along the floor of the nasal cavity and parallel to the roof of the mouth.
- The bottom of the nasal cavity is formed by the superior aspect of the palatine bone, which forms the hard palate below the nose.
- Beneath the olfactory bulb is the cribriform plate, which forms the boundary between the superior aspect of the nasal cavity and the brain. During head injuries or facial trauma, damage to the cribriform plate may occur. For this reason, nasal intubation and nasogastric tube insertion are absolutely contraindicated because neural tissue can be injured.

Nasal cavity openings (sinuses, ducts, and tubes)

- The frontal, ethmoid, maxillary, and sphenoid sinuses are four paired paranasal sinuses that drain into the nasal cavity.
- The *frontal sinuses* are located above the eyes, the *ethmoidal sinuses* are located between the eyes, the *maxillary sinuses* are located under the eyes (these are the largest paranasal sinuses), and the *sphenoid sinuses* are located behind the eyes.
- The frontal, ethmoid, and maxillary sinuses drain onto the lateral wall of the nasal cavity, whereas the sphenoid sinuses drain onto the posterior roof.
- Each sinus communicates with the nasal cavity via a *sinus ostium*. This opening has a higher percentage of cilia than the surrounding mucosa and allows for the drainage of sinus fluid into the nasal cavity. Nasal mucosal swelling can lead to blockage of the sinus ostium and fluid accumulation within the sinus cavity, causing pressure, pain, and sinusitis.
- Several possible functions of the paranasal sinuses have been suggested, which include the following: (1) a decrease in frontal skull weight, (2) increase in voice resonance, (3) insulation from rapid temperature fluctuations within the nasal cavity, (4) regulation of intranasal gas pressures, (5) humidification and heating of inhaled air, and (6) immunological defense.
- The *nasolacrimal duct* opens into the inferior meatus of the nasal cavity and drains tears from the eyes.
- The *eustachian tube* opens in the nasopharynx and allows the middle ear to equalize with atmospheric pressure.
- Prolonged nasotracheal intubation can lead to obstruction of the paranasal sinuses and sinus infection.
- Swelling within the nasal cavity can obstruct eustachian drainage, and upper airway infection can spread into the middle ear. Either may cause diminished hearing and/or pain.

Vascular supply

- The nasal cavity receives blood from both the internal and external carotid arteries (Fig. 1.1). The rich blood supply promotes rapid humidification and heating of inhaled air.
- The internal carotid artery bifurcates to become the ophthalmic artery, which then divides into the anterior and posterior *ethmoidal arteries*. The ethmoidal arteries enter the nasal cavity through the cribriform plate and supply blood to the superior, middle, and anterior portions of the nasal cavity.
- The external carotid artery gives rise to the maxillary artery. It then branches into the *sphenopalatine* and *descending palatine arteries*. The descending palatine artery branches into the *greater palatine artery* once it passes through the greater palatine foramen, and it supplies the hard palate. This artery travels anteriorly through the hard palate and passes through the incisive canal (pathway between the oral and nasal cavities) to anastomose with the sphenopalatine artery and supply blood to the nasal septum.
- The sphenopalatine artery passes through the sphenopalatine foramen and then branches into the *posterior lateral nasal arteries*, which then spread anteriorly over the nasal turbinates and meatuses to anastomose with the ethmoidal arteries and the nasal portion of the greater palatine artery. The sphenopalatine and nasal arteries supply the posterior, inferior, and middle portions of the nasal cavity.
  - Epistaxis (nosebleeds) is most often caused by the sphenopalatine artery and may require surgical ligation for hemostasis.

Location	Vascular Innervation (Arterial)	Nervous Innervation
Nasal	***Internal Carotid*** ↓ Ophthalmic a. ↓ Anterior & Posterior Ethmoidal a. ***External Carotid*** → Maxillary a. ↓ Sphenopalatine a. ↓ Posterior Lateral Nasal a. ***External Carotid*** → Descending Palatine a. ↓ Greater Palatine a.	***Olfactory*** (cranial nerve I) ***Trigeminal*** (cranial nerve V) → Maxillary n. ↓ Nasopalantine n. Maxillary n. ↓ Greater Palantine n. ↓ Lateral Posterior Inferior Nasal n. ***Trigeminal*** (cranial nerve V) → Ophthalmic n. ↓ Nasociliary n. ↓ Anterior & Posterior Ethmoidal n. ***Facial (cranial nerve VII)*** ↓ Postganglionic Parasympathetic innervation
Oral	***External Carotid*** → Maxillary a. ↓ Greater & Lesser Palantine a. Superior & Inferior Alveolar a. Buccal a. ***External Carotid*** → Lingual a. ***External Carotid*** → Facial a. ↓ Submental a.	***Trigeminal (cranial nerve V)*** → Maxillary n. ↓ Greater & Lesser Palatine n. Nasopalatine n. Superior Alveolar n. ***Trigeminal (cranial nerve V)*** → Mandibular n. ↓ Lingual n. Buccal n. Inferior Alveolar n. ***Facial (cranial nerve VII)*** ↓ Chorda Tympani n. ***Vagus (cranial nerve X)*** ***Glossopharngeal (cranial nerve IX)*** ***Hypoglossal (cranial nerve XII)***
Pharyngeal	***External Carotid*** → Lingual a. / Facial a. / Maxillary a. / Ascending pharyngeal arteries a. ***Subclavian a.*** ↓ Inferior thyroid a.	***Trigeminal (cranial nerve V)*** ↓ Maxillary n. ***Glossopharngeal (cranial nerve IX)*** ↓ Pharyngeal plexus ***Vagus (cranial nerve X)*** ↓ Pharyngeal plexus Superior (internal) laryngeal n. Recurrent laryngeal n. Arnold's n.
Laryngeal	***External Carotid*** ↓ Superior Thyroid a. ↓ Superior Laryngeal a. ↓ Cricothyroid a. ***Subclavian a.*** ↓ Inferior thyroid a. ↓ Inferior Laryngeal a.	***Vagus (cranial nerve X)*** → Superior laryngeal n. / Recurrent laryngeal n.

Fig. 1.1 Vascular and nervous innervation of the oral, nasal, pharyngeal, and laryngeal regions.

Nervous supply

- The functions of nervous innervation within the nasal cavity are smell and sensory (e.g., pain and temperature).
- The *olfactory nerve* (cranial nerve [CN] I) controls the sense of smell. The bulb of this nerve sits on the superior surface of the cribriform plate within the cranial vault. The cribriform plate is a porous bone that allows the nerves of the olfactory bulb to pass through and innervate the nasal cavity to provide the sensation of smell. The olfactory nerve branches are covered and protected by the superior nasal turbinates, and they are located in the upper-third area of the nasal cavity. Some of the olfactory nerve endings innervate the middle turbinate.
- The maxillary and ophthalmic nerve branches of the *trigeminal nerve* (CN V) provide general pain and temperature sensation to the nasal mucosa, maxilla, sinuses, and palate.
- The *nasopalatine nerve* is a branch of the maxillary nerve that enters the nasal cavity through the sphenopalatine foramen. The nasopalatine nerve innervates the nasal septum posteriorly below the orifice of the sphenoid sinus and runs obliquely downward and forward through the septum to pass through the roof of the mouth at the incisive canal, where it then innervates structures of the oral cavity.
- The ophthalmic nerve branches into the *nasociliary nerve* within the orbit of the eye, and the nasociliary nerve then divides into the *anterior* and *posterior ethmoidal nerves*. These nerves innervate the ethmoid sinuses, the anterior septum, and the skin and lateral sides of the nose.
- The anterior ethmoidal nerve innervates the middle and anterior ethmoid sinuses. It enters and descends within the nasal cavity from a superior and anterior position to provide sensory fibers in the anterior septum and lateral portion of the nose.
- The posterior ethmoidal nerve innervates the sphenoid and posterior ethmoid sinuses.
- The *greater palatine nerve* is a division of the maxillary nerve that carries sensory information and passes through the pterygopalatine fossa and pterygopalatine ganglion. As the greater palatine nerve exits the pterygopalatine fossa, it enters the greater palatine canal to innervate the mucosa of the posterior hard palate. While traveling in the canal, it branches off into the *lateral posterior inferior nasal branches* to innervate the nasal cavity.
- The lateral, posterior, and inferior nasal branches of the greater palatine nerve exit the greater palatine canal through the palatine bone to innervate the posterior and inferior nasal cavities; lateral walls; and superior, middle, and inferior nasal turbinates.
- The frontal, maxillary, ethmoid, and sphenoid sinuses are all innervated by the maxillary and ophthalmic nerve branches of the trigeminal nerve.

KNOWLEDGE CHECK

1. Which arteries originate from the internal carotid artery and supply the superior, middle, and anterior portions of the nasal cavity?
   a. Ethmoidal
   b. Sphenopalatine
   c. Maxillary
   d. Descending palatine
2. Which are the largest nasal turbinates?
   a. Superior
   b. Middle
   c. Lateral
   d. Inferior

Answers can be found in Appendix A.

Mouth and Oral Cavity

Oral cavity structures

Hard palate, soft palate, and uvula

- The roof of the mouth comprises the hard and soft palates. The *hard palate* is a bony plate in the roof of the mouth that separates the nasal cavity from the oral cavity. Within the nasal cavity superiorly, it is covered by respiratory mucosa (ciliated, pseudostratified columnar epithelium), whereas within the oral cavity inferiorly, it is covered by oral mucosa (stratified squamous epithelium). The soft palate continues posteriorly from the hard palate and ends at the uvula.
- The *soft palate* is a muscular structure that can either move downward to seal off the oral cavity from the pharynx or rise to occlude the nasopharynx during oropharyngeal swallowing.
- The *uvula* is a projection from the posterior soft palate. It contains muscle fibers that allow it to shorten or broaden, facilitating closure of the soft palate against the posterior pharyngeal wall, thus sealing off the nasopharynx during swallowing. It also contains serous glands that produce thin saliva that lubricates the throat. Additionally, the uvula is considered an accessory speech organ.

Tongue, cheeks, oral cavity floor, and glands

- The floor of the mouth consists of the tongue, bilateral mylohyoid muscles, geniohyoid muscles, and salivary glands and ducts.
- The *tongue* is a large, muscular, flexible organ located within the oral cavity. Inferiorly and posteriorly, the tongue is anchored to the hyoid bone, whereas inferiorly and anteriorly, it is connected to the floor of the mouth by the frenulum. The tongue is covered with specialized mucosa that forms tiny bumps called *papillae*. On the surface of the papillae are thousands of nerve endings that make up taste bud receptors. As such, the tongue has a primary role in taste, mastication, swallowing, and speech.
- The cheeks form the lateral portion of the oral cavity. The insides of the cheeks are lined with buccal mucosa that functions to maintain moisture by secreting mucin (the main part of mucus). The *buccinator muscles* are located laterally and anteriorly at either side of the face between the maxilla and mandible. These muscles provide structure to the cheeks and assist with mastication and swallowing. The space between the teeth and gums and inside the cheek is known as the *vestibule* or *buccal cavity*.
  - When relaxed and positioned posteriorly in the oral and pharyngeal spaces, the tongue is a primary cause of airway obstruction.
  - Macroglossia is an enlarged tongue that can result from congenital, inflammatory, traumatic, cancerous, and metabolic causes. Macroglossia is an indication of a potentially difficult airway.
- The *mylohyoid paired muscles* form a muscular diaphragm that attaches to the right and left sides of the mandible and to the body of the hyoid bone. They provide structural support to the floor of the mouth. Functionally, the mylohyoid muscles elevate the hyoid bone and tongue, which assists with swallowing and speaking.
- The *geniohyoid muscles* are cordlike muscles that are located on the superior surface of the oral cavity floor's muscular diaphragm (mylohyoid muscles). Anteriorly, they attach to the inside center of the mandible and run posteriorly to the body of the hyoid bone. These muscles help provide anterior movement of the larynx during swallowing.
- The *submandibular* and *sublingual glands* are located on the floor of the mouth. The submandibular glands are located below the lower jaw. They secrete saliva into the oral cavity through the submandibular duct, which opens at the base of the tongue on either side of the frenulum. The sublingual glands are located just beneath the tongue and anterior to the submandibular glands. These are the smallest major salivary glands and produce 3%–5% of saliva in the mouth. The secretion of saliva occurs from several small sublingual ducts known as *ducts of Rivinus*. Some of these small ducts join the submandibular duct for saliva drainage.
- The *parotid glands* are the largest salivary glands. They are located on either side of the mouth, anterior to each ear. Their function is to secrete saliva through the parotid ducts into the mouth to facilitate mastication, swallowing, and digestion. The parotid ducts are long excretory ducts that pierce each buccinator muscle and then open into the mouth, opposite each second molar on the inside of the cheek.

Skeletal framework of the oral cavity and teeth

- The maxilla, palatine, and temporal bones are all paired.
- The mandible, sphenoid, and hyoid bones are unpaired.
- The upper teeth are fixed to elevated arches of alveolar bone in the maxilla, whereas the lower teeth are fixed to elevated arches of alveolar bone in the mandible.
- Gingiva (gums) are specialized oral mucosa that cover the alveolar bone and surround the teeth.
- If the teeth are removed, the alveolar bone is reabsorbed, and the arches disappear.
- The teeth are notable by their position and function. From anterior to posterior, the teeth consist of incisors, canines, premolars, and molars.
- An adult has 32 complete teeth, each identified by a number starting with the upper right "wisdom" molar on the maxilla. The upper 16 are counted from right to left on the maxilla, and the lower 16 continue from left to right on the mandible. As such, the upper four incisors (from right to left) consist of teeth numbers 7, 8, 9, and 10, whereas the lower four incisors (from left to right) consist of teeth numbers 23, 24, 25, and 26.

Vascular supply

- The majority of arterial blood to the oral cavity is supplied by arteries branching from the *external carotid artery* (see Fig. 1.1).
- Veins generally follow the arteries within the oral cavity and have the same names. Venous drainage

from the palate is via the pterygoid venous plexus, whereas drainage from the tongue goes into the internal jugular vein.

- The *greater* and *lesser palatine arteries* arise from the maxillary artery. The greater palatine artery supplies the hard palate, whereas the lesser palatine artery supplies the soft palate.
- The maxillary artery branches into the *superior* and *inferior alveolar arteries*, which provide blood supply to the upper and lower teeth.
- *Lingual arterial branches* supply blood to the tongue. The deep lingual artery supplies the anterior tongue, whereas the dorsal lingual arteries supply the posterior tongue. The sublingual artery provides blood to the floor of the mouth and the sublingual gland.
- *Submental arteries* supply the submandibular and sublingual glands.
- Blood supply to the parotid salivary glands is from branches of the external carotid artery as well as the superficial temporal arteries.
- The *buccal artery* provides blood supply to the lateral cheek portions of the oral cavity.

Nervous supply

- The *trigeminal nerve* divides into the *maxillary* and *mandibular nerve branches*, which provide sensory information to the oral cavity.
- The maxillary branch divides into the *greater* and *lesser palatine* and *nasopalatine nerves*, which innervate the hard and soft palates.
- The mandibular branch gives rise to the *lingual* and *buccal nerves*. The lingual nerve provides sensory innervation to the floor of the oral cavity and anterior two-thirds of the tongue, whereas the buccal nerve innervates the skin and mucosa of each cheek.
- Special sensory taste fibers called *chorda tympani* arise from the facial nerve and innervate the anterior two-thirds of the tongue.
- The *superior* and *inferior alveolar nerves* arise from the maxillary and mandibular branches of the trigeminal nerve. The alveolar nerves create the *dental plexus*, which innervates the teeth.
- The *inferior alveolar nerve* innervates the mylohyoid muscles.
- The lingual, palatine, nasopalatine, and alveolar nerves provide sensory innervation to the gingiva (gums).
- The *lingual nerve* provides sensation to the anterior two-thirds of the tongue, whereas the *glossopharyngeal nerve* provides sensory innervation to the posterior third. The *facial nerve* carries taste sensations to the central nervous system (CNS). Finally, the *hypoglossal nerve* provides all motor function for the tongue (except for the palatoglossal muscle, which is innervated by the vagus nerve).
- The *vagus nerve* innervates the muscles of the soft palate.

KNOWLEDGE CHECK

1. Which nerve provides sensory innervation to the posterior third of the tongue?
   a. Hypoglossal
   b. Glossopharyngeal
   c. Lingual
   d. Trigeminal
2. Which is considered a paired bone within the oral cavity?
   a. Mandible
   b. Maxilla
   c. Sphenoid
   d. Hyoid

Answers can be found in Appendix A.

Pharynx

Nasopharynx, oropharynx, and hypopharynx

- The *pharynx* is a hollow muscular tube that connects the oral and nasal cavities to the larynx and esophagus. It expands from the base of the skull to the bottom of the cricoid cartilage. It is divided into the nasopharynx, oropharynx, and laryngopharynx (hypopharynx).
- The *nasopharynx* extends from the base of the skull to the upper surface of the soft palate. This area functions to conduct air during inhalation and then funnel it toward the larynx. The eustachian (auditory) tubes open into the nasopharynx.
- The *oropharynx* is posterior to the oral cavity and extends from the soft palate to the superior border of the epiglottis. The posterior third of the tongue is the anterior border of the oropharynx. It plays a role in both the voluntary and involuntary phases of swallowing and conducts airflow to the larynx.
- The *laryngopharynx* or *hypopharynx* is the most caudal portion of the pharynx. It begins with the inferior border of the epiglottis and extends to the pyriform sinuses and cricopharyngeus muscle. Similar to the oropharynx, the laryngopharynx facilitates the passage of food and air.

    - The *pyriform sinuses* are spaces formed between muscle fibers that are attached to the thyroid cartilage and are adjacent to each side of the inferior border of the cricoid cartilage.
- The *superior*, *middle*, and *inferior pharyngeal muscles* are arranged in sequence and contract from top to bottom to constrict the pharyngeal lumen and propel food boluses and liquid inferiorly into the esophagus.
    - The superior pharyngeal constrictor functions within the oropharynx, whereas the middle pharyngeal constrictor acts on the upper portion of the laryngopharynx.
    - The inferior pharyngeal constrictor, the thickest of the three constrictor muscles, acts on the lower laryngopharynx and has two sections. The superior section is the thyropharyngeus, which attaches to the thyroid cartilage. The inferior section is the cricopharyngeus, which attaches to the cricoid cartilage.
- The *stylopharyngeus*, *salpingopharyngeus*, and *palatopharyngeus muscles* function to elevate the pharynx and larynx to facilitate swallowing.
    - The salpingopharyngeus muscle opens the eustachian tube during swallowing to equalize the pressure between the atmosphere and the auditory canal.

Lingual, palatine, tubal, and pharyngeal tonsils (Waldeyer tonsillar ring)

- The lingual, palatine, tubal, and pharyngeal tonsils, also known as the *Waldeyer tonsillar ring*, are a collection of tonsillar lymphatic tissues that surround the upper pharynx. The function of this lymphatic tissue is to provide an immunological response to pathogens that are ingested or inhaled.
    - The *lingual tonsil* makes up the inferior part of the ring and sits at the posterior base of the tongue in the oropharynx.
    - The *palatine tonsils* sit between the palatoglossal and glossopharyngeal arches on each side of the oral cavity. These form the anterior lateral part of the ring and are the tonsils seen on each side of the tongue during oral examination.
    - The posterior lateral portion is formed by the *tubal tonsils*, which are located in the nasopharynx next to where each eustachian tube opens.
    - The superior part of the Waldeyer tonsillar ring is the *pharyngeal tonsil*, also called the *adenoid tonsil*. The adenoids are located posterior to the uvula on the posterior roof of the nasopharynx.
- Lingual tonsillar hypertrophy can be a source of airway obstruction that is difficult to assess externally. This condition is frequently realized during laryngoscopy, causing unanticipated difficulty with viewing the glottic opening and supporting structures.
- Chronic viral or bacterial infection of the palatine tonsils can lead to inflammation and hypertrophy. This can cause upper airway obstruction requiring tonsillectomy.
- Bleeding as a result of a tonsillectomy can be from the external palatine vein or the tonsillar branch of the facial artery.
- Recurrent viral infections of the adenoid tonsil can lead to chronic pathological enlargement, causing obstruction of the eustachian tube openings. This prevents normal drainage and equalization with atmospheric pressure within the middle ear. These conditions are ideal for infection and can lead to chronic otitis media.

Upper esophageal sphincter

- This area is formed by the *cricopharyngeus muscle* to serve as a valve at the top of the esophagus.
- The most inferior pharyngeal structure is the cricopharyngeus muscle, also known as the *inferior pharyngeal sphincter*.
- When the cricopharyngeus muscle contracts, it has two major functions: (1) to prohibit air from entering the esophagus during breathing and (2) to protect against reflux and aspiration of esophageal contents.

Vascular supply

- The *external carotid* artery provides most of the blood supply to the pharynx (see Fig. 1.1).
- The branches of the external carotid artery that deliver blood to the pharynx include the *lingual*, *facial*, *maxillary*, and *ascending pharyngeal arteries*.
- The *subclavian artery* provides some perfusion via the pharyngeal branches of the *inferior thyroid artery*.
- Venous drainage is facilitated by the pharyngeal venous plexus, which then drains into the internal jugular vein.

Nervous supply

- The *maxillary division* of the *trigeminal nerve* (CN V) provides sensory innervation to the nasopharynx.
- Sensory innervation to the oropharynx is provided by the *glossopharyngeal nerve* (CN IX) via the *pharyngeal plexus*.
- Sensory innervation to the laryngopharynx is provided by the *vagus nerve* (CN X) via the *pharyngeal plexus* and some branches of the *superior (internal) laryngeal nerve*.

- The *pharyngeal plexus* is a network of nerves formed by the pharyngeal branches from both the *glossopharyngeal* (CN IX) and *vagus* (CN X) nerves.
- The internal branch of the superior laryngeal nerve (SLN), which is a branch of the vagus nerve, provides sensory innervation from the epiglottis to the base of the tongue (oropharynx).
- The *vagus nerve* (CN X) provides motor function to the majority of muscles located in the pharynx, including the superior and middle pharyngeal constrictors, the salpingopharyngeus, and the palatopharyngeus muscles.
  - A branch of the vagus nerve, called the *recurrent laryngeal nerve* (RLN), has both sensory and motor functions. It provides sensory innervation below the level of the vocal cords and motor innervation to the majority of the intrinsic muscles of the larynx except for the cricothyroid muscle. The external branch of the SLN innervates the cricothyroid muscle.
  - Another branch of the vagus nerve, known as the *Arnold nerve*, innervates the external auditory canal as well as some parts of the laryngopharynx. Stimulation of this nerve within the ear canal can result in coughing.
- The *glossopharyngeal nerve* (CN IX) provides motor innervation directly to the stylopharyngeus muscle causing a widening of the pharynx, which helps with swallowing and speech.

KNOWLEDGE CHECK

1. The artery that provides the majority of the blood supply to the pharynx is the ________ artery.
   a. subclavian
   b. common carotid
   c. transverse cervical
   d. external carotid
2. Damage to which nerve would cause motor dysfunction to the pharyngeal muscles?
   a. Glossopharyngeal
   b. Vagus
   c. Hypoglossal
   d. Facial
3. Which pharyngeal muscle is innervated by the glossopharyngeal nerve?
   a. Salpingopharyngeus
   b. Cricopharyngeus
   c. Stylopharyngeus
   d. Palatopharyngeus

Answers can be found in Appendix A.

Larynx

- The larynx, also known as the *voice box*, assists with breathing and phonation, provides the cough reflex, and protects the trachea and lower airways against aspiration.
- There are several anatomical structures that merit definition:
  - The *rima glottidis* or glottis is the opening between the vocal cords and the arytenoid cartilages. It is also known as the *laryngeal opening* or *glottic opening*.
  - The *aryepiglottic folds* establish the lateral borders of the laryngeal inlet and assist with physiologic closure of the glottis. They are bound by the epiglottis anteriorly and by the arytenoid cartilages posteriorly. Both the cuneiform and corniculate cartilages are embedded within the posterior aspect of the aryepiglottic folds.
  - The *false vocal cords* are also known as the *vestibular folds* or *ventricular folds*. They consist of mucous membranes with embedded fibrous tissue. The false cords are located laterally and superiorly to each vocal cord. These folds function in concert with other laryngeal structures to maintain breathing; prevent food, liquid, and other foreign substances from entering the airway during swallowing; and contribute to deep sonorous phonations. They are composed of skeletal muscle and are paralyzed by neuromuscular blocking agents.
  - The *true vocal cords*, also known as the *vocal folds*, are flat bands that are pearly white and contain a vocal ligament surrounded by mucous membranes. Anteriorly, they attach to the thyroid cartilage, and posteriorly, they attach to the arytenoid cartilages. Their outer edges attach to intrinsic laryngeal muscles, whereas their inner edges form the rima glottis. These cords are the major source of speech from air movement, oscillation, and vibration.

Hyoid bone

- The hyoid bone is not anatomically a part of the larynx, although the larynx is suspended from this bone. The hyoid bone is a U-shaped bone situated in the base of the mandible in the anterior portion of the neck in front of the third cervical vertebra and superior to the thyroid cartilage. It is suspended in place by multiple muscles and ligaments.
- Physiologically, the hyoid bone assists with breathing, swallowing, and speech.

- The middle pharyngeal constrictor, hypoglossal, and genioglossus muscles attach to the hyoid bone from the oral and pharyngeal cavities.
- Suprahyoid muscle attachments include the digastric, stylohyoid, geniohyoid, and mylohyoid muscles.
- Infrahyoid muscle attachments include the thyrohyoid, omohyoid, and sternohyoid muscles.
- The three main ligaments that support the hyoid bone are the stylohyoid ligament, the thyrohyoid membrane, and the hyoepiglottic ligament.

Single laryngeal cartilages (*Fig. 1.2*)

Epiglottic cartilage

- The epiglottis is a single leaflike cartilage that is positioned superiorly to the glottic opening and projects upward behind the tongue and hyoid bone. It forms the anterior aspect of the laryngeal inlet (glottic opening) and functions to protect the inlet by closing over the glottic aperture during swallowing.
- The epiglottis has a lingual and a laryngeal surface. The lingual surface is covered with a mucous membrane and cellular structure that protects it from the digestive tract. It is innervated by the glossopharyngeal nerve (CN IX), which provides the afferent response for the gag reflex. The laryngeal surface is composed of a cellular structure that is consistent with the respiratory tract, including goblet cells for secreting mucus. The SLN, a branch of the vagus nerve (CN X), provides efferent motor innervation for the protective cough reflex.
- The space between the base of the tongue and the epiglottis is known as the *superior vallecula*, whereas the space between the epiglottis and true vocal cords is called the *inferior vallecula*.
- The epiglottis is a primary anatomical landmark identified during direct or video laryngoscopy. It has also been termed *epiglotoscopy*.
- Epiglottitis is an acute inflammation of the epiglottis (especially in children) that obstructs the pharynx and laryngeal opening. It can cause severe respiratory distress and is considered a medical emergency.

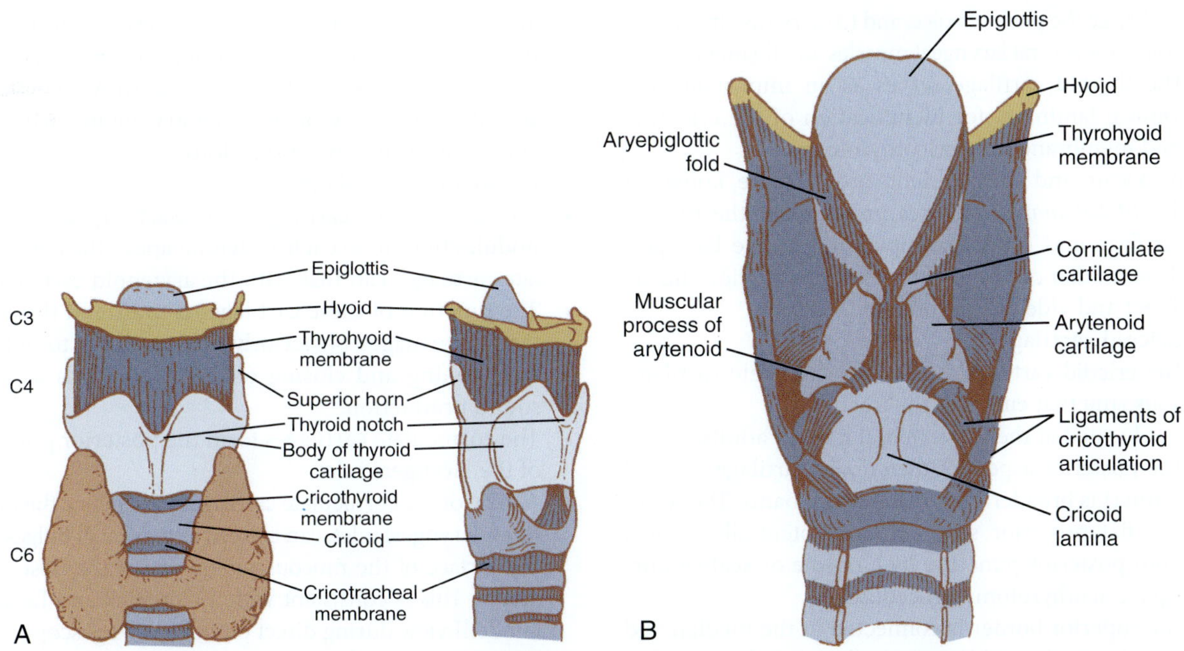

Fig. 1.2 (A) Anterior view of the laryngeal cartilages. External frontal *(left)* and anterolateral *(right)* views of the larynx. Notice the location of the cricothyroid membrane and thyroid gland in relation to the thyroid and cricoid cartilages in the frontal view. The horn of the thyroid cartilage is also known as the *cornu*. In the anterolateral view, the shape of the cricoid cartilage and its relation to the thyroid cartilage are shown. (B) Posterior view of laryngeal cartilages. Cartilages and ligaments of the larynx are seen posteriorly. Notice the location of the corniculate cartilage within the aryepiglottic fold. (Modified from Ellis H, Feldman S. *Anatomy for Anaesthetists*. 6th ed. Blackwell Scientific; 1993; Hagberg CA, Artime CA, Aziz MF. *Hagberg and Benumof's Airway Management*. 5th ed. Elsevier; 2023.)

It is commonly caused by a *Haemophilus influenzae* bacterial infection. Signs and symptoms include fever, sore throat, difficulty swallowing, excessive drooling, stridorous breathing, dyspnea, and a "cherry red" epiglottis. Management of this condition includes antibiotics, inhaled racemic epinephrine, intravenous (IV) steroids, and tracheal intubation or even tracheostomy in emergency situations.

Thyroid cartilage

- The largest cartilage within the laryngeal skeleton is the thyroid cartilage. It is formed by two lamina that fuse at the center, forming the laryngeal prominence ("Adam's apple"). The thyroid cartilage is located between the C4 and C5 vertebral levels.
- The entire superior border is an anchor point for the *thyrohyoid membrane*, which connects to the hyoid bone, whereas the inferior border is an anchor point for the *cricothyroid ligaments* and *membrane*, which connect to the cricoid cartilage.
- The primary functions of the thyroid cartilage are to (1) protect the vocal folds (vocal cords), (2) alter position to change the pitch of voice, and (3) serve as attachment points for several laryngeal muscles and ligaments.
- The thyroid cartilage serves as an important anatomical landmark for identification of the cricothyroid membrane for a cricothyrotomy.
- Backward and upward rightward pressure, known as the *BURP maneuver*, uses pressure on the thyroid cartilage and causes manipulation of the laryngeal skeleton that can improve the vocal cord view during direct and video laryngoscopy.

Cricoid cartilage

- The cricoid cartilage is the only complete cartilaginous ring that encircles the trachea.
- It is located at the C6 vertebral level in adults.
- The posterior aspect of the cricoid cartilage (cricoid lamina) is broader than the anterior band. The wider and flat posterior segment can potentially protect from posterior puncture by a needle or scalpel during a cricothyrotomy procedure.
- The superior border is connected to the median and lateral cricothyroid ligaments, forming the cricothyroid membrane.
- This is a durable cartilage that consists of a considerable amount of collagen, which can become calcified and ossified with advanced age.
- Cricoid cartilage functions include (1) serving as an attachment point for the cricothyroid, posterior cricoarytenoid, and lateral cricoarytenoid muscles; (2) supporting arytenoid cartilages (arytenoid articular surface) and ligaments that open and close the airway; and (3) speech production.
- The cricoid cartilage is the primary anatomical landmark for the application of cricoid pressure during the Sellick maneuver. It is also used to help identify the cricothyroid membrane for cricothyrotomy.

Paired laryngeal cartilages (see Fig. 1.2)

Arytenoid cartilages

- These are three-sided, pyramid-shaped cartilages that attach to the vocal folds (vocal cords) and function to facilitate vocal cord movement.
- The arytenoid cartilages assist with vocal cord tensing, relaxation, and approximation.
- These cartilages articulate with the superior and posterolateral aspect of the cricoid cartilage (arytenoid articular surface) that forms the cricoarytenoid joints. These joints allow the arytenoid cartilages to come together, move apart, rotate, and tilt both anteriorly and posteriorly.
- The arytenoid cartilages are anatomical landmarks that can be seen when performing a direct laryngoscopy. A Cormack and Lehane grade IIb view is consistent with a view of only the arytenoid cartilages and a posterior view of the glottis.

Corniculate cartilages

- The corniculate cartilages are elastic-type conical nodules that sit on each arytenoid apex. The corniculate cartilages can fuse with the arytenoid cartilages.
- The function of these cartilages is to extend the arytenoid cartilages posteriorly and medially to aid in the opening and closing of the vocal cords and in sound production.
- The corniculate cartilages form the posterior portion of the laryngeal inlet.
- A view of the corniculate cartilages, and hence the posterior laryngeal inlet, can be seen as two small bulges on the surface of the mucous membrane of the posterior glottis. This is consistent with a Cormack and Lehane Grade II view during direct or video laryngoscopy.

Cuneiform cartilages

- The cuneiform cartilages are a pair of elongated yellow elastic cartilages that sit in the aryepiglottic fold and form the lateral aspect of the laryngeal inlet (glottic opening).
- They are positioned immediately above and move with the arytenoid cartilages.

- During direct or video laryngoscopy, these can be seen laterally on the laryngeal inlet as two small bulges on the surface of the mucous membrane.
- They reinforce the aryepiglottic folds and function to support the vocal folds and lateral aspects of the epiglottis.

Laryngeal musculature

Extrinsic musculature

- These muscles connect the larynx to the hyoid bone and function to stabilize the larynx and move it superiorly and inferiorly during phonation, breathing, and swallowing (Box 1.1).
- The suprahyoid muscles and stylopharyngeus muscle (a pharyngeal muscle) elevate the larynx, whereas the infrahyoid muscles depress the larynx (except for the thyrohyoid muscle). The thyrohyoid muscle depresses the hyoid bone, causing the larynx to elevate.
- Suprahyoid muscles include the digastric, stylohyoid, geniohyoid, and mylohyoid.
- Infrahyoid muscles (also known as the *strap muscles*) include the thyrohyoid, omohyoid, sternohyoid, and sternothyroid muscles.

Intrinsic musculature

- These are smaller muscles that connect to the individual structures of the larynx and control (1) vocal fold adduction (close), (2) vocal fold abduction (open), and (3) vocal fold (cord) tension (Table 1.1).

BOX 1.1 Extrinsic Muscles of the Larynx

Muscles That Elevate the Larynx

Suprahyoid Muscles
- Stylohyoid
- Digastric
- Mylohyoid
- Geniohyoid

Pharyngeal Muscle
- Stylopharyngeus

Infrahyoid Muscle
- Thyrohyoid: depresses hyoid, causing laryngeal elevation

Muscles That Depress the Larynx

Infrahyoid Muscles
- Omohyoid
- Sternohyoid
- Sternothyroid

From Tarrazona V, Deslauriers J. Glottis and subglottis: a thoracic surgeon's perspective. *Thorac Surg Clin.* 2007;17:561–570.

- The overall functions of the intrinsic laryngeal musculature are to open the vocal cords during inspiration, close them during swallowing, and alter their tension during phonation. This is accomplished by intrinsic laryngeal muscular contraction, which alters both the muscular and vocal process positions on the arytenoid cartilage, resulting in vocal fold changes in length, tension, shape, and spatial orientation.
- The *laryngeal inlet* is where the pharynx meets the larynx. It is bordered anteriorly by the epiglottis, laterally by the aryepiglottic folds, and posteriorly by the arytenoid and corniculate cartilages and interarytenoid folds. The musculature that surrounds the inlet provides some degree of closure for airway protection during swallowing. The *aryepiglottic* and *oblique arytenoid muscles* constrict the laryngeal inlet, whereas the *thyroepiglottic muscle* widens the inlet (Fig. 1.3).

Intrinsic laryngeal adductor muscles. The intrinsic laryngeal musculature consists of the following:

- *Lateral cricoarytenoid* muscles adduct and lengthen the vocal cords to the greatest degree. This action causes a narrowing of the rima glottis (glottic closure), causing a modulation of tone and volume during phonation. They are innervated by the RLN.
- The *thyroarytenoid externus* and *internus (vocalis)* muscles adduct and shorten the vocal cords (releasing vocal cord tension), leading to a lower resonant speech. They are innervated by the inferior portion of the RLN.
- The *transverse* and *oblique arytenoids (interarytenoid)* muscles adduct the arytenoid cartilages, causing closure of the posterior rima glottis and a narrowing of the vocal cords. These are the only unpaired intrinsic laryngeal muscles. They are innervated by the inferior portion of the RLN.

Intrinsic laryngeal abductor muscles

- *Posterior cricoarytenoid* muscles abduct the vocal folds. These are the only muscles that open and widen the vocal folds and rima glottis, and they are principally responsible for glottic opening. They are innervated by the inferior portion of the RLN.

Intrinsic laryngeal tensor muscles

- *Cricothyroid* muscles tighten and adduct the vocal cords, resulting in increased tension. This action increases the resonant frequency of the vocal cords and helps with forceful speech. They are innervated by the external branch of the SLN.

TABLE 1.1 Intrinsic Muscles of the Larynx

Muscles Involved	Nervous Innervation	Main Function
Posterior cricoarytenoids	Recurrent laryngeal nerve	Abduction of vocal cords
Lateral cricoarytenoids	Recurrent laryngeal nerve	Adduction and lengthening of arytenoids causing glottis closure
Interarytenoid (transverse and oblique arytenoids)	Recurrent laryngeal nerve	Closing of posterior commissure of the glottis causing vocal cord narrowing
Thyroarytenoids and vocalis	Recurrent laryngeal nerve	Shortening (reduced tension) and adduction of vocal cords
Aryepiglottic	Recurrent laryngeal nerve	Constriction of laryngeal vestibule
Cricothyroids	Superior laryngeal nerve (external branch)	Adduction and increasing tension of vocal cords

From Tarrazona V, Deslauriers J. Glottis and subglottis: a thoracic surgeon's perspective. *Thorac Surg Clin.* 2007;17:561–570.

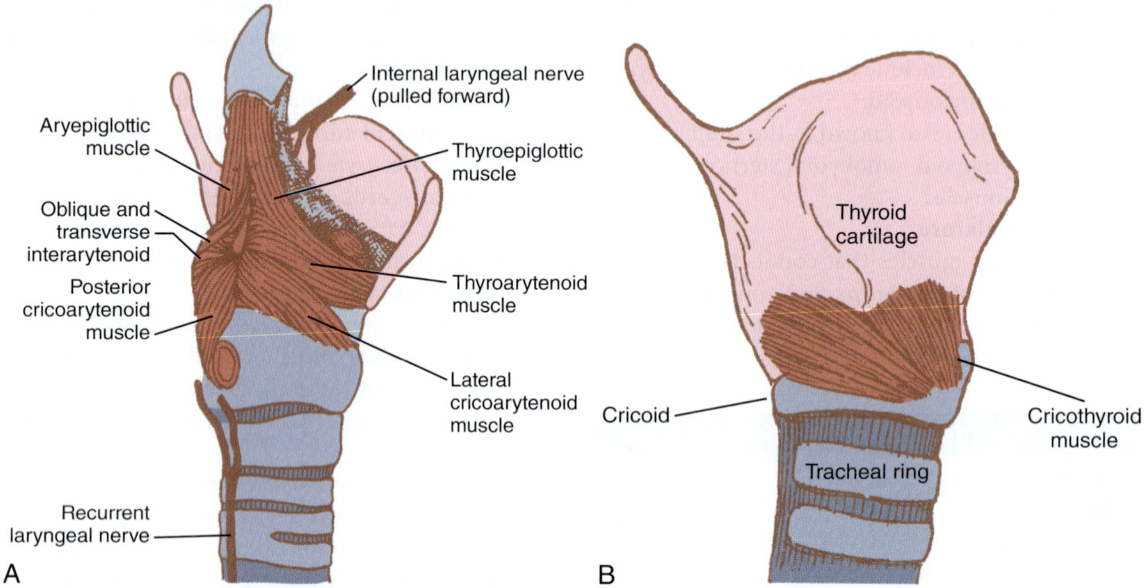

Fig. 1.3 Posterior view of the larynx showing the laryngeal cartilages and muscles. (A) Intrinsic muscles of the larynx and their nerve supply. (B) The cricothyroid muscle and its attachments. (Modified from Ellis H, Feldman S. *Anatomy for Anaesthetists*. 6th ed. Blackwell Scientific; 1993; Hagberg CA, Artime CA, Aziz MF. *Hagberg and Benumof's Airway Management*. 5th ed. Elsevier; 2023.)

Arterial supply

- There are two main arterial supplies to the larynx: the superior and inferior laryngeal arteries (see Fig. 1.1).
- The venous supply mirrors that of the arterial blood supply.
- The *superior laryngeal artery* is a branch of the *superior thyroid artery*, which comes from the *external carotid artery*. The superior laryngeal artery meets with the internal branch of the SLN and courses through the thyrohyoid membrane to innervate and source the supraglottic structures. The *cricothyroid artery* is a major branch of the superior laryngeal artery and courses inferiorly along the thyroid cartilage to supply the cricothyroid muscle and joint.
- The *inferior laryngeal artery* is a branch of the *inferior thyroid artery*, which comes from the thyrocervical trunk of the *subclavian artery*. This artery travels

with the RLN in the tracheoesophageal groove and supplies the infraglottic regions of the larynx.

- Both the superior and inferior laryngeal arteries anastomose with each other to form a complex meshwork of arterial blood supply to the larynx.

Nervous supply

- Eight to 10 nerve fiber roots originate within the nucleus ambiguus (located within the medulla) and combine to form the efferent motor fibers of the vagus nerve. The vagus nerve exits the base of the skull and descends in the carotid sheath. It then provides two major nerve branches that innervate the larynx:
  - Superior laryngeal nerve (SLN)
  - Recurrent laryngeal nerve (RLN)
- There are two *SLNs* that pass bilaterally on each side of the larynx.
  - Provide sensory innervation from the glottic and supraglottic structures of the larynx (oropharynx)
  - Provide motor innervation to the cricothyroid muscle
- *RLNs* are branches of the vagus nerve. The left RLN loops around the aortic arch, and the right RLN loops around the subclavian artery. Both RLNs ascend in each tracheoesophageal groove to innervate the laryngeal structures.
  - Each supplies sensory input from mucous membranes below the vocal cords.
  - Provide sensory, secretory, and motor fibers to the cervical regions of the esophagus and trachea
  - Provide motor innervation to all the intrinsic muscles of the larynx except the cricothyroid muscle
  - This nerve provides motor innervation to the posterior cricoarytenoid muscles, which are the only muscles that abduct (open) the vocal cords.
  - Damage to the RLN can result in vocal cord dysfunction and airway obstruction.

KNOWLEDGE CHECK

1. The inferior laryngeal artery is a branch of the:
   a. external carotid artery.
   b. internal carotid artery.
   c. subclavian artery.
   d. deep cervical artery.
2. Vocal cord movement is primarily facilitated by which cartilage(s)?
   a. Cricoid
   b. Cuneiform
   c. Arytenoid
   d. Thyroid
   e. Corniculate
3. Which intrinsic laryngeal muscle is innervated by the external superior laryngeal nerve (SLN)?
   a. Lateral cricoarytenoid
   b. Cricothyroid
   c. Posterior cricoarytenoid
   d. Thyroarytenoid
4. Damage to which nerve can cause vocal cord dysfunction and airway obstruction?
   a. Recurrent laryngeal
   b. Superior laryngeal
   c. Pharyngeal plexus
   d. Inferior alveolar

Answers can be found in Appendix A.

Lower Airway (Below Cricoid Cartilage)

Trachea

- The trachea begins at the level of the sixth cervical vertebra and ends at the level of the fifth thoracic vertebra opposite the manubriosternal junction (sternal angle). Thus half of the trachea is intrathoracic, and the other half is extrathoracic.
- The adult carina can move as much as 5 cm superiorly from its normal resting position because both ends of the trachea are connected to mobile structures.
- The tracheobronchial tree receives sympathetic stimulation from the first through fifth thoracic ganglia. Branches of the vagus nerve provide parasympathetic innervation. Carinal stimulation results in an extreme sympathetic response because of its extensive sensory innervation.
- With flexion or extension of the head, an in situ ETT tip can move an average of 3.8 cm and as much as 6.4 cm. In young infants and children, even ETT movements as small as 1 cm can cause extubation or bronchial intubation.
- An adult trachea has an inner diameter of approximately 1.5 to 2.5 cm and a length of roughly 10 to 12 cm.
- Sixteen to 20 hyaline C-shaped cartilage rings surround the trachea from top to bottom. The opening of the C faces posteriorly. These cartilages provide anterior and lateral protection and structure to the trachea.

- The only complete circular cartilage within the trachea is the cricoid cartilage, which is located at the top of the trachea.
- The cricoid cartilage is connected to the trachea by the cricotracheal membrane at the level of the sixth cervical vertebra.
- The trachealis muscle connects the posterior ends of the incomplete C-shaped cartilaginous tracheal rings at the back of the trachea adjacent to the esophagus. The function of this smooth muscle is to constrict the trachea and forcefully expel air during coughing.
- The trachea is considered a conductive region of the respiratory system, and it is responsible for bulk gas movement.
- *Tracheitis* is inflammation of the trachea. One of the more common causes is a bacterial *Staphylococcus aureus* infection. Signs and symptoms include inspiratory stridor, croupy cough, fever, malaise, dizziness, throat irritation, and labored breathing. This condition is particularly dangerous in young children because of their smaller tracheal lumens. Treatment consists of antibiotic therapy and possible admission to the intensive care unit with intubation and airway management.
- *Tracheomalacia* is a weakening of the tracheal cartilages. This condition can lead to tracheal collapse and airway obstruction (especially during increased exhalation airflow). Tracheomalacia can occur in children as a result of a congenital anomaly (e.g., tracheoesophageal fistula or esophageal atresia) or sustained external compression. In adults, it can result from chronic infection of the trachea or from prolonged intubation. Treatment includes airway management using continuous positive airway pressure (CPAP) or bilateral positive airway pressure (BiPAP) and may necessitate surgery.
- *Tracheotomy* or *tracheostomy* is a surgical incision in the anterior neck between the hyaline cartilages used to access the inner trachea. This opening bypasses laryngeal access to the trachea and allows for the placement of a tracheotomy tube to facilitate breathing. Indications for this procedure include a need for long-term mechanical ventilation or in acute emergencies when tracheal access is necessary as a result of severe upper airway obstruction.

Bronchi

- At the carina, the trachea divides into the right and left mainstem bronchus.
- The right bronchus splits at an approximate 25-degree angle and the left at a 45-degree angle. Because of the less acute angle, endobronchial intubation or aspiration of foreign material is more likely to enter the right bronchus.
- The right upper lobe bronchus divides from the right mainstem bronchus at an estimated 90-degree angle at only 2.5 cm from the trachea in most adults. Thus when a patient is in the supine position, it is more likely that aspirated foreign material or fluids will enter the right upper lobe.
- In roughly 10% of the adult population, the right upper lobe separates from the right mainstem bronchus by less than 2.5 cm. In this population, the right upper lobe could be occluded by a right-sided double-lumen tube bronchial cuff, a bronchial blocker, or an ETT that has been placed into the right mainstem bronchus. Also, in 2%–3% of the population, the right upper lobe opens into the trachea, which may make occlusion of the right upper lobe difficult during right-sided lung surgery.
- The left mainstem bronchus extends approximately 5 cm before branching to the left upper lobe.
- From the mainstem bronchi, the bronchopulmonary tree divides into lobar (secondary) and segmental or intrasegmental (tertiary) bronchi.
- From the right mainstem bronchus, the lobular divisions include the upper (superior), middle, and lower (inferior) lobes, and the left divides into the upper (superior) and lower (inferior) lobes (Fig. 1.4).
- Segmental divisions of the right superior lobe include the apical, posterior, and anterior segments; those of the right middle lobe divide into the lateral and

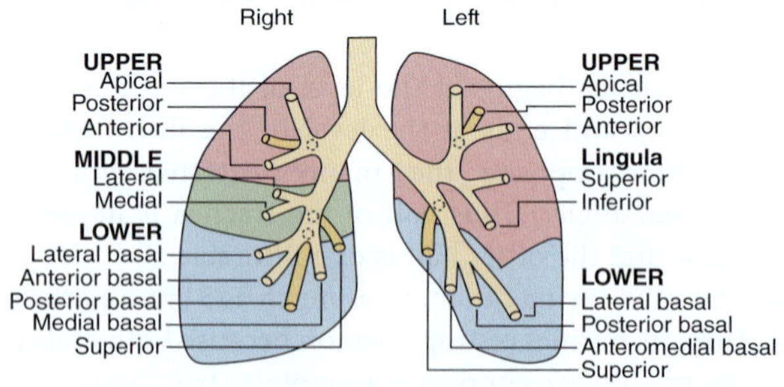

Fig. 1.4 Lobes and bronchopulmonary segments of the lungs. *Red,* Upper lobes; *blue,* lower lobes; *green,* right middle lobe. The 19 major lung segments are labeled. (From Lumb AB, Thomas CR. *Nunn and Lumb's Applied Respiratory Physiology.* 9th ed. Elsevier; 2021.)

BOX 1.2 Lung Lobes and Segments

Right Lung

Right Upper Lobe (Three Segments)

1. Apical
2. Anterior
3. Posterior

Right Middle Lobe (Two Segments)

1. Medial
2. Lateral

Right Lower Lobe (Five Segments)

1. Superior
2. Anterior basal
3. Posterior basal
4. Lateral basal
5. Medial basal

Left Lung

Left Upper Lobe (Four Segments)

1. Apical posterior
2. Anterior
3. Superior lingual
4. Inferior lingual

Left Lower Lobe (Four Segments)

1. Superior
2. Anteromedial basal
3. Posterior basal
4. Lateral basal

From Elisha S, Heiner JS, Nagelhout JJ. *Nurse Anesthesia*. 7th ed. Elsevier; 2023.

medial segments; and the right inferior lobe comprises the superior, anterior basal, lateral basal, medial basal, and posterior basal segments (Box 1.2).

- Segmental divisions of the left superior lobe contain the apical posterior (fused into one segment), anterior, and lingual (superior and inferior) segments; those of the inferior lobe include the superior, anteromedial basal, lateral basal, and posterior basal segments.
- Each bronchus is lined with pseudostratified, ciliated, columnar epithelial cells; longitudinal elastic fibers; smooth muscle; abundant mucoserous glands; and hyaline cartilages that provide support. As the bronchi divide deeper into the lung, hyaline cartilages exist only as irregular plates, and there is an increase in smooth muscle.
- Each bronchus is considered a conductive region of the respiratory system and is responsible for gas movement.

Bronchioles Extending to Terminal Bronchioles

- Bronchioles subdivide after the third-generation bronchi (tertiary bronchi).
- Bronchioles lack supportive cartilages and glands in their submucosa and instead contain a higher proportion of smooth muscle and ciliated cuboidal epithelium that provides structure. They range from 0.6 to 1 mm in diameter.
- Three to four bronchiolar generations exist until the terminal bronchioles. The terminal bronchioles are the final conductive airway generations and are incapable of gas exchange.

Respiratory Bronchioles and Alveolar Ducts

- Respiratory bronchioles follow the terminal bronchioles and are considered transitional airways. They not only facilitate gas movement but also are the first site in the tracheobronchial tree where limited gas exchange begins to occur.
- Two to three generations of respiratory bronchioles exist in the average adult before transitioning to alveolar ducts.
- Several generations of alveolar ducts are present, which provide multiple openings into alveolar sacs. Gas exchange occurs within alveolar ducts. The last alveolar duct divisions transition into alveolar sacs and open into alveolar clusters.
- The bronchioles contain cellular components of inflammation and immunity. In the early stages of inflammation, several biochemical mediators are released from these cells and are involved in the antibody-mediated hypersensitivity reactions that stimulate the contraction of bronchial smooth muscle.
- *Bronchiolitis* is an inflammation of the bronchioles that usually occurs in young children around 3–6 months of age. Viruses, such as the respiratory syncytial virus and influenza, are the usual causes. Treatment is primarily focused on symptom management, allowing the virus to run its course. In severe cases, the airway may need to be supported with intubation and mechanical ventilation.
- *Bronchospasm* is a sudden constriction of the smooth muscle within the walls of the bronchioles. This results in an acute narrowing and obstruction of the small bronchial lumens. The primary trigger is immune system activation (specifically the complement system) with degranulation of basophils and mast cells as a result of exposure to environmental triggers.

Bronchospasm is a symptom associated with asthma, chronic bronchitis, anaphylaxis, aspiration, pulmonary edema, light anesthesia, airway management, and other conditions that affect the lungs. Acute treatment consists of the administration of β_2-agonists (albuterol), muscarinic acetylcholine receptor antagonists, increasing volatile agent concentration (if under general anesthesia), and epinephrine if needed (see Bronchospasm and Bronchoconstriction in the Airway Complication section).

- *Bronchiolitis obliterans* can occur in adults and is characterized by scarring and fibrosis within the bronchioles, causing severe respiratory compromise and difficulty breathing. Causes include exposure to toxic vapors, chronic viral infections, rheumatoid arthritis (RA), and organ transplant. Signs and symptoms usually progress slowly over several weeks and can include a dry cough, wheezing, shortness of breath, and fatigue. Treatment includes oxygen therapy, steroid administration, and bronchodilator therapy. Lung transplant is considered in some severe cases.
- *Bronchiectasis* is a condition of abnormal bronchial dilation. Chronic bronchial inflammation can lead to both elastic and muscular destruction of the bronchial walls, leading to permanent dilation. This condition can be caused by airway obstruction from a mucus plug, atelectasis, foreign body aspiration, infection, cystic fibrosis, tuberculosis, or congenital weakness of the bronchial wall. Systemic disorders such as rheumatoid disease, inflammatory bowel disease, or immunodeficiency syndromes can also cause bronchiectasis. Signs and symptoms include a chronic productive cough, lower respiratory tract infections, purulent sputum production, alterations in pulmonary function tests (PFTs; decreased forced vital capacity and expiratory flow rate), hypoxemia, and/or respiratory distress. Treatment includes antibiotics, bronchodilators, supplemental oxygen, chest physiology, and pulmonary resection in select individuals.

Alveoli

- The alveoli are the primary sites for oxygen and carbon dioxide gas exchange.
- There are approximately 25 million alveoli at birth and 300–500 million alveoli in the average adult.
- Alveolar type I cells (pneumocytes) provide structure to the alveoli. Type II alveolar cells secrete surfactant. Surfactant is a lipoprotein that coats the inner surface of the alveoli, causing a reduction in surface tension at end expiration; prevents lung collapse; and facilitates lung expansion.
- The alveolar–capillary membrane consists of an alveolar epithelial layer and a thin elastic basement membrane (consisting of alveolar type I cells), an interspace, and a capillary endothelium with a thin basement membrane. It is possible for both basement membranes to fuse together, allowing for more rapid gas exchange between the alveoli and pulmonary capillaries.
- *Pores of Kohn* are microscopic passages within the alveoli that allow air to pass through the alveolar septum into adjacent alveoli, thus promoting collateral ventilation with an even distribution of air. They only open during deep spontaneous respirations; consequently, during mechanical ventilation or hypoventilation, the lungs generally do not benefit from their effect.
- Alveoli contain cellular components of inflammation and immunity. Alveolar macrophages are the primary immune system cells involved with the ingestion and removal of foreign material within the alveoli.
- Pulmonary capillaries form a dense network within the alveolar walls, creating an almost continuous thin film of blood surrounding the alveoli. Blood is spread within the pulmonary capillary bed over 70–100 m^2 of alveolar surface area. This exposes large quantities of blood to the gases within the alveoli.
- *Atelectasis* is the collapse of alveoli within the lung. It can occur as a result of compression, absorption, resorption, or impaired surfactant production. *Compression atelectasis* is caused by external compression on the lungs from a tumor, fluid, or air in the pleural space or from abdominal distention. Anesthesia with muscle paralysis relaxes the diaphragm and mediastinum, allowing mediastinal tissues and abdominal organs to exert pressure on the lungs. Mechanical ventilation causes a mechanical compression in the dependent and caudal areas of the lungs. *Absorption atelectasis* occurs when high concentrations of oxygen are administered, washing out the nitrogen within the alveoli. Because oxygen absorbs into the bloodstream rapidly, there is no nitrogen left within the alveoli to stent it open, thus causing an absorption atelectasis. *Resorption atelectasis* occurs because of hypoventilation or an obstruction that prevents air from reaching the alveoli. The gases within the alveoli are absorbed into the surrounding areas, and the alveoli collapse.

- *Decreased surfactant* leads to increased surface tension within the alveolar wall, promoting collapse. Some of the reasons this can occur include lung prematurity in infants, acute respiratory distress syndrome (ARDS), mechanical ventilation, and aspiration. Surgery, especially those surgeries that involve the thorax and upper abdomen, promotes atelectasis from a multitude of causes, including pain, lack of position changes, secretions that pool in dependent lung regions, and compression of lung tissue. Furthermore, patients who receive anesthesia are likely to have some degree of atelectasis, especially if they are receiving mechanical ventilation.
- Treatment for atelectasis in an awake patient includes deep breathing exercises with an incentive spirometer, frequent position changes, and early ambulation. For patients under anesthesia who are receiving mechanical ventilation, decreasing atelectasis includes the use of positive end-expiratory pressure (PEEP), pulmonary recruitment breaths delivered over several seconds, and inhaled bronchodilators.

KNOWLEDGE CHECK

1. The right mainstem bronchus bifurcates from the carina at which angle?
   a. 5 degrees
   b. 25 degrees
   c. 45 degrees
   d. 90 degrees
2. Which is a segmental bronchus of the right middle lobe?
   a. Superior
   b. Lateral
   c. Anterior
   d. Posterior
3. A patient is admitted to the hospital with a dry cough, fatigue, and respiratory distress. Several weeks ago, he was exposed to a textile fire with toxic fumes. Which disease process is most probable?
   a. Bronchiolitis
   b. Pneumonia
   c. Bronchiolitis obliterans
   d. Bronchiectasis
4. Which type of atelectasis most commonly occurs during general anesthesia?
   a. Compression
   b. Absorption
   c. Resorption
   d. Impairment

Answers can be found in Appendix A.

PHYSIOLOGIC CONCEPTS

Resistance to Breathing

- Airway resistance is the opposition that airflow encounters from anatomic and pathophysiologic causes as it travels from the upper airway to the alveoli. It is influenced by forces of friction or obstruction within the airway. It can be measured using body plethysmography. The nasal cavity, pharynx, and larynx comprise approximately 40% of the total airway resistance in a healthy individual.
- Laminar and turbulent flow are the major determinants of resistance. *Laminar flow* is characterized by lower pressures that consist of the orderly and parallel movement of molecules. In contrast, *turbulent airflow* involves higher pressures because molecules are moving in varying directions, which greatly increases resistance. True laminar flow occurs in the smaller airways because the diameters of the tubes are reduced, and linear velocity is low. Turbulent flow exists with higher gas flow rates and generally occurs in the large airways. Airflow moving past the frequent branches within the airway results in turbulence and is what causes breath sounds on auscultation.
- Poiseuille's law focuses on resistance to laminar flow. Resistance is directly proportional to the length of a tube. Therefore the longer the tube, the more resistance occurs. Conversely, resistance is inversely proportional to the radius of the tube. Thus doubling the radius of a tube will decrease resistance up to 16 times. A clinically applicable example would be the administration of a bronchodilator. Administration of a bronchodilator causes bronchodilation, which increases the radius, causing decreased airflow resistance. Viscosity also plays a role. The more viscous the gas or liquid, the more internal friction will occur, resulting in more resistance.
- Resistance to inspiration occurs because of the lungs' inherent elastic recoil, the frictional resistance of lung tissues, and the resistance to airflow caused by the multiple branches within the lung pathways. Airflow resistance is greatest in the small airways because of their small diameter (radius). However, the net total resistance is low because of the significantly high number of small airways with parallel pathways. In other words, as the airways branch below the main bronchi, there is more cross-sectional area for air to travel, resulting in air pressure decreases and a more

laminar flow. Most resistance to airflow occurs from singular narrowed portions of the airway (e.g., glottis), in the trachea and main bronchi because of turbulent flow, and in the medium-sized bronchi because they have the ability to vary their diameters according to smooth muscle tone. After initial inhalation, increasing lung volumes do exert a retractive or stenting force on airway tissues, causing reduced airflow resistance, which then facilitates continued inhalation.

- Upper airway obstruction (e.g., tracheal stenosis, a laryngeal mass, partially closed glottis, or kinked ETT) causes extreme airflow resistance. Reducing flow velocity and gas density may help improve airflow past the obstruction. For example, reducing inspiratory flow rates or the inspiratory/expiratory ratio can decrease inspiratory pressures and promote a more laminar flow. In addition, the density of the gas can be reduced to promote better flow. Helium is significantly less dense than air and diminishes airflow resistance threefold compared with air. Thus heliox (70% helium and 30% oxygen) can be used in the setting of upper airway obstruction because of its decreased density. However, the fraction of inspired oxygen (FIO_2) is limited to approximately 30%, which may negate the advantages of improved airflow.

- During expiration, air pressure and flow are greatest at the alveolar level and gradually decline as the flow reaches the mouth and nose. During normal quiet breathing, the pressures inside the smaller airways (bronchioles and alveoli) are greater than the dynamic forces of intrapleural pressure (which are negative). Thus during a normal expiration, the combination of elastic recoil of the lung and negative intrapleural pressure maintains airway patency and promotes airflow movement toward the mouth and nose and into the atmosphere. However, during forced expiration, when the muscles of the chest and abdomen contract, air is forcefully expelled from the lungs. It is possible that this greater force causes the smaller airways to collapse, resulting in air trapping. Reasons for small airway collapse are (1) a significantly more positive intrapleural pressure from the forceful muscle contraction, causing compression on small airways, and (2) the lack of cartilage within the bronchioles and decreased elasticity of pulmonary tissue from disease (emphysema) and/or advanced age.

Pulmonary Compliance and Airway Pressures

Airway pressures measured during positive-pressure ventilation are related to the compliance of the lung and include the peak airway and plateau pressures. Pulmonary compliance represents lung elastic tissue distensibility: the ability of the lungs to stretch and expand. It is calculated by dividing the change in volume by the change in pressure. Pulmonary compliance can be either static or dynamic.

- *Static lung compliance* is the pressure required to maintain pulmonary volume when there is no gas flow. It is directly related to the compliance of the respiratory system. Static lung compliance (Cstat) is linked to the plateau pressure (Pplat) and is measured at the end-inspiratory point of the plateau pressure: $Cstat = V_T/(Pplat - PEEP)$.
- *Dynamic lung compliance* is the pressure measured during gas flow or during an active inspiration. Dynamic lung compliance is always lower than or equal to static lung compliance, meaning the pressures are either greater than or equal to those of static lung compliance. It is correlated to peak airway pressure: $Cdyn = V_T/(Ppeak - PEEP)$.
  - ***Peak airway pressure*** is the highest (peak) airway pressure reached during inspiration. It is designated as *PIP* or *Ppeak* and should be kept less than 40 cm H_2O during the mechanical ventilation of healthy patients. Low PIP can lead to hypoventilation and atelectasis, whereas high PIP can cause barotrauma and compromise hemodynamics. Bronchospasm and plugging of the bronchioles cause a decrease in dynamic lung compliance and a consequent increase in peak airway pressures but do not affect the static lung compliance and plateau pressures.
  - ***Plateau pressure*** is the pressure applied to the small airways and alveoli during inspiration. It is measured at end inspiration during the inspiratory pause after these airways have equilibrated with gases. Plateau pressure is designated *Pplat*. Without respiratory disease, the plateau pressure is only slightly lower (approximately 2–5 cm H_2O) than PIP. The reason peak pressure can decrease to a plateau value is because of the redistribution of gas from stiffer alveoli (large alveoli that have limited expansion) to more compliant alveoli

(smaller alveoli that can expand more). As gas redistributes within the small airways (alveoli, alveolar ducts, and respiratory bronchioles), less pressure is required to hold the same amount of gas, resulting in a small pressure reduction and a plateau pressure. Lung protection strategies aim to keep the plateau pressure less than 30 cm H_2O to prevent volutrauma and overdistention of the alveoli. Tension pneumothorax, atelectasis, pulmonary edema, and pneumonia all reduce both static and dynamic lung compliance and increase both peak and plateau pressures.

- ***Airway pressures and compliance applications.*** PIP and plateau pressure rise together in situations that affect both the respiratory conduction areas and the gas exchange areas. Examples include higher V_T, pulmonary edema, pleural effusion, peritoneal gas insufflation, tension pneumothorax, Trendelenburg position, ascites, obesity, pregnancy, endobronchial intubation, and atelectasis. In these circumstances, both static and dynamic lung compliance decrease. Conditions where the PIP rises with no change in plateau pressure are associated with a decrease in dynamic compliance (i.e., decreased gas flow) but no change in static compliance. Examples include a kinked ETT, excessive secretions in the upper airway, bronchospasm, or airway compression. A pulmonary embolus does not change resistance and would have no effect on static or dynamic compliance.

Lung Volumes, Functional Residual Capacity, and Closing Capacity

Lung Volumes

There are four lung volumes. All but the *residual volume* can easily be measured with spirometry (Fig. 1.5 and Table 1.2).

1. *V_T* occurs during normal quiet breathing and is estimated to be approximately 500 mL in an average-sized adult. V_T fluctuates in accordance with physiologic demands. For example, it can increase with relaxation and during deep sleep. In contrast, it can decrease during times of stress, nervousness, or fear.
2. *Inspiratory reserve volume* is the maximum volume of air that can be inhaled after a normal V_T breath. This volume is dependent on patient effort, and the estimated volume is between 3000 and 3300 mL.

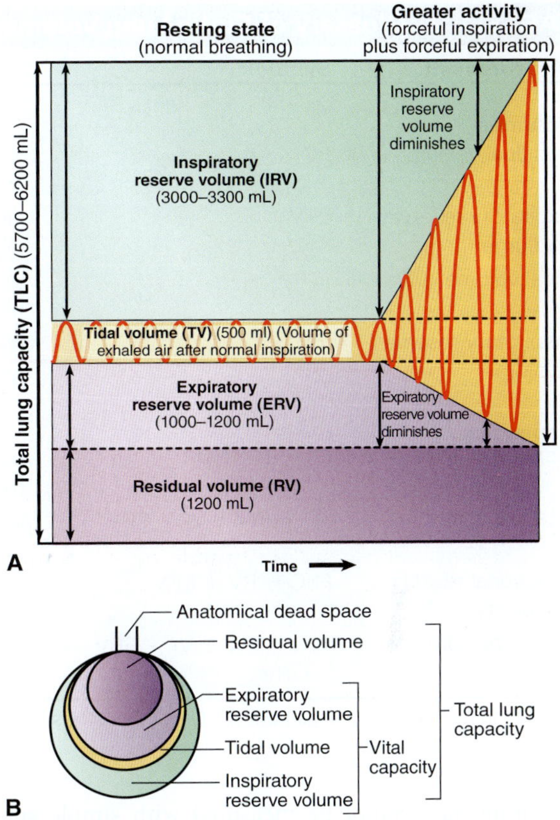

Fig. 1.5 Pulmonary ventilation volumes. (A) A tracing like that produced with a spirometer. (B) The pulmonary volumes as relative proportions of an inflated balloon. During normal, quiet breathing, approximately 500 mL of air is moved into and out of the respiratory tract, an amount called the *tidal volume*. During forceful breathing (like that during and after heavy exercise), an extra 3300 mL can be inspired (the inspiratory reserve volume), and an extra 1000 mL or so can be expired (the expiratory reserve volume). The largest volume of air that can be moved in and out during ventilation is called the *vital capacity*. Air that remains in the respiratory tract after a forceful expiration is called the *residual volume*. (From Patton KT, Bell F, Thompson T, et al. *The Human Body in Health and Disease*. 8th ed. Elsevier; 2024.)

3. *Expiratory reserve volume* is the volume of gas that can be forcefully exhaled after a normal V_T breath. This volume is estimated to be between 1000 and 1200 mL.
4. *Residual volume* is the volume of gas left within the lung after a forced exhalation. Residual volume does not fluctuate with mood or sleep, but it can be affected by body habitus, pathophysiological conditions, anesthesia, and surgery. This is the only lung

TABLE 1.2 Glossary of Static Lung Volumes and Capacities

Measurement	Symbol	Definition	Capacity (mL)
Volumes			
Residual volume	RV	Volume of air remaining in the lungs after maximum respiration	1200
Expiratory reserve volume	ERV	Maximum volume of air expired from the resting end-expiratory level	1200
Tidal volume	V_T	Volume of air inspired or expired with each breath during quiet breathing	500
Inspiratory reserve volume	IRV	Maximum volume of air inspired from the resting end-inspiratory level	3100
Capacities			
Inspiratory capacity	$IC = IRV + V_T$	Maximum volume of air inspired from the end-expiratory level (the sum of IRV and V_T)	3600
Vital capacity	$VC = IRV + V_T + ERV$	Maximum volume of air expired from the maximum inspiratory level	4800
Functional residual capacity	$FRC = RV + ERV$	Volume of air remaining in the lungs at the end-expiratory level (the sum of RV and ERV)	2400
Total lung capacity	$TLC = IRV + V_T + ERV + RV$	Volume of air in the lungs after maximum inspiration (the sum of all volumes)	6000

From Elisha S, Heiner JS, Nagelhout JJ. *Nurse Anesthesia.* 7th ed. Elsevier; 2023.

volume that cannot be measured with simple spirometry, but it can be approximated using an inert gas dilution method or a nitrogen washout technique. The most accurate method for measuring residual volume uses body plethysmography. Residual volume is estimated to be approximately 1200 mL in an adult.

Lung capacities consist of two or more lung volumes.

- *Inspiratory capacity* is made up of both the inspiratory reserve volume and V_T and is estimated to be between 3500 and 3800 mL in the adult.
- *Vital capacity* includes the inspiratory reserve volume, V_T, and expiratory reserve volume and has an estimated volume between 4500 and 5000 mL in the adult.
- *Functional residual capacity (FRC)* consists of the residual volume and the expiratory reserve volume and is estimated to be approximately 2200–2400 mL in the adult. This is the lung volume that remains after a normal V_T breath. Small airways maintain their patency by both lung recoil forces and chest wall expansive forces that are in equal opposition to each other and are connected by the pleural surfaces. In addition, alveolar air pressure and alveolar surfactant act to maintain alveolar patency and combine with chest elastic and recoil forces to create FRC. The volume within the FRC can saturate hemoglobin with oxygen during apnea.
  - Several factors negatively affect FRC. Conditions such as obesity, pregnancy, alterations in position (supine, Trendelenburg, lithotomy, etc.), general anesthesia, mechanical ventilation, intrinsic restrictive lung diseases (pulmonary edema, ARDS, aspiration, pneumonia, pulmonary fibrosis, alveolar proteinosis, sarcoidosis, etc.), and extrinsic restrictive diseases (ascites, scoliosis, flail chest, pneumothorax, pleural effusion, spinal cord damage, Guillain-Barré syndrome, etc.) can all reduce FRC.
- *Total lung capacity* includes the inspiratory reserve volume, V_T, expiratory reserve volume, and residual volume and is estimated to be approximately 5700–6200 mL in the adult.

Closing Volume and Closing Capacity

Closing volume is the volume within the lung where the small airways begin to close during exhalation. During expiration, the distending force of air on smaller airways incrementally decreases. This facilitates airway collapse. For most of a healthy adult's life, this is a volume that is lower than residual volume and is not clinically relevant. Normally, this begins to occur in the bases of the lung. Closing capacity is the sum of the closing volume and residual volume. Closing capacity can increase in certain conditions, such as smoking, chronic obstructive pulmonary disease (COPD), obesity, pregnancy, supine position, asthma and bronchospasm, atelectasis, pneumonia, and pulmonary edema.

Oxygen and Carbon Dioxide Transport

Physiologic Dead Space

Physiologic dead space is the sum of anatomic dead space and alveolar dead space. This is gas that does not participate in gas exchange at the alveolar–capillary membrane. With no pulmonary disease, physiologic dead space is equal to anatomic dead space, which consists of the gas volume that travels through the conducting airways (upper airway, trachea, main bronchi, segmental bronchi, and bronchioles). Approximately one-third of the inspiratory volume is anatomic dead space. Alveolar dead space includes gases in nonperfused alveoli. A clinically relevant example of physiologic dead space is the difference between the blood partial pressure of CO_2 ($Paco_2$) and the end-tidal CO_2 ($ETco_2$). The $Paco_2$ is higher than the $ETco_2$ because of CO_2 dilution within the conducting airways. In patients free of pulmonary dead space or pulmonary shunt, the $Paco_2$ value is estimated to be 5 mm Hg higher than the $ETco_2$.

- *Alveolar dead space* includes anything that interrupts perfusion, such as pulmonary embolus, hydrostatic pressure failure (e.g., severe hypotension), obliteration of pulmonary capillaries (e.g., COPD), pulmonary vascular vasoconstriction, and high intrathoracic pressure compressing pulmonary vasculature or inhibiting venous return (e.g., PEEP, excessive positive-pressure ventilation).
- *Mechanical dead space* comprises anything artificially used for ventilation. Both an ETT and a tracheal tube will reduce dead space within the upper airway because the volume within these tubes (because of their limited lengths and diameters) is less than the volume within the upper airway. Extensions or Y-pieces added to the circuit and attached to the ETT would increase the amount of mechanical dead space.

Oxygen Transport and Delivery

Oxygen is transported and delivered almost exclusively by hemoglobin. A small amount of O_2 is dissolved within the blood plasma. Approximately two-thirds of every breath reaches the terminal airways to participate in alveolar ventilation in normal lungs. The majority of O_2 within the alveoli diffuses through the alveolar epithelium, across the interstitial space, and through the capillary endothelium; crosses a small amount of plasma; and enters the red blood cells (RBCs) to combine with hemoglobin. A small amount of O_2 diffuses into the plasma and maintains an arterial O_2 partial pressure (Pao_2). The majority of O_2 is bound to and transported to body cells by hemoglobin. Hemoglobin can hold and carry 1.36 mL of O_2 per gram. Thus, by taking the hemoglobin value and multiplying it by the total percentage O_2 saturation (Sao_2) and O_2 carrying constant and then adding it to the amount of O_2 dissolved in the blood plasma, a calculation can be made for O_2-carrying capacity:

$$\text{Cao}_2\ (\text{concentration of arterial oxygen}) = (\text{Pao}_2 \times 0.003) + (1.36 \times \text{Hgb} \times \text{Sao}_2)$$

A calculation of total O_2-carrying capacity from someone breathing room air with an Sao_2 of 98%, a Pao_2 of 100 mm Hg, and a normal hemoglobin of 15 g/dL shows the following:

$$\text{Cao}_2 = (100\ \text{mm Hg} \times 0.003) + \left(1.36 \times \frac{15\ \text{g}}{\text{dL}} \times 0.98\right) = 20\ \text{mL O}_2$$

Thus, 20 mL of O_2 is transported on hemoglobin per 100 mL of blood. Assuming a cardiac output of 5 L/min, the total O_2 transported would equal 1000 mL/min. In order to calculate how much oxygen is delivered to the body cells, a venous blood gas is required. Assuming normal venous blood gas values of Svo_2 of 70% and Pvo_2 of 40 mm Hg, a calculation can be made using the same formula:

$$\text{Cvo}_2\ (\text{concentration of venous oxygen}) = (40\ \text{mm Hg} \times 0.003) + \left(1.36 \times \frac{15\ \text{g}}{\text{dL}} \times 0.72\right) = 15\ \text{mL O}_2$$

Subtracting 15 from 20 demonstrates that approximately 5 mL of O_2 per 100 mL of blood (one-fourth, or 250 mL/min total) is picked up and used by the body cells. Factors that can reduce oxygen delivery to the body cells are (1) a decrease in oxygen supply within the lungs (i.e., hypoventilation or pulmonary obstruction), (2) a decrease in cardiac output (i.e., pump failure), (3) a decrease in O_2-carrying capacity (i.e., hemorrhage or anemia), and (4) an increase in O_2 consumption without an adequate supply (i.e., hypermetabolic states).

Carbon Dioxide Transport and Removal

Carbon dioxide is transported within the blood in three ways: (1) 5%–10% is dissolved in blood plasma; (2) 5%–10% undergoes a rapid nonenzymatic reaction to combine with terminal amine groups of plasma proteins and become carbamino compounds, and about 15%–20% combines with hemoglobin to form carbaminohemoglobin compounds; and (3) an estimated 65%–75% is transported in the form of bicarbonate (Fig. 1.6). Within the RBC, CO_2 interacts with carbonic anhydrase and

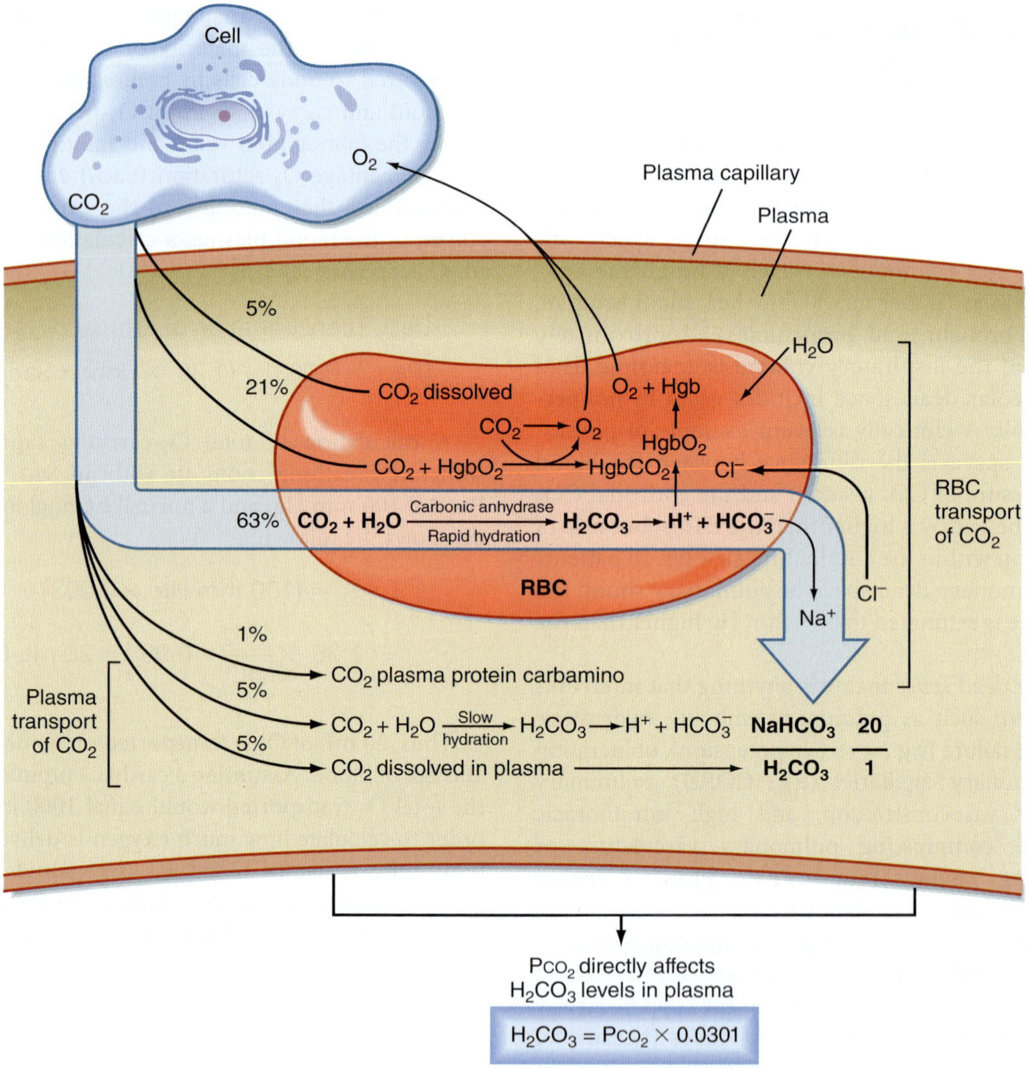

Fig. 1.6 Mechanisms of CO_2 transport in blood. The predominant mechanism by which CO_2 is transported from tissue cells to the lung is in the form of bicarbonate anion (HCO_3^-). *H_2CO_3,* Carbonic acid; *HgbO,* oxyhemoglobin; *$NaHCO_3$,* sodium bicarbonate; *RBC,* red blood cell. (From Koeppen BM, Stanton BA. *Berne & Levy Physiology*. 8th ed. Elsevier; 2024.)

combines with water to form carbonic acid. Carbonic acid then dissociates into bicarbonate (HCO_3^-) and hydrogen (H^+) ions. As bicarbonate leaves the RBC, it is exchanged with chloride ions (Cl^-) to maintain electrical neutrality. This is known as the *chloride shift* or the "hamburger shift." This process is then reversed within the RBC when bicarbonate reaches the lungs, resulting in CO_2 and H_2O. Carbon dioxide then diffuses out of the RBC and into the alveoli to be exhaled.

Oxyhemoglobin Dissociation Curve

The oxyhemoglobin dissociation curve is a graphic depiction of how blood and hemoglobin carry and release oxygen. The curve plots the O_2 saturation of hemoglobin on the vertical axis against the oxygen tension on the horizontal axis. As the partial pressure of oxygen increases, the hemoglobin becomes increasingly saturated with oxygen. Hemoglobin's affinity for oxygen is influenced by *pH*, *Paco₂*, *temperature*, and *2,3-diphosphoglycerate* (produced in RBCs in response to anemia/hypoxia). The curve may shift to the left or the right, depending on these changes. The steep decline in the curve facilitates the unloading of O_2 at the peripheral capillaries, whereas the flat portion of the curve represents the loading of O_2 onto hemoglobin in the pulmonary capillaries. Thus, in the pulmonary capillaries, where Pao_2 is high, hemoglobin binds O_2, whereas in the peripheral capillaries, where Pao_2 is low, hemoglobin releases O_2. Hypoxia is defined as a Pao_2 less than 80 mm Hg. An O_2 saturation of 90% via pulse oximetry correlates to a Pao_2 of 60 mm Hg, which signifies moderate hypoxia.

- The *Bohr effect* describes the impact that $Paco_2$ and H^+ ions have on the hemoglobin molecule and the oxyhemoglobin dissociation curve. Both a low pH (acidosis) and high $Paco_2$ (hypercapnia) shift the curve to the right because the excess H^+ ions affect the amino acids of hemoglobin, lowering its affinity for O_2. The Bohr effect is also the reason why hemoglobin will deliver and release O_2 more readily to highly metabolic cellular areas that have higher concentrations of CO_2, such as the heart and brain.
- The *Haldane effect* describes how environments with a low Pao_2 will cause a leftward shift in the CO_2 dissociation curve, allowing the removal of more CO_2. Deoxygenated hemoglobin (located in peripheral capillaries of rapidly metabolizing tissues) is a weak acid and a better proton acceptor than oxygenated hemoglobin. Thus, it will more readily bind to the free H^+ ions produced by the dissociation of carbonic acid within the RBC at the peripheral capillaries, allowing the transport of more CO_2 in the form of bicarbonate (see Fig. 1.6) back to the lungs. In contrast, the oxygenation of hemoglobin that occurs in the lungs reduces hemoglobin's affinity for CO_2, causes a rightward shift in the CO_2 dissociation curve, and promotes CO_2 removal.

Irritant Receptors and Creation and Management of Secretions

Irritant Receptors in Upper Airway and Tracheobronchial Tree

Mechanical or chemical irritation of the nasal mucosa, upper airways, or tracheobronchial tree induces coughing and sneezing reflexes. Nasal mucosal irritant receptors mediate their sensory response via the trigeminal and olfactory nerves, causing reflexive sneezing, bronchoconstriction, and increased blood pressure. Upper airway and tracheobronchial tree mucosal irritant receptors are sensory mediated by the vagus nerve and reflexively stimulate coughing and bronchoconstriction.

Juxtacapillary Receptors

Juxtacapillary (J) receptors are located within the alveolar septum and are juxtaposed to pulmonary capillaries. They are sensory cells that are stimulated by pulmonary capillary engorgement or increased pulmonary interstitial volume (i.e., pulmonary edema), pulmonary emboli, or specific chemicals in the pulmonary circulation. The J receptors send afferent stimuli via the vagus nerve to the respiratory centers in the medulla in order to stimulate tachypnea and/or dyspnea.

Mucus Creation and Management

Mucus is created by goblet cells and serous cells within seromucous glands that exist in both the upper and lower airways. Goblet cells are present in the surface epithelium of airway and lung tissue. Seromucous glands are contained within the connective tissue layer just beneath the respiratory mucosal epithelium. Mucus is made up of water, carbohydrates, glycoproteins, proteins derived from plasma, lipids, and products of cell death such as DNA. Mucus also contains antibacterial components such as lysosomes, lactoferrin, and antibacterial proteins and peptides. Lymphocytes also help with immunologic defense. Approximately 2 L of mucus is produced per day by the respiratory tract. The purpose of mucus is to trap dust particles, bacteria, and other inhaled debris so that they can be transported and expelled from the airway.

Mucus management

- Cilia in the upper and lower airways transport mucus toward the pharynx so that it may be swallowed and then digested in the stomach. This process is rarely noticeable unless there are large inhaled particles or large amounts of mucus. Larger particles generally become trapped in the nose and stimulate the sensory endings of irritant receptors, causing the sneeze reflex to expel the particles and mucus.
- The mucosal epithelium at the terminal bronchiole level is thin, with few ciliated cells and no goblet cells. Bacteria and debris that pass in these areas are removed by macrophages within the alveoli or expelled through coughing.
- Respiratory mucosal irritation and inflammation cause an increase in mucus production. The combination of inflammation and increased mucus production triggers the cough reflex to expel these secretions as sputum.
- Sputum production is associated with several airway diseases and activities, such as bronchitis, COPD, and smoking. Smoking destroys ciliated cells, allowing mucus to accumulate in the tracheobronchial tree. Smoking and pulmonary disease frequently cause chronic coughing because of increased sputum production from the proliferation of goblet cells and the hypertrophy of submucosal mucus-producing glands.
- Laryngoscopy and tracheal intubation cause irritation and inflammation of airway tissue and an increase in mucus production. Mechanical stimulation from laryngoscope blades, video laryngoscopes, and other airway devices triggers an increase in secretions that can inhibit adequate viewing of airway structures. Thus, the immediate availability and use of suction equipment is important for timely removal of these secretions. In addition, secretions of varying volumes are frequently present upon the removal of an ETT or supraglottic airway device (SAD), necessitating removal by suctioning and patient coughing to prevent airway obstruction.

Cardiovascular Response to Airway Management

- The mechanisms that stimulate the hemodynamic response to laryngoscopy and intubation are not completely understood. A sympathetic discharge (increased heart rate and blood pressure), most likely triggered by sensory stimulation from the upper airway, is frequently observed. This response can be attenuated by the administration of a β-blocking agent (e.g., esmolol). Other pharmacologic agents that help blunt this response include IV administration of an opioid and/or propofol prior to airway manipulation.
- Sensory information from airway stimulation is transmitted to the medulla of the brainstem via the glossopharyngeal nerve, the internal branch of the SLN, and the RLN. The medulla then regulates sympathetic outflow to the heart and adrenal medulla via preganglionic cholinergic fibers from the spinal cord. Efferent sympathetic outflow directly to the heart occurs from spinal cord levels T1–T5. The adrenal medulla receives sympathetic outflow from T8–T11 via the greater and lesser splanchnic nerves, causing chromaffin cells to release epinephrine and norepinephrine into the bloodstream. Total thoracolumbar blockade has been shown to diminish sympathetic outflow and the hemodynamic response to airway management. However, lower spinal cord injuries appear to allow some degree of sympathetic discharge to the heart and adrenal medulla, depending on the site of injury.

KNOWLEDGE CHECK

1. Using a bronchodilator to improve gas flow is an example of which physical law?
   a. Bernoulli's
   b. Boyles's
   c. Poiseuille's
   d. Charles's
2. In which condition does peak inspiratory pressure rise while the plateau pressure remains unchanged? *(Select all that apply.)*
   a. Tension pneumothorax
   b. Atelectasis
   c. Kinked endotracheal tube
   d. Bronchospasm
   e. Mucus plug
   f. Pulmonary edema
3. Which lung capacity delays the onset of hypoxia during apnea?
   a. Inspiratory
   b. Total lung
   c. Functional residual
   d. Closing

KNOWLEDGE CHECK—cont'd

4. The majority of carbon dioxide is transported in the blood
   a. in a dissolved state.
   b. as bicarbonate.
   c. bound to hemoglobin.
   d. bound to plasma proteins.
5. A primary mechanism for endogenous mucus management is facilitated by which type of cell?
   a. Ciliated
   b. Goblet
   c. Serous
   d. Lymphocyte

Answers can be found in Appendix A.

PATHOPHYSIOLOGIC CONCEPTS

Anaphylaxis

- Anaphylaxis is a severe type I hypersensitivity reaction that typically manifests within minutes of an antigen exposure in sensitive individuals. Signs and symptoms include angioedema, systemic vasodilation, hypotension, dysrhythmias, bronchospasm, and extravasation of fluids and proteins. This critical event affects the airway in several ways.
- *Identification:* Respiratory symptomatology for anaphylaxis includes airway obstruction from angioedema of the tongue, oropharynx, and larynx. This may appear as swelling in the neck, tongue, uvula, and laryngeal structures, with altered voice and/or inspiratory stridor. Other respiratory symptoms can include bronchospasm with or without wheezing, chest tightness, cough, rhinitis, nasal congestion, and rhinorrhea.
- *Differential diagnosis:* Signs and symptoms associated with anaphylaxis (specific to the airway) can resemble many of the critical events that affect both the upper and lower airways, lead to airway obstruction, and cause hypoxia. Angioedema that develops within the upper airway could be mistaken for laryngospasm, hematoma of the soft tissue surrounding the larynx, laryngeal mass, sublingual mass, Ludwig angina, or vocal cord dysfunction causing stridor. Lower airway obstruction with bronchospasm and wheezing can be caused by asthma, aspiration of foreign material, light anesthesia, pneumothorax, or pulmonary edema.

  It is possible that angioedema can be triggered directly by a medication or as a result of a genetic fault instead of an allergic reaction. Medications that can activate drug-induced angioedema include angiotensin-converting enzyme inhibitors, angiotensin 2 receptor blockers, and ibuprofen or other nonsteroidal antiinflammatory drugs (NSAIDs). Hereditary angioedema can be caused by an infection or injury, surgery or dental treatment, stress, pregnancy, or medications such as contraceptive pills.
- *Management and treatment:* Anaphylaxis-induced angioedema and airway obstruction can occur rapidly and be life threatening. Management includes discontinuation of the offending source (e.g., medication), suspension of anesthetic agents (e.g., volatile agents), administration of 100% oxygen, prompt airway intervention with ETT intubation, and adequate IV access for the administration of epinephrine. Subsequent treatments to decrease the immune response and manage associated symptoms include histamine-blocking agents (e.g., diphenhydramine, famotidine), additional vasopressors (e.g., norepinephrine, vasopressin), bronchodilators (e.g., albuterol, terbutaline), and corticosteroids (e.g., hydrocortisone).

Asthma

Asthma is a chronic inflammatory disorder of the tracheobronchial tree caused by inflammatory mediators. Several inflammatory mediators have been linked with asthmatic exacerbations, including eosinophils, mast cells, neutrophils, macrophages, and leukotrienes. The pathophysiology that results leads to constriction of both the large and small airways (bronchoconstriction), increased capillary permeability, vasoconstriction, and increased secretions from mucous glands. Chronic inflammation of the airways can produce airway remodeling that manifests as mucus hypersecretion, smooth muscle hypertrophy, fibrosis, and angiogenesis. Asthma can result from an allergic or nonallergic component, be exercised induced, or develop from occupational irritants or infection. However, all types of asthma result in some degree of airflow obstruction. Status asthmaticus is refractory to bronchodilator therapy and is an emergency.

- *Identification:* Signs and symptoms include coughing, wheezing, chest tightness, airflow obstruction, tachypnea, and dyspnea.
  - During anesthesia, a slanted or "shark-fin" appearance is noted on the $ETco_2$ waveform, indicating expiratory obstruction. Wheezing may or may

not be present. A decreasing saturation reflects poor oxygen exchange and hypoxemia. Increased mucus production can occur, and high inspiratory pressures are generally noted.

- Diagnosis of asthma is based on history and physical exam and is supported by diagnostic testing that consists of PFTs that show increases in residual volume, FRC, and total lung capacity because of gas trapping beyond the closed airways. The hallmark PFT from an asthma exacerbation is a reduced peak expiratory airflow rate. Values that fall below 50% of the predicted forced expiratory volume indicate severe bronchoconstriction. Eosinophilia is common in both the sputum and blood samples of patients with asthma.
- *Differential diagnosis:* Bronchoconstriction and wheezing are the primary signs associated with asthma and other respiratory comorbidities. Thus, the differential diagnosis as a result of wheezing could include pneumothorax, chronic bronchitis, endobronchial intubation, ETT obstruction, anaphylaxis, pulmonary aspiration, or pulmonary edema.
- *Management and treatment:* The goals for management include a reduction in airflow obstruction, corticosteroid supplementation, and prevention of symptom exacerbation.
  - Short-acting β_2-agonists are used for acute asthmatic symptom relief, and the use of this treatment more than 2 days per week indicates poor control. Patients demonstrating inadequate control of symptoms are placed on inhaled corticosteroids. Additional treatments depend on severity of symptoms and patient response to medications. Leukotriene receptor antagonists, long-acting β_2-agonists, mast cell stabilizers (cromolyn), theophylline, inhaled anticholinergic (ipratropium), and oral corticosteroids can be used for management.
  - Preoperative management assesses the level of asthma control, medication use, previous hospitalizations or intubations, and overall pulmonary function. Short-acting bronchodilators, corticosteroids, and anxiolytics can be given in the immediate preoperative area to help prevent an exacerbation of symptoms. Medications that release histamine, such as atracurium, mivacurium, and morphine, should be avoided. Additionally, medications that can influence a bronchospasm, such as β-blockers, prostaglandins, and ergot derivatives, should also be avoided.
  - Propofol can be used for routine anesthesia induction in the asthmatic population because it is unlikely to induce wheezing. Both lidocaine and opioids have been shown to blunt airway hyperactivity. If the patient exhibits active asthma symptoms, then ketamine can be considered because it is the only induction medication that has bronchodilating properties. Extubation should occur when deemed safe by the anesthesia provider. Deep extubations avoid mechanical bronchial stimulation by the ETT. Anticholinesterase agents have the potential to cause bronchospasm; thus, the lowest possible dose for reversal of neuromuscular blockade should be considered. Sugammadex does not exhibit cholinergic actions and may be the reversal agent of choice in patients with reactive airways.
  - Intraoperative bronchospasm can be managed by increasing the level of inhalation agent (as long as no hypotension is present) and rapidly increasing the anesthetic depth with propofol or ketamine. During acute episodes, 100% oxygen should be administered, and a β_2-agonist should be given. If bronchospasm persists in adult patients, then epinephrine boluses (10 mcg IV) can be given in increments until symptoms subside. Hydrocortisone IV (100–200 mg) helps reduce future exacerbations and decreases pulmonary inflammation. Magnesium IV (1–2 gm) and an inhaled anticholinergic can be considered if symptoms persist. Finally, aminophylline IV can be considered if the patient remains intubated.

Carbon Dioxide Abnormalities

Carbon dioxide abnormalities include anything that causes abnormal gas exchange or an excess production/absorption of carbon dioxide (CO_2). Abnormal or altered gas exchange can result from hypoventilation, ventilation–perfusion imbalances, pulmonary shunting, or diffusion abnormalities. Sources of excess CO_2 production or absorption within the body include hypermetabolic production, CO_2 absorption, and environmental exposure.

Abnormal CO_2 Exchange

- *Hypoventilation* can result from a brainstem injury, medications (e.g., general anesthetics, muscle relaxants, opioids), or medical conditions (e.g., neuromuscular disorders, COPD, obesity). The amount of retained CO_2 increases within the blood if CO_2 is not delivered to the lungs, diffused at the alveolar–capillary membrane, and exhaled out of the body. $Paco_2$ values above 50 mm Hg are significant and require treatment. Values that exceed 70 mm Hg lead to respiratory acidosis and activation of the sympathetic nervous system; they can be life threatening.
- *Pulmonary perfusion imbalances* or physiologic dead space can be a consequence of hypotension (e.g., heart failure, hypovolemia, and other shock states), pulmonary emboli, or lung tissue damage (e.g., emphysema). Airways are open and available for the ventilation of CO_2, but blood flow (and thus CO_2) is not delivered to the alveoli.
- *Pulmonary shunting* relates to alveoli that receive perfusion but do not receive adequate ventilation. Blood flowing past areas of nonfunctional lung tissue is unable to deliver and release CO_2 and pick up O_2. The result is blood returning to the left heart, with increases in CO_2 and decreases in O_2, which is then pumped out to body organs and tissues. The larger the shunt, the lower the Pao_2 and the higher the $Paco_2$, which increases the degree of respiratory acidosis and hypoxemia. Examples of pulmonary shunt include pneumonia, pulmonary edema, tissue trauma causing alveolar swelling, atelectasis, bronchospasm, mucus plugging or other airway obstructions, and pulmonary arteriovenous fistula.
- *Diffusion limitations* relate to the movement of gases across the thin membrane that separates the alveoli from the pulmonary capillaries. These limitations usually relate to the diffusion of O_2 only because the diffusion of CO_2 occurs very rapidly as a result of its increased solubility. In healthy individuals, the alveolar–capillary membrane functions very well for O_2 diffusion because it is very thin (0.1–0.5 μm) and has a large surface area (70–100 m^2). Diffusion limitations occur when there is (1) an increased thickness of the membrane (e.g., pulmonary edema, interstitial pulmonary fibrosis, chronically increased pulmonary vascular resistance), (2) a loss of surface area for diffusion (e.g., emphysema, surgical removal of lung tissue, lung tissue trauma, pulmonary cancer), (3) a reduced concentration of alveolar partial pressure of O_2 (e.g., hypoventilation, inhalation of CO, or any pathophysiologic process that limits alveolar ventilation), and (4) an increase in blood velocity limiting the time for O_2 to diffuse.

Excess CO_2 Production/Absorption

Increased $Paco_2$ can cause tachypnea, tachycardia, cardiac dysrhythmias, and altered levels of consciousness. Excessively high concentrations can cause convulsions, coma, and death.

- Hypermetabolic states such as fever, sepsis, malignant hyperthermia, and thyrotoxicosis can produce excess CO_2. Identification of the particular cause is essential for appropriate treatment and can include specific antibiotic administration for sepsis, dantrolene sodium for malignant hyperthermia, and antithyroid medications with β-blockade for thyrotoxicosis. Hemodynamic, electrolyte, and acid–base management may be required in any of these conditions.
- Absorption of excess CO_2 can result from CO_2 insufflation during laparoscopic procedures. Increasing the respiratory rate and V_T (if peak inspiratory pressure is not excessive) and monitoring the $ETco_2$ gas concentration are the usual methods for managing this situation.
- Exposure to high CO_2 levels can occur during anesthesia or as a result of environmental causes. Rebreathing exhaled CO_2 or unscavenged CO_2 from exhausted soda lime during anesthesia is a possible complication. Modern anesthesia machines monitor the fraction of inspired CO_2 and will sound an alarm if there is an elevation above the zero level. Replacing exhausted soda lime and increasing oxygen flow rates are methods to decrease the rebreathing of exhaled CO_2 in these situations. Environmental exposure to CO_2 is rare but can occur if an excess of CO_2 is in a confined space. Symptoms of CO_2 toxicity include dyspnea, cough, dizziness, chest pain, and headache. Solid carbon dioxide (dry ice) can cause cryogenic burns from direct contact, and when warmed rapidly, it releases large amounts of CO_2. If released in a confined space, this can lead to asphyxia from CO_2 inhalation and toxicity. Immediate removal from this environment, O_2 therapy, and in severe cases, assisted ventilation are necessary treatment options.

Conditions Associated With Difficult Airway Management

There are many congenital and acquired conditions that are associated with difficult airway management. For a list of more common congenital and acquired conditions, see Table 1.3.

Congenital Conditions and Associated Features

Congenital conditions that are present from birth are either inherited or caused by environmental factors. Associated features common to congenital conditions are the reasons for airway difficulty. These features include the following:

- *Micrognathia:* Also called *mandibular hypoplasia* or *hypognathia*, micrognathia is an incomplete development or underdevelopment of the mandible. It can be one of several parts of a craniofacial abnormality and can interfere with feeding and breathing in neonates. It is associated with difficult direct laryngoscopy and intubation in pediatric and adult patients. This feature often self-corrects as the child grows.
- *Retrognathia:* This condition presents with a retrusion (backward recession) of either the mandible or maxilla. This more often affects the mandible and results in an overbite. This feature is associated with a malocclusion of the jaw that can result in feeding problems as a neonate and in teeth crowding with biting difficulties, causing a temporomandibular joint (TMJ) disorder as an adult. Sleep apnea can result from tongue occlusion because of the recessed position of the mandible. This feature is frequently associated with difficult laryngoscopy and intubation in both children and adults.
- *Prognathia:* In this condition, either the mandible or maxilla protrudes forward. Prognathia is associated with malocclusion of the jaw, resulting in misalignment of the top and bottom teeth. It can cause problems with mastication and speech.
- *Mandibular hypoplasia:* This is incomplete or underdevelopment of the lower jaw (see earlier micrognathia description). It can result from abnormal congenital development or acquired (e.g., traumatic) conditions such as Pierre Robin sequence and Treacher Collins syndrome. Mandibular hypoplasia is associated with difficult intubation.
- *Maxillary hypoplasia:* This is incomplete or underdevelopment of the upper jaw. It results in backward displacement of the mandible (midface retrusion), creating the illusion of mandibular protrusion. This condition can be associated with Crouzon syndrome, Angelman syndrome, and fetal alcohol syndrome.
- *Macroglossia:* This is an abnormally large tongue. True macroglossia can be a result of muscular hypertrophy or a vascular malformation and is usually present secondarily to a congenital or acquired disorder. *Pseudomacroglossia* refers to a normally sized tongue that appears large because of an abnormally small orofacial structure. Macroglossia can cause excessive drooling, eating difficulties, speech impairments, snoring, airway obstruction, and stridorous breath sounds. Frequently, the tongue is noted to protrude from the mouth. Congenital and acquired conditions associated with macroglossia include Down syndrome, Beckwith-Wiedemann syndrome, amyloidosis, hemangioma, congenital hypothyroidism, trauma, cancer, endocrine disorders, and inflammatory or infectious processes. Macroglossia can interfere with direct laryngoscopy, SAD placement, and bag-mask ventilation.
- *Glossoptosis:* This is a retraction and downward displacement of the tongue toward the pharynx. Glossoptosis is a known feature of Pierre Robin sequence and Down syndrome. This condition can severely impede direct visualization of the vocal cords during direct laryngoscopy.
- *Microstomia:* This condition results in a small oral aperture that can result in difficulties with alimentation and dental care. It can be a feature of acquired conditions, such as burns or facial scleroderma, or it can result from congenital disorders, such as Freeman-Sheldon syndrome or arthrogryposis multiplex congenita. A small oral opening can cause difficulty with the insertion of any airway device.
- *Microcephaly:* This condition results in a smaller-than-normal head. The brain does not develop properly, and the consequences are intellectual disability, poor motor and speech, abnormal facial features, seizures, and dwarfism.
- *Cervical spine abnormalities:* These abnormalities include an abnormally developed cervical spine, fusion of two or more cervical vertebrae, or stiff cervical joints, and they result in decreased cervical range of motion. Several congenital disorders are associated with limited mobility of the cervical spine. Down syndrome, Hurler syndrome, Hunter syndrome, and

TABLE 1.3 Conditions Associated With Difficult Airway Management

Pathologic Conditions	Associated Features Affecting Airway Management
Congenital Conditions	
Pierre Robin sequence	Cleft palate, retrognathia, micrognathia, glossoptosis
Treacher Collins syndrome	Mandibular hypoplasia, malar (zygomatic) hypoplasia, choanal atresia
Goldenhar syndrome	Hemifacial macrosomia; mandibular hypoplasia; vertebrae may be incomplete, fused, or underdeveloped
Klippel-Feil syndrome	Fusion of two or more cervical vertebrae, limited neck range of motion, short neck
Down syndrome	Macroglossia, microcephaly, cervical spine abnormalities, obstructive sleep apnea, dental anomalies
Mucopolysaccharidosis I and II (Hurler syndrome and Hunter syndrome, respectively)	Macroglossia, odontoid hypoplasia, dwarfism, dental anomalies, stiff joints, obstructive airway disease, recurrent respiratory infections
Beckwith-Wiedemann syndrome	Macroglossia, microcephaly
Cri du chat syndrome	Microcephaly, retrognathia, micrognathia, stridor (high-pitched voice), short neck
Cherubism	Mandibular and maxillary fibrous tissue overgrowth, abnormal dentition
Acquired Infections	
Epiglottitis	Epiglottal and laryngeal edema
Laryngotracheobronchitis (croup)	Laryngeal and subglottic edema
Laryngeal papillomatosis	Obstructive papillomas within the larynx and upper airway
Oral/retropharyngeal abscesses	Distortion and/or stenosis of airway tissues, trismus
Ludwig angina	Floor of the mouth soft-tissue inflammation causing airway distortion and/or stenosis, trismus
Acquired Arthritis	
Rheumatoid arthritis	Limited cervical spine range of motion, atlantoaxial instability, temporomandibular joint ankyloses, cricoarytenoid arthritis
Ankylosing Spondylitis	Cervical spine and temporomandibular joint ankyloses/immobility, limited chest expansion
Acquired Tumors	
Cystic lipoma, adenoma, goiter	Altered airway anatomy, stenosis
Carcinoma of the tongue, larynx, or thyroid	Altered airway anatomy, stenosis, fixation of larynx or surrounding tissues
Other Acquired Conditions	
Trauma	Head, neck, and/or facial tissues can be distorted by trauma, edema, and/or hemorrhage; any bony structure can be unstable (facial, mandibular, cervical); laryngeal structures can be damaged or distorted
Burns	Airway edema, bronchospasm, smoke inhalation (decreased Pa_{O_2})
Radiation	Edema, fixation of tissue, friable tissue, impaired lymphatic drainage
Morbid obesity	Thick neck with redundant tissue, large tongue, obstructive sleep apnea
Acromegaly	Macroglossia, prognathism, vocal cord swelling

Pa_{O_2}, Arterial O_2 partial pressure.

Morquio syndrome are associated with cervical spine instability. Klippel-Feil syndrome is characterized by a fusion of two or more cervical vertebrae. A characteristic of Goldenhar syndrome is cervical hemivertebrae or underdeveloped vertebrae. In-line stabilization, limited cervical motion, and neutral head positioning during airway manipulation and laryngoscopy should be performed in these patient populations.

- *Craniofacial macrosomia:* This condition refers to abnormal smallness of the craniofacial structures, causing facial asymmetry. It can affect one or both sides of the face and frequently includes mandibular and/or maxillary hypoplasia. Ear anomalies are often present as part of this condition. A cleft lip and/or palate can also be a feature of this condition. Alterations in facial structure can lead to difficulty with bag-mask ventilation, direct laryngoscopy, and orotracheal intubation.
- *Cleft palate:* This is the result of a failure of the roof of the mouth (hard palate) to close during fetal development. This cleft produces a hole between the oral and nasal cavities; can result in feeding problems, speech problems, and hearing problems; and is frequently associated with other anomalies. Care should be taken during direct laryngoscopy to avoid lodging the airway device within the cleft.
- *Choanal atresia:* This condition results in congenital narrowing or closure of the posterior nasal cavity (choana) that causes difficulty breathing. The obstruction is caused by bone and soft tissue and is believed to be a result of failed canalization (tunneling) of the nasal fossae during fetal development.
- *Dental anomalies:* These comprise deviations of dental tissue enamel, dentin (hard bony tissue that forms the bulk of tooth beneath the enamel), or cementum (portion of periodontium that attaches the root of the tooth to the alveolar bone). They can occur as a result of congenital or acquired factors. Anomalies can manifest as variations of tooth size, number, and shape. Dental anomalies can alter the space within the oral cavity, and if any teeth are loose and become dislodged during airway management, they can cause severe airway obstruction.
- *Goiter:* This is an abnormal enlargement of the thyroid gland. It can be the result of an iodine deficiency or overproduction (Graves disease) or underproduction (Hashimoto disease) of thyroid hormone. Goiter can also be caused by nodules that develop within the gland. Symptoms can include swelling at the base of the neck, feeling of tightness within the throat, coughing, hoarseness, difficulty swallowing, and/or difficulty breathing. Goiter usually occurs in people over 40 years of age, but it can occur in youth, infancy, or at birth.
- *Laryngomalacia:* This is a congenital softening of the upper laryngeal tissues. The lack of rigidity of the upper laryngeal cartilage can lead to the arytenoid cartilages, as well as the mucosa over these cartilages, collapsing into the airway, causing a partial obstruction during inhalation and thus producing stridorous breathing. This condition is the most common cause of chronic stridorous breathing in infancy. It most often resolves on its own, with less than 15% of patients requiring surgery because of feeding or breathing inadequacies. Laryngomalacia can also be seen in older patients with neuromuscular conditions that cause the throat muscles to become weak.
- *Tracheal cartilaginous anomalies:* There are several tracheal cartilage pathological phenotypes, which include the following:
  1. *Tracheomalacia:* Weakness or softening of the cartilage rings, allowing the trachea to collapse during breathing or pressure.
  2. *Tracheal stenosis:* Narrowing of the tracheal lumen; instead of the normal C-shaped cartilage with intervening tissues that allow expansion, the cartilages are O-shaped and unable to grow.
  3. *Tracheal agenesis:* Complete absence of tracheal cartilages below the larynx.
  4. *Tracheal cartilaginous sleeve:* Cartilage rings are fused together, with a loss of intercartilage ligaments and soft tissue (essentially the entire trachea is cartilage).
  5. *Tracheoesophageal fistula:* Failure of the foregut tube to separate into the trachea and esophagus during fetal development results in an abnormal connection between the esophagus and the trachea; the most common type is an esophageal atresia with a distal tracheoesophageal fistula.

Acquired Conditions and Associated Features

Acquired conditions develop as a result of infection, environment, trauma, pathology, or other miscellaneous reasons (see Table 1.3). Similar to congenital conditions, acquired conditions have associated features that can affect airway management, including:

- *Epiglottic, laryngeal, and subglottic edema*
  - *Acute epiglottitis* occurs as a result of epiglottic inflammation and swelling. It usually has a rapid onset and is caused by a bacterial infection. Signs and symptoms of acute epiglottitis include fever, difficulty swallowing, drooling, hoarse voice, and stridorous breathing. This is an emergent condition because an inflamed epiglottis can cause a complete glottic obstruction. Prompt airway control and intubation with an ETT are essential. If swelling makes intubation impossible, then an emergency cricothyrotomy is necessary.
  - *Laryngeal edema* most often occurs as a result of intubation and damage to the laryngeal mucosa. Signs include stridorous breathing and an increased respiratory effort. Reintubation with a smaller ETT, IV steroid administration, nebulized epinephrine, and inhaled helium/oxygen mixtures are treatment options for postextubation laryngeal edema. If risk factors for laryngeal swelling are present (e.g., traumatic intubation or intubation for extended periods of time), then a leak test should be performed prior to extubation. Laryngeal edema can also result from an allergic reaction (see Anaphylaxis section), hereditary or acquired angioedema, or trauma to the larynx. General treatment for these conditions consists of IV epinephrine, C1 esterase inhibitors (angioedema), airway management, and treatment of any other accompanying sign or symptom.
  - *Subglottic edema* occurs below the larynx. This can occur as a result of acute laryngotracheobronchitis (croup), prolonged or traumatic intubation, bronchoscopy, or anaphylaxis. Signs and symptoms include hoarseness, sore throat, stridor, cough, hemoptysis, and/or dyspnea. Airway considerations should include a smaller-than-normal ETT, nebulized racemic epinephrine, IV steroids, and/or cool mist humidification.
- *Tracheal or subglottic stenosis:* Narrowing of the trachea resulting from an injury or illness after birth. Symptoms include stridor, cough, wheeze, dyspnea, asthma that responds poorly to treatment, chest congestion, and frequent infections (e.g., pneumonia, upper respiratory infections). Management includes bronchoscopy and several procedural (tracheal dilation with balloon or dilator) and surgical options (laser surgery, tracheal stent, or tracheal reconstruction).
- *Obstructive sleep apnea:* The pathogenesis of obstructive sleep apnea (OSA) is not completely understood. However, it is known that several upper airway pharyngeal dilator muscles (tensor palatine, genioglossus, and hyoid muscles) can relax and allow airway tissue to collapse against the posterior pharyngeal wall during a sleep or sedated state. Repeated collapse of the pharyngeal airway results in hypopnea and/or apnea. This leads to both hypercapnia and hypoxemia with frequent sympathetic nervous system activation. Consequently, each of these events is associated with cortical arousal, causing an individual with OSA to cycle between sleep and wakeful states, thus prohibiting deeper levels of sleep. Obese adults with large neck circumferences are likely to have some degree of OSA. Children with adenotonsillar hypertrophy, altered craniofacial development (e.g., Pierre Robin sequence, Treacher Collins syndrome, or Crouzon syndrome), or neuromuscular anomalies (e.g., cerebral palsy, encephalopathy) are at risk of experiencing OSA. Airway-related complications related to OSA include airway obstruction, hypoxemia, regurgitation, pulmonary aspiration, laryngospasm, and bronchospasm. The STOP-BANG scoring system is a good predictor of severe OSA (Box 1.3). Patients should be encouraged to use their CPAP machines before and after surgery if available.
- *Submandibular space infections:* These are infections and acute cellulitis of the soft tissues of the submandibular, sublingual, suprahyoid, and floor of the mouth spaces. Ludwig angina is a bacterial infection causing severe cellulitis that occurs on the floor of the mouth below the tongue. Causes include dental infections (commonly second and third mandibular molars), an extension of peritonsillar cellulitis, poor dental hygiene, tooth extractions, and trauma (e.g., mandibular fractures or floor of mouth lacerations). Signs and symptoms include pain in the involved teeth or area, firmness of the sublingual tissues and the suprahyoid soft tissues on external examination, drooling, trismus, dysphagia, stridor from laryngeal edema, and elevation of the posterior tongue causing obstruction of the posterior oral pharynx. These infections can cause severe airway obstruction (especially Ludwig angina) within hours and require

BOX 1.3 Sleep Apnea Assessment

STOP-BANG Scoring System

STOP

1. *Snoring:* Do you snore loudly (louder than talking or loud enough to be heard through closed doors)?
2. *Tiredness:* Do you often feel tired, fatigued, or sleepy during the daytime?
3. *Observed apnea:* Has anyone observed you stop breathing during your sleep?
4. *Pressure:* Do you have or are you being treated for high blood pressure?

BANG

5. *Body mass index (BMI):* Greater than 35 kg/m^2?
6. *Age:* Older than 50 years?
7. *Neck circumference:* Measured around laryngeal prominence (Adams apple)
   For male, is your shirt collar 17 inches/43 cm or larger?
   For female, is your shirt collar 16 inches/41cm or larger?
8. *Gender:* Male?

Risk of Obstructive Sleep Apnea

OSA—Low Risk: Yes to 0–2 questions
OSA—Intermediate Risk: Yes to 3–4 questions
OSA—High Risk: Yes to 5–8 questions
or Yes to 2 or more of 4 STOP questions + male sex
or Yes to 2 or more of 4 STOP questions + BMI > 35 kg/m^2
or Yes to 2 or more of 4 STOP questions + neck circumference 17 inches/43 cm in male or 16 inches/41 cm in female

immediate airway intervention to prevent total obstruction. Because of the potential for difficult intubation, the anesthetist should consider asleep or awake intubation using video laryngoscopy or flexible nasal endoscopy (e.g., fiberoptic intubation) in the operating room. If the condition is advanced with severe airway obstruction, then a surgical airway should be immediately available. Further treatment includes incision and drainage and antibiotic therapy.

- *Oral and retropharyngeal abscesses:* Oral or dental abscesses are frequently the result of a bacterial infection. Common dental abscesses include both periapical (infection within a dead tooth) and periodontal (infection alongside a living tooth within the periodontium) abscesses. Pain and swelling are the most common signs and symptoms of dental abscesses. These abscesses do not typically cause upper airway distortions or obstructions unless the infection spreads to the surrounding soft tissue and/or lymph nodes within the neck.
- *Retropharyngeal abscesses* are most often caused by bacterial infections of the tonsils, throat, sinuses, adenoids, or nose. Trauma from a sharp object (e.g., fish bone) can also lead to a retropharyngeal abscess. These are more common in children ages 1–8 because the lymph nodes at the back of the throat do not begin to disappear until 4–5 years of age. Symptoms include pain and difficulty swallowing, excessive drooling, fever, stiff neck, and stridor. Complications from these abscesses can include abscess rupture into the airway, causing severe obstruction, hemorrhage around the abscess, pneumonia, laryngospasm, blood clot formation within the jugular veins, and sepsis. Retropharyngeal abscesses can lead to severe airway obstructions, especially in pediatric patients, who have small airway diameters. Prompt treatment with antibiotics, airway management, and surgical incision and drainage generally leads to good outcomes.
- *Laryngeal papillomas:* These are caused by human papillomavirus and can occur in children and adults. They are characterized by benign tumors within the upper airway and trachea. These tumors often form on the vocal cords themselves, leading to symptoms of hoarseness, voice changes, stridor, cough, and dyspnea. Progression of the disease with excessive tumor growth can lead to dysphagia, pneumonia, ARDS, failure to thrive in children, and recurrent upper respiratory infections. The symptomatology of laryngeal papillomas can be confused with asthma, croup, and bronchitis. Primary treatment is surgical removal of the tumors, and often repeated treatments are needed throughout the lifespan. Smaller ETTs are recommended to avoid premature tumor avulsion (with potential airway obstruction) and vocal cord trauma.
- *Trismus:* This is a term for limited mouth opening. Normal mandibular movement for mouth opening is 4 cm, normal lateral movement is 1 cm, and normal protrusive movement is 1 cm. Trismus causes a limitation in all movements of the mandible. The most common cause of trismus is inflammation of the soft tissue surrounding an impacted third molar (pericoronitis). Other causes include mastication muscle inflammation; peritonsillar, retropharyngeal, or parapharyngeal abscesses; TMJ dysfunction; submucous fibrosis; zygomatic arch fracture; radiation therapy of

the head and neck; tetanus; malignant hyperthermia; seizures; stroke; and succinylcholine-induced masseter muscle spasm. Treatment involves management of the underlying condition, physical therapy, range-of-motion devices, warm compresses, and pharmacological therapy (e.g., NSAIDs and muscle relaxants).

- *TMJ ankylosis:* TMJ is the result of a pathologic condition causing abnormal stiffening and immobility of one or both of the temporomandibular joints. Both joints represent a functional unit; thus even if there is injury to only one TMJ, it will affect the other side. TMJ ankylosis is most commonly a consequence of trauma or infection that results in a fusion of the mandibular head (condyloid process) to the mandibular fossa of the skull, causing decreased range of motion. The lack of adequate mouth opening interferes with mastication, oral hygiene, and speech and can potentially be life threatening in an airway emergency. Other causes include previous TMJ surgery, congenital deformities, and RA. Those patients with long-term RA may develop severe TMJ destruction, resulting in airway obstructions that resemble micrognathia or OSA syndrome.
- *Rheumatoid arthritis:* RA is a systemic autoimmune disorder that primarily affects joints. It can affect the joints of the airway and cervical spine by causing cricoarytenoid and/or cricothyroid arthritis, TMJ arthritis, and anterior atlantoaxial subluxation. There is a high prevalence of laryngeal involvement in patients with RA. These patients can present with ventilation and intubation difficulties (e.g., narrowed glottis aperture, laryngeal deviation, laryngospasm, cricoarytenoid joint fixation). Because of the potential for developing laryngeal mucosal edema, extubation is a critical period that can result in postextubation stridor, laryngospasm, and airway obstruction. Patients with progressive RA frequently have coexisting TMJ immobility with limited mouth opening and micrognathism. Patients with RA (especially severe peripheral rheumatoid involvement) should be suspected of having atlantoaxial instability. Because of the many potential causes of airway difficulty in patients with RA, serious consideration should be given to airway management strategies that employ minimal manipulation of the cervical spine, spontaneous ventilation, and video laryngoscopy using fixed or flexible techniques. Care should be taken if a flexible laryngoscopy technique is used because blind passage of an ETT through the vocal cords can be traumatic.
- *Ankylosing spondylitis:* This is a form of arthritis that primarily affects the spine, but it can affect other joints, such as the shoulders, hips, TMJ, and even the cricoarytenoid joints. Ankylosing spondylitis is characterized by long-term inflammation that leads to fusion and rigidity of joints (again primarily of the spine) as well as osteoporosis. These patients are at risk for neurological deficits because airway manipulation and even a small amount of neck extension of a fixed cervical spine can lead to cervical fractures and spinal nerve root compression. Thus, great care should be taken not to move the cervical spine during airway manipulation. Another airway consideration is that normal chest expansion can be compromised as a result of ankylosis of thoracic vertebrae.
- *Cervical spine instability:* Acquired cervical spine instability is the result of trauma to the head and/or neck. This condition can be diagnosed by history, clinical evaluation, radiography, computed tomography (CT), or a combination of these. Immediate airway intervention should occur in patients who present with high cervical spine injuries (above C5) or evidence of respiratory failure. The primary goal during airway manipulation is to avoid any further deterioration of neurologic function. This is accomplished by maintaining physiologic spinal alignment and spinal immobilization during airway manipulation. Manual in-line stabilization of the head and neck should be performed no matter the airway management technique chosen. Direct laryngoscopy and intubation with removal of the anterior cervical collar using manual in-line stabilization has demonstrated minimal cervical movement. Rigid and flexible video laryngoscopy are popular options that limit the degree of cervical movement. Also, the use of an SAD that facilitates intubation is an option. Finally, emergency cricothyrotomy equipment should be readily available.
- *Atlantoaxial instability (subluxation):* The subluxation most often involves the atlanto-occipital joint (C1 and C2). It can be a result of a bone or ligament abnormality. The most common abnormalities involve the transverse ligament and the odontoid process. The transverse ligament holds the odontoid process of C2 against the anterior arch of C1. Both the transverse ligament and odontoid process are the primary restraints against anterior–posterior subluxation or dislocation. Symptoms occur when the posterior arch of C1 or the odontoid process of C2 impinges on the

spinal cord or spinal nerve roots. Neck pain, limited neck mobility, fatigue, abnormal gait, torticollis (head tilt), sensory deficits, lack of coordination, spasticity, and hyperreflexia are all potential symptoms of atlantoaxial instability.

Causes of Upper and Lower Airway Obstruction

Upper Airway Obstructions

The upper airway consists of the air conduction passages that extend from the nasal and oral openings to the larynx. Thus, upper airway obstructions can be caused by trauma, pathology, or foreign bodies within the oral or nasal, oropharyngeal, and/or pharyngeal and laryngeal spaces.

- *Obstructions of the nasal and oral cavities.* A complete upper airway obstruction would be unlikely if it occurred solely within either the oral or nasal cavities because the alternate air conduction cavity would provide a conduit for oxygenation and ventilation. However, severe trauma to the face that causes bleeding and a disruption of normal anatomic structures could cause total airway obstruction in these areas. Furthermore, severe burns and airway swelling could also cause similar problems. Appropriate management for these problems focuses on support of spontaneous ventilation and awake intubation (if possible) or a rapid-sequence induction with intubation. Front-of-neck access should always be considered and be readily available at the bedside if initial airway management plans fail. Premature neonates with congenital anomalies that result in anatomic distortions of the face and associated macroglossia (e.g., Treacher Collins syndrome, Pierre Robin syndrome, mucopolysaccharidosis) can result in severe upper airway obstructions. Awake intubation with spontaneous ventilation is the preferred method of airway management for these patients.
- *Obstructions of the oropharyngeal cavity.* The tongue has been recognized as the most common cause of upper airway obstruction, especially in supine individuals with little or no muscle tone. A simple head tilt with a chin lift or anterior mandibular jaw thrust usually relieves a tongue-induced upper airway obstruction. Sleep apnea is a significant cause of upper airway obstruction. The most common cause of OSA is obesity (body mass index [BMI] > 30 kg/m^2). Obesity with excess upper airway tissue results in a decreased amount of oropharyngeal cavity space. Relaxation and subsequent posterior collapse of the tongue and soft palate tissues while in a supine position cause oropharyngeal obstruction. A mandibular jaw thrust maneuver can relieve an acute obstruction, whereas chronic management consists of CPAP support.
  - Trauma to the oropharyngeal cavity with tissue disruption can cause airway obstruction. Infective processes such as an abscess (e.g., peritonsillar) can lead to airway obstructions in this space. Ludwig angina (angina Ludovici) is a cellulitis and swelling in the floor of the mouth that can affect the base of the tongue, causing total airway obstruction. Identification of the obstruction and prompt airway intervention are crucial in these situations.
- *Obstructions of the pharyngeal and laryngeal cavities.* Obstructive conditions that affect the pharyngeal and laryngeal cavities can be caused by laryngeal muscle spasms, foreign bodies, angioedema, infection, trauma, surgical complications, or pathology.
  - *Laryngospasm* causing glottic closure must be managed to prevent hypoxia. Prompt identification, CPAP, deepening the plane of anesthesia, stimulation of the laryngospasm notch (jaw thrust with pressure just posterior to mandibular angles), and sometimes IV or intramuscular (IM) succinylcholine are all management strategies for laryngospasm.
  - *Foreign bodies*, such as teeth or other objects, aspirated into the pharyngeal cavity generally cause partial airway obstructions, whereas those aspirated into the laryngeal cavity (smaller space) are more likely to cause complete airway obstruction. The Heimlich maneuver has been used to relieve such obstructions. This maneuver violently removes air from the lungs to forcefully expel acute foreign bodies from the larynx.
  - *Angioedema* causes swelling of the soft tissue of the pharyngeal and/or laryngeal spaces. Identification of the underlying cause (e.g., allergic, drug induced, idiopathic, or hereditary) is important in order to administer the correct treatment and relieve the swelling.
  - *Infections* can lead to swelling and airway obstruction. Epiglottitis and laryngotracheobronchitis (croup) are two pathophysiologic conditions that can cause severe airway obstruction in pediatric populations. Identification of the offending pathogen is important so that the correct IV antibiotics

can be administered. Additional treatments include cool mist humidifiers and IV steroids. Tracheal intubation should be considered in situations where swelling could lead to life-threatening airway obstructions.

- *Airway trauma* within the pharyngeal and laryngeal areas can lead to airway obstruction. Airway tissue can be damaged, causing swelling or complete disruption of the air conduction passage. Hemorrhage or hematomas can occur as a result of trauma, exacerbating or even producing obstruction.
- *Surgical complications* as a result of neck surgery can produce swelling, hemorrhage, and/or hematomas within the pharyngeal and laryngeal spaces. Many times, these complications occur in the postoperative period and may require airway management outside the operating room.
- Pathology such as a tumor or cyst can be a source of airway obstruction. These obstructions can rapidly worsen when pathology induces swelling and/or distorts normal anatomic structures and necessitates immediate airway management.
- Goals for airway management are similar to those already discussed and focus on supporting spontaneous ventilation and awake intubation or, when indicated, rapid-sequence induction. Front-of-neck access (e.g., cricothyrotomy) equipment should be readily available in the event that primary and secondary airway plans fail and there is an inability to ventilate the patient.

Lower Airway Obstruction

Air passages from the trachea down to the alveoli comprise the lower airway. Obstructions in these areas can result from blockage of the trachea, bronchi, bronchioles, and alveoli or from extrapulmonary causes.

- ***Tracheal obstructions.*** Causes of obstruction within the trachea can occur from aspirated foreign bodies, trauma, surgery, or pathology.
  - *Aspirated foreign bodies* into the trachea can cause complete airway obstruction (especially in young children) but more often result in partial airway obstruction. It is possible for an aspirated foreign body to cause trauma and swelling to the airway and laryngeal tissues. Patients with stridorous breathing after foreign body aspiration have the potential to worsen and progress to complete obstruction. General anesthesia with promotion of spontaneous respiration and tracheal foreign body retrieval by an ear, nose, and throat (ENT) surgeon are generally warranted in these situations.
  - *Trauma* to the trachea can cause tracheal laceration, dissection, hemorrhage, and/or hematoma. Any trauma to the neck may result in tracheal damage. If the trachea is found to be lacerated or transected, an ETT should be immediately placed past the laceration or used as a bridge from one end of the transection to the other. It is possible for the lower part of the trachea to retract into the thorax after tracheal transection. Retrieval can be accomplished using Kelly forceps or a surgical clamp. Hemorrhage can be managed using suction and intubation with the ETT extending past the area of trauma. A hematoma can swell to cause a complete tracheal obstruction and needs to be identified and evacuated as soon as possible. A serious possible complication of neck surgery (e.g., carotid endarterectomy or thyroid or neck tumor removal) is the development of a hematoma that can compress the trachea, leading to stridor, dyspnea, altered airway anatomy, and difficult or impossible airway management.
  - Tracheal surgery can lead to tracheomalacia (softened trachea), which can collapse and obstruct as a result of respiratory forces within the thorax.
  - Pathology within the trachea can be a result of angioedema or a tracheal tumor. Pharyngeal and laryngeal cavity obstructions can cause angioedema and should be identified to correctly manage this complication. Tracheal tumors can prevent a normal-size ETT from fitting correctly. Consideration for an awake intubation with a smaller ETT may be warranted in these situations.
  - Airway management for tracheal obstructions can be challenging, and an ENT surgeon or other competent surgeon should be available and ready to perform a tracheostomy as a primary airway.
- ***Bronchi obstructions.*** It is possible for a main bronchus to become obstructed by aspiration of a foreign body. This is an airway emergency that requires bronchoscopy and, in rare cases, surgical intervention. Great care should be taken to keep the patient as calm as possible and to maintain spontaneous respirations.
- ***Bronchiolar and alveolar obstructions.*** Obstructive problems within the bronchiolar and alveolar sections of the respiratory tree are most often the

result of a pathophysiologic process. These can include ARDS, aspiration pneumonia, anaphylaxis, asthma, bronchospasm, COPD, pulmonary edema, sarcoidosis, or any other lung pathology. Acute trauma to the lungs can result in anatomic destruction and hemorrhage within the pulmonary tissues, producing a lower airway obstruction. Inhalational injuries caused by smoke, chemicals, or very hot steam can result in bronchiolar–alveolar swelling and damage, resulting in an obstruction.

The primary management of many of these obstructive pathophysiologic conditions is to provide respiratory support and treatment of the cause.

- ***Extrapulmonary obstructions.*** These types of respiratory obstructions tend to be more restrictive in nature and occur outside the lung's conducting airways in the lung pleura or chest wall. These conditions are liable to restrict lung expansion, resulting in decreased lung volumes, causing dyspnea, tachypnea, increased work of breathing, and potentially inadequate ventilation and oxygenation. Morbid obesity (BMI > 30 kg/m^2), term pregnancy, thoracic trauma (e.g., pneumothorax, fractured ribs or sternum, pulmonary contusion), severe ascites, thoracic cage abnormalities (e.g., kyphosis or scoliosis), and diaphragmatic hernia are all examples of extrapulmonary obstructions.

Hypoxia

Hypoxia and Hypoxemia

Hypoxia is a broad term used to describe a lack of oxygen at the tissue level. Quantitatively, hypoxia is defined as Pao_2 less than 80 mm Hg. It can be localized or affect the entire body. *Hypoxemia* is an abnormally low content of oxygen in the blood. Generalized hypoxia is usually a result of hypoxemia and occurs when there is ventilation or perfusion mismatch or when there is decreased environmental oxygen (e.g., high altitude, underwater diving, carbon monoxide poisoning). Local hypoxia can occur with the use of a peripheral tourniquet or in pathophysiologic states of decreased blood flow to tissues (e.g., diabetes, peripheral artery disease, frostbite).

Hypoxia—Differential Diagnosis

The differential diagnosis for hypoxia can be determined by identifying the underlying cause, which can be ischemic, hypoxemic, anemic, or histotoxic.

- *Ischemic hypoxia:* This is associated with insufficient blood supply to body organs and/or tissues. It can result from pump failure (e.g., congestive heart failure [CHF], myocardial infarction [MI], trauma, or cardiac tamponade), pulmonary or peripheral embolism, peripheral vascular disease, sickle cell crisis, or any hypotensive cause (i.e., hemorrhage, sepsis, anaphylaxis, neurogenic shock, anesthesia overdose).
- *Hypoxemic hypoxia:* This condition is defined as a deficiency of oxygen in arterial blood. It can occur as a result of an airway obstruction, decreased respiratory drive, ventilation–perfusion mismatch, hypoventilation, or decreased environmental oxygen.
  - *Airway obstruction* leads to hypoxia when there is a blockage within the upper or lower airway. Upper airway obstructions can be caused by the tongue; a foreign body; thick, copious mucus; laryngospasm; RLN damage; hemorrhage; hematoma; tumor; tissue trauma; tissue swelling; and/or an infective process such as an abscess. Lower airway obstructions are a consequence of foreign bodies, mucus, asthma, bronchospasm, lung inflammation (e.g., ARDS, aspiration, chronic bronchitis, cystic fibrosis), infection (e.g., pneumonia), trauma, pneumothorax, hemothorax, and/or tension pneumothorax.
  - *Decreased respiratory drive* can result from respiratory alkalosis, alterations in nerve transmission (e.g., neurogenic shock, phrenic nerve damage), local anesthesia systemic toxicity, high spinal anesthetic, CNS depression (e.g., opioid overdose, general anesthetics, head trauma, stroke), or respiratory muscle incompetence or failure (e.g., diaphragmatic trauma, phrenic nerve paralysis, intercostal nerve paralysis).
  - *Ventilation–perfusion mismatch* examples include pulmonary embolism, pulmonary vasoconstriction, pulmonary edema, alveolar or bronchiolar tissue damage (e.g., aspiration, ARDS, trauma), any type of airway obstruction, asthma and bronchospasm, atelectasis, infection (e.g., pneumonia), COPD, and/or any hypotensive cause. All of these either influence the diffusion of oxygen into the blood or prevent blood from acquiring oxygen, resulting in hypoxemia and hypoxia.
  - *Hypoventilation* can result from pathophysiologic causes (e.g., stroke, MI, severe acidosis, hypocarbia), respiratory depressant medications (e.g., opioids), inadequate reversal of neuromuscular blockade, iatrogenic causes (i.e., high spinal

anesthetic, complications of regional anesthesia in the neck, or local anesthetic systemic toxicity [LAST]), brain trauma, or from ventilator dysfunction (e.g., low respiratory rate, low respiratory volume, circuit disconnect).
- Examples of *decreased environmental oxygen* are high altitude, underwater diving, and any situation in which there is a low concentration of oxygen (e.g., carbon monoxide leak; hypoxic gas mixture; anesthesia equipment malfunction, such as circuit disconnect or gastric tube malplacement into the trachea with active suctioning).

- *Anemic hypoxia:* This is an inadequate amount of functional hemoglobin (and thus oxygen-carrying capacity) in the blood. Acutely, this can result from hemorrhage and massive blood loss; chronically, this can result from iron deficiency, chronic kidney disease, thalassemia, and sickle cell disease. However, both carbon monoxide poisoning and methemoglobinemia also represent this type of hypoxia because these molecules bind tightly to hemoglobin, causing its oxygen-carrying capacity to be severely decreased.
- *Histotoxic hypoxia:* This is an inability of body cells to effectively utilize oxygen. Cyanide poisoning is a well-known cause of this type of hypoxia because of its ability to inactivate cellular oxidative phosphorylation enzymes (specifically cytochrome oxidase), effectually inhibiting the cells' ability to use oxygen and synthesize adenosine triphosphate. Hydrogen sulfide poisoning is another example of histotoxic hypoxia.

BOX 1.4 Management of Hypoxia

- Administer 100% oxygen.
- Determine and treat the specific cause of hypoxia.
- Provide manual ventilation, confirm airway patency, and increase minute ventilation as needed.
- Perform endotracheal intubation and confirm correct placement.
- Verify pulse oximetry reading.
- Obtain arterial blood gas values.
- Administer bronchodilators as needed.
- Consider CPAP if the patient is not intubated.
- Consider PEEP if the patient is intubated.
- Perform cardiac resuscitation per American Heart Association ACLS/PALS protocol as necessary

Miscellaneous Treatments

- Consider suctioning trachea, bronchial lavage, corticosteroid, and/or antibiotics for gastric aspiration.
- Promote peripheral perfusion with inotropic and vasopressive medications and assess lactic acid values.
- Confirm adequate hemoglobin concentration and consider blood transfusion.
- Administer methylene blue IV 1 to 2 mg/kg over 5 min for hypoxia caused by methemoglobinemia.
- Descend to lower altitude for high-altitude hypoxia.
- Provide hyperbaric oxygen therapy for carbon monoxide or cyanide poisoning.
- Consider hydroxocobalamin or sodium thiosulfate for cyanide poisoning.

ACLS/PALS, advanced cardiac life support/pediatric advanced life support; *CPAP,* continuous positive airway pressure; *PEEP,* positive end-expiratory pressure.

Hypoxia Management and Treatment

The overall aim of management and treatment of hypoxia is to identify the underlying cause, correct it, and promote adequate oxygenation of the tissues. Ensuring a patent airway, using high concentrations of oxygen, and promoting good circulation are paramount when managing hypoxia (Box 1.4).

Pulmonary Edema

The anatomic layers that divide the alveoli from the pulmonary capillary consist of the alveolar epithelium (of type I cells), alveolar epithelial basement membrane, interstitial space, capillary endothelial basement membrane, and capillary endothelium. These layers vary depending on where they are located within the lung. For example, because each main bronchus and pulmonary artery enters the lung cavity at the hilum, they intussuscept the pleura (or fold over and make a pocket), creating a surrounding connective tissue sheath. This is the interstitial space, and it contains connective tissue fibrils, elastic fibers, fibroblasts, macrophages, and lymphatics until the terminal bronchioles. There are no lymphatics at the alveolar–capillary membrane. This space decreases in thickness as it travels nearer the alveoli. At the alveolar–capillary generation, the epithelial and endothelial basement membranes fuse together, creating a minimal interstitial space without interstitial fluid. This allows for faster diffusion of gases. Between each capillary endothelial cell is a gap or junction that is a potential pathway for fluid to travel from the intravascular space to the interstitial space or from the interstitial space to the intravascular space.

- *Identification:* The signs and symptoms of pulmonary edema include dyspnea, tachypnea, dizziness, fatigue, rales or crackles on auscultation, decreasing oxygen saturation, and hypoxemia. A chest x-ray can demonstrate pulmonary infiltrates. An echocardiogram (ECG) can identify decreased cardiac function.
- *Differential diagnosis and causes:* The symptomatology associated with pulmonary edema can be similar to that of bronchospasm, foreign body aspiration of a particulate that reaches the alveolar level, atelectasis, pneumonia, cerebral vascular accident, and a severe anxiety attack. Pulmonary edema can result from many causes, including heart failure, negative pressure against a closed glottis, alveolar damage from aspirated material, kidney injury, high altitude, transfusion-related acute lung injury (TRALI), eclampsia, ARDS, sepsis, trauma, inhalation injury, infection, and radiation to the lung.
- *Management and treatment:* The primary goal is to address and manage the underlying cause, followed by (1) improvement of oxygenation using oxygen therapy combined with BiPAP or CPAP, with intubation reserved only for severe cases; (2) maintenance of adequate perfusion with inotropes such as dobutamine if there is evidence of decreased organ perfusion; and (3) reduction of excess extracellular fluid by limiting IV fluids and using diuretics such as furosemide. Nitrates can be considered in cardiogenic pulmonary edema to decrease preload and afterload. High-altitude pulmonary edema is managed with oxygen and acetazolamide, and the definitive treatment is descent to a lower altitude.

KNOWLEDGE CHECK

1. Which medication should be administered first to treat anaphylaxis?
   a. Albuterol
   b. Diphenhydramine
   c. Norepinephrine
   d. Epinephrine
2. Which is an appropriate initial treatment for an acute intraoperative bronchospasm as a result of asthma? *(Select all that apply.)*
   a. Propofol
   b. Albuterol
   c. Succinylcholine
   d. Magnesium
   e. Epinephrine
   f. Atropine
3. Which condition limits diffusion of gas at the alveolar–capillary membrane?
   a. Bronchospasm
   b. Hyperventilation
   c. Glottic obstruction
   d. Interstitial edema
4. A primary concern surrounding airway management for cervical spine instability is to
   a. minimize neck movement.
   b. administer a corticosteroid.
   c. intubate after the patient is in a deep plane of anesthesia.
   d. avoid succinylcholine.
5. Which anatomic structure is most likely to cause complete airway obstruction?
   a. Oral cavity
   b. Pharynx
   c. Larynx
   d. Trachea
6. Which condition is an example of anemic hypoxia?
   a. CHF
   b. Pneumonia
   c. Cyanide poisoning
   d. Methemoglobinemia
7. A patient who is having an open bowel resection has received 2 units of packed RBCs for a hemoglobin value of 7 g/dL intraoperatively. The patient's blood pressure is 152/91 mm Hg, heart rate is 95 beats/min, oxygen saturation is 89%, and $ETco_2$ is 38 mm Hg. Ventilator settings include volume control ventilation of 600 mL V_T and a respiratory rate of 10 breaths/min. Peak inspiratory pressures have become slightly elevated over the last hour, from 26 mm Hg to 32 mm Hg. Auscultation of the chest reveals fine crackles. The most likely differential diagnoses based on this information include which of the following? *(Select all that apply.)*
   a. Atelectasis
   b. Pulmonary edema
   c. MI
   d. Anaphylaxis
   e. Mucus plug in the endotracheal tube
   f. Bronchospasm

Answers can be found in Appendix A.

AIRWAY BLOCKS

Effective anesthesia within the airway is essential for a successful awake intubation. Anesthesia to the nasal septum, nasal wall, and nasopharynx interrupts nerve transmission from the anterior ethmoidal, nasopalatine, and sphenopalatine nerves that originate from the ophthalmic and maxillary divisions of the trigeminal nerve (Fig. 1.7). Blockade of the glossopharyngeal nerve effectively anesthetizes the oropharynx and laryngopharynx. Finally, nervous innervation of the hypopharynx and subglottic regions of the larynx occurs from branches of the vagus nerve. Local anesthetic blockade of the SLN (internal and external branches) affects the epiglottis, cricothyroid muscle, and mucous membranes at the entrance of the larynx and the vocal cords. Anesthesia of the RLN affects sensation below the vocal cords as well as the intrinsic muscles of the larynx, with the exception of the cricothyroid muscle.

Medications That Facilitate Airway Anesthesia

- *Lidocaine:* An amide local anesthetic used for topical and infiltration anesthesia. Lidocaine is used frequently by anesthesia providers for anesthetizing the airway because of its rapid onset, short duration of action, and low threshold for causing methemoglobinemia. The most effective solutions for topical anesthesia are the 4% aqueous solution and 5% paste.
- *Benzocaine (HurriCaine spray or Cetacaine spray):* Benzocaine is an ester local anesthetic used for topical anesthesia. Frequently provided in a 20% solution that is used as a spray to provide topical anesthesia to the oral mucosa, it comes flavored in a water-soluble polyethylene glycol base (HurriCaine spray; Beutlich Pharmaceuticals, Bunnell, FL) or can be combined with other substances and local anesthetics (e.g., Cetacaine spray; Cetylite, Pennsauken, NJ). Benzocaine can cause methemoglobinemia, especially when combined with lidocaine.
- *Prilocaine:* This is an amide local anesthetic used for topical anesthesia. Pseudocholinesterase deficiency may affect the metabolism of this local anesthetic. Prilocaine appears to be the local anesthetic most likely to cause methemoglobinemia.
- *Phenylephrine spray:* This is a selective α_1-adrenergic receptor agonist of the phenethylamine class that causes vasoconstriction. Vasoconstriction of nasal

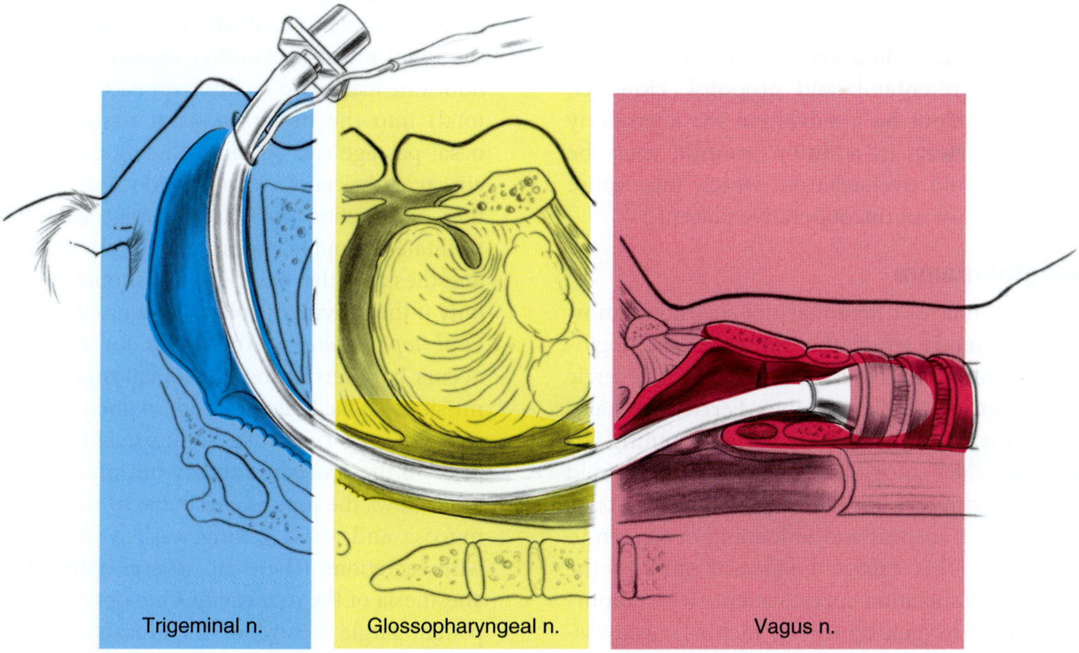

Fig. 1.7 Cranial nerve innervation of the upper airway. *n,* Nerve. (From Farag E, Mounir-Soliman L, eds. *Brown's Atlas of Regional Anesthesia.* 5th ed. Elsevier; 2017.)

blood vessels increases the airway lumen diameter and reduces postcapillary venule fluid exudation. It is sprayed topically into each nasal passage to decrease blood flow to prevent or decrease bleeding during nasal instrumentation and intubation.

- *Oxymetazoline spray:* This is a selective α_1-adrenergic receptor agonist and α_2-adrenergic receptor partial agonist that causes vasoconstriction. In addition to the α_1-adrenergic receptor vasoconstriction, local administration of this drug results in vasoconstriction from direct endothelial postsynaptic α_2-adrenergic receptor stimulation (opposite of central α_2-adrenergic receptor action). It is sprayed topically into each nasal passage to decrease blood flow to prevent or decrease bleeding during nasal instrumentation and intubation.
- *Glycopyrrolate:* This is an anticholinergic medication that is useful as an antisialagogue. The drying of mucosal secretions within the upper airway facilitates and potentiates the action of topically administered local anesthetics and decreases the amount of local anesthetic that is washed into the stomach. Administration of 0.2 mg IV is recommended 15–20 minutes before administering topical anesthesia.
- *Sedation medications:* Several different anesthetic medications have been used to reduce anxiety and help facilitate an awake intubation procedure. Examples include midazolam, ketamine, dexmedetomidine, remifentanil, and propofol. However, sedation should not be a substitute for a properly anesthetized airway. In addition, caution must be exercised to avoid oversedation, which may cause hypoventilation or an uncooperative patient.

Methemoglobinemia

Methemoglobinemia is a hereditary or acquired (most common) condition in which the iron within hemoglobin is oxidized from the ferrous form (Fe^{2+}) to the ferric form (Fe^{3+}), causing methemoglobin. Ferric iron has a decreased affinity for oxygen, whereas the remaining ferrous iron within the hemoglobin molecule tends to hold on to oxygen with greater affinity. What results is decreased oxygen transport and unloading of oxygen to tissues and cells. This causes a leftward shift in the oxyhemoglobin dissociation curve. Patients with comorbidities that affect oxygen transport, such as cardiovascular disease, anemia, pulmonary disease, or abnormal hemoglobin (i.e., carboxyhemoglobin, sickle cell), may experience symptoms at lower methemoglobin levels. Signs and symptoms of methemoglobinemia can include headache, mental status changes, anxiety, fatigue, exercise intolerance, shortness of breath, seizures, coma, and/or death. Treatment consists of removing the offending agent, providing high concentrations of supplemental oxygen, and administering methylene blue in a 1–2-mg/kg IV dose over 5–10 minutes.

Topical Anesthesia

The goal of topical anesthesia is to provide anesthesia to the nasopharynx, oropharynx, and hypopharynx in order to facilitate awake intubation in those patients who present with recognized difficult airways.

- *Nasal topicalization:* The objective is to anesthetize the branches of the trigeminal nerve that innervate the nasopharynx. This can be completed by first decreasing the blood flow to the nasopharynx using vasoconstrictors such as phenylephrine or oxymetazoline. One to two sprays of either vasoconstrictor is recommended into each nasal passage, with the patient instructed to inhale as the spray is administered. Pledgets soaked with lidocaine 4% solution can be placed into the preferred nasal passage for intubation. Each pledget should be advanced slowly to avoid nasal trauma and then should be left in the nasopharynx for up to 1 minute to facilitate transfer of the lidocaine to the nasal mucosa. Another option is to atomize the lidocaine using two or three sprays of 4% (up to 2 mL total) into the preferred nasal passage. Finally, the nasal passage can be dilated using a nasopharyngeal airway. Lubrication with 5% lidocaine paste will further anesthetize the nasal passage as well as help facilitate nasopharyngeal airway placement. Topical anesthesia of the nasopharynx should be performed only if the provider is planning a nasal intubation.
- *Oral topicalization:* Anesthesia for the oropharynx occurs by interrupting glossopharyngeal nerve transmission. To facilitate oral topical anesthesia, glycopyrrolate 0.2 mg IV can be administered 15–20 minutes prior to the procedure to dry out mucosal secretions. This allows the topical anesthetic to reach more of the mucosa and avoid getting washed into the stomach with secretions. There are several options for topical anesthesia of the oral cavity. One option is to have the patient gargle 2–3 mL of 4% lidocaine for 30 seconds. Another is to provide nebulized 4% lidocaine. However, when providing lidocaine via this route, the

oxygen flows should be minimized to prevent the local anesthetic from entering the lungs. Another disadvantage when using the nebulizer is the lengthy time required to effectively anesthetize the mucosa. Perhaps the most effective method for oral cavity topical anesthesia is the use of an atomization device. These are available in commercially disposable models that have directional flow tips or as a simple, malleable straw-type device. If using an atomizer, such as the MADgic device (Teleflex, Morrisville, NC), deposit an initial 2 mL of 4% lidocaine into the oral cavity (Fig. 1.8). Allow the patient to recover and then deposit an additional 2–3 mL of 4% lidocaine further down the oropharynx into the hypopharynx by retracting the patient's tongue and slowly advancing the atomizer. Finally, if available, apply 5% lidocaine paste (thumbnail-sized dollop) to the end of a tongue blade and place this onto the back of the patient's tongue, near the base of both the right and left tonsillar pillars. Allow the tongue blade to rest on the posterior tongue for a minimum of 1 minute while rotating it from side to side, allowing the medication to melt onto the tongue and then drip down into the hypopharynx.

- *Laryngeal topicalization:* Effective topical anesthesia for the larynx and trachea targets the SLN and RLN. This can be accomplished by atomizing 2–3 mL of 4% lidocaine directly onto the vocal cords and surrounding anatomy. The patient will likely cough, and it is possible the atomization device will need to be withdrawn. To complete topicalization of the airway, advance the atomization device directly to the entrance of the vocal cords and deposit 2 mL of lidocaine 4% directly into the trachea. This technique allows for a total of 8–10 mL of lidocaine 4% and a small amount of lidocaine 5% paste to be administered topically. Lidocaine toxicity is a rare potential complication; however, the majority of topical anesthesia is not absorbed by the mucosa and into the bloodstream. It is prudent to avoid any subsequent IV lidocaine. It is also important to continuously monitor the patient for signs and symptoms of local anesthetic systemic toxicity and avoid further administration of local anesthetic if signs and symptoms are observed.

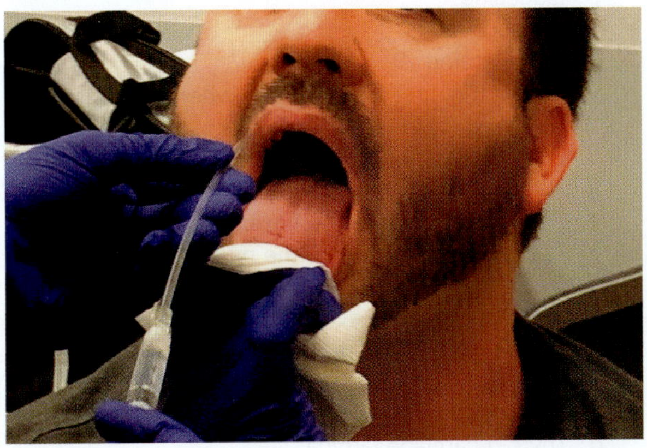

Fig. 1.8 Oral topical anesthesia with atomization device.

Glossopharyngeal Block

The goal of the glossopharyngeal block is to anesthetize the lingual branch of the glossopharyngeal nerve, which supplies sensory innervation to the posterior third of the tongue. Have the patient open their mouth, and displace the patient's tongue to the opposite side with a tongue blade. With the tongue moved to the opposite side, a canal or gutter is formed. Insert a 23- or 25-gauge spinal needle approximately 0.25–0.5 cm deep, where the gutter meets the base of the palatoglossal arch, and aspirate for air. If air is aspirated, the needle is too deep and should be withdrawn until no air is aspirated. If blood is obtained, withdraw the needle and reposition it more medially. This is done to avoid intracarotid injection. After correct positioning, 1–2 mL of 2% lidocaine is injected, and the block is then repeated on the opposite side (Fig. 1.9).

Superior Laryngeal Nerve Block

Locate the greater cornu of the hyoid bone, which lies beneath the angle of the mandible and can be palpated

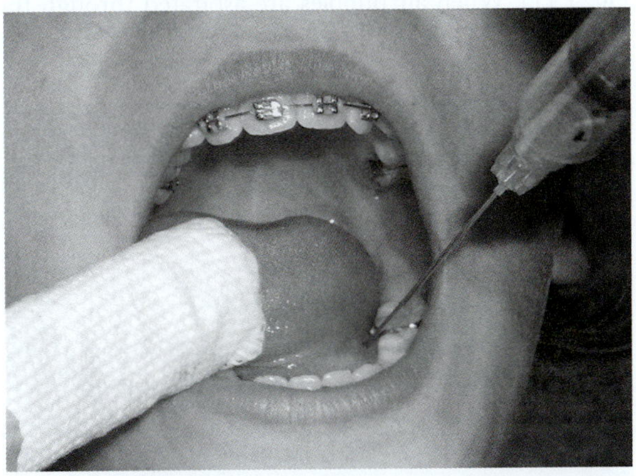

Fig. 1.9 Glossopharyngeal nerve block. (From Elisha S, Heiner JS, Nagelhout JJ. *Nurse Anesthesia*. 7th ed. Elsevier; 2023.)

with the thumb and index finger on either side of the anterior neck as a rounded structure. Once located, displace the hyoid bone toward the side that is being injected, and insert the needle perpendicular to the skin to make contact with the inferior border of the greater cornu. Position the needle to the caudal edge of the hyoid bone, where it then meets the thyrohyoid membrane. Resistance may be appreciated as the tip of the needle contacts the thyrohyoid membrane. This site approximates the area where the SLN pierces the thyrohyoid membrane. Aspirate for air or blood. If air is aspirated, the needle has been placed too deeply and is in the pharynx; the tip of the needle should be withdrawn and repositioned. The same should occur if blood is aspirated. Inject 1 mL of local anesthetic (e.g., lidocaine 2%) just above the thyrohyoid membrane. Then advance the needle an additional 2–3 mm through the membrane, and inject 2 mL of local anesthetic (Fig. 1.10). The procedure is then repeated on the other side.

Transtracheal Block

The goal of the transtracheal block is to anesthetize the vocal cords and upper trachea by injecting local anesthetic through the cricothyroid membrane. To administer the block, first palpate the cricothyroid membrane with the index and middle fingers and localize the skin. Attach a 22-gauge needle or a 24-gauge angiocatheter to a syringe containing 3–5 mL of either lidocaine 2% or 4%. Stabilize the laryngeal cage with the nondominant hand, and use the dominant hand to insert the needle at the midline at a 90-degree angle to the skin through the cricothyroid membrane while continuously aspirating (Fig. 1.11). When air bubbles are aspirated through the solution, the tip of the needle is in the tracheal lumen. If using an angiocatheter, the catheter is advanced into the tracheal lumen, and the needle is withdrawn, which may produce coughing. Injection of the contents into the tracheal lumen will cause coughing and atomize the local anesthetic onto the vocal cords and upper trachea. Care must be taken to stabilize the needle so as not to tear the tracheal mucosa or dislodge the needle and risk puncture during patient coughing. Use of the softer angiocatheter rather than the needle may decrease trauma.

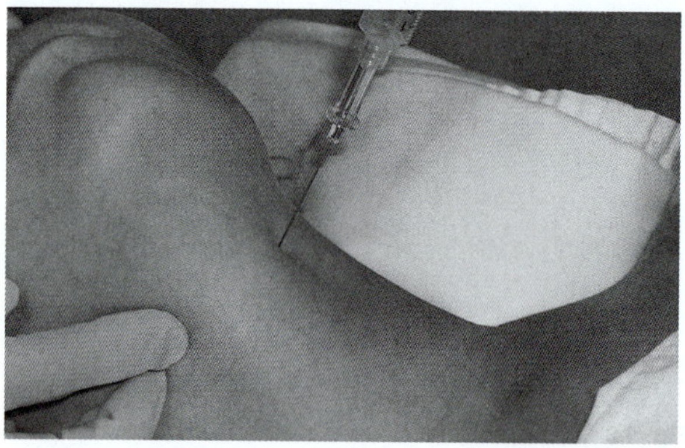

Fig. 1.10 Superior laryngeal nerve block. (From Elisha S, Heiner JS, Nagelhout JJ. *Nurse Anesthesia*. 7th ed. Elsevier; 2023.)

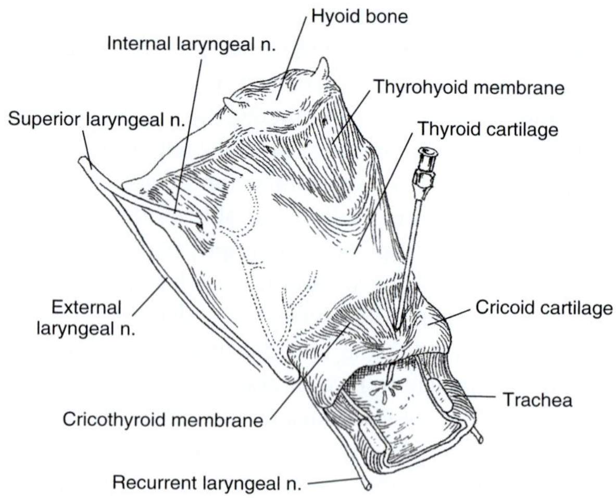

Fig. 1.11 Transtracheal injection. *n*, Nerve. (From Elisha S, Heiner JS, Nagelhout JJ. *Nurse Anesthesia*. 7th ed. Elsevier; 2023.)

KNOWLEDGE CHECK

1. Which medication is most likely to cause methemoglobinemia?
   a. Prilocaine
   b. Lidocaine
   c. Benzocaine
   d. Mepivacaine
2. Which is the first intervention when anesthetizing the nasal cavity?
   a. Dilate the nares with a nasopharyngeal airway.
   b. Have the patient inhale atomized lidocaine.
   c. Cautiously advance the flexible endoscope.
   d. Apply oxymetazoline to the nasal passage.
3. Which is the primary landmark for placement of a superior laryngeal block?
   a. Cricothyroid membrane
   b. Thyrohyoid membrane
   c. Greater cornu of the hyoid bone
   d. Thyroid cartilage lamina

Answers can be found in Appendix A.

AIRWAY ASSESSMENT

It is well known that individual airway assessments can be poor and unreliable predictors of actual difficulty. There is no single examination that consistently demonstrates a high sensitivity and specificity with minimal false-positive or false-negative reports of airway difficulty. The most effective way to assess an airway involves the use of multiple airway tests to identify a potential difficult airway (Table 1.4).

External Assessment

External observations are perhaps the best airway assessments. A patient who appears to have a difficult airway probably does. An external assessment takes into account facial and neck anatomy and pathology. Examples can include a protruding tumor of the jaw or neck; mandibular hypoplasia (short chin); large, thick neck; limited mouth opening; trauma to the face or neck; or devices that limit airway accessibility (e.g., cervical collar or halo traction device).

Neck Circumference

Obesity, and more specifically an increased neck circumference (greater than 43 cm [17 in] measured circumferentially at the thyroid cartilage), is a strong predictor of intubation difficulty. Redundant tissue is more difficult to displace during laryngoscopy, especially when there is decreased muscle tone. A history of snoring is another indicator that excessive airway tissue may obstruct glottic views during intubation procedures and increase the difficulty of ventilation.

Thyromental Distance

The thyromental distance (TMD) is a measurement of the thyromental space (Fig. 1.12). This space is an available pliable compartment, directly anterior to the larynx, where the tongue can be displaced during laryngoscopy to improve the direct line of sight with the glottic opening. The thyromental space is bordered laterally by the neck, superiorly by the mentum, and inferiorly by the semifixed hyoid bone. The TMD is measured from the thyroid notch to the lower border of the mentum (at the chin) when the patient's head is extended and the mouth is closed. A TMD *less* than 6 cm, or three ordinary fingerbreadths, is associated with a higher incidence of difficult direct laryngoscopy and intubation. Conditions such as radiation or pathologic factors (e.g., tumors) may cause the thyromental space to become noncompliant, whereas mandibular hypoplasia does not allow submental space for the tongue. A noncompliant or small thyromental space prevents tongue displacement during direct laryngoscopy, causing it to protrude into the pharyngeal space. A malpositioned

TABLE 1.4 Components of the Preoperative Airway Physical Examination

Airway Examination Component	Indication of Airway Difficulty
Length of upper incisors	Relatively long
Relation of maxillary and mandibular incisors during normal jaw closure	Prominent "overbite" (maxillary incisors anterior to mandibular incisors)
Relation of maxillary and mandibular incisors during voluntary protrusion (ULBT)	Inability to protrude mandibular incisors anterior to maxillary incisors
Interincisor distance	Less than 3 cm
Visibility of uvula	Not visible when tongue is protruded with patient in sitting position (e.g., Mallampati class III or greater)
Shape of palate	Highly arched or very narrow
Compliance of mandibular space	Stiff, indurated, occupied by mass, or noncompliant
Thyromental distance	Less than three ordinary fingerbreadths
Length of neck	Short
Thickness of neck	Thick (greater than 43 cm)
Range of motion of head and neck	Patient cannot touch tip of chin to chest or cannot extend neck

ULBT, Upper lip bite test.
From Berkow LC. Strategies for airway management. *Best Pract Res Clin Anaesthesiol.* 2004;18:531–548.

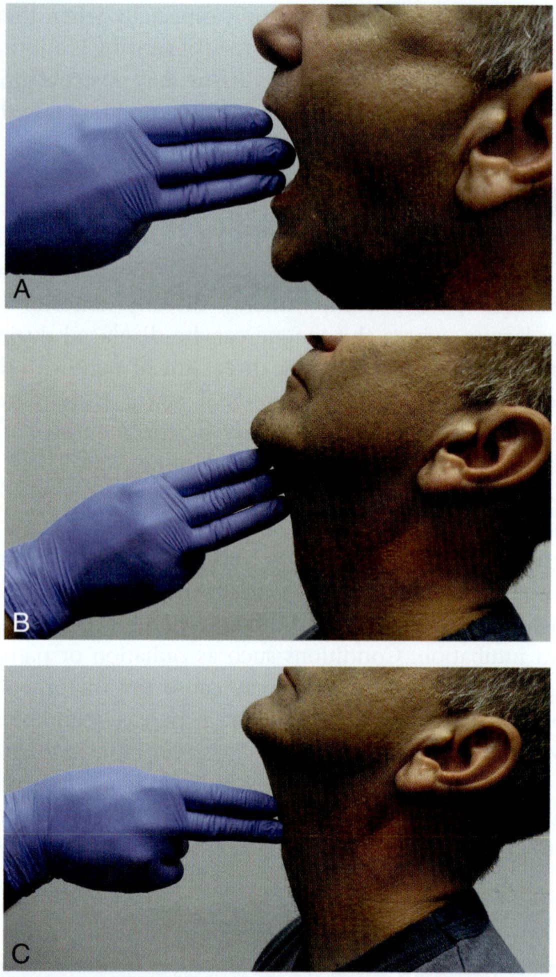

Fig. 1.12 3-3-2 assessment. (A) Mouth opening (distance between upper and lower incisors) at least three fingerbreadths. (B) Mentum (protruding part of chin) to thyroid notch, also known as *thyromental distance*, at least three fingerbreadths. (C) Thyroid notch to hyoid bone at least two fingerbreadths.

tongue that does not fit into the thyromental space can obstruct the operator's line of sight with the glottic opening during direct laryngoscopy. Conversely, assessment of a long TMD (greater than 9 cm) may also indicate a potentially difficult laryngoscopy and intubation. Difficulty is due to a large hypopharyngeal tongue, caudal larynx, and longer mandibulohyoid distance.

Atlanto-Occipital Joint Mobility

The atlanto-occipital joint provides the highest degree of mobility in the neck, with a normal head extension of up to 35 degrees. The full range of neck flexion and extension varies from 90 to 165 degrees. Proper atlanto-occipital joint mobility is required for positioning the head in an extended position for airway management. Extension of the head and neck improves direct laryngoscopic views by promoting displacement of the tongue and better aligning the oral, pharyngeal, and laryngeal axes. Evaluation of atlanto-occipital joint extension is conducted with the patient seated in an upright neutral position; the patient is then asked to lift the head back with the chin up as far as possible. If the patient demonstrates substantial or complete immobility of the atlanto-occipital joint, then significant compromise with direct laryngoscopy should be anticipated. Furthermore, cervical spine diseases such as cervical pathology (e.g., degenerative disease, rheumatic disease, ankylosing spondylitis, neurologic pathology, trauma, or a previous surgical intervention) or spinal abnormalities (e.g., Down syndrome, fused cervical vertebrae) may lead to difficult laryngoscopy and difficult airway management in general.

Mallampati Classification

Mallampati classification is a commonly used technique to assess mouth opening, the size of the tongue in relation to the size of the oropharynx, and posterior oropharyngeal structures. To perform this assessment, the patient is instructed to sit upright, extend the neck, open the mouth as much as possible, protrude the tongue, and avoid phonation. There are four Mallampati classes (Fig. 1.13):

- *Class I:* Full visualization of the entire oropharynx, including soft palate, uvula, fauces (archway between oral and pharyngeal cavities), and tonsillar pillars (pharyngopalatine arch)
- *Class II:* Visualization of the soft palate, fauces, and uvula
- *Class III:* Visualization of the soft palate and base of the uvula
- *Class IV:* Visualization of the hard palate only

A combination of higher Mallampati classification, decreased TMD, and limited interincisor opening is a strong predictor of both laryngoscopic and intubation difficulty.

Interincisor Gap (Mouth Opening)

Interincisor gap (mouth-opening) assessment is important because most airway adjuncts are placed through

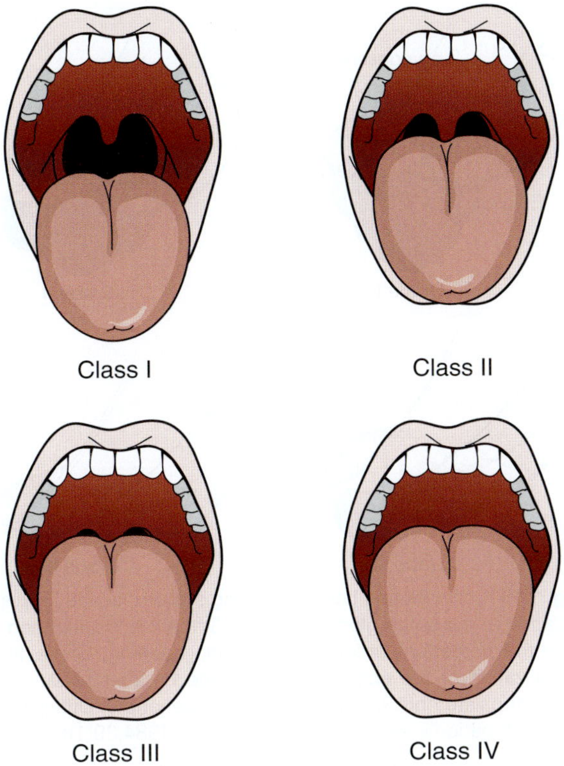

Fig. 1.13 Mallampati classification for difficult intubation. (From Hornacky A, Phillips N. *Berry & Kohn's Operating Room Technique*. 15th ed. Elsevier; 2025.)

the mouth. A small interincisor gap can cause difficulty with laryngoscopy and SAD placement. An adequate interincisor opening is at least two to three average fingerbreadths, or a minimum of 4 cm. An increase in maxillary incisor length can reduce the interincisor gap and create a sharper angle between the oral and glottic openings. Furthermore, prominent incisors or "buck teeth" increase the risk of dental damage from any device inserted into the airway. Finally, loose or awkward teeth can impede the placement of a laryngoscope blade, video laryngoscope, and ETT or create an obstruction in the event a tooth is dislodged and falls posteriorly and caudally into the laryngeal opening or trachea.

Mandibular Protrusion Test

The mandibular protrusion test is also known as the *upper lip bite test* (ULBT). This assessment demonstrates the patient's ability to extend the mandibular incisors anteriorly and past the maxillary incisors. The primary purpose of this exam is to assess the mobility of the patient's TMJ function and forward subluxation of the jaw. Difficulty with laryngoscopy arises when the patient is unable to protrude the mandibular incisors past the maxillary incisors. Decreased mandibular movement impairs the ability to place an oral airway, prevents an adequate jaw thrust to relieve a soft-tissue obstruction, and enforces malplacement of the tongue, leading to an obstructed view of the glottic opening. The assessment includes three classes, with ULBT class C indicating a potentially difficult laryngoscopic view, whereas class A would indicate an adequate view using conventional laryngoscopy (Fig. 1.14).

- *Class A:* Patient can protrude the lower incisors anteriorly past the upper incisors and can bite the upper lip above the vermilion border (line where the lip meets the facial skin).
- *Class B:* Patient can move the lower incisors in line with the upper incisors and bite the upper lip below the vermilion border but cannot protrude lower incisors beyond that point.
- *Class C:* Lower incisors cannot be moved in line with the upper incisors and cannot bite the upper lip.

Cormack and Lehane Grading

Cormack and Lehane grading is an objective scoring system used to describe laryngoscopic difficulty by directly evaluating pharyngeal structures, glottic structures, and most importantly, the glottic opening. The assessment can be used during direct or video laryngoscopy. There are four different grades of view (Fig. 1.15). The Grade II score was modified into two parts because there was a large amount of subjectivity with the initial grading. Difficulty with intubation is assumed to increase as the grades rise in number:

- *Grade I:* Widest or full view of the glottic opening.
- *Grade IIa:* Partial view of the glottis; anterior commissure is not seen.
- *Grade IIb:* Only the posterior portion of the glottic opening can be visualized or only the arytenoid cartilages.
- *Grade III:* Only the epiglottis can be visualized; no portion of the glottic opening can be seen.
- *Grade IV:* Epiglottis cannot be seen; the only view is of the soft palate.

Percentage of Glottic Opening

Percentage of glottic opening (POGO) is assessed when looking at the glottic opening directly or during

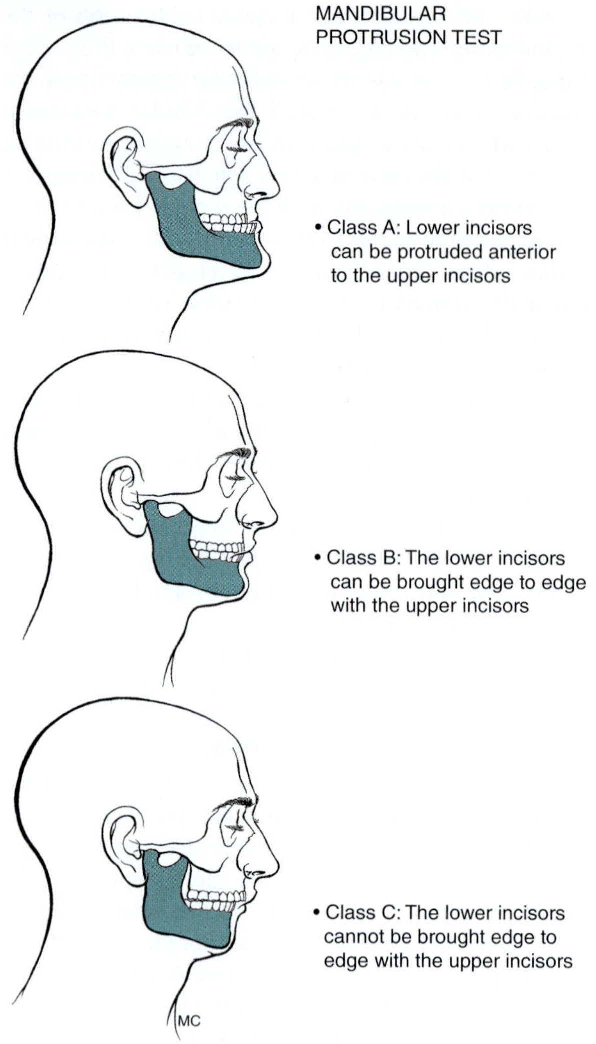

Fig. 1.14 Mandibular protrusion test classes A, B, and C (also known as the *upper lip bite test*). (Modified from Munnur U, de Boisblanc B, Suresh MS. Airway problems in pregnancy. *Crit Care Med.* 2005;33(suppl 10):S259–S268.)

videolaryngoscopy. It is defined as the linear span from the anterior commissure to the interarytenoid notch. A POGO score of 100% is a full view of the anterior commissure and every glottic structure up to the interarytenoid notch. A POGO score of 0% indicates that no portion of the glottic opening (including the interarytenoid notch) is visualized. Objective scoring between 0% and 100% is dependent on the judgment of the person performing the laryngoscopy.

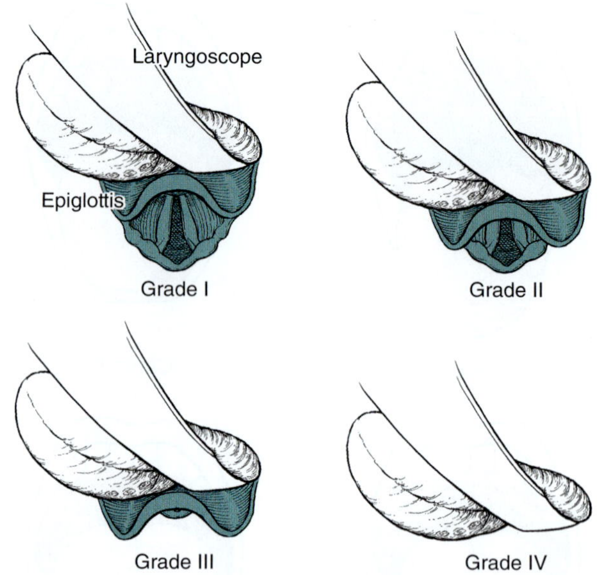

Fig. 1.15 Cormack and Lehane grading system. Grade I is visualization of the entire glottic opening. Grade II is visualization of only the posterior portion of the glottic opening. Grade III is visualization of the epiglottis only. Grade IV is visualization of the soft palate only. (From Cormack RS, Lehane J. Difficult tracheal intubation in obstetrics. *Anaesthesia.* 1984;39:1105–1111.)

Previous Difficult Airway

One of the best assessments for determining a patient's airway status is to ask the patient about a history of a difficult airway or to review previous anesthesia records that explain why the patient was perceived as challenging and what interventions were used. Prior history of difficult airway management is a predictor of future difficulties with airway management. This may change if a patient has had surgery to remove an obstructive tumor of the face or neck or if the patient has lost a significant amount of weight in the facial and neck areas.

Ultrasonography of the Airway

There are several ultrasound assessments that can be applied to the airway. There is emerging evidence that ultrasound can be used to predict a difficult Cormack-Lehane grade. Ultrasound can also be used to evaluate pathology within the airway and help influence airway management choices. It can be used to predict the diameter of the trachea or bronchi as well as the localization of the trachea. Ultrasound has been used to identify the cricothyroid cartilage and cricothyroid membrane in patients who are severely obese or when it is challenging to identify the anatomy with surface landmarks and palpation alone. Ultrasonography can also be used to identify anatomic structures within the neck to help facilitate airway blocks. Finally, it can be used to confirm ETT placement.

Lingual Tonsillar Hypertrophy

Lingual tonsillar hypertrophy is most frequently seen in patients who had a tonsillectomy as a child, heavy smokers, patients with uncontrolled gastroesophageal reflux disease (GERD), and perimenopausal females. Lingual tonsillar hyperplasia (see later Lingual tonsillar hyperplasia subsection) is usually a result of a chronic low-grade infection of the lingual tonsils. This condition most commonly occurs in adults. Hypertrophy and hyperplasia are among the most common causes of an unidentified difficult laryngoscopy and intubation. This condition is difficult to assess externally, and unless there is suspicion of the condition, it frequently goes unrecognized. The hypertrophic lymphoid tissue at the base of the tongue acts to obstruct direct views during laryngoscopy. Furthermore, the fragile tissue can bleed easily, causing further viewing obstructions. Flexible intubation with an endoscope, bougie stylets, and/or video laryngoscopy can be considered for management of a patient with this condition.

KNOWLEDGE CHECK

1. A minimum neck circumference of ___ cm is associated with difficult intubation.
   a. 33
   b. 43
   c. 53
   d. 63
2. During direct laryngoscopy, the epiglottis is visualized, but the laryngeal opening is not seen. Which view is consistent with this assessment?
   a. Grade I
   b. Grade II
   c. Grade III
   d. Grade IV
3. Which airway abnormality is the most common reason for an unanticipated difficult airway?
   a. Mandibular hypoplasia
   b. Lingual tonsillar hypertrophy
   c. Glossoptosis
   d. Laryngeal stenosis

KNOWLEDGE CHECK—cont'd

4. Which single preoperative airway assessment can predict difficult airway management?
   a. Mallampati evaluation
   b. Prior difficult airway
   c. Lingual tonsillar hypertrophy
   d. TMD

Answers can be found in Appendix A.

AIRWAY EQUIPMENT, MANAGEMENT OF DEVICES, AND PROCEDURES

Oxygen Delivery Devices and Anesthesia Circuits

Several oxygen delivery devices are routinely used during anesthesia practice, such as nasal cannulas, simple facemasks, nonrebreathing facemasks, and anesthesia facemasks attached to ventilation circuits.

- *Nasal cannulas:* These are generally used to deliver oxygen at lower flow rates. The nasal cannula can provide an FiO_2 of approximately 24% at 1 L of flow. The FiO_2 increases by about 4% for each additional liter of flow, so at 6 L of oxygen flow, a patient would receive approximately 44% FiO_2. Ultimately, oxygen delivery depends on the patient's respiratory effort and pattern. Higher flows for prolonged periods can dry nasal mucosal membranes, leading to mucosal irritation, epistaxis, and/or ear tenderness.
- *Simple facemasks:* These provide a larger reservoir for oxygen delivery of approximately 100–200 mL to the patient. There are no valves; however, the mask contains side ports that allow for the entrainment of room air and for exhaled gases to be expired. The mask does require a minimum flow rate of 5 L/min in order to prevent the accumulation and rebreathing of exhaled CO_2. Recommended flow rates range from 5 to 8 L, with FiO_2 values approximating 40% with a 5 L/min flow rate and up to 60% with an 8 L/min flow rate. Similar to the nasal cannula, effective oxygen delivery is consistent with the patient's overall respiratory effort.
- *Nonrebreathing facemasks:* These employ a reservoir bag with a 600- to 1000-mL capacity. Nonrebreather masks also have three unidirectional valves. Two are located on the sides of the mask to prevent room air from entering and act as a one-way valve for exhaled CO_2. The third is placed between the mask and the reservoir bag to prevent exhaled CO_2 from entering.

Thus, when a patient inhales, oxygen from the reservoir bag will pass through the third unidirectional valve into the mask and then the patient's airway. These masks are used to provide FiO_2 concentrations of 80%–90% and require flow rates of 10–15 L/min. If oxygen is not flowing through this system, the patient is at risk of rebreathing significant amounts of CO_2. Finally, as with previous oxygen delivery devices discussed, the patient's respiratory effort is a primary determinant of actual oxygenation.

- *Anesthesia facemasks:* Anesthesia facemasks are single-use transparent plastic masks that contain a body, a seal, and a connection point. The body determines the facemask shape and is the point where the airway provider holds the mask. The seal forms the rim of the mask, contains an air-filled cushion, and is the part that contacts the patient's face, thus "sealing" the airway mask with the patient. The connector contains a 22-mm female adaptor. Many anesthesia masks contain a collar with hooks that allow the application of retaining straps in order to hold the mask in place. Anesthesia masks provide oxygen delivery to a patient who is spontaneously breathing, allow for assisted spontaneous ventilation, and are the means to provide controlled ventilation via positive pressure, as long as the contact seal with the patient is suitable. Complications of a malpositioned anesthesia facemask include skin and ocular injuries. Retaining straps can cause facial nerve injury. Aggressive positive-pressure ventilation with an anesthesia facemask can lead to gastric distention, vomiting, and even aspiration.
- *Anesthesia circle system:* When applied to an anesthesia circuit, a facemask with appropriate seal becomes an anesthesia circle system. A circle system is a closed system that permits the delivery of precise amounts of inhaled gases and anesthetics while preventing the rebreathing of carbon dioxide. The anesthesia circuit is composed of disposable tubing that contains an inspiratory and expiratory limb as well as an anesthesia ventilation reservoir bag. As part of the anesthesia circle system, gases in the inspiratory limb advance toward the patient, and gases exhaled from the patient travel away in the expiratory limb. Each limb has a unidirectional valve that allows the gases to flow precisely in this sequence. All expiratory gases then pass through carbon dioxide–absorbent granules that remove the gas from the system. Gases enter the circle system via the fresh gas delivery hose and common gas outlet. The circle system allows for the use of low fresh gas flows and the rebreathing of inhaled anesthetics and other mixed gases. As long as the carbon dioxide–absorbent granules are unexhausted, no rebreathing of carbon dioxide occurs. Gases exit the system via the adjustable pressure-limiting (APL) valve during manual ventilation or via the ventilator relief valve during mechanical ventilation and then enter a scavenging system. The APL valve has the ability to create an adjustable leak during manual ventilation. When completely open, gases pass into scavenging because this is the path of least resistance. When the APL valve is adjusted into a more closed position, a resistance is created that is sufficient to force gas into the airway and inflate the lungs during manual ventilation. If more than 1–3 mm Hg of inspired CO_2 is detected on capnography, then the fresh gas flow should be increased to a minimum of 5–8 L/min in order to dilute the exhaled CO_2 and send it to the scavenger system.
- *Supraglottic airway devices:* SADs are airway adjuncts that provide ventilation above the glottic opening. These include laryngeal mask airways (LMAs), Esophageal-Tracheal Combitubes (Medtronic, Minneapolis, MN), King Laryngeal Tube (LT) airways (King Systems, Noblesville, IN), Air-Q (Cookgas, El Paso, TX), Ambu airways (Ambu Inc., Columbia, MD), and several other models (Table 1.5). Indications for SAD include (1) rescue ventilation for difficult mask ventilation and failed intubation, (2) an alternative to endotracheal intubation for elective surgery in the operating room, and (3) as a conduit to facilitate endotracheal intubation. These devices are well tolerated by patients because they follow the same inherent pathway as the airway and require minimal tissue distention within the hypopharyngeal space. They have proven to be valuable tools for airway management, especially in patients who are difficult to ventilate and/or intubate. A significant concern with the use of SADs is the possibility of aspiration once these devices are in place. High airway ventilation pressures can lead to gastric insufflation. These devices can also be malpositioned or cuffs can be overinflated, resulting in airway tissue trauma or failure to ventilate the patient. Finally, pathophysiologic diseases that require high peak airway pressures for ventilation, such as asthma,

TABLE 1.5 Comparison of Various Supraglottic Airway Devices

Device	Primary Function	Special Considerations
LMA Unique	Single-use, basic LMA	Least expensive LMA product; can place ETT through lumen
LMA Supreme	Second-generation SAD; includes a second lumen for gastric tube placement and gastric suctioning	Can ventilate at higher peak inspiratory pressures (up to 30 cm H_2O); allows for gastric suctioning; rigid design facilitates insertion and placement; incorporates a bite block
Flexible LMA	Airway lumen is flexible.	Lumen can be moved out of the way when surgery is performed on the face and neck.
Fastrach LMA	SAD designed to facilitate intubation through the airway lumen	Can be used for supraglottic ventilation and/or intubation; rigid design to facilitate insertion and placement; guiding handle at proximal end; incorporates an epiglottic elevating bar at mask end; guided ramp built into floor of mask aperture
Air-Q	SAD designed to facilitate intubation through the airway lumen	Can be used for supraglottic ventilation and/or intubation; oval-shaped laryngeal mask; is nonrigid and does not contain an epiglottic elevating bar; does allow for a removable stylet; comes in pediatric sizes
I-gel	Second-generation SAD; includes a gastric channel for tube placement, gastric suctioning, and early warning of regurgitation	Mask is a noninflatable gel-like material that creates a contact seal with tissues; incorporates a bite block
King LTS-D	Second-generation SAD; includes a second lumen for gastric tube placement and suctioning; used frequently in prehospital settings	Does not have a mask that covers laryngeal opening; instead has two balloons that seal the hypopharynx from the esophagus and oropharynx
Ambu airways	Ambu AuraGain is a second-generation SAD. Ambu AuraFlex has a flexible airway lumen. The Ambu Aur-i allows for tracheal intubation.	Various options for airways and procedures

ETT, Endotracheal tube; *LMA,* laryngeal mask airway; *SAD,* supraglottic airway device.
All devices are single-use and used for supraglottic ventilation.

COPD, or an airway tumor, may render SADs ineffective as a ventilation device.

- Second-generation SADs are recommended in difficult airway situations and for patients who may have a history of GERD. These newer models (1) attempt to reduce the risk of aspiration by incorporating a channel for gastric decompression and suctioning of secretions, (2) have reinforced tips that prevent folding, (3) incorporate improved cuff designs to help create a better cuff seal with higher ventilation pressures, and (4) are more rigid in their design to prevent rotation and facilitate easier insertion.
- Intubating SADs provide supraglottic ventilation and then facilitate either a blind or flexible endoscopically guided intubation through the barreled airway channel. A common indication for an intubating SAD is when difficulty with facemask ventilation and/or with tracheal intubation occurs but supraglottic ventilation is adequate. Intubating SADs allows for continued ventilation and volatile anesthesia delivery until tracheal intubation is accomplished.
- Supraglottic tubes (Esophageal-Tracheal Combitube; King LT airway) are placed blindly through the mouth and are positioned into the esophagus. These tubes have a distal balloon to occlude the esophagus, as well as a larger proximal balloon to occlude the posterior oropharynx. Between the two balloons is a ventilation port at approximately the level of the laryngeal opening.

These devices can be used for both rescue and routine management, but are primarily used for prehospital airway emergencies.

Intubation Stylets

Intubation stylets are devices placed either directly or blindly into the trachea to facilitate intubation.

- The Trachlight (Laerdal Medical Corporation, Wappingers Falls, NY) is a lighted stylet that uses a bright light source that does not require low ambient light for optimum performance to transilluminate the neck. It is inserted into the mouth, blindly advanced, and rotated toward the anterior neck. As the light source enters the glottic opening, a well-defined, circumscribed glow is noticed below the thyroid prominence and can be readily seen on the anterior neck. The ETT is then advanced over the stylet and into the trachea. Esophageal placement results in a much more diffuse transillumination of the neck without this circumscribed glow. It can be used in patients with a small oral opening or minimal neck manipulation and can be used in both the anticipated and unanticipated difficult airway when conventional laryngoscopy has failed. The risk of injury or failure is increased because of the blind insertion, and the device is contraindicated in patients with any upper airway anomaly, such as foreign body, tumor, polyps, epiglottitis, laryngeal trauma, or soft-tissue injuries. Placement may be more difficult in patients with short, thick necks or redundant soft tissue, and the device should be avoided in the "can't ventilate, can't intubate" scenario.
- The Eschmann stylet (e.g., bougie stylet) is a 15-French flexible intubation stylet 60 cm in length with a 40-degree bend at the distal tip (Fig. 1.16). It is used when the glottic opening is difficult to visualize (i.e., Cormack and Lehane grade IIa, IIb, or III). Initial visualization of the epiglottis or posterior arytenoid cartilages is important for correct placement; however, it is not essential to visualize the glottic opening for proper placement, although it does help. The stylet is advanced behind the epiglottis in an anterior direction and then advanced into the glottic opening. Feeling the stylet "bounce" along the tracheal rings as it progresses farther down the trachea is confirmation of placement, but it is not always felt. The stylet should be advanced until the 25-cm marking is at the lip, where the stylet is then held in place. An ETT is inserted over the stylet and then passed into the trachea. If resistance is felt during advancement, the ETT can be rotated 90 degrees to the left (counterclockwise) and then advanced. An alternative technique is to advance the ETT over the stylet until the ETT is in the oropharynx. Direct or video laryngoscopy is then performed while an assistant holds the stylet in place in the trachea. The ETT is then advanced through the glottic opening and into the trachea. Care should be taken not to advance the stylet too far into the trachea and risk a bronchial or distal tracheal puncture. The intubation stylet may be used during several potential clinical scenarios, including but not limited to (1) aiding advancement and delivery of an ETT during video laryngoscopy, (2) guiding ETT placement during difficult tracheal intubation, (3) being left in situ during tracheal extubation, and (4) facilitating advancement and delivery of a tracheal tube during open surgical cricothyrotomy.

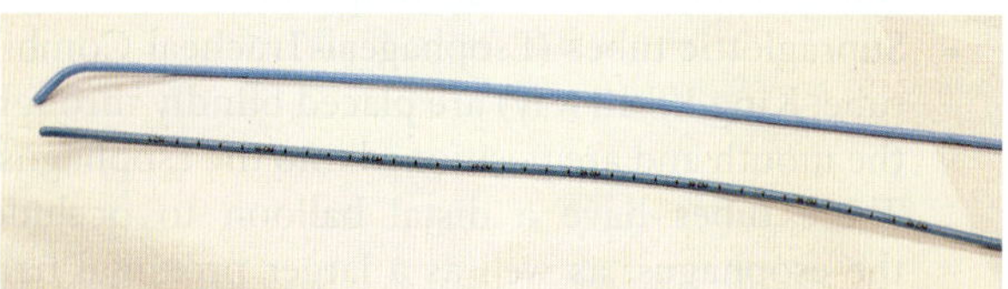

Fig. 1.16 Eschmann stylet or gum elastic bougie. (From Elisha S, Heiner JS, Nagelhout JJ. *Nurse Anesthesia*. 7th ed. Elsevier; 2023.)

- Airway exchange catheters (AECs) facilitate the interchange of an ETT and/or extubation of the trachea. These catheters are capable of gas exchange using either jet ventilation or oxygen insufflation from an adapter and bag mask. The AEC is introduced through an existing ETT with the distal tip placed above the carina. Once in place, the ETT can be removed, and a new ETT is placed over the AEC, which acts as a stylet guide into the trachea. If the new ETT encounters resistance or "hang-up" during advancement, attempting to withdraw it 2–3 cm and rotating it 90 degrees may facilitate passage. An alternative technique is to place the new ETT over the AEC and advance it until the ETT is in the oropharynx, then use a laryngoscope or video laryngoscope to displace tissue and facilitate advancement. The AEC can be left in the trachea after extubation of a difficult airway in the event that the patient requires reintubation. Care should be taken not to advance the AEC distally into either of the mainstem bronchi or to exert excessive force that could result in tracheal or bronchial mucosal damage or perforation. If jet insufflation is used with the AEC, then muscular paralysis should be considered to prevent glottic closure and allow for gas egress.

Flexible Intubating Bronchoscopes and Fiberoptic Stylets

Intubating scopes can be either flexible or rigid and assist with the placement of ETTs through video-assisted confirmation. These devices can be used during routine airway management, but they are more frequently employed when the airway is expected to be difficult or during management of an unanticipated difficult airway. Previously referred to as *fiberoptic scopes*, flexible intubating bronchoscopes now incorporate distal cameras with light-emitting diode (LED) lights instead of fiberoptic light sources.

- A flexible intubating bronchoscope can be used to evaluate an airway, facilitate intubation in a patient with a difficult airway, check ETT placement, change an existing ETT, and/or perform postextubation evaluations. Flexible intubating scopes now incorporate a small camera at the distal end of the flexible tip that transmits images to an external screen for viewing. Housed within the flexible intubating scope handle and scope shaft are working channels that can facilitate oxygen delivery, act as suction ports, or be used to instill local anesthetics. The handle contains a lever for controlling the distal end of the scope through one plane (either up or down). Light and video are supplied to an external source for viewing.
- Limitations with flexible intubating bronchoscopes include the following:
  - Impaired viewing due to fogging, blood, or secretions. Soaking the scope in warm saline, the use of an antifog liquid, or placing the scope in the buccal mucosa inside the patient's lip for 5 seconds before use may help prevent fogging. Copious secretions or blood can obstruct the operator's view. This may be prevented with the instillation of oxygen at 10–15 L/min through one of the side channels or with effective suctioning.
  - Flexible intubating scopes should be used with extreme caution in patients with epiglottitis, laryngotracheitis, or bacterial tracheitis because inexperienced operation and aggressive contact with inflamed tissue may cause a partial obstruction to convert into a total airway obstruction.
  - Caution should be exercised in patients with airway burns because of the restricted size and the hyperirritability of the airway.
  - Use is limited in airway trauma. The presence of blood, tissue, and mucus in the airway may obscure the lens and make visualization impossible. If significant soft-tissue trauma is present, edema of the tissues can prevent adequate visualization of the larynx and trachea.
  - Lack of patient cooperation in awake patients may make use of flexible scopes difficult or impossible.
  - During hypoxic situations, in which both intubation and ventilation have failed and immediate airway access is required, it may be prudent to attempt a different airway technique because of time constraints.
- Indications for the use of flexible intubating bronchoscopes include the following:
  - *An anticipated difficult airway:* These patients usually include a history of intubation difficulty and upper airway obstructions such as angioedema, tumors, abscesses, hematomas, Ludwig angina, or lingual hyperplasia.
  - *Cervical spine immobilization:* Examples are patients with traumatic cervical injuries, an unstable cervical spine, or a cervical spine with a severely decreased range of motion.
  - *Anatomic abnormalities of the upper airway:* Patients with a restricted mouth opening or hypoplastic mandible or who are morbidly obese may fall into this category.
  - *Failed intubation attempt, but ventilation possible with a mask or SAD device:* In these unanticipated difficult airway situations, the operator has time to set up and perform the flexible intubation technique. Use of a specialized oral airway (i.e., Ovassapian or Williams airway) or SAD can direct the flexible endoscope toward the larynx.
  - *Surgery to the face or jaw:* Some surgeries require nasal intubation. Flexible intubating endoscopes can be used to intubate the trachea through the nasal passages.
  - *Physiologic difficult airway:* Examples include patients experiencing severe hypotension that limits the use of anesthetic agents or those with severe respiratory distress with limited respiratory

reserves who are at risk of critical hypoxemia and desaturation during any apneic period. Awake intubation using a flexible intubating scope may be the best option for these patients.

- A suction device must be accessible whenever flexible intubation is used. Medications should also be readily available and include local anesthetics, resuscitation drugs, induction agents, and neuromuscular blocking agents. The operator can perform the technique either at the head of the bed with the patient in the supine position or from the front with the patient in a sitting position. The frontal approach with the patient sitting upright may help prevent tissues from falling against the posterior pharynx and impeding views, promote the patient's natural breathing, and decrease anxiety in an awake patient (Fig. 1.17).
- Flexible intubation bronchoscopy is performed by first loading an ETT onto the shaft of the scope. The scope is then inserted through either the mouth or the nose and advanced to the posterior pharynx. The larger the ratio between the flexible scope shaft and the internal diameter size of the ETT, the more the potential for "hang-up" with the ETT on airway structures. Manipulation of the scope is accomplished within two planes by adjusting the lever on the handle up or down and by rotating the scope laterally (right or left) with the wrist. The dominant hand holds the handle with the arm bent and resting on the operator's shoulder while the other hand holds the distal portion of the scope to keep the shaft in a straight, taut position (see Fig. 1.17). Care must be taken to keep the scope in the patient's midline while the tip is advanced toward the epiglottis. The operator should be able to visualize the different oral and pharyngeal airway structures if not using an oral guide. If at any point the view is lost, the scope should be retracted until identifiable airway anatomy is visualized. Insufflation of oxygen through the suction port not only aids in the oxygenation of the patient but also helps clear debris and keep the optics clear. Once the laryngeal opening is visualized, the tip of the scope is passed through the glottic opening and advanced until the tracheal rings come into view. The ETT is then advanced downward into the trachea, with the scope used as a stylet. If "hang-up" is encountered, the ETT should be slightly retracted 1–2 cm, rotated 90 degrees counterclockwise, and then advanced. The ETT should never be forced into the airway because this may cause trauma. After the ETT is advanced into the trachea, the operator can verify placement by visualization of the carina distal to the end of the ETT.

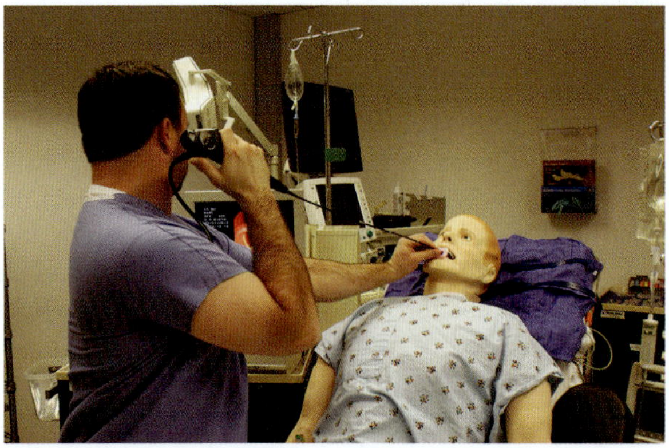

Fig. 1.17 Flexible intubation bronchoscopy (frontal approach) on a mannequin. (From Elisha S, Heiner JS, Nagelhout JJ. *Nurse Anesthesia*. 7th ed. Elsevier; 2023.)

- Rigid and malleable fiberoptic stylet devices can be used in difficult airway situations, when intubation has failed, or during routine airway management. These devices provide the operator with an indirect view of the glottic opening through a transmitted image via a fiberoptic bundle that is enclosed in a rigid or malleable stylet. These stylets allow viewing around the base of the tongue, which makes them suitable for patients with limited cervical spine mobility, patients with limited mouth opening, and patients with altered oral and pharyngeal anatomy. Examples of semirigid (malleable) fiberoptic stylets include the Shikani optical stylet (Calrus Medical, Minneapolis, MN) and the Levitan first-pass success scope (Calrus Medical). Rigid stylets include the Bonfils Retromolar Intubation Fiberscope (KARL STORZ Endoscopy-America, Inc., El Segundo, CA) and the Bullard laryngoscope (Olympus America, Center Valley, PA). Indications and limitations with the use of these devices are similar to those of flexible intubation endoscopes.

Direct Laryngoscopy and Tracheal Intubation

Also known as *standard laryngoscopy*, direct laryngoscopy remains a cornerstone of traditional airway management.

- Optimal head and neck positioning are important for successful direct laryngoscopy and tracheal intubation. This can be accomplished by using pillows, towels, or blankets or by using the operating room table's positioning functions in order to align the tragus of the ear with the patient's sternum. Flexion of the neck and extension of the atlanto-occipital joint, or "sniffing position," provides proper alignment of the oral, pharyngeal, and tracheal axes (Fig. 1.18). Manipulation of the head and neck must be used with caution in patients with decreased cervical range of motion caused by degenerative disease, rheumatic disease, neurologic pathology, trauma, or previous surgical intervention.

- Preoxygenation and denitrogenation increase the oxygen concentration within the lungs to avoid or delay arterial desaturation prior to the induction of anesthesia and during subsequent apneic periods. Preoxygenation is the administration of oxygen and should include 100% inspired oxygen, a tight mask seal, and instructing the patient to breathe at normal V_T for 3–5 minutes while providing a minimum fresh gas flow of at least 5 L/min. Denitrogenation is the act of removing nitrogen from the lungs that is a result of breathing room air. The process involves using high concentrations of oxygen to wash out the nitrogen contained in lungs, resulting in a higher alveolar oxygen concentration. Signs of adequate preoxygenation are a respiratory bag that moves with each inspiration/expiration, a well-defined $ETco_2$ waveform, and a fraction of expired oxygen that increases up to 90%. If time is limited, a patient can be instructed to take eight vital capacity breaths within 60 seconds before the induction of anesthesia.
- Direct laryngoscopy is accomplished by displacing the tongue from right to left, advancing the laryngoscope into the hypopharynx, and elevating the epiglottis using either a curved blade or a straight blade in the operator's left hand. The use of the curved (e.g., Macintosh) laryngoscope blade requires the anesthetist to (1) place the

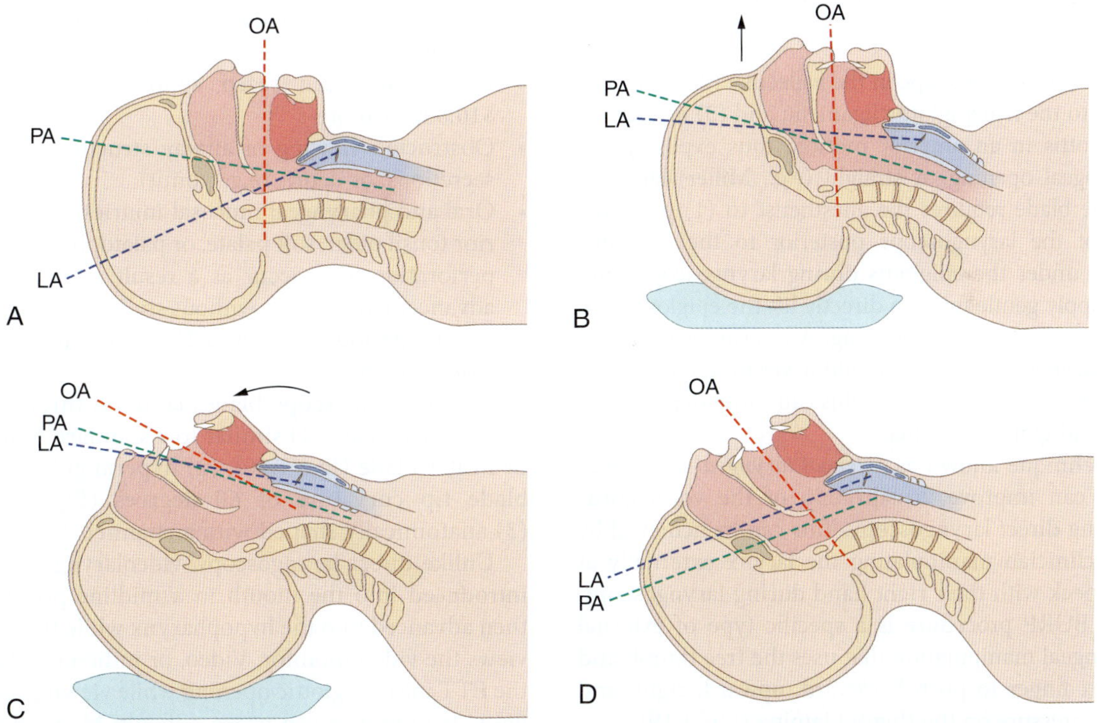

Fig. 1.18 Oral axis *(OA)*, pharyngeal axis *(PA)*, and laryngeal axis *(LA)* for intubation. (A) Nonaligned position. (B) Head resting on a pad causes flexion of the neck and aligns the PA and LA. (C) Head resting on pad causes flexion of the neck, and neck extension into the sniffing position aligns the OA, PA, and LA. (D) Extension of the neck without head elevation aligns the PA and LA but not the OA. (From Miller RD, Pardo MC, eds. *Basics of Anesthesia*. 6th ed. Elsevier; 2011.)

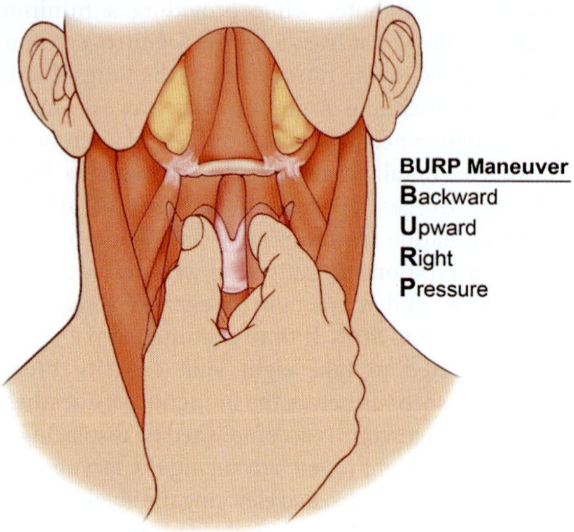

Fig. 1.19 External laryngeal manipulation using the backward and upward rightward pressure (BURP) maneuver. (Reproduced with permission from Baylor College of Medicine. Drawn by Creative Services. In Hagberg CA, Artime CA, Aziz MF. *Hagberg and Benumof's Airway Management*. 5th ed. Elsevier; 2023.)

tip of the laryngoscope in the vallecula; (2) apply tension to the hyoepiglottic ligament; and (3) elevate the epiglottis in an anterior motion, thus exposing the laryngeal opening. A straight (e.g., Miller) laryngoscope blade requires the anesthetist to (1) place the tip of the laryngoscope posterior to the epiglottis (e.g., under the epiglottis during laryngoscopy) and (2) apply gentle force to directly lift the epiglottis and expose the laryngeal opening. A levering action with the laryngoscope blade should never be applied to the patient's dentition because this can cause dental damage and gingival trauma.

- A technique known as *external laryngeal manipulation* can improve visualization of the vocal cords during direct laryngoscopy. This can be achieved by the clinician manipulating the larynx externally at the neck with their right hand during laryngoscopy. The BURP procedure is a specific type of external laryngeal manipulation that uses the free thumb and index finger to push backward, upward, right, and with pressure on the thyroid lamina (Fig. 1.19).

Video Laryngoscopy

Video laryngoscopes contain a light source and a distal micro video camera on the end of the device, which enables the transmission of video images to an external viewing screen. Glottic visualization is indirectly accomplished and tracheal intubation performed while the operator views an external video monitor. Video laryngoscopy is a popular choice for anticipated difficult airways and as a rescue strategy for unexpected difficult airways.

Video laryngoscopy advantages:

- Magnification of the airway, allowing visualization of airway structures in greater detail.
- Blade design and anterior angulation, along with placement of the video camera on the distal portion of the blade, permit the operator to visualize structures that would otherwise be difficult or impossible to see under direct laryngoscopy.
- The external monitor displays a larger view of airway anatomy and allows other practitioners to visualize airway anatomy and understand current airway conditions.
- The recording capabilities allow for education, documentation, and research.

Disadvantages of video laryngoscopy include the following:

- Cost, which can reach approximately $5000 to $10,000 or more
- Obstructed viewing of airway structures by blood, secretions, or debris (e.g., vomit)
- Oral and pharyngeal mucosal injuries, such as anterior tonsil pillar, soft palate, or palatopharyngeal arch perforation, can occur as a result of indirect ETT advancement with or without stylets, especially during the period when the ETT is not viewed on the video screen.

Video laryngoscope blades come in three separate designs which are (1) similar to a standard Macintosh or Miller blade (Fig. 1.20), (2) hyperangulated with a blade tip curvature of 60 degrees (Fig. 1.21), or (3) anatomically shaped with a channel (Fig. 1.22).

Unlike direct laryngoscopy, videolaryngoscopes are introduced into the mouth in a midline position and then advanced into the hypopharynx while the operator views the video monitor. Video, or indirect, delivery of the ETT into the glottic opening while viewing an external video monitor can prove difficult. Manipulation of the ETT in an up-and-down and side-to-side motion can help with placement. Furthermore, rigid stylets are commercially available to help mold the ETT into a hyperangulated tip. An Eschmann stylet (bougie) can

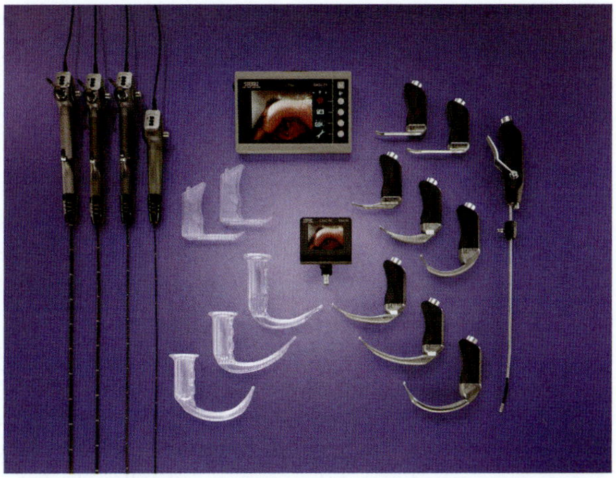

Fig. 1.20 The C-MAC video laryngoscope with option for fiberoptic bronchoscope addition. (Copyright © KARL STORZ SE & Co. KG, Germany.)

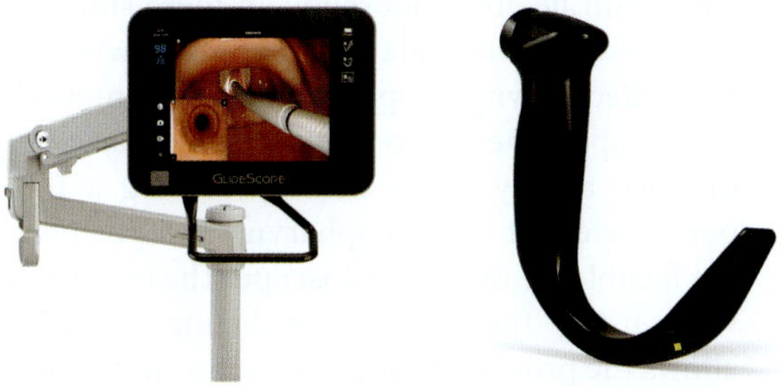

Fig. 1.21 The Glidescope Core and the Glidescope Spectrum single-use video laryngoscope. (Courtesy of Verathon, Inc.)

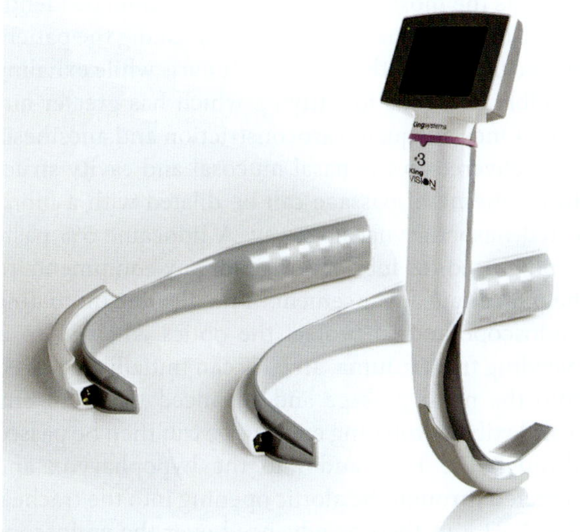

Fig. 1.22 King Vision with channel blade feature. (Courtesy Ambu.)

also be used to facilitate ETT delivery. Many video laryngoscope devices are available. Some of the more popular models include the GlideScope (Verathon Medical, Bothell, WA); C-MAC (KARL STORZ Endoscopy-America, Inc.); McGrath (Medtronic); and channel scope devices such as the Pentax Airway Scope (Pentax Medical, Montvale, NJ), the Res-Q-Scope II (Res-Q-Tech-NA Inc., Woodstock, Ontario, Canada), and the King Vision (King Systems).

Awake Intubation

Awake intubation is the process by which an ETT is placed into the trachea while a patient is adequately spontaneously breathing. This can be accomplished while the patient is completely awake or sedated. A recognized or anticipated difficult airway is the primary indication for this procedure. An awake intubation has several benefits, which include the following: (1) upper pharyngeal muscle tone is maintained, which preserves the patency of the upper airway; (2) spontaneous ventilation continues uninterrupted; (3) visualization of airway structures may be easier because laryngeal anatomy remains in its primary anatomical position (in the anesthetized and paralyzed individual, the larynx can move into a more anterior position); (4) aspiration is less likely in the awake state; and (5) neurological symptoms can be monitored in patients with cervical pathology.

- *Preparation:* Preparation for an awake intubation includes educating the patient regarding what to expect, removal and drying of secretions, anesthetizing the patient's airway, and providing adequate sedation if needed. There are times when a patient may cough during topicalization of the airway, and this should be communicated to the patient at the beginning. Once the airway is fully topicalized, the patient may lose the subjective sensation of airflow, which can lead to a feeling of not breathing. Education about and anticipation of this potential sensation can help relieve anxiety. Topical anesthesia, nerve blocks, or a combination of the two can be used to anesthetize a patient's airway. Either atropine or glycopyrrolate can be administered 15–20 minutes before the procedure to limit secretions. Radiation can cause fibrosis and loss of mucus-producing glands; thus, drying of the airway can be extensive with the use of an antisialagogue in this patient population. If an antisialagogue is not used, another option is to suction and apply gauze pads to remove existing secretions immediately prior to anesthetizing the airway. Administration of light sedation may help reduce the patient's stress and provide for a calmer environment. Several options exist, including midazolam, ketamine, remifentanil, or dexmedetomidine. However, carefully titrated amounts that avoid any respiratory depression should be used.

- *Oral awake intubation:* This can be accomplished using a flexible intubating endoscope (more commonly known as a *fiberoptic scope*), a video laryngoscope, or both. The use of an oral airway guide, such as an Ovassapian or Williams airway (Fig. 1.23), can help with oral flexible endoscopic delivery toward the laryngeal opening. The key to any awake intubation is sufficient anesthesia of the upper airway mucosa. Either a frontal (see Fig. 1.17) or head-of-the-bed approach can be used to intubate using the flexible intubating endoscope. The advantages of the head-of-the-bed approach include familiarity with intubating from this position, and the airway anatomy view is similar to direct laryngoscopy. The advantages of intubating from the frontal approach with the patient in the sitting position include the following: the frontal appoach (1) allows airway anatomy to remain in its anatomic position; (2) prevents airway structures from falling against the posterior pharyngeal wall; (3) permits easier ventilation in the upright position; and (4) may help reduce patient anxiety because the patient will be at eye level with the provider performing the procedure.
    - It is important to always keep the airway anatomy in view when using flexible endoscopy. Once the laryngeal opening is visualized, the scope is advanced into the trachea, and the ETT is passed over the scope and into the trachea. The ETT should be positioned 2–3 cm above the carina.
    - Video laryngoscopy can also be used as an intubation device during an awake intubation. The key is gentle, guided placement of the video laryngoscope blade. The operator is positioned on a step stool to the left of a patient in the sitting position who has an anesthetized airway. The operator holds the video laryngoscope in the left hand and uses the right hand to guide the laryngoscope blade behind the patient's tongue and then gently engages the base of the tongue and vallecula. Intubation can proceed once adequate visualization of the vocal cords is seen.
    - There may be times when the operator has difficulty with flexible endoscopy. In these situations, the operator can use a dual approach with both the video laryngoscope and flexible intubating endoscope. The video laryngoscope can gently displace airway tissue while providing a third-person view of the hypopharynx and position of the flexible intubating endoscope. The first-person view using the flexible intubating endoscope allows the provider to drive the scope in the direction of the trachea and deliver the ETT.
- *Nasal awake intubation:* This is accomplished using a flexible intubating endoscope. The nasal passage that permits the most amount of airflow should be identified. The procedure can be done by asking the patient to occlude either the right or left naris while exhaling forcibly and thus identifying which has greater airflow. Once adequate vasoconstriction and anesthesia are delivered to the nasal mucosal and cavity structures, the nasal passage can be dilated with a lubricated nasopharyngeal airway. A lidocaine 5% paste can be used for lubrication of airway equipment. To help facilitate advancement of the flexible intubating endoscope and to protect the optics when there is bleeding from trauma, an ETT can initially be placed into the nasal passage and advanced to 13–14 cm. The flexible intubating endoscope can then be passed through the ETT and into the hypopharynx and directed through the glottic opening into the trachea. The ETT can then be advanced over the endoscope and into the trachea.

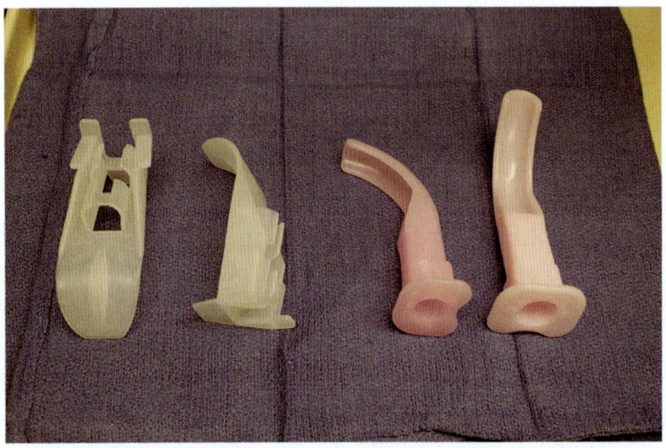

Fig. 1.23 Ovassapian *(left)* and Williams *(right)* airways. (From Elisha S, Heiner JS, Nagelhout JJ. *Nurse Anesthesia*. 7th ed. Elsevier; 2023.)

Subglottic Interventions and Emergency Front-of-Neck Access

These interventions consist of airway access through the cricothyroid membrane or the trachea. Cricothyrotomy techniques are performed by perforation or incision of the cricothyroid membrane, thereby establishing airflow into the trachea. The cricothyroid membrane is a fibroelastic membrane located inferior to the thyroid cartilage and superior to the cricoid cartilage. Perhaps the most common error during the management of the failed airway (i.e., cannot intubate and cannot ventilate) is the hesitation or indecision to rapidly move to front-of-neck access when other noninvasive methods of ventilation have proven unsuccessful. A lack of decisiveness and/or persistent attempts at laryngoscopy can result in hypoxemia and brain injury or death.

Needle Cricothyrotomy With Transtracheal Jet Ventilation

This procedure is performed using a needle (e.g., 16-gauge angiocatheter or Ravussin needle) or a venous or arterial angiocatheter. IV angiocatheters are at risk of softening and kinking at body temperature; thus, consideration should be given to catheters designed specifically for an airway cricothyrotomy. Ventilation through a needle cricothyrotomy catheter requires a jet injector powered by an oxygen source in order to generate the airway pressures needed to oxygenate the lungs. A needle cricothyrotomy with transtracheal jet ventilation (TTJV) can be used in a failed airway. However, many believe this specific technique should be reserved for those airways in which the anatomy is less favorable for placement of a surgical cricothyrotomy (e.g., small children less than 10 years old) or as a temporary means of ventilation until a more definitive airway can be established. The needle cricothyrotomy procedure can be accomplished quickly using a large-bore catheter inserted through the cricothyroid membrane at a 90-degree angle to the neck and directly toward the posterior cricoid wall. Confirmation of placement can be seen as air bubbles that are aspirated into a syringe half-filled with saline. The catheter is then held in place and attached to a high-flow oxygen insufflation device or transtracheal jet ventilator (Fig. 1.24). Once attached to the transtracheal jet ventilator, inspiratory pressures should not exceed 50 psi on the regulator, and in most instances, a minimum of 20–25 psi is sufficient. A 1-second inspiration at 25 psi with a rate of 20 breaths per minute delivers a 285-mL V_T or 5.7 L/min of oxygen. It may be difficult to determine bilateral breath sounds and bilateral chest rise in an adult. Exhalation occurs passively through the upper airway. Obstructions to passive exhalation or excessively large V_T result in hyperinflation, barotrauma, and incomplete exhalation of CO_2, and this has been shown to be a common occurrence with needle cricothyrotomy. Several options are available to help the airway remain open for the exhalation of ventilated gases and include the placement of bilateral nasal airways or an oral airway, a jaw thrust maneuver, or placement of a supraglottic airway. Finally, after successful placement of a needle cricothyrotomy and during TTJV, it is possible that the high tracheal pressures generated can potentially stent open the glottis, thus making direct laryngoscopy and identification of airway structures easier. Complications associated with the use of TTJV include barotrauma, hypoxemia, subcutaneous emphysema, pneumothorax, pneumomediastinum, hypercarbia, high intrathoracic pressures, esophageal puncture, tracheal puncture, airway mucosal damage, blood or mucus obstruction, catheter kinking, and inadvertent catheter removal.

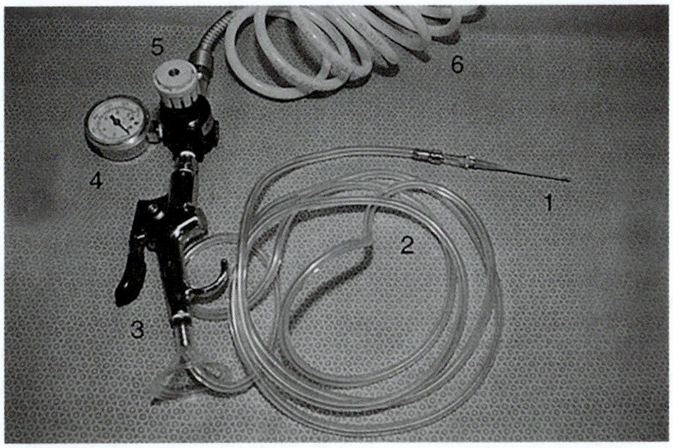

Fig. 1.24 Transtracheal jet ventilation system assembly: *(1)* IV angiocatheter; *(2)* small-bore tubing assembly with Luer lock fitting; *(3)* manual on/off valve; *(4)* pressure gauge (e.g., psi); *(5)* adjustable pressure regulator; and *(6)* high-pressure hose assembly, with Diameter Index Safety System oxygen fitting *(not shown)*. (From Elisha S, Heiner JS, Nagelhout JJ. *Nurse Anesthesia*. 7th ed. Elsevier; 2023.)

Surgical Cricothyrotomy

A surgical cricothyrotomy is accomplished by making an incision through the cricothyroid membrane and inserting a cuffed tracheostomy tube or an ETT into the trachea. Most airway algorithms and strategies recommend this procedure as a last effort to provide airway access and ventilation when it has failed with other, more conventional and less invasive methods. A surgical airway can be performed using a commercially available kit (i.e., Cook Melker cricothyrotomy kit, Cook Medical, Bloomington, IN; Quicktrach II, VBM Medical, Inc; Pertrach, Tri-anium Health Services, Dublin, OH; or Portex cricothyrotomy kit, Smiths Medical, Minneapolis, MN); with a conventional cricothyrotomy tray; or with a scalpel, bougie stylet, and ETT. Indications for cricothyrotomy include but are not limited to the following: (1) failed airway (cannot intubate and cannot ventilate); (2) traumatic injuries to the maxillofacial, cervical spine, head, or neck structures that make intubation through the nose or mouth difficult to impossible; (3) immediate relief of an upper airway obstruction (i.e., hemorrhage, massive regurgitation, edema, infection, or foreign body); and (4) the need for a definitive airway for neck or facial surgery, assuming intubation is not possible because of some structural abnormality that is congenital or acquired. Absolute contraindications to surgical cricothyrotomy are rare. However, infants and small children less than 10 years of age should not receive a needle cricothyrotomy in failed airway situations because the anatomy of the child's larynx is small, pliable, and movable. Instead, a surgical airway should be performed by an ENT surgeon. Relative contraindications for cricothyrotomy include preexisting laryngeal or tracheal diseases such as tumors, infections, or abscesses in the location of the cricothyroid membrane; distortion of neck anatomy (e.g., hematoma); bleeding diathesis; and history of coagulopathy. The use of ultrasound to identify sonoanatomy can help locate laryngeal, cricoid, and cricothyroid anatomy in those patients in whom physical palpation is difficult. Complications of a surgical cricothyrotomy include false passage of the tracheostomy tube or ETT, subcutaneous emphysema, pneumothorax, pneumomediastinum, hypercarbia, neck tissue trauma, esophageal puncture, airway mucosal damage, blood or mucus obstruction, and hypoxemia. There are several different techniques for performing a surgical cricothyrotomy that include a traditional open technique, a wire-guided technique, and the bougie technique. The procedural method chosen depends on the equipment or kits available and the provider's familiarity with the specific equipment and procedure. A wire-guided cricothyrotomy, also known as the *Seldinger technique*, is demonstrated in Figs. 1.25–1.30. A technique that relies on equipment found in most operating rooms is the bougie or finger-scalpel-bougie technique (Fig. 1.31). A vertical cut-down incision through the skin and adipose tissue from the thyroid notch extending caudad several centimeters (or three fingerbreadths) allows palpation of the cricothyroid membrane through the incision when difficult to palpate externally. Once located with the provider's nondominant index finger, a transverse incision is made through the membrane to each lateral border of the cricothyroid cartilage. The provider then advances the index finger through the incision to the inside border of the cricothyroid cartilage. A bougie is then advanced into the trachea while the provider's finger acts as a guide. The tube is then passed over the bougie and into the trachea. A potentially serious complication associated with this technique is a false passage of the bougie and/or tube through a dissected pretracheal fascial layer of tissue. This can occur with even minor force. Verification of correct placement should be performed and can be accomplished with visual bilateral chest rise and auscultation, sustained positive ET_2, and/or visual confirmation of tracheal anatomy using a flexible intubating endoscope or other optical device through the tube.

Retrograde Intubation

A retrograde wire-guided intubation may be considered when intubation has failed but ventilation is possible. Indications can include impaired visualization of the vocal cords from blood, secretions, or anatomic anomalies; airway tumors; an unstable cervical spine; or upper airway trauma. A commercial kit is available for retrograde intubation, or the practitioner can choose to insert a "J-wire" via a cricothyrotomy and pass the device cephalad into the oropharynx. This procedure is performed by inserting a 14- to 18-gauge IV catheter or a Cook needle through the cricothyroid membrane and directing it cephalad. After aspiration of air is confirmed, a wire is then inserted through the needle and advanced cephalad until it can be visualized in the posterior pharynx. It is then either advanced through the mouth or retrieved using Magill forceps. The distal end of the wire is secured with a clamp at the neck to prevent the wire from being pulled into the trachea prematurely. An ETT is then directed over the wire and passed into

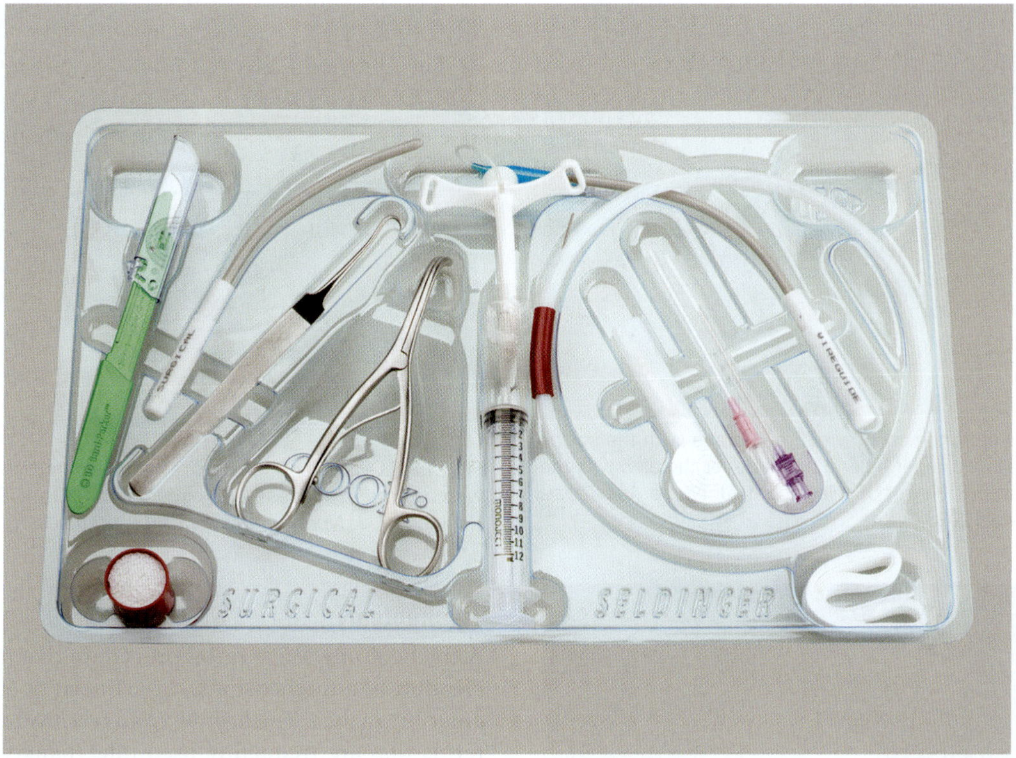

Fig. 1.25 Melker cricothyrotomy set. Options for open surgical *(tray left)* or wire-guided *(tray right)* techniques. (From Cook Medical Incorporated.)

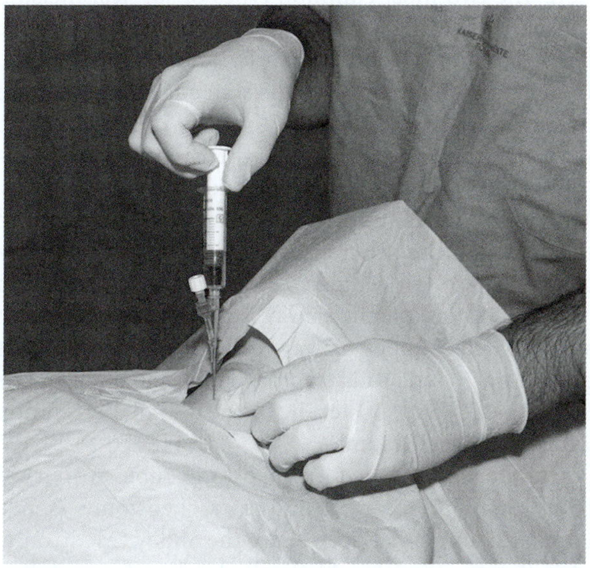

Fig. 1.26 Needle inserted through the cricothyroid membrane at a 90-degree angle. Aspiration of air confirms tracheal placement. (From Elisha S, Heiner JS, Nagelhout JJ. *Nurse Anesthesia*. 7th ed. Elsevier; 2023.)

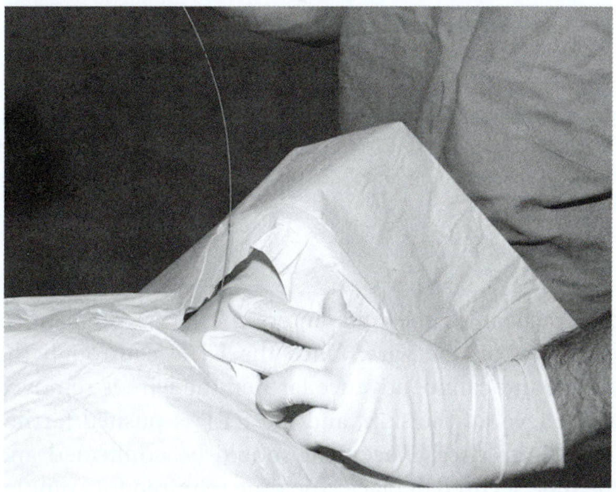

Fig. 1.27 A guidewire is threaded through a needle or catheter and placed in the trachea. Once guidewire is placed through the needle and into the trachea, remove the needle or catheter over the guidewire. (From Elisha S, Heiner JS, Nagelhout JJ. *Nurse Anesthesia*. 7th ed. Elsevier; 2023.)

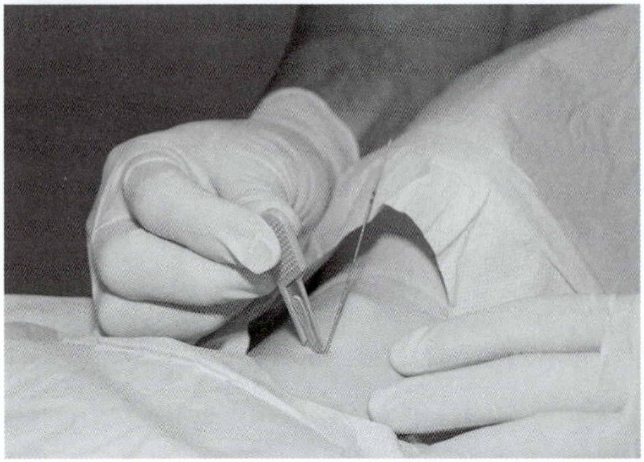

Fig. 1.28 Puncture the cricothyroid membrane with the scalpel provided to allow a larger hole to be made for the airway catheter. (From Elisha S, Heiner JS, Nagelhout JJ. *Nurse Anesthesia*. 7th ed. Elsevier; 2023.)

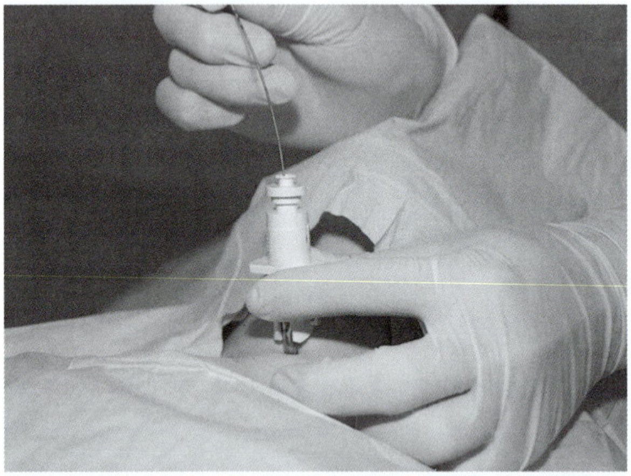

Fig. 1.29 Thread airway catheter/dilator set over the guidewire, through the cricothyroid membrane, and into the trachea. (From Elisha S, Heiner JS, Nagelhout JJ. *Nurse Anesthesia*. 7th ed. Elsevier; 2023.)

the trachea. As the tube enters the larynx, tension is increased on the wire. Once the ETT is through the larynx and cannot advance farther, the wire is removed at the level of the skin, and the ETT is pushed farther into the trachea. Placement should be confirmed and the tube secured in place. The time required for completion and the potential difficulty of wire or suture retrieval and then ETT passage limit the usefulness of this technique.

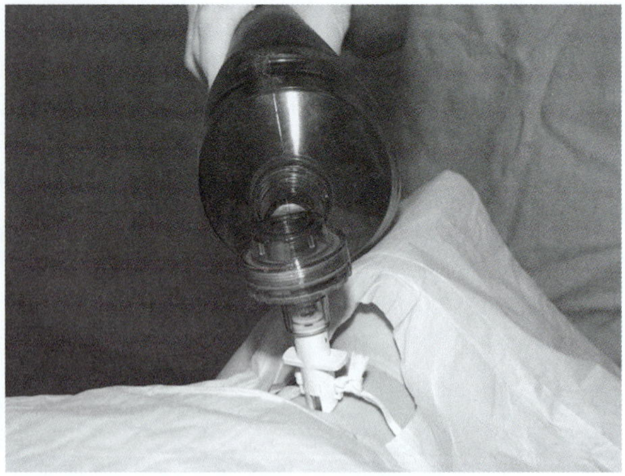

Fig. 1.30 Dilator and guidewire removed together. Ventilate with bag mask or anesthesia circuit. (From Elisha S, Heiner JS, Nagelhout JJ. *Nurse Anesthesia*. 7th ed. Elsevier; 2023.)

Tracheotomy

A tracheotomy is a surgical procedure that involves the creation of a tracheostomy, or artificial opening in the anterior trachea. *Tracheotomy* and *tracheostomy* are two terms that are frequently used interchangeably. A tracheotomy can be either temporary or permanent and can be placed either percutaneously or by surgical incision. The two most common types of surgical incision consist of a vertical slit incision or a Bjork flap. The Bjork flap tracheotomy is done by suturing an inverted, U-shaped flap of trachea to the skin edge. The standard tracheotomy is performed at the level of the fourth to sixth tracheal rings and below the isthmus of the thyroid gland. This procedure can take up to 30 minutes. Tracheotomies are traditionally done by a surgeon with the patient under general anesthesia, although in emergencies these procedures are performed rapidly in order to restore patent airway access in someone with an obstructed upper airway. Complications with this procedure include RLN trauma, damage to large vessels in the neck, and posterior tracheal wall perforation with esophageal trauma.

Tracheostomy tubes. Tracheostomy tubes are curved tubes that are inserted into a tracheostomy stoma. Popular commercial devices are the Shiley (Medtronic) and Portex (Smiths Medical) tracheostomy tubes. These devices consist of an outer cannula with a flange or neck plate, an inner cannula, and an obturator.

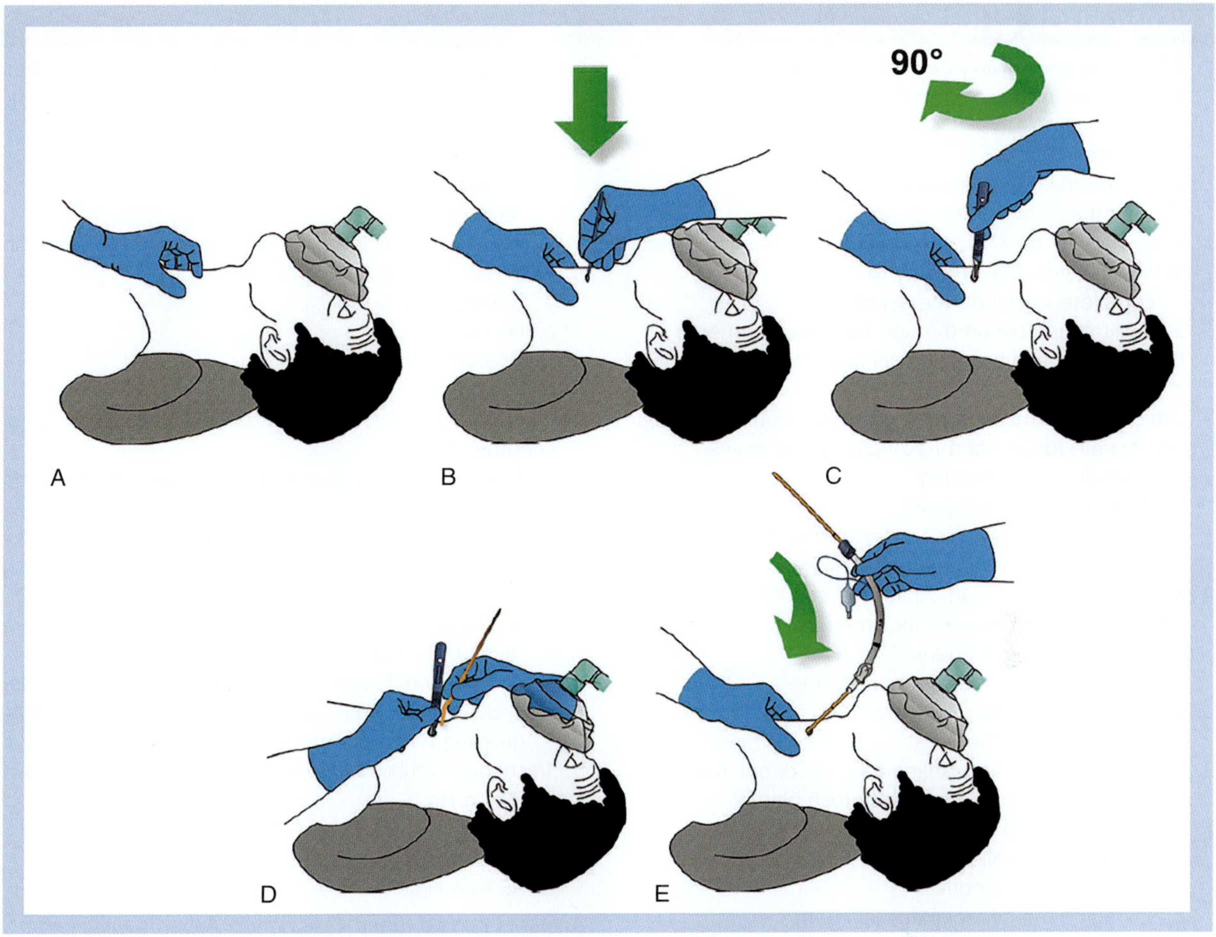

Fig. 1.31 Bougie or finger, scalpel, bougie cricothyrotomy technique. (A) Identify cricothyroid membrane. (B) Stabilize laryngeal cage and make transverse stab incision through cricothyroid membrane to lateral border of cricoid cartilage. (C) Rotate scalpel and continue incision to opposite border. (D) Remove scalpel and insert index finger of nondominant hand through incision to dilate tissues. Pass bougie under the pad of the index finger into the trachea. (E) Railroad 6.0 endotracheal tube or tracheotomy tube over bougie and into trachea. Remove bougie, confirm tube placement, and ventilate. (From Frerk C, Mitchell VS, McNarry AF, et al. Difficult Airway Society 2015 guidelines for management of unanticipated difficult intubation in adults. *Br J Anaesth*. 2015;115:827–848.)

The neck plate has lateral holes to secure the device with cloth ties or Velcro straps around the neck. The inner cannula fits inside the outer cannula and locks in place to prevent it from being displaced during coughing. These tubes are disposable or reusable and can be removed to facilitate cleaning and the removal of mucus. The obturator has a blunted tip to prevent airway trauma during insertion. They are resistant to kinking and can be rigid or flexible, depending on the needs of the patient. They are either cuffed or uncuffed. Cuff inflation pressures should be monitored when using a cuffed tracheostomy tube because tracheal capillary perfusion pressure is 25–30 mm Hg. Thus, pressures of 15–20 mm Hg should be assessed and maintained in order to prevent tracheal capillary compression with resulting decreased mucosal blood flow.

KNOWLEDGE CHECK

1. Which oxygen delivery device is associated with insufflation of air in the stomach?
   a. Nasal cannula
   b. Simple facemask
   c. Nonrebreather facemask
   d. Anesthesia facemask
2. A primary benefit of second-generation supraglottic airway devices is their ability to
   a. completely occlude the esophagus.
   b. facilitate intubation through the airway lumen.
   c. adjust the position of the airway lumen.
   d. suction gastric contents.
3. Which airway management situation would be most appropriate for use of a Trachlight airway device?
   a. A small mouth opening
   b. A penetrating neck injury
   c. An awake intubation on a recognized difficult airway
   d. A Cormack and Lehane grade of IV
4. A clinical situation that limits the use of the flexible intubating bronchoscopes includes:
   a. oromaxillofacial surgery.
   b. patient in severe respiratory distress.
   c. penetrating injury to the jaw.
   d. fixed flexion of the neck.
5. Which is the primary maneuver for direct laryngeal visualization when using a Macintosh blade?
   a. Lifting the epiglottis
   b. Engaging the vallecula
   c. Displacing the tongue
   d. Engaging the hyoepiglottic ligament
6. The hyperangulation of video laryngoscopy blade tips is angled to approximately what degree?
   a. 45 degrees
   b. 60 degrees
   c. 75 degrees
   d. 90 degrees
7. Which opioid provides the safest profile for sedation when conducting an awake intubation?
   a. Remifentanil
   b. Fentanyl
   c. Hydromorphone
   d. Morphine
8. Which patient would most benefit from a surgical cricothyrotomy?
   a. A 5-year-old with severe obstructing epiglottitis who has an O_2 saturation of 70%
   b. A 67-year-old patient after carotid endarterectomy with an expanding hematoma that is obstructing the airway
   c. A 76-year-old patient with pneumonia and severe respiratory distress who has an O_2 saturation of 84%
   d. A 27-year-old patient with an impaled knife just above the thyroid cartilage and who has audible gurgling when breathing
9. Tracheotomy tube cuff pressure should be maintained at
   a. 8 mm Hg.
   b. 18 mm Hg.
   c. 28 mm Hg.
   d. 38 mm Hg.

Answers can be found in Appendix A.

AIRWAY MANAGEMENT CONCEPTS

Cricoid Pressure/Rapid-Sequence Intubation

Rapid-sequence induction with cricoid pressure is performed on individuals who are at risk for aspiration. The purpose of cricoid pressure, also referred to as the *Sellick maneuver*, is to apply external anterior pressure to the cricoid cartilage, causing posterior displacement of the cricoid lamina against the cervical vertebrae in an effort to occlude the esophagus and prevent regurgitation and possible aspiration of stomach contents during the induction of general anesthesia. Cricoid pressure has remained a standard of anesthetic practice despite the limited evidence supporting its efficacy. A rapid-sequence induction is used in patients who are considered to have full stomachs and at risk for aspiration. The optimal amount of force on the cricoid cartilage necessary to effectively occlude the esophagus without obstruction of the trachea is considered to be approximately 4 kg of force (e.g., 40 N). It is possible that cricoid pressure can interfere with laryngeal visualization during laryngoscopy and impede ventilation through a facemask or SAD. Furthermore, radiologic and magnetic resonance imaging have shown that the esophagus can naturally be found lateral to the cricoid ring in more than 50% of patients. With the application of laryngeal or cricoid pressure, the esophagus may lateralize in up to 90% of patients.

A list of risk factors for gastric aspiration can be found in Box 1.5. Rapid-sequence induction includes adequate preoxygenation and denitrogenation followed by induction with a general anesthetic agent and neuromuscular blocking agent in rapid sequence. Ventilation is withheld

BOX 1.5 Risk Factors for Gastric Aspiration

Surgical/Patient Populations	Pathophysiologic Conditions	Other Causes
Emergency surgery	Gastrointestinal obstruction	Full stomach
Trauma	Ascites	Difficult airway management
Obstetrics	Diabetic gastroparesis	High gastric pressure with low esophageal sphincter tone
Obesity	Gastroesophageal reflux	Impaired airway reflexes
	Hiatal hernia	Depressed level of consciousness
	Peptic ulcer disease	Opioid administration
	Head injury	Cricoid pressure
	Seizures	Residual neuromuscular relaxation
	Nausea and vomiting	
	Cardiac arrest	

Modified from Elisha S, Heiner JS, Nagelhout JJ. *Nurse Anesthesia*. 7th ed. Elsevier; 2023.

as long as patient oxygen saturation remains adequate. It is acceptable to ventilate a patient, especially those patients at risk for rapid desaturation, as long as inspiratory pressures and respiratory rates are kept low. Tracheal intubation is performed as soon as the patient is rendered unconscious and is fully paralyzed.

Preoxygenation, Denitrogenation, and Apneic Oxygenation

- Preoxygenation is the process of providing 100% FiO_2 in order to increase the alveolar concentration of oxygen. Adequate preoxygenation is accomplished by (1) flushing the anesthesia circuit with high concentrations of O_2, (2) ensuring a complete seal exists with no leak to air between the anesthesia facemask and the patient, and (3) providing an 8–10-L/min flow of O_2 for 3–5 minutes while the patient maintains a spontaneous breathing pattern. If time is limited, another technique for preoxygenation is to provide a complete seal between the anesthesia mask and the patient, increase the O_2 flow to 10 L/min, and then have the patient take eight vital capacity breaths immediately prior to induction. Desaturation can be delayed with adequate preoxygenation in healthy individuals for up to 5 minutes. Preoxygenation is mandatory when performing rapid-sequence induction.
- Denitrogenation is the washout of nitrogen from the lungs. This is the true measure of adequate preoxygenation. Although a patient's oxygen saturation may reach 100%, this is not a measure of complete denitrogenation because O_2 can bind to hemoglobin fairly rapidly. The true measure of adequate denitrogenation is when the fractional exhaled portion of O_2 is 90% or greater. It is not uncommon for the terms *preoxygenation* and *denitrogenation* to be used interchangeably.
- Apneic oxygenation (also called *apneic mass-movement oxygenation*) is a strategy to provide a patient with oxygen during times of apnea, and more specifically during intubation of the trachea. Even without lung expansion and diaphragmatic movements, alveoli will continue to receive oxygen if a higher oxygen concentration gradient exists in the upper respiratory areas. Approximately 230–250 mL/min of oxygen diffuses from the alveoli into the bloodstream during apnea, whereas only 8–21 mL/min of carbon dioxide is transferred into the alveoli. The body tissues buffer the remaining carbon dioxide for a short amount of time. This O_2–CO_2 difference is the result of blood gas solubility and hemoglobin's affinity for oxygen and causes the alveoli's net pressure to become slightly subatmospheric. This subatmospheric pressure gradient facilitates gas to flow from the pharynx down into the alveoli. Apneic oxygenation can sustain a patient's PaO_2 for significant amounts of time without ventilation. However, the patient's alveolar CO_2 concentration will rise because it is not exhaled. Hypercapnia and acidosis are probable if either spontaneous or assisted breaths are not administered within a reasonable amount of time. The process of providing apneic oxygenation during an intubation procedure requires a patent upper airway and a nasal cannula. A nasal cannula is placed under an anesthesia facemask during preoxygenation and set to a high flow rate

(15 L/min or higher); thus during apnea, the high concentration of oxygen can reach the hypopharynx and become entrained into the trachea. The effects of such high nasal cannula oxygen flows can be minimized as long as this technique is used for short-term apneic episodes. Apneic oxygenation is a technique for oxygenation in patients who are at risk for rapid desaturation during apnea. Examples of patients that may benefit from apneic oxygenation include patients who are obese, pregnant, pediatric, or elderly. Patients with lung disease (e.g., ARDS, pneumonia) may also benefit from apneic oxygenation during intubation.

Expected and Unexpected Difficult Airway and Algorithms

- A patient with an expected difficult airway (Box 1.6), as determined by the provider, demonstrates one or more indicators of challenge or difficulty with facemask ventilation, laryngoscopy and intubation, supraglottic airway ventilation, and/or cricothyrotomy. The specific assessments that help identify problems with these methods of airway management have been discussed earlier. When difficulty is anticipated, the airway provider must have an initial strategy planned, followed by several other strategies to be immediately implemented in the event the initial strategy fails. Awake intubation after anesthetizing the patient's airway is recommended by many airway algorithms because it preserves spontaneous ventilation. Good communication of events with the operating room team allows for shared awareness and immediate help.
- An unexpected difficult airway (see Box 1.6) is also called the *unanticipated difficult airway*. In this situation, the airway provider does not expect to have or does not anticipate having difficulty with facemask ventilation, laryngoscopy, intubation, or other airway management techniques. Difficulty with the airway is usually encountered after the patient is anesthetized. There are many causes of unanticipated difficulty, such as a compressive tumor, aspiration, mucosal swelling, trauma, or pathology such as enlarged lymphoid tissue at the base of the tongue (e.g., lingual tonsillar hyperplasia). Without prior airway imaging, a hypertrophic lingual tonsil is usually discovered during

BOX 1.6 Difficult Airway Management

General Considerations and Management Strategies

- Conduct a thorough airway assessment and consider factors that may indicate the following:
  1. Difficult mask ventilation
  2. Difficult laryngoscopy and intubation
  3. Difficult supralaryngeal airway use and/or placement
  4. Difficult cricothyrotomy placement
- Obtain and review previous anesthesia records to assess potential for difficult ventilation/intubation.
- Formulate alternative plans in the event that difficult ventilation/intubation occurs.
- Have various airway adjuncts immediately available.
- Provide adequate preoxygenation.
- Achieve an ideal airway positioning.
- Consider administering glycopyrrolate.
- Do not delay an emergency cricothyrotomy if unable to intubate and ventilate and patient oxygen saturation is decreasing.
- Communicate clearly with other operating room personnel.

Anticipated Difficult Airway

- Anesthetize the airway using local anesthesia (i.e., topical, infiltration, and or field block).
- Perform awake flexible endoscopic (fiberoptic) intubation with spontaneous ventilation.
- Perform awake video laryngoscopy with spontaneous ventilation.
- Titrate sedative medications carefully to avoid hypoventilation or apnea.

Unanticipated Difficult Airway

- Call for help.
- Maintain spontaneous ventilation.
- If muscle relaxant (rocuronium or vecuronium) has already been administered, provide mask ventilation and consider use of an oropharyngeal airway.
- Consider immediate reversal with sugammadex 16 mg/kg IV.
- If ventilation by mask is inadequate, place a supraglottic airway (SGA) for ventilation.
- *If ventilation is adequate*, consider intubation through the SGA, video laryngoscopy for intubation, or flexible endoscopic intubation.
- Limit direct and or video laryngoscopy (three attempts maximum).
- *If ventilation is inadequate, intubation is unsuccessful, and hypoxia exists*, verbalize "failed airway" and do not delay an emergency cricothyrotomy.

laryngoscopy by a failure to visualize the glottic opening and a description of a Cormack and Lehane grade III or IV airway. Lingual tonsillar hyperplasia is believed to be the most common cause of unanticipated difficulty with laryngoscopy and intubation. Although lingual tonsillar hyperplasia is often asymptomatic, there are indicators that may alert the anesthetist to the presence of this potential obstruction, which include sore throat, dysphagia, globus sensation, snoring, feeling of a lump in the throat, and OSA.

- Airway algorithms and strategies are tools that help airway providers establish plans for safe airway care in the face of both expected and unexpected difficult airways. Multiple difficult airway algorithms exist, such as the American Society of Anesthesiologists' difficult airway algorithm and the Difficult Airway Society's difficult intubation guidelines (Figs. 1.32 and 1.33). Many of the guidelines suggested in difficult airway algorithms are based on expert opinions in the field of airway management, but they lack empirical evidence. An understanding of how these algorithms and strategies function is important for proper use because in an acute difficult airway situation, the provider should already have decided on several preset strategies and plans for managing any type of failure that could occur. Review and simulated patient experiences should be routinely undertaken to ensure continued competency with potential alternate airway management strategies.

Airway Management Outside the Operating Room

In non–operating room anesthesia (NORA) settings, equipment and personnel may not be readily available or educated to manage a difficult airway. Therefore, this can lead to the potential for poor airway outcomes. Whether providers find themselves in the intensive care unit, emergency department, radiology suite, or any other location in the hospital, a keen awareness of the anatomically difficult airway, as well as the physiologic and situationally difficult airway, is necessary to effectively manage airways in these locations, especially because help may not be immediately available. Portable airway boxes or kits can be prepared that allow the provider several options for laryngoscopy, video laryngoscopy, bag-mask ventilation, supraglottic ventilation, and cricothyrotomy. As discussed previously, a good understanding of airway algorithms and strategies is important for appropriate decision making. Furthermore, proper monitoring of patients in need of airway management and ongoing ventilation outside the operating room is essential, especially pulse oximetry and $ETco_2$ monitoring.

Tracheal Extubation Techniques

- Tracheal extubation can be performed with the patient deeply anesthetized (e.g., Guedel stage III) or fully awake. Complications of tracheal extubation, such as laryngospasm and bronchospasm, are increased when extubation is performed during Guedel stage II of anesthesia (e.g., excitatory plane). Advantages of an anesthetized or "deep" extubation include decreased cardiovascular stimulation, decreased coughing, and no patient straining or bucking, whereas the disadvantages include absent or obtunded airway reflexes and increased risks of aspiration, airway obstruction, and hypoventilation. Advantages of an awake extubation include the full return of airway reflexes, decreased risk of aspiration, and patient cooperation. The disadvantages of an awake extubation involve an increase in cardiovascular stimulation, coughing, and straining or flailing. Patients at risk for aspiration or with a history of difficult intubation should be extubated when airway reflexes return and they can ventilate spontaneously without difficulty. Increased cardiovascular stimulation during awake tracheal extubation can be minimized using β-blockers, calcium channel blockers, and vasodilators. Coughing and straining can be lessened by using IV or laryngeal topical local anesthetics and opioids, although caution should be exercised with the use of opioids and their penchant for causing hypoventilation.
- Tracheal extubation of the difficult airway should command the same attention as intubation. Effective strategies for tracheal extubation in high-risk patients include the following: (1) use of an airway exchange catheter; (2) extubation over a flexible intubating scope, which allows visual assessment of laryngeal and tracheal tissues—this technique is useful when supraglottic or laryngeal tissue injury, tracheomalacia, or paradoxical vocal cord motion is a concern; (3) extubation through a supraglottic airway, which can occur through an LMA Classic, Supreme, or Fastrach (Teleflex); or (4) simply leaving an ETT in place until extubation criteria are met and the ETT is safe to remove. An AEC is generally well tolerated and allows the patient to continue spontaneous ventilation, phonation, and clearance of secretions. It can be left in

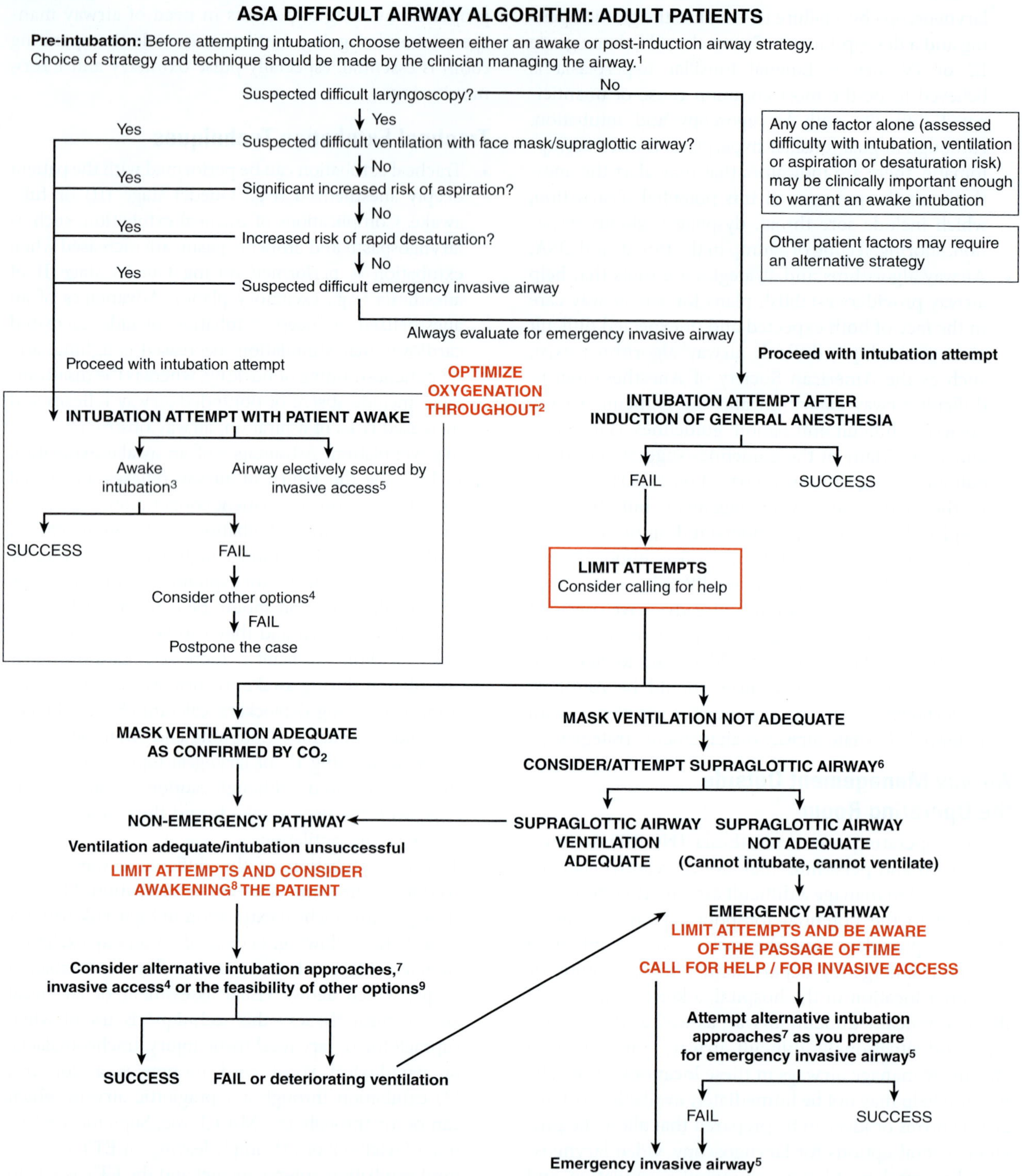

Fig. 1.32 The American Society of Anesthesiologists' difficult airway algorithm. *LMA*, Laryngeal mask airway. (From Apfelbaum JL, Hagberg CA, Connis RT, et al. 2022 American Society of Anesthesiologists Practice Guidelines for Management of the Difficult Airway. *Anesthesiology*. 2022;136(1):31-81.)

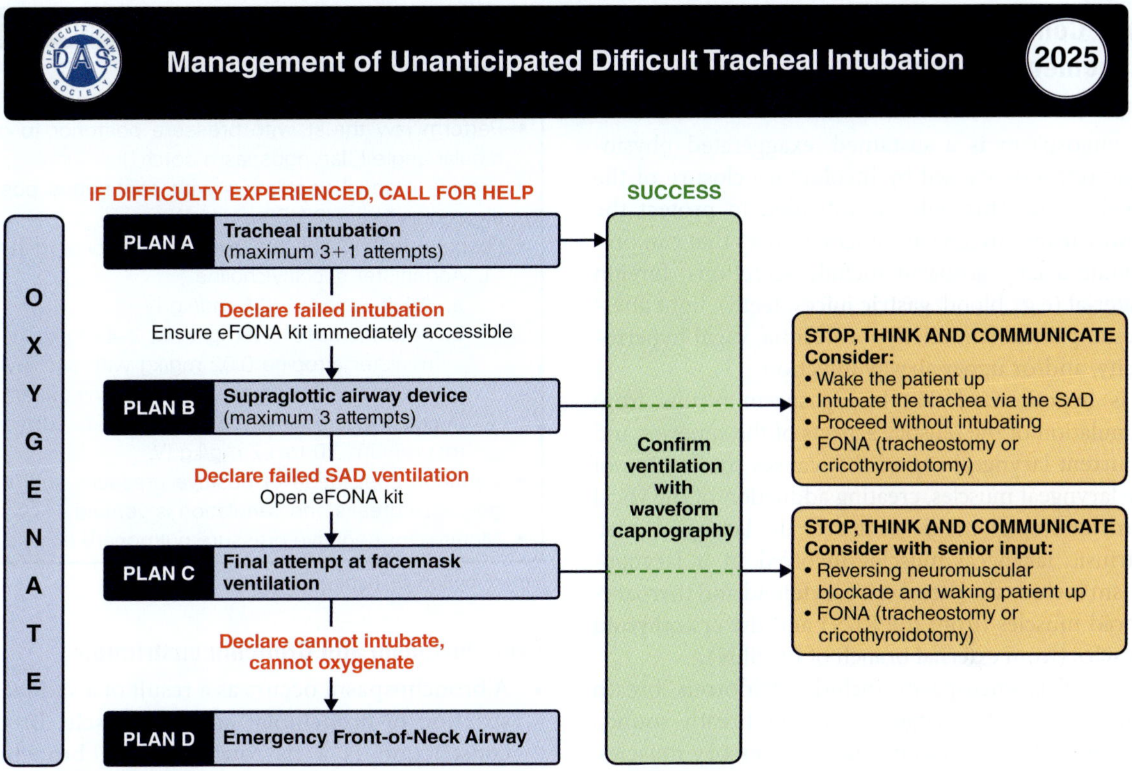

Fig. 1.33 The Difficult Airway Society's unanticipated difficult tracheal intubation guidelines. *eFONA,* Emergency front of neck access; *FONA,* front of neck access; *SAD,* supraglottic airway device. (From Ahmad I, El-Boghdadly K, Iliff H, et al. Difficult Airway Society 2025 guidelines for management of unanticipated difficult tracheal intubation in adults. *Br J Anaesth.* Published online November 7, 2025.)

place until it is determined that reintubation is not necessary. A plan for failed extubation and the need for emergent reintubation should be discussed with the operating room team prior to extubation of the difficult airway. These plans can include the use of SADs, video laryngoscopy, and cricothyrotomy.

KNOWLEDGE CHECK

1. Which patient conditions are at high risk for aspiration? *(Select all that apply.)*
   a. Occipital tumor
   b. Gastritis
   c. Intestinal obstruction
   d. Subdural hematoma
   e. Cholelithiasis
   f. Ascites
2. Which is a measure of adequate denitrogenation?
   a. Oxygen saturation of 100%
   b. Respiratory rate of 16–20 breaths/min
   c. Fraction of exhaled O_2 of 90%
   d. Oxygen flow at 8 L/min
3. Which factor has been found to be the most common cause of an unanticipated difficult laryngoscopy and intubation?
   a. Lingual tonsillar hyperplasia
   b. Mallampati class III assessment
   c. Mandibular hypoplasia
   d. Excessive neck tissue
4. Which extubation technique should be avoided when removing an ETT from a patient with a difficult airway?
   a. Extubation over an airway exchange catheter
   b. Deep plane of anesthesia extubation
   c. Extubation through a supraglottic device
   d. Awake extubation with patient cooperation

Answers can be found in Appendix A.

Airway Complications (Identification and Management of Each)

Laryngospasm

- Laryngospasm is a sustained, exaggerated physiologic response caused by involuntary closure of the vocal cords. This reflex is intended to protect the airway from foreign substances. Causes that can precipitate a laryngospasm include secretions, foreign material (e.g., blood, gastric juices, teeth), light anesthesia, painful stimuli, hypocalcemia, vagal hypertonicity, and/or upper airway infection.
- It is hypothesized that laryngospasm results from stimulation of the sensory aspects of the superior and recurrent laryngeal nerves that causes contraction of the laryngeal muscles, creating adduction of the vocal cords and epiglottic descent over the laryngeal inlet. Intrinsic laryngeal muscles involved in a laryngospasm include the lateral cricoarytenoid and thyroarytenoid muscles (from the RLN) and the cricothyroid muscles (from external branch of the SLN).
- Signs of laryngospasm include stridorous breath sounds (partial laryngospasm), no breath sounds (complete laryngospasm), use of accessory muscles, absence of air movement with respiratory effort, paradoxical thoracic movement, airway obstruction, decreasing oxygen saturation, absent capnogram, and bradycardia (late sign).
- Complications include hypoxemia, vacuum-induced (negative-pressure) pulmonary edema, hypoxemia, ischemic brain damage, and death.
- Management strategies consists of stimulus removal, suctioning of secretions, mandibular (jaw) thrust with pressure posterior to the condylar processes of the mandible (laryngospasm notch), positive pressure equal to 15–30 cm H_2O, 100% oxygen, deepening the anesthesia plane with small doses of propofol, and/or succinylcholine (0.1 mg/kg IV in adult patients and 1–2 mg/kg IV or 3–4 mg/kg IM in pediatric patients). In the pediatric population, atropine (0.02 mg/kg) should be administered in combination with succinylcholine to avoid the potential for bradycardia (Box 1.7).
- Persons with substantial muscle mass who experience laryngospasm can generate significant inspiratory force, leading to negative-pressure pulmonary edema with even one or two breaths. Laryngospasm can occur in up to 10% of pediatric general anesthesia cases.

BOX 1.7 Management of Laryngospasm

- Provide Fio_2 100%.
- Place an oral airway and confirm airway patency.
- Perform jaw thrust with pressure posterior to mandibular angle ("laryngospasm notch").
- Provide manual ventilation with continuous positive airway pressure (20–30 cm H_2O).
- For persistent, inadequate ventilation and/or oxygenation:
  1. Administer succinylcholine.
     a. Adult dose 0.1–0.5 mg/kg IV
     b. Pediatric dose 1–2 mg/kg IV, 3–4 mg/kg IM (administer atropine 0.02 mg/kg with succinylcholine to avoid bradycardia in pediatric patients)
  2. If succinylcholine is contraindicated, administer rocuronium 1.0 to 1.2 mg/kg IV.
- Continue application of positive pressure until laryngospasm breaks and ventilation is verified.
- Monitor for negative-pressure pulmonary edema.

Fio_2, Fraction of inspired oxygen.

Bronchospasm and Bronchoconstriction

- A bronchospasm occurs as a result of a sudden constriction of bronchiolar smooth muscle. Bronchoconstriction is a narrowing of the bronchi and bronchioles and can occur as a result of (1) smooth muscle constriction, (2) inflammation of the bronchi and bronchiolar walls, and/or (3) excessive mucus production. Several disorders can result in a bronchospasm caused by bronchoconstriction, including anaphylaxis, asthma, aspiration, foreign body, COPD, endobronchial intubation, ETT obstruction, exercise, emotions (anxiety), pneumothorax, and/or pulmonary edema.
- Active wheezing, coughing, dyspnea, tachypnea with labored breathing, and at times hypoxia are signs of an active bronchospasm or bronchoconstriction. Under anesthesia, the signs may show an altered upward sloping of the expiratory limb of the $ETco_2$ waveform, increased peak airway and plateau pressures, wheezing, decreasing oxygen saturation, and/or hypoxia.
- Treatment for acute bronchospasm aims at identifying the primary cause and correcting it and administering albuterol, inhaled or IV corticosteroids, inhaled anticholinergics, and IV or IM epinephrine in an emergency (Box 1.8). Bronchospasm during general anesthesia is treated initially by deepening the level of anesthesia using inhalation agents,

BOX 1.8 Management of Bronchospasm

- Maintain a secure and patent airway.
- Provide FiO_2 100%.
- Manual ventilation with a bag mask or anesthesia circuit.
- Identify and treat the underlying mechanical or pathological cause.

Mild to Moderate Bronchospasm (Adequate Ventilation With Acceptable Oxygen Saturation)

- Increase anesthetic depth.
- Increase inhalational anesthetic concentration.
- Administer albuterol via nebulizer or metered dose inhaler (if intubated, consider administration through ETT).

Severe Bronchospasm (Difficult or Inability to Ventilate and Associated With Hypoxia)

1. Call for help.
2. Stop surgery.
3. Provide treatment as indicated previously.
4. Administer beta agonist and anticholinergic bronchodilators.
5. Medications for life-threatening bronchospasm: Epinephrine IV bolus 10–100 mcg IV bolus; epinephrine IV infusion 1–4 mcg/min
   a. Terbutaline (0.25–0.5 mg subcut)
   b. Magnesium sulfate (25–40 mg/kg IV)
   c. Aminophylline (loading dose 6 mg/kg IV, IV infusion 0.5–0.7 mg/kg/h)
6. Administer corticosteroids (hydrocortisone 100 mg IV).
7. Evaluate peak inspiratory pressures and consider pressure support ventilation with prolonged expiratory times.
8. Obtain arterial blood gas values to direct treatment.

ETT, Endotracheal tube; *FiO_2,* fraction of inspired oxygen.

propofol, and/or ketamine and increasing the FiO_2 to 100%. A short-acting β_2-agoinist (albuterol) is then administered through the anesthesia circuit closest to the patient. Incremental bolus doses of epinephrine (10 mcg at a time) can be given as long as symptoms persist and no cardiac anomalies are present. For life-threatening bronchospasm, epinephrine (bolus doses titrated up to 100 mcg IV) should be given and repeated as needed. Corticosteroids (hydrocortisone 100 mg IV) are also administered to decrease bronchiolar inflammation. Because the onset of action of corticosteroids is a minimum of 1 hour, it should not delay treatment with inhalation agents and epinephrine. If bronchospasm persists, terbutaline (0.25–0.5 mg subcut), aminophylline (loading dose 6 mg/kg IV, IV infusion 0.5–0.7 mg/kg/h), and magnesium sulfate (25–40 mg/kg IV) can be considered. Mechanical ventilation strategies should allow for longer expiratory times and avoid lung volumes and plateau pressures that cause lung hyperinflation and barotrauma.

Hemorrhage in the Airway

- Airway hemorrhage is the result of trauma or pathology. Trauma can occur as a result of prehospital circumstances (e.g., penetrating or blunt force trauma) or iatrogenic causes (e.g., persistent laryngoscopy attempts, forceful insertion of airway adjuncts such as a supraglottic airway, bronchoscopy procedure). Pathological causes of airway hemorrhage can include cervical or neck masses or lesions with vessels that rupture. Bleeding can occur within the nasal, oral, and hypopharyngeal cavities; can occur within the fibrous tissues of the skin and muscle of the neck, leading to a hematoma; can come from the lungs; or can come from the esophagus (e.g., esophageal varices).
- Signs and symptoms of airway hemorrhage include hemoptysis, choking, gagging, expanding neck mass, airway obstruction, decreased oxygen saturation, and/or decreasing hemoglobin level. Recognition of hemorrhage is paramount to adequate treatment. Identification can include visualization of blood in the airway itself, hemoptysis, external or internal trauma, decreased hemoglobin value, or visualization using an endoscope within the esophagus or lung.
- Treatment includes prompt recognition, suctioning of blood from the airway, immediate rapid-sequence induction, ligation, clamping or pressure on the hemorrhaging vessel(s), hematoma evacuation, and blood transfusion as needed. In acute situations where the airway is rapidly filling with blood, leading to airway obstruction and aspiration, it may be difficult to visualize the glottic opening for intubation. If this occurs, it is important to have at least two suction setups available. Initially suction the airway, and then leave the first suction in place to the left side of the mouth. The anesthetist can then advance the laryngoscope or video laryngoscope with the left hand while using a second suction device in the right hand to continue suctioning. This is termed *laryngoscopy lead by suction.* An additional maneuver can

be performed by a second provider pressing on the chest during laryngoscopy. This may push air up through the glottis and create air bubbles as a signal for anatomic orientation of the glottic opening. Intubation can then occur. If the ETT is found to be in the esophagus, it should be left in place (especially if the bleeding is esophageal in nature). This can serve to orient the position of the esophagus in further laryngoscopy attempts. For hemorrhage below the upper airway, a surgeon is required to locate and stop the bleeding. Lung hemorrhage generally requires lung isolation with a double-lumen ETT or bronchial blocker followed by a bronchoscopy, thoracoscopy, or thoracotomy. Esophageal hemorrhage requires intubation and then ligation of the vessels using an upper esophageal endoscopy. If intubation fails and ventilation is not possible using a facemask or supraglottic airway, then an emergency cricothyrotomy should always be part of the airway management strategy and be immediately available.

Airway Trauma

- Airway trauma can be penetrating or blunt and result in hemorrhage; mucosal inflammation or ulceration; dental damage; laceration of lip, tongue, turbinate, or mucosa; dislocation or fracture of the mandible; fracture of the maxilla or facial bones; retropharyngeal dissection; laryngeal trauma; tracheal or esophageal laceration; or external trauma to the face and/or neck.
- Dental injury is the most common type of airway trauma, according to anesthesia-related closed claims databases. The maxillary central incisors are the most at risk for dental trauma during laryngoscopy and intubation. Risk factors for dental trauma include (1) preexisting dental pathology (e.g., carious teeth, periodontitis, paradentosis, or fixed dental work) and (2) one or more indicators of difficult laryngoscopy and intubation (e.g., upper incisor protrusion).
- The patient's history of the specific mechanism of injury is important for recognition of airway structures that could potentially be traumatized. Assessment of dentition and the complete airway is necessary in order to formulate an appropriate plan to avoid airway trauma.
- Management of dental damage should concentrate on the removal of any free tooth or teeth from the airway to avoid foreign body aspiration. An incident report should be completed, detailing all events that led to the damage. Management of an airway that has sustained significant trauma consists of maintaining spontaneous ventilation in patients with a patent airway. During airway trauma situations in which a patient is breathing with minimal or no discomfort, an ETT should be placed without obtunding the patient's ventilatory effort using awake intubation techniques while maintaining a patent open airway. Rapid airway control using either intubation or front-of-neck access (i.e., cricothyrotomy) occurs when airway obstruction is noted. Rapid-sequence induction should occur in crash airway situations to obtain the best possible first-pass view. Front-of-neck access should occur when airway trauma is severe enough that intubation through the glottis is not possible. When managing the patient with a traumatic airway, both laryngoscopy and video laryngoscopy should be available, along with methods to provide supraglottic ventilation. Front-of-neck access should be prepared in advance of airway manipulation, available at the bedside, and immediately performed in the event of laryngoscopy and ventilation failure to avoid critical hypoxemia.

Vomiting and Aspiration

- Aspiration consists of the passage of fluid or solid material that has been regurgitated up the esophagus and down into the trachea and/or lungs, causing obstruction, infection, and ultimately, impaired ventilation with hypoxemia. This can occur as a result of an impaired swallowing effort (e.g., Parkinson disease, multiple sclerosis, stroke) or a suppressed cough reflex (e.g., anesthesia administration, substance abuse, neurotrauma, CNS abnormalities). While the patient is in the upright or supine position, the right lung is more susceptible to being contaminated with gastric contents. This occurs because the angle of the right main bronchus is straighter than that of the left main bronchus, allowing easier passage of foreign material.
- The degree of pulmonary damage from aspiration depends on (1) the type of material aspirated (liquid or solid), (2) the acidity of the aspirate (pH less than 2.5), and (3) the quantity that was aspirated (more than 30 mL). Solid material can cause bronchial inflammation and airway obstruction, leading to distal airway collapse, whereas acidic material (solid or fluid) can chemically burn lung parenchyma, causing

pneumonitis. The pathophysiologic changes that occur in the bronchi and bronchioles as a result of aspiration include inflammation, excess mucus production, loss of ciliary function, and bronchospasm. Acidic aspirate that reaches the alveoli causes damage to the alveolocapillary membrane, resulting in hemorrhagic pneumonitis; alveolar type II cell and surfactant destruction; pulmonary edema; and stiff, noncompliant lungs that can rapidly progress to ARDS.

- Signs and symptoms in an awake patient include choking, coughing, gagging, vomiting, fever, dyspnea, wheezing, and infection (e.g., pneumonia). Signs in an anesthetized patient include hypotension, wheezing, presence of stomach contents in the hypopharynx, low oxygen saturation, high peak airway pressures, hypoxemia, and infiltrates seen on a chest radiograph.
- Preventive treatment in patients considered to have a full stomach includes (1) ASA fasting guidelines before surgery and anesthesia; (2) administration of a gastrokinetic medication (e.g., metoclopramide 10 mg IV), an antacid (e.g., bicitrate 30 mL PO), and a histamine 2 antagonist (e.g., famotidine 20 mg IV or cimetidine 300 mg IV); and (3) consideration of orogastric or nasogastric tube placement to facilitate the removal of stomach contents. A rapid-sequence induction with cricoid pressure is recommended for patients who require a general anesthetic and who are at risk for aspiration. Treatment of a patient who has aspirated includes lateral head positioning (assuming there is no trauma to the cervical spine) and immediate suctioning of the airway. Intubation followed by prompt suctioning through the endotracheal tube before positive-pressure ventilation may remove any aspirate while still in the trachea. Supplemental oxygen, mechanical ventilation, PEEP, and/or CPAP should be used if there is evidence of hypoxemia based on clinical assessment and blood gas analysis. Antibiotic therapy is only used if there is evidence of infection or fecal material is present. If a specific pathogen is identified, a broad-spectrum antibiotic that is effective against gram-negative rods, anaerobes, and *Bacteroides fragilis* can be administered. Diuretics can be administered for pulmonary edema unless hypovolemia exists. Steroid administration is controversial and may contribute to a bacterial superinfection. Steroid use has been discouraged during the initial treatment of aspiration.

Acute Pulmonary Edema

- Pulmonary edema occurs when fluid accumulates within the pulmonary interstitium and alveoli. The etiology of pulmonary edema can occur from high pulmonary capillary hydrostatic pressures (e.g., cardiogenic pulmonary edema), increased permeability of the capillary membranes (e.g., noncardiogenic pulmonary edema) from a strong inspiratory effort against an obstructed upper airway (e.g., negative-pressure pulmonary edema from laryngospasm, foreign body, or upper airway tumor), or a disproportionate amount of interstitial and/or alveolar fluid (e.g., inadequate lymphatic drainage). Cardiogenic pulmonary edema can be caused by myocardial dysfunction (i.e., ischemia or infarction) or fluid overload, such as CHF, renal insufficiency, or massive fluid resuscitation. Causes of noncardiogenic pulmonary edema include ARDS, sepsis, pneumonia, pulmonary aspiration, traumatic lung contusions, TRALI, pulmonary embolisms, and neurogenic causes (i.e., stroke, neurotrauma, intracerebral hemorrhage).
- Signs and symptoms of acute pulmonary edema include rales, wheezing, and/or rhonchi; bronchospasm; hypotension or hypertension; tachycardia; decreased O_2 saturation; dyspnea; hypoxemia; and pulmonary congestion with interstitial infiltrates on chest x-ray. If the patient is on a ventilator, then high PIP, decreased V_T, and decreased lung compliance may be observed. One of the primary signs that helps differentiate cardiogenic pulmonary edema from noncardiogenic pulmonary edema is an increase in cardiac filling pressures (e.g., increased central venous pressure [CVP], pulmonary capillary wedge pressure, and jugular venous distention). Finally, a patient who experiences a laryngospasm (especially patients with a large muscle mass) and exerts a respiratory effort against a closed glottis is at high risk for developing negative-pressure pulmonary edema. Pink, frothy sputum that is suctioned from the ETT is common after this type of event.
- Management of acute pulmonary edema includes prompt recognition, treatment of the offending cause, and supportive ventilation measures with 100% Fio_2. Intubation may be needed in patients exhibiting decreased respiratory efforts and tachypnea. Mechanically ventilated patients should receive PEEP and pressure control ventilation. Serial arterial blood gas (ABG) tests, chest radiography, and ECG

should be performed to guide therapy. Diuretics (furosemide 10–20 mg IV) may help reduce pulmonary congestion. An upright seated position or reverse Trendelenburg position is recommended if in the operating room. If the patient is not hypotensive, then a nitroglycerin infusion of 0.25–1 mcg/kg/min may help reduce cardiac stress. Support cardiovascular function with inotropic agents (i.e., dopamine 3–10 mcg/kg/min, dobutamine 5–10 mcg/kg/min, milrinone 0.25–0.75 mcg/kg/min, or epinephrine 10–200 mcg/kg/min). Hemodynamic monitoring with an arterial line and CVP should accompany inotropic agent use. Bronchospasms can be managed with albuterol. Finally, airway obstruction should be alleviated as soon as possible in patients who generate enough force to cause negative-pressure pulmonary edema (i.e., rapid treatment of laryngospasm with succinylcholine 10–100 mg IV). Care for these patients includes continued intubation with oxygen therapy and PEEP or noninvasive respiratory support with CPAP, postoperative monitoring for 12–24 hours, suctioning of secretions, diuretic therapy, chest radiography, and expert consultation.

Mucus Plug

- Mucus plug is an accumulation of mucus that occurs in the airway as a result of an ineffective cough and/or thick mucus production. It can result in pulmonary and ETT obstruction. Certain pathophysiologic conditions, such as asthma, COPD, and cystic fibrosis, cause excess mucus production that can predispose an individual to development of a mucus plug. Artificial ventilation with an ETT and poor suctioning can also lead to the formation of a mucus plug within the ETT.
- Signs of a mucus plug in the awake, spontaneously ventilating patient include decreased cough effort and airway obstruction accompanied by dyspnea, tachypnea, cyanosis, decreased pulse oximetry, and hypoxemia. Patients who are under anesthesia and ventilated with an ETT exhibit higher-than-normal PIP and plateau pressures, decreased inspiratory volumes, possible upward-sloping or absent $ETco_2$ capnography, atelectasis, hypoxemia, decreased pulse oximetry, hypercarbia, and/or complete airway obstruction.
- A mucus plug should be suspected anytime there is an ETT obstruction. Mucus that causes total airway obstruction is a lethal problem if not identified and corrected quickly. Immediate ETT suctioning is required, and if this does not alleviate the problem, reintubation with a new ETT may be necessary. Ventilation with 100% Fio_2 should be administered during the management of a mucus plug. A partial mucus plug is managed with ETT suctioning to remove the plug and then with alveolar recruitment maneuvers to improve ventilation and decrease atelectasis.

Esophageal Intubation

- Esophageal intubation occurs when an ETT is placed into the esophagus rather than the trachea during an intubation procedure. It can also occur as a result of ETT displacement from the trachea and into the esophagus during patient positioning, during head and neck manipulation, or after the removal of devices from the esophagus (e.g., transesophageal echocardiography [TEE] probe, nasogastric tube). During difficult intubation procedures in which difficulty is encountered with glottic visualization, the possibility of inadvertently placing the ETT into the esophagus increases significantly. Unrecognized esophageal intubation can lead to severe hypoxemia and death.
- Signs of esophageal intubation include no chest rise, absent breath sounds, absent or inconsistent $ETco_2$ waveforms, cyanosis, hypoxia, a decreasing pulse oximetry value (delayed sign), and/or positive auscultation of air entering the stomach. Unrecognized esophageal intubation will result in hypoxemia, hypercarbia, airway trauma from repeated laryngoscopy attempts, hyperdynamic response (e.g., hypertension and tachycardia are compensatory signs associated with hypoxia; bradycardia and hypotension are late signs of hypoxia), myocardial ischemia/infarction, and/or cerebral ischemia.
- It is imperative that confirmation of ETT placement within the trachea be promptly verified after intubation. This can occur by visualization of the ETT passing through the vocal cords, condensation inside the ETT upon exhalation, equal and bilateral auscultated breath sounds, symmetrical chest rise, adequate anesthesia bag compliance, and consistent $ETco_2$ capnography. Flexible endoscopy through the ETT to visualize the carina of the trachea is a sensitive indicator for ETT placement confirmation. Video laryngoscopy is another sensitive indicator for correct ETT placement. ETT placement should also be verified after each change in patient position or ETT manipulation.

- If esophageal intubation occurs, then the ETT should be removed so that bag-mask ventilation with 100% FiO_2 can be performed. Reintubation should occur with a clean ETT and with video laryngoscopy or a different airway adjunct. The provider should also routinely have a supraglottic device available.

Endobronchial Intubation

- Endobronchial intubation occurs when an ETT is placed either intentionally or unintentionally into a mainstem bronchus or segmental bronchus. What results is ventilation of one lung or lung segment and hypoventilation of the opposite lung. Endobronchial intubation may occur during any intubation procedure and is sometimes difficult to identify. It often occurs within the right mainstem bronchus and is more common in infants and children because of the relatively short distance between the glottis and the carina. Another situation in which endobronchial intubation may occur is intubation through a tracheostomy. Endobronchial intubation may also occur following extreme flexion of the neck because the tip of the ETT can move an average of 3.8 cm (and up to 6 cm) toward the carina when the neck is moved from full extension to full flexion. Certain surgeries, such as neurosurgery, ENT, or thoracic surgery, sometimes require flexion or extension of the neck or surgical manipulation of the upper airway, trachea, and/or bronchi.
- Signs and symptoms associated with endobronchial intubation include a deep ETT insertion depth (i.e., greater than 24 cm at the lip in the adult patient), increased PIP, asymmetrical chest expansion, unilateral breath sounds (decreased breath sounds on the nonventilated side), a possible altered $ETCO_2$ waveform, and hypoxemia. Review of a chest radiograph demonstrates the tip of the ETT at or below the level of the carina. What can result is barotrauma from the high peak airway pressures in the affected lung, atelectasis of the nonaffected lung, and inadequate ventilation.
- When endobronchial intubation is discovered, the tube should be immediately moved into the correct position. The ETT cuff should be deflated and the tube carefully withdrawn back into the trachea. Suctioning through the ETT should be considered. The insertion depth should be verified at or less than 24 cm at the lip. The cuff should then be reinflated and the lungs hyperinflated with 100% FiO_2 in order to sufficiently expand any atelectatic areas. Inspiratory pressures should be monitored. Placement should be verified with bilateral, equal, and symmetrical chest rise with equal breath sounds on auscultation, and the ETT should be resecured.

Pulmonary Embolism

- An embolism is a foreign substance or blood clot that travels through the circulatory system and then lodges and obstructs an artery. A pulmonary embolism is either a partial or complete blockade of the arterial system within the pulmonary circulation. A pulmonary embolism can result from a thrombus, fat, amniotic fluid, gas (e.g., CO_2 or air), or tumor. An embolism can be caused by a deep vein thrombosis that can occur as a result of immobility and or hypercoagulability during surgery; in the postpartum patient; in the elderly; in the obese patient; in those who have prolonged immobilization, a history of CHF or recent MI, or circulatory insufficiency in the lower extremities; or in patients who may be in a hypercoagulable state. Fat emboli can occur from long bone or pelvic fractures, reaming of bone marrow, or high-pressure injections into bone marrow during orthopedic procedures. Amniotic fluid embolisms that enter the maternal circulation can occur during or shortly after vaginal or cesarean births. A gas embolism occurs when air or gas enters the circulation. Situations in which this can occur are during CO_2 insufflation for laparoscopic surgery or when venous sinuses or vessels are open to the air, such as in a sitting craniotomy.
- Signs and symptoms of a pulmonary embolism include dyspnea, pleuritic chest pain, hypoxemia, hemoptysis, rales, crackles, wheezes, and atelectasis. Cardiovascular signs and symptoms include hypotension (which can be severe), tachycardia, and ECG changes (ST-wave changes, bradycardia, pulseless electrical activity, right bundle branch block, asystole). Additional signs that can help in the differential diagnosis of patients under general anesthesia include altered or absent $ETCO_2$ waveform on capnography and increased CVP and pulmonary arterial (PA) pressures. Fat emboli typically do not manifest until 24–72 hours after trauma or insult. Signs of fat emboli are a petechial rash on the upper torso and neck, thrombocytopenia, and/or fat globules in the urine or sputum. Amniotic fluid embolisms are

associated with high mortality and can cause cardiogenic shock, respiratory failure, disseminated intravascular coagulation, seizures, and coma.

- A positive D-dimer blood test indicates a potential pulmonary embolism and is positively diagnosed with a physical assessment and pulmonary angiography, a spiral CT scan with contrast, or a ventilation/perfusion scan.
- Medical management focuses on respiratory and cardiovascular support and consultation with pulmonary and critical care experts. Severe pulmonary embolisms that cause cardiovascular collapse require cardiopulmonary resuscitation with consideration of emergent cardiopulmonary bypass, extracorporeal membrane oxygenation, or pulmonary embolectomy. Invasive monitors such as an arterial line, TEE, CVP, and PA catheter can help guide management strategies. If a pulmonary embolism is suspected, then intubation should be considered. Ventilation strategies include high FiO_2 values and PEEP. $ETCO_2$ values are unreliable, and routine ABG values should guide ventilation and oxygenation strategies. Intravascular volume should be expanded with IV crystalloid infusions. Inotropic bolus doses of ephedrine 5–20 mg IV or epinephrine 10–100 mcg IV bolus may help correct hypotension during initial presentation. Other inotropic infusions such as dopamine, dobutamine, milrinone, or epinephrine may be needed. Heparin therapy (5000 unit bolus IV followed by 1000 units/h infusion) can be started if the patient is not bleeding. Heparin therapy may even be used preemptively in high-risk populations. An inferior vena cava filter is another treatment option for prevention of pulmonary embolism in high-risk patients.

Pneumothorax

- A pneumothorax occurs when the pleural cavity is exposed to the atmosphere or if there is a rupture of a bronchus, alveolus, or emphysematous bulla. Situations causing pleural cavity exposure include penetrating thoracic trauma, traumatic rib fractures, central line placement (subclavian or internal jugular approach), peripheral nerve blocks on or near the chest (e.g., intercostal, paravertebral, supraclavicular, infraclavicular, or stellate ganglion blocks), high PIP and barotrauma, and surgical procedures near the pleural cavity (e.g., mediastinoscopy, esophageal surgery, or upper abdominal laparoscopy). A tension pneumothorax is the progressive buildup of air within the pleural space with no escape. What results is a buildup in pressure and cardiorespiratory compromise from compression of mediastinal structures and the contralateral lung.
- Signs and symptoms include dyspnea, tachypnea, cough, chest pain, hypotension, tachycardia, hypoxemia, cyanosis, and asymmetrical chest rise. Hyperresonance during percussion occurs on the affected side. Hypercarbia and high PIP with a decrease in pulmonary compliance and low V_T are signs of a pneumothorax in the anesthetized and ventilated patient. Subcutaneous emphysema that reaches the neck and face is possible if the open pleural cavity communicates with the tissue layers of the skin. Signs of a tension pneumothorax include tracheal deviation; neck vein distention; severe cyanosis and hypotension; and even a bulging hemidiaphragm, which would only be visible during abdominal laparoscopy or open abdominal surgery.
- Confirmation of a pneumothorax is the initial step toward management (Box 1.9). Diagnosis is confirmed by chest auscultation; chest radiography; chest percussion; palpation for tracheal deviation; and elimination of other possible differential diagnoses, such as an obstructed ETT and endobronchial intubation. Treatment for a pneumothorax consists of providing 100% FiO_2, avoiding use of nitrous oxide, and placement of a chest tube by a surgeon. Cardiovascular support should be provided until resolution of the pneumothorax, with a crystalloid fluid bolus, IV vasopressors and inotropes (effects may be delayed if there is decreased venous return from pneumothorax compression), invasive monitoring, and decreasing or discontinuing of cardiac depressive and anesthetic medications. If a tension pneumothorax is suspected, a needle thoracostomy should be performed as a temporizing measure until a chest tube can be inserted. Needle thoracostomies are performed with a large-bore IV catheter (14-gauge or larger). The needle is inserted on the affected side at either the second intercostal space at the midclavicular line or in the fourth intercostal space at the midaxillary line.

Airway Fire

- An airway fire can result in an airway burn that can be either thermal or chemical, and it can result in

BOX 1.9 Management of a Pneumothorax

- Administer 100% oxygen.
- Maintain airway patency (endotracheal intubation if respiratory distress occurs).
- Provide needle decompression on affected side: large-bore IV in second intercostal space at the midclavicular line or fourth intercostal space at the midaxillary line.
- Place chest tube on affected side.
- Obtain arterial blood gas values.
- Obtain chest radiograph and chest computed tomographic scan.
- Ventilation strategy for acute lung injury:
  - Provide low tidal volume to avoid volutrauma (4–6 mL/kg).
  - Adjust respiratory rate to maintain normocarbia.
  - Minimize peak airway pressures to avoid barotrauma (< 40 cm H_2O).
  - Use PEEP (minimum 10 cm H_2O).
- Obtain complete blood count and coagulation studies.
- Monitor and treat anemia and hypovolemia in the event of hemothorax.
- Avoid nitrous oxide administration.
- Provide cardiovascular support with fluids and inotropic agents.
- Assess for decreased venous return.
- Perform cardiac resuscitation per American Heart Association ACLS/PALS protocol as necessary

ACLS/PALS, advanced cardiac life support/pediatric advanced life support; *IV,* intravenous; *PEEP,* positive end-expiratory pressure.

damage to the airway mucosa anywhere between the mouth and alveoli. Causes of an airway burn include ignition of an ETT from a laser, ignition of inhalation anesthetic gases or high concentrations of oxygen near the airway, or ignition from the inhalation of hot gases. Those at risk of an airway fire and burn include patients undergoing laser surgery in the pharynx, larynx, or tracheobronchial tree; patients undergoing tracheostomy or external head and neck surgery using electrocautery; or patients with an acute burn from the environment.

- Signs of an airway fire include actual visualization of the ignition of the ETT, operating room surgical drapes, or patient hair and skin or visualization of the fire within the surgical field or breathing circuit. It is also possible to smell smoke or burning material. Signs of an airway burn and damage include edema, charred mucosa within the airway, singed hairs within or around the airway, decreased oxygen saturation, diminished pulmonary compliance, bronchospasm, pulmonary edema, and/or ARDS.
- Management of an airway fire initially starts with fire prevention (Box 1.10). Operating room teams should receive fire safety training and assess fire risk before every surgery. To prevent high concentrations of oxygen from accumulating under drapes or in the patient's airway, providers should use vented surgical drapes and administer the lowest acceptable concentration of FiO_2 (e.g., 21%–30%) during any surgery near the head or neck. If laser surgery within the airway is planned, then a specialized laser ETT should be used with methylene blue–colored saline infused into the ETT cuff. Prior to any laser or electrocautery of the airway, the surgeon can suction the oropharynx. The surgeon may also use a scalpel or scissors to enter the airway during a tracheotomy. Treatment for an acute airway fire that results in an airway burn is to stop the flow of oxygen by either disconnecting the circuit from the ETT or turning off the oxygen. The fire should be directly extinguished with saline, and the ETT should be removed from the airway. Reintubation should occur as soon as possible because airway edema can occur rapidly (should consider the use of an airway exchanger and/or a smaller-sized ETT). Use 100% FiO_2 during reintubation as long as the fire is extinguished. Direct assessment of the extent of airway damage can occur during reintubation and immediately thereafter with a flexible endoscope. Remove any remaining foreign material from the airway. Airway supportive care can be provided with mechanical ventilation using PEEP as tolerated and lung-protective tidal volumes. Corticosteroids such as hydrocortisone (100 mg IV) and a nebulized racemic epinephrine treatment can be used. Consultation with a burn specialist for advanced treatment is necessary.

Upper Airway Edema (Angioedema)

- The most common types of upper airway edema are laryngeal edema and angioedema. Laryngeal edema is a complication of tracheal intubation (see later Postoperative Stridor subsection). Angioedema is swelling within the deep skin layers, such as the dermis, subcutaneous tissues, and mucosal and

BOX 1.10 Prevention and Management of Airway Fire

Prevention of Airway Fire

- Provide fire training to staff and assess fire risk to the patient prior to any surgical procedure.
- Used vented drapes and low oxygen flow rates during sedation if the patient's head is covered and electrocautery is used.
- Administer lowest possible FiO_2 between 21% and 30% oxygen concentration.
- Cover facial hair or other body hair with water-soluble gel.
- Have sterile saline or water available to extinguish fire.
- Avoid petroleum-based ointments in surgical area (i.e., ophthalmic ointment).
- Encourage surgeon to actively suction surgical gas/smoke.
- Moisten sponges that are used near ignition sources (especially near the airway).
- Protect the patient's eyes with wet gauze and laser goggles.
- Display fire precaution signs inside and outside operating room.
- Allow sufficient time for flammable skin preparations to dry.

Airway Fire

- Call for help.
- ***Shut off medical gases*** (i.e., disconnect circuit, turn off oxygen flow, and discontinue ventilation).
- ***Extinguish airway fire with sterile saline or water.***
- ***Remove tracheal tube and flammable material from airway.***
- Verify fire is extinguished.
- Reestablish ventilation with bag mask or anesthesia circuit and reintubate.
- Verify degree of injury using fiberoptic bronchoscope.
- Consider IV/inhaled corticosteroids/inhaled racemic epinephrine.
- Consult burn specialists for advanced treatment

Operating Room Fire

- Activate the fire alarm/notify surgical team members.
- Call for help.
- ***Immediately remove burning drapes and all flammable material from the patient.***
- Extinguish fire with CO_2 extinguisher, sterile saline, or water.
- If fire engulfs the patient, disconnect breathing circuit, stop oxygen flow, and manually ventilate with bag-valve device.
- Verify that the fire is extinguished.
- Remove the patient from the operating room and close doors.
- Turn off the gas supply to operating room suite.
- Administer total IV anesthesia until the surgery can be completed.
- Save involved materials and devices and report all fires to the hospital's risk management department.

FiO_2, Fraction of inspired oxygen; IV, intravenous.

submucosal tissues. Angioedema can result from an allergen (e.g., insect bite, food, pollen, or animal dander) or medication (e.g., antibiotics, muscle paralytics, aspirin, NSAIDs, and angiotensin-converting enzyme inhibitors). It can also be hereditary in nature, which results in low C1 esterase inhibitor protein levels. This type may manifest spontaneously throughout the patient's life. Angioedema most commonly affects the face and neck, but it can also occur in the limbs, genitals, and bowels.

- Signs and symptoms of angioedema can occur rapidly and can be a result of an anaphylactic reaction (see earlier Anaphylaxis section). Several signs and symptoms can manifest, which include swelling of the soft tissues of the face and eyes, causing difficulty with vision; laryngeal swelling, resulting in a hoarse voice; throat swelling; bronchospasm; hypotension; tachycardia; and urticaria.
- Primary treatment for angioedema of the upper airway is preservation of a patent airway. Intubation should occur as soon as possible when angioedema threatens to occlude the upper airway. Allergic angioedema can be treated with epinephrine injections, administration of corticosteroids (e.g., hydrocortisone 100 mg IV), and histamine receptor blockade (e.g., diphenhydramine 25–50 mg IV). Secondary treatment is aimed at identifying and removing the cause. Hereditary angioedema is specifically treated by administering C1 inhibitor concentrates (e.g., Cinryze [Shire, Lexington, MA], recombinant C1 inhibitor), an antiinflammatory medication such as icatibant, and/or fresh frozen plasma.

Recurrent Laryngeal Nerve Damage

- The RLN supplies nervous innervation to the majority of the laryngeal muscles. Injury to this nerve is a potential complication as a result of thyroid and parathyroid surgery, other neck procedures, or tumor compression. The right RLN is more susceptible to injury during thyroid surgery because it passes close to the bifurcation of the inferior thyroid artery.

- Unilateral damage to the RLN can cause paralysis of the posterior cricoarytenoid muscle on the surgical side, resulting in loss of abduction. The affected vocal cord then assumes a paramedian position. Symptoms manifest as hoarseness and dyspnea during physical activity. Bilateral nerve damage can lead to loss of bilateral vocal cord abduction, leading to dyspnea, stridor, and even complete obstruction.
- Management of unilateral RLN damage is supportive with supplemental oxygen administration and monitoring. Patients with bilateral RLN damage may require emergency intubation or a tracheostomy if the obstruction is severe.

Postoperative Stridor

- Stridor is the high-pitched sound of rapid and turbulent air flowing past a narrowed or partially obstructed upper airway. Stridor can occur from obstruction of the vocal cords, epiglottis, pharynx, or extrathoracic trachea. Postoperative stridor is a concerning sign and is likely due to vocal cord injury, swelling, spasm, or paralysis. Injury to the vocal cords can occur from trauma during laryngoscopy and intubation, injury to the RLN after neck or thoracic surgery, inadequate reversal of neuromuscular blockade, or pathology affecting the RLN (e.g., airway tumors). Stridor can also occur as a result of swelling of extrathoracic tracheal and/or upper airway mucosa or an airway mass impinging on airway structures and obstructing airflow (e.g., vocal cord polyps, laryngeal tumor, or expanding neck hematoma).
- Signs and symptoms include a high-pitched inspiratory sound, inspiratory retractions of the neck and/or chest, accessory muscle use, decreased inspiratory volumes, tachypnea, dyspnea, restlessness, hypoxemia, decreased O_2 saturation, cyanosis, and hypercarbia.
- Management consists of providing 100% FiO_2, suctioning secretions, and administering CPAP with assisted ventilation as needed in the awake patient (Box 1.11). Any degree of neuromuscular blockade should be reversed, and the impact of respiratory depressant drugs should be assessed. Patients with decreasing levels of consciousness due to hypoxia should receive airway support with a jaw thrust, oral or nasal pharyngeal airway, and emergency reintubation. Front-of-neck access should be immediately available in the event of airway failure. An expanding hematoma requires emergency surgery. If swelling or edema of airway anatomy is present, dexamethasone 10 mg IV, nebulized racemic epinephrine, and/or cool mist humidification is indicated. The potential for foreign bodies and retained gauze or throat pack should be evaluated. Finally, the patient should be referred to an otorhinolaryngologist for evaluation.

BOX 1.11 Management of Postoperative Stridor

- **Provide supplemental humidified oxygen and increase FiO_2 as needed.**
- Consider racemic epinephrine treatment.
- Assess airway patency, quality of breathing, and hemodynamic stability.
- Consider CPAP in the adult patient.
- Secure IV access.
- Administer corticosteroid (e.g., hydrocortisone 100 mg IV).
- Assess for residual neuromuscular blockade.
- Support ventilation with bag mask as needed.
- Provide a calm, nonthreatening environment to prevent anxiety and agitation, which may worsen airway resistance and work of breathing.
- Consider reintubation with a smaller endotracheal tube.

CPAP, Continuous positive airway pressure; *FiO_2,* fraction of inspired oxygen.

Vocal Cord Granulomas, Lesions, or Tumors

- Vocal cord granulomas are masses that grow on laryngeal cartilages as a result of irritation or injury. They are frequently the result of long-term intubation. The most frequent site is the vocal process of the arytenoids because the ETT is positioned directly between the vocal cords. Vocal cord lesions are noncancerous growths that include nodules, polyps, and cysts. These are associated with excessive vocal use or trauma. Laryngeal tumors are the result of head and neck cancers, and most form within the squamous cells that line the inside of the larynx.
- Signs and symptoms associated with vocal cord granulomas, lesions, or tumors include voice changes, hoarseness, stridor, dyspnea, tachypnea, coughing, feeling a lump in the throat, neck pain, airway

obstruction, low oxygen saturation, and potentially hypoxemia.

- Management of vocal cord granulomas, lesions, and tumors depends on the cause, how big the obstruction is, and what symptoms are occurring. The patient should be referred to a speech-language pathologist for any voice-related change. Medical management for reflux, allergies, stress, smoking, or any other medical problem is necessary before granulomas and lesions will heal. If the lesion or granuloma is large enough, it may require surgical removal (i.e., laser surgery). Laryngeal tumors and cancers can be treated with radiation therapy, chemotherapy, and/or surgery.

Lingual Tonsillar Hyperplasia

- Hyperplasia of the lingual tonsils consists of enlarged, rounded masses of lymphoid tissue on the dorsal surface at the base of the tongue. The lingual tonsils are surrounded by the vallate papillae anteriorly, the epiglottis posteriorly, and the tonsillar pillars laterally. A primary cause of hyperplasia (which is an increase in the number of lingual tonsillar cells) is usually a chronic low-grade infection of the lingual tonsils, and this condition most commonly occurs in adults. Lingual tonsillar hypertrophy (which is an increase in the size of lingual tonsillar cells) is most frequently seen in patients who had a tonsillectomy as a child, heavy smokers, patients with uncontrolled GERD, and perimenopausal females. Both hyperplasia and hypertrophy of the lingual tonsil are frequently unrecognized. Both conditions are a primary cause of unexpected difficult laryngoscopy, intubation, and mask ventilation. Difficulty with airway management occurs after the induction of anesthesia and the administration of muscle paralysis, causing the tissue to relax and severely obstruct the laryngeal opening.
- Lingual tonsillar hyperplasia is often asymptomatic; however, there are signs that indicate the potential for airway difficulty and obstruction. These include sore throat, dysphagia, nonproductive cough caused by irritation, globus sensation, snoring, feeling of a lump in the throat, and OSA.
- Ideally, management of this condition involves recognizing the possibility of hypertrophy or hyperplasia and evaluating for the condition using flexible endoscopy at the base of the tongue. However, this condition is difficult to assess externally. Thus, if the provider encounters an unexpected difficult or impossible laryngoscopic view of the vocal cords or difficulty with facemask ventilation, then lingual tonsillar hyperplasia should be ruled out as a potential cause, and efforts to secure the airway via front-of-neck access may be necessary.

KNOWLEDGE CHECK

1. Which laryngeal muscles are innervated by the external branch of the SLN during laryngospasm?
   a. Cricothyroid
   b. Lateral cricoarytenoid
   c. Posterior cricoarytenoid
   d. Thyroarytenoid
2. Which is a primary treatment for moderate to severe bronchospasm under general anesthesia?
   a. Magnesium 2 gm IV
   b. Ketamine 200 mg IV
   c. Epinephrine 20 mcg IV
   d. Terbutaline 250 mcg subcut
3. If the ______ nerve is damaged during thyroidectomy, it can result in stridor, hoarseness, and possibly respiratory difficulty.
   a. RLN
   b. internal branch of the SLN
   c. external branch of the SLN
   d. glossopharyngeal nerve
4. Which would be considered a noncardiogenic cause of pulmonary edema?
   a. Pulmonary embolism
   b. Excess fluid infusion
   c. CHF
   d. Myocardial ischemia
5. Which is considered a specific sign associated with pulmonary fat embolism?
   a. Dyspnea
   b. Hypotension
   c. Seizures
   d. Petechiae
6. Which intervention should be avoided in a patient with a pneumothorax?
   a. 1000-mL bolus of lactated Ringer solution
   b. Epinephrine 50 mcg IV
   c. Hydrocortisone 100 mg IV
   d. Nitrous oxide greater than 30%

KNOWLEDGE CHECK—cont'd

7. The initial treatment when managing an intraoperative airway fire is to
   a. pour saline on the fire.
   b. remove the ETT.
   c. stop oxygen flow.
   d. remove all surgical drapes.
8. A primary treatment for a patient with hereditary angioedema is
   a. plasmapheresis.
   b. β-blocker therapy.
   c. infusion of fresh frozen plasma.
   d. nebulized racemic epinephrine.
9. A patient has stridorous breathing, dyspnea, tachypnea, neck pain, and a globus feeling within the neck. Which of the potential diagnoses is most probable?
   a. RLN damage
   b. Lingual tonsillar hyperplasia
   c. Vocal cord tumor
   d. Laryngospasm

Answers can be found in Appendix A.

2

Pharmacology

GENERAL PRINCIPLES OF PHARMACODYNAMICS AND PHARMACOKINETICS

Pharmacodynamics

- *Pharmacodynamics* is the study of the biochemical and physiologic effects of drugs (especially pharmaceutical drugs). Pharmacodynamics places emphasis on dose–response relationships—that is, the relationships between drug concentration and effect.

Important Pharmacodynamic Concepts

- *Agonist:* An agonist is a substance that binds to a specific receptor and triggers a response within the cell. It mimics the action of an endogenous ligand (e.g., hormone or neurotransmitter) that binds to the same receptor. In adequate concentrations, it can cause maximal activation of all receptors (a full agonist).
- *Antagonists:* An antagonist is a drug that has affinity for the receptor but no efficacy. It does not activate the receptor to produce a physiologic action. By occupying the receptor, it may block an endogenous chemical response and physiologic change. Antagonists commonly have a higher affinity for a given receptor than do agonists. Types of antagonism include pharmacologic, in which competitive antagonism is reversible and noncompetitive antagonism is irreversible, requiring synthesis of new receptors to reestablish homeostasis. Pharmacokinetic, chemical, and physiologic antagonism may also occur.
- *Affinity or potency:* When considering agonists, the term *potency* is used to differentiate between different agonists that activate the same receptor and can all produce the same maximal response (efficacy) but at differing concentrations. The most potent drug requires the lowest dose.
- *Efficacy or intrinsic activity:* The efficacy of a drug is its ability to produce the desired response expected by stimulation of a given receptor population. It refers to the maximum possible effect that can be achieved with the drug. The term *intrinsic activity* is often used instead of *efficacy*, although this more accurately describes the relative maximum effect obtained when comparing compounds in a series.
- *Partial agonist:* A partial agonist activates a receptor but cannot produce a maximum response. It may also be able to partially block the effects of full agonists. It is postulated that partial agonists possess both agonist and antagonist properties; thus, the term *agonist-antagonist* has been used. A partial agonist has a lower efficacy than a full agonist.
- *Inverse agonist:* A drug or endogenous chemical that binds to a receptor, resulting in the opposite action of an agonist. Using the two-state model, inverse agonists appear to bind preferentially to the inactivated receptor. They may have a theoretical advantage over antagonists in situations in which a disease state is partly due to an upregulation of receptor activity.
- *Spare receptor concept:* The relationship between the number of receptors stimulated and the response is usually nonlinear. A maximal or near-maximal response can often be produced by activation of only a fraction of the receptors present. An example can be found in the neuromuscular junction. Occupation of more than 70% of the nicotinic cholinergic muscle receptors by an antagonist is necessary before there is a reduction in response, implying that a maximal response is obtained by activation of only 30% of the remaining number of receptors.

- *Tolerance:* Individual variation can result in a situation in which an increasing concentration of drug is required to produce a given response. This usually results from its chronic exposure to the agonist. Very rapid development of tolerance, frequently with acute drug administration, is referred to as *tachyphylaxis.* The underlying mechanism is not clear. Common causes include up- or downregulation, enzyme induction, depleted neurotransmitter, protein conformational changes, and changes in gene expression.
- *Ligand:* In biochemistry, a ligand is a molecule that can bind and form a complex with a receptor to produce a biologic response. Ligands are endogenous chemicals, such as neurotransmitters and hormones, or are exogenously administered drugs.
- *Quantal drug response:* Using dose–response curves, the actions of a drug can be quantified and expressed as the effective dose, ED_{50}; toxic dose, TD_{50}; and lethal dose, LD_{50}. The therapeutic index is the LD_{50}/ED_{50}.
- *Receptor adaptation or homeostasis:* The number and activity of a receptor population may increase or decrease in response to (usually) chronic drug administration. *Upregulation* is the process by which a cell increases the number of receptors to a given drug. *Downregulation* is the process by which a cell decreases the number of receptors for a given drug in response to chronic stimulation. β-Adrenergic receptors, for example, upregulate in the presence of antagonists and downregulate in the presence of agonists.
- *Tachyphylaxis:* This is acute tolerance, the rapid appearance of a progressive decrease in response to a given dose of a drug after continuous administration.
- *Ceiling effect:* The *ceiling effect* of a drug refers to the dose beyond which there is no increase in effect. Additional dosing often leads to adverse effects.
- *Therapeutic window:* The dosage range of a drug that provides safe, effective therapy with minimal adverse effects

Pharmacokinetics

- *Pharmacokinetics* is a branch of pharmacology dedicated to determining the fate of substances administered to a living organism: evaluation of the absorption, distribution, metabolism, and excretion of a drug.

Binding of Drugs to Plasma Proteins

- Plasma albumin is most important and is a source of species variation; β-globulin and α_1-acid glycoprotein also bind some drugs that are bases.
- Plasma albumin mainly binds drugs that are acidic. α_1-Acid glycoprotein mainly binds drugs that are basic. Saturable binding sometimes leads to a nonlinear relationship between dose and free (active) drug concentration.
- Extensive protein binding slows drug elimination (metabolism and excretion by glomerular filtration).
- Competition between drugs for protein binding can lead to clinically important drug interactions, but this is uncommon.

Movement of Drugs Across Cellular Barriers

- To traverse cellular barriers (e.g., gastrointestinal [GI] mucosa, renal tubule, blood–brain barrier, placenta), drugs must cross lipid membranes.
- Drugs cross lipid membranes mainly by passive diffusional transfer or by carrier-mediated transfer.
- The main factors that determine the rate of passive diffusional transfer across membranes are a drug's lipid solubility and the concentration gradient.
- Most drugs are weak acids or weak bases; their state of ionization varies with pH according to the Henderson-Hasselbalch equation.
- With weak acids or bases, only the uncharged species (the protonated form for a weak acid; the unprotonated form for a weak base) can diffuse across lipid membranes; this gives rise to pH partition or ion trapping.
- The term *pH partition* means that weak acids tend to accumulate in compartments of relatively high pH, whereas weak bases do the reverse.
- Carrier-mediated transport involves solute carriers, including organic cation transporters and organic anion transporters, and P-glycoproteins (P for permeability, also referred to as *adenosine triphosphate [ATP]-binding cassette transporters*) in the renal tubule, blood–brain barrier, and GI epithelium. These are important for determining the distribution of some drugs, are prone to genetic variation, and are targets for drug interactions. Many are chemically related to endogenous substances.
- Drugs that have a very low lipid solubility, including those that are strong acids or bases, are generally poorly absorbed from the gut.

- A few drugs (e.g., levodopa) are absorbed by carrier-mediated transfer.
- Absorption from the gut depends on many factors, including the following:
  - GI motility and pH
  - Particle size
  - Physicochemical interaction with gut contents (e.g., chemical interaction between calcium and tetracycline antibiotics)
- Bioavailability is the fraction of an ingested dose of a drug that gains access to the systemic circulation. It may be low because absorption is incomplete or because the drug is metabolized in the gut wall or liver before reaching the systemic circulation.
- Bioequivalence implies that if one formulation of a drug is substituted for another, no clinically untoward consequences will occur.

Routes of Administration

- See Table 2.1.

Drug Distribution

The major compartments are as follows:

- Plasma (5% of body weight)
- Interstitial fluid (16% of body weight)
- Intracellular fluid (35% of body weight)
- Transcellular fluid (2% of body weight)
- Fat (20% of body weight)
- Volume of distribution (V_d) is defined as the volume of plasma that would contain the total body content of a drug at a concentration equal to that in the plasma.
- Water-soluble drugs are mainly confined to plasma and interstitial fluids; most do not enter the brain after acute dosing (e.g., neuromuscular blocking agents).
- Lipid-soluble drugs reach all compartments and may accumulate in fat (e.g., induction agents, narcotics).
- For drugs that accumulate outside the plasma compartment (e.g., in fat or by being bound to tissues), V_d may exceed total body volume.

TABLE 2.1 Routes of Administration

Route	Bioavailability	Comments
Intravenous	100% (by definition)	Most rapid onset; allows for titration of doses; suitable for large volumes
Intramuscular	75%–100%	Moderate volumes feasible; may be painful
Subcutaneous	75%–100%	Smaller volumes than intramuscular; may be painful; suitable for implantation of pellets
Oral	5%–100%	Most convenient and economical; first-pass effect may be significant; requires patient cooperation
Rectal	30%–100%	Less first-pass effect than oral; useful in pediatric patients
Inhalation	5%–100%	Common anesthetic use for inhalation drugs, steroids, bronchodilators, and occasionally resuscitative drugs; very rapid onset (parallels intravenous administration)
Sublingual	60%–100%	Lack of first-pass effect; absorbed directly into systemic circulation
Intrathecal	Low (intentionally)	Specialized application, such as with local anesthetics and analgesics, chemotherapy, and antibiotic administration; circumvents blood–brain barrier
Topical	80%–100%	Includes skin; cornea; and buccal, vaginal, and nasal mucosae. Dermal application results in slow absorption; used for lack of first-pass effect; prolonged duration of action.
Intranasal	Up to 95%	Rich vascular plexus provides a direct route into the blood; best for lipid-soluble agents; mist or atomized formulation is most effective; 0.25–0.3 mL ideal or up to <1 mL of highly concentrated preparation; avoids gastrointestinal destruction and first-pass metabolism; may rapidly achieve therapeutic brain and spinal cord (central nervous system) drug concentrations.
Intraosseous	Up to 100%, depending on site	Recommended for emergency access when an intravenous line cannot be established, such as during resuscitation or in pediatrics

From Elisha S, Heiner JS, Nagelhout JJ. *Nurse Anesthesia*. 7th ed. Elsevier; 2023.

TABLE 2.2 **Tissue Groups Based on Perfusion**[a]

Characteristic	Vessel-Rich	Muscle	Fat	Vessel-Poor
Percentage of body weight	10%	50%	20%	20%
Percentage of cardiac output	75%	19%	6%	0
Perfusion (mL/min per 100 g)	75	3	3	0

[a]The vessel-rich group represents the central compartment, and the muscle, fat, and vessel-poor groups are peripheral compartments.

From Elisha S, Heiner JS, Nagelhout JJ. *Nurse Anesthesia*. 7th ed. Elsevier; 2023.

- For many drugs, disappearance from the plasma follows an exponential time course characterized by the plasma half-life.
- Plasma half-life is directly proportional to the V_d and inversely proportional to the overall rate of clearance.
- With repeated dosage or sustained delivery of a drug, the plasma concentration approaches a steady value within four or five plasma half-lives. Complete elimination of a drug from the body takes four or five half-lives.
- A two-compartment model is often needed. In this case, the kinetics are biexponential. The two components roughly represent the processes of transfer between plasma and tissues or distribution (α phase) and elimination from the plasma (β phase).
- Some drugs show nonexponential "saturation" kinetics with important clinical consequences, especially a disproportionate increase in steady-state plasma concentration when the dose is increased (Table 2.2).

Drug Metabolism

- Phase I reactions involve oxidation, reduction, and hydrolysis and usually form more chemically reactive products, sometimes pharmacologically active, toxic, or carcinogenic products. Phase I reactions often involve a monooxygenase system in which cytochrome enzymes play a role (Box 2.1).
- Phase II reactions are conjugation (e.g., glucuronidation) of a reactive group (often inserted during phase I reaction) and usually form inactive and polar products that are readily excretable in urine.
- Some conjugated products are excreted via bile, reactivated in the intestine, and then reabsorbed through enterohepatic circulation (e.g., narcotics, benzodiazepines).

BOX 2.1 **Common Anesthesia-Related Drugs That Undergo Phase 1 Hydrolysis**

Catalyzed by Pseudocholinesterase
- Succinylcholine
- Mivacurium
- Cocaine
- Procaine
- Chloroprocaine
- Tetracaine
- Neostigmine (partial pathway)
- Edrophonium (partial pathway)

Nonspecific Esterase-Dependent
- Remifentanil
- Atracurium (partial pathway)
- Cisatracurium (partial pathway)
- Esmolol (RBC esterase)
- Aspirin
- Clevidipine

RBC, Red blood cell.

- Induction of enzymes by other drugs and chemicals can greatly accelerate hepatic drug metabolism. It can also increase the toxicity of drugs with toxic metabolites and is an important cause of drug interactions, such as in enzyme inhibition.
- Some drugs show rapid "first-pass" hepatic metabolism and therefore poor oral bioavailability because of presystemic metabolism in the liver or intestinal wall when they are administered orally (Table 2.3).

Summary of Pharmacokinetic Principles

- Clinical pharmacokinetics is the discipline that describes the absorption, distribution, metabolism, and elimination of drugs in patients who require drug therapy.

TABLE 2.3 Pharmacokinetic Metrics for Describing Drug Offset

Parameter	Definition	Advantages	Limitations
Terminal half-life	Time taken for drug concentration in the blood to fall by one-half of the current value	• Easily understood • Simple to calculate • Useful for describing drug disposition in a one-compartment model	• One-compartment models rarely used for describing the kinetics of anesthetic drugs • Not "context sensitive" with respect to infusion duration • Not informative with respect to actual duration of action
Context-sensitive decrement times	Time required for drug concentration to decrease by a given percentage after termination of an infusion of a given duration	• Can be calculated for the central (plasma) or a peripheral effect compartment • Context sensitivity allows rational drug selection based on anticipated infusion duration	• Decrement curves are generated by kinetic-dynamic simulation using known models • Impractical to attempt clinical validation, owing to vast numbers of patients required • An arbitrary decrement time (particularly if relating to plasma concentration) may not relate to actual recovery time
Mean effect time	Calculation of the average recovery time, based on the probability of drug effect as a function of drug concentration and time	• An extension of the context-sensitive half-time—for example, estimates of C_{90}, the concentration at 90% recovery, which considers the probability of drug effect, in addition to pharmacokinetic parameters	• Calculation requires knowledge of the concentration–effect relationship and the variance of drug concentration • Useful for quantifying the duration of drug effect when dealing with "response or no response" binary data

Adapted from Rigby-Jones AE, Sneyd JR. Pharmacokinetics and pharmacodynamics—is there anything new? *Anaesthesia.* 2012;67(1):5–11; Minto CF, Schnider TW. Contributions of PK/PD modeling to intravenous anesthesia. *Clin Pharmacol Ther.* 2008;84(1):27–38; Bailey JM. Context-sensitive half-times: what are they and how valuable are they in anaesthesiology? *Clin Pharmacokinet.* 2002;41(11):793–799.

- Clearance is the most important pharmacokinetic parameter because it determines the steady-state concentration for a given dosage rate. Physiologically, clearance is determined by blood flow to the organ that metabolizes or eliminates the drug and the efficiency of the organ in extracting the drug from the bloodstream.
- The dosage and clearance determine the steady-state concentration.
- The fraction of drug absorbed into the systemic circulation after extravascular administration is defined as its *bioavailability.*
- Pharmacokinetic models are useful for description of data sets; prediction of serum concentrations after several doses or different routes of administration; and calculation of pharmacokinetic constants such as clearance, V_d, and half-life. The simplest example uses a single compartment to represent the entire body.
- The V_d is a proportionality constant that relates the amount of drug in the body to the serum concentration. The V_d is used to calculate the loading dose of a drug that will immediately achieve a desired steady-state concentration. The value of the V_d is determined by the physiologic volume and how the drug binds in blood and tissues. The V_d determines the loading dose.
- Half-life is the time required for serum concentration to decrease by one-half after absorption and distribution are complete. Half-life is important because it determines the time required to reach steady state and the dosage interval. Half-life is a dependent kinetic variable because its value depends on the values of clearance and V_d.

- The half-life determines the time to reach steady state and the time for "all" drug to be eliminated from the body. Complete elimination of a drug from the body takes four or five half-lives.
- If a drug obeys first-order pharmacokinetics, a simple ratio of dosage to steady-state concentration can be used to estimate a new dosage if the clearance has not changed.
- Phenytoin is an example of a drug that obeys the Michaelis-Menten model rather than first-order pharmacokinetics. In this case, as plasma concentration increases, the clearance decreases, and the half-life becomes longer.
- *Cytochrome P450* is a generic term for the group of enzymes responsible for most drug metabolism oxidation reactions. Several cytochrome P450 isozymes have been identified, including CYP1A2, CYP2C9, CYP2C19, CYP2D6, CYP2E1, and CYP3A4.
- Factors to be taken into consideration when deciding on the best drug dose for a patient include age, sex, weight, ethnic background, other concurrent disease states, and other drug therapy.
- The principal transport protein involved in the movement of drugs across biologic membranes is P-glycoprotein. P-glycoprotein is present in many organs, including the GI tract, liver, and kidney.

Elimination of Drugs by the Kidney

- Most drugs, unless highly bound to plasma protein, cross the glomerular filter freely.
- Many drugs, especially weak acids and weak bases, are actively secreted into the renal tubule and therefore are more rapidly excreted.
- Lipid-soluble drugs are passively reabsorbed by diffusion across the tubule and are not efficiently excreted in the urine.
- Because of the pH partition, weak acids are more rapidly excreted in alkaline urine, and vice versa.
- Several important drugs are removed predominantly by renal excretion and are liable to cause toxicity in elderly persons and patients with renal disease.
- There are instances of clinically important drug interactions due to one drug reducing the clearance of another. Examples include diuretics increasing the effects of lithium. Another example is that indomethacin increases the toxicity of methotrexate. These are less common than interactions due to altered drug metabolism.

Pharmacogenomics

- *Pharmacogenomics* is the study of how genes affect a person's response to drugs. This field of study combines pharmacology (the science of drugs) and genomics (the study of genes and their functions) to develop effective, safe medications and doses that will be tailored to a person's genetic makeup.

Drug Interaction Terminology

- See Table 2.4.

TABLE 2.4 Drug Interaction Terminology

Drug Interaction	Explanation	Viewed as an Equation
Addition	The combined effect of two drugs acting via the same mechanism is equal to that expected by simple addition of their individual actions. Example: midazolam plus diazepam	1 + 1 = 2
Synergism	The combined effect of two drugs is greater than the algebraic sum of their individual effects. Example: midazolam plus propofol	1 + 1 = 3
Potentiation	The enhancement of the action of one drug by a second drug that has no detectable action of its own Example: penicillin plus probenecid	1 + 0 = 3
Antagonism	The action of one drug opposes the action of another. Example: fentanyl plus naloxone	1 + 1 = 0

From Elisha S, Heiner JS, Nagelhout JJ. *Nurse Anesthesia*. 7th ed. Elsevier; 2023.

KNOWLEDGE CHECK

1. A drug that is highly ionized (99%) at body pH will
   a. be water soluble.
   b. be lipid soluble.
   c. have a high oral bioavailability.
   d. easily penetrate the blood–brain barrier.
2. An increase in the number and activity of the drug-metabolizing enzymes in the liver is referred to as
   a. enzyme induction.
   b. functional tolerance.
   c. kinetic tolerance.
   d. upregulation.
3. Which enzyme is inhibited by etomidate, leading to prolonged decreases in cortisol secretion?
   a. Aminolevulinic acid (ALA) synthetase
   b. Pseudocholinesterase
   c. Methionine synthetase
   d. 11β-hydroxylase
4. Which enzyme system is responsible for most drug metabolism via oxidation reactions?
   a. Pseudocholinesterase
   b. Cytochrome P450
   c. Organic cation transporters
   d. Glucuronic transferase
5. A drug is eliminated from the body after how many half-lives?
   a. Three
   b. Five
   c. Seven
   d. Nine
6. What is the pharmacologic definition of a drug that is an agonist?
   a. Binds to a specific receptor and triggers a response in the cell
   b. Interacts within the cellular lipid bilayer to inhibit an action
   c. Breaks down the ligand into an inactive state
   d. Metabolizes the activity of a drug during oxidation and reduction reactions

Answers can be found in Appendix A.

INHALATION ANESTHETICS

Anesthetic Implications

- Inhalation agents remain the most commonly administered class of drugs used to maintain general anesthesia.
- The ease of administration of all ether-based volatile anesthetics, with or without N_2O, lends them to common use among a diverse surgical population.
- All inhalation agents (except nitrous oxide) are contraindicated in patients who are susceptible to malignant hyperthermia (MH) (Table 2.5 and Box 2.2).
- Central nervous system (CNS) effects are summarized in Tables 2.6 and 2.7.
- Cardiac effects are summarized in Table 2.8.
- Metabolism, select effects, and advantages and disadvantages of the inhalation anesthetics are listed in Tables 2.9–2.11.

Nitrous Oxide

- Nitrous oxide has a niche role as a supplement to the more potent anesthetics.
- Its use has declined in recent years in the United States.

TABLE 2.5 Select Characteristics of Inhalation Anesthetics

Characteristics	Nitrous Oxide	Isoflurane	Desflurane	Sevoflurane
Molecular formula	N_2O	$C_3H_2ClF_5O$	$C_3H_2F_6O$	$C_4H_3F_7O$
Ostwald blood–gas partition coefficient (37°C)	0.47	1.43	0.42	0.68
Oil–gas partition coefficient	1.4	99	18.7	50
Saturated vapor pressure (mm Hg, at 20°C)	Gas	238	669	157
Molecular weight (g/mol)	44.01	184.49	168.04	200.05
Preservative	None	None	None	None

From Elisha S, Heiner JS, Nagelhout JJ. *Nurse Anesthesia*. 7th ed. Elsevier; 2023.

BOX 2.2 Mechanisms of Action of Inhalation Anesthetics

- No single comprehensive or unitary theory of exactly how anesthetic medications exert their physiologic effects has been empirically determined. The effects of the inhalation anesthetics cannot be explained by a single mechanism. Multiple targets contribute to the sedation, unconsciousness, amnesia, immobility, and analgesic actions of anesthetics.
- The most likely targets include tandem pore potassium channels; voltage-gated sodium channels; NMDA receptors; and the pentameric ligand-gated ion channels (pLGICs), including glycine receptors (GlyRs) and $GABA_A$ receptors.
- The potency of general anesthetics correlates with their solubility in oil, which is expressed as the oil/gas solubility coefficient of the anesthetic (Meyer-Overton rule). The more lipid soluble the anesthetic, the higher the potency.
- Mutational analysis using transgenic and knock-in/knockout mice is being used to identify the role of specific types of proteins, ion channels, and other actions of general anesthetics.
- Important actions of inhaled anesthetics are associated with altered activity of neuronal ion channels, particularly the fast synaptic neurotransmitter receptors such as nicotinic acetylcholine, GABA, and glutamate receptors. Anesthetics affect neuronal ion channels by binding directly to protein sites.
- The immobilizing effect of inhaled anesthetics involves actions in the spinal cord. These involve modulation of ion channels, reduced spontaneous action potential firing of spinal neurons via glycine, effects on $GABA_A$ receptors and NMDA receptors, and depression of motor neurons (perhaps via hyperpolarization).

GABA, γ-Aminobutyric acid; *$GABA_A$*, γ-aminobutyric acid A; *NMDA*, *N*-methyl-D-aspartate.
From Forman SA. Molecular approaches to improving general anesthetics. *Anesthesiol Clin.* 2010;28(4):761–771.

- Chronic exposure to N_2O can lead to inactivation of the vitamin B_{12} cofactor for the enzyme methionine synthetase. This may disrupt deoxyribonucleic acid (DNA) synthesis and is thought to be related to the teratogenic and immunosuppressant effects (Fig. 2.1).
- Nitrous oxide is an antagonist at the *N*-methyl-D-aspartate (NMDA) receptor and thus is a potent analgesic.
- Nitrous oxide has been implicated in increasing the incidence of postoperative nausea and vomiting (PONV).
- Nitrous oxide had been used to promote the "second-gas effect" with extremely lipid-soluble inhalation agents such as halothane, which has a blood gas solubility of 2.4. The rationale was that nitrous oxide would increase the speed of alveolar uptake of halothane. With modern inhalation agents such as sevoflurane, the blood gas solubility (0.60) closely approximates nitrous oxide (0.42). Therefore nitrous oxide does not play a role in a "second-gas effect."
- Nitrous oxide is highly diffusible, and therefore it is implicated in increasing the mass of air-filled spaces within the body (e.g., bowels, inner ear), and as such, its use may be limited, depending on the surgical procedure.
- N_2O has a significant negative impact on the environment by trapping thermal radiation from escaping from Earth's surface. Its tropospheric lifetime is approximately 120 years.
- Current concerns exist regarding inhalation agents and N_2O administration to infants and children during brain development (Table 2.12; see Table 2.11).
- The contraindications to the use of nitrous oxide are listed in Table 2.13.

Inhalation Agents

- Inhalation anesthetics are frequently coadministered with intravenous (IV) sedative hypnotics, opiates, muscle relaxants, and other agents to provide for safe operative conditions. All of the inhalation agents are vaporized from liquid to gas for inhalation, cause myocardial depression and vasodilation in a dose-dependent manner, inhibit hypoxic pulmonary vasoconstriction, and are triggers for MH. The three inhalation agents used in the United States are sevoflurane (Ultane), desflurane (Suprane), and isoflurane (Forane).
- Sevoflurane is currently the most widely used inhalation anesthetic agent. Its advantages include a rapid onset and offset due to its low blood gas solubility, along with ease of rapidly changing the anesthetic depth. It is very useful for induction in pediatric patients without initial IV access because it has a pleasant odor and causes minimal airway

TABLE 2.6 **Effect of Various Anesthetic Agents on Neurophysiologic Monitoring of Evoked Potentials**

Drug Name	Drug Class	Effect on SSEPs	Effect on MEPs	Length of Emergence	Approximate $CST_{1/2}$ (min) at 2/4/6 h and B:GC for Volatile Agents	Clinical Advantages Relating to Intraoperative Neurophysiologic Monitoring	Disadvantages
Propofol	GABA agonist	↓	↓	+++	15/20/30	Titratable, smooth emergence	Accumulation, slow wake-up
Etomidate	GABA agonist	↑↑	–	++ Fast emergence after a single dose, but accumulates with prolonged infusion	5/10/20	Titratable, hemodynamically stable	Adrenal suppression, PONV, myoclonic seizures
Midazolam	Benzodiazepine	↓	–	+++	40/60/65	Amnestic	Prolonged emergence
Ketamine	NMDA antagonist	↑	–/↓	+++	15/30/40	Analgesic, amnestic, sympathomimetic, hemodynamically stable	Hallucinations
Fentanyl	Opioid synthetic	–/↓	↓	+++	40/160/240	Analgesic	Accumulation, respiratory depression
Remifentanil	Opioid synthetic	–/↓	–/↓	+	7/7/7	Potent analgesic	Hyperalgesic effect after discontinuation
Sufentanil	Opioid synthetic	–/↓	↓	++	15/20/30	Potent analgesic	Respiratory depression
Dexmedetomidine	α_2-Agonist	–/↓	–/↓	+++		Sedative-hypnotic with preserved respiratory drive, awake intubation	Bradycardia and heart block

Isoflurane	Inhalational	↓↓	↓↓↓	+++	1.4	Low cost; reduced $CMRO_2$ of CNS	
Sevoflurane	Inhalational	↓↓	↓↓	++	0.65	Mask induction	Emergence delirium
N_2O	Inhalational	↓↓	↓↓	+	0.47	Rapid elimination, analgesic effect	Synergistic effect on signal depression with evoked potentials, PONV
Desflurane	Inhalational	↓↓	↓↓	+	0.42	Rapidly titratable, fast elimination	Emergence delirium, bronchospasm
Rocuronium	NDMR	–	↓↓↓	N/A	N/A	Relatively short half-life and quick elimination after IOA with low doses	Interindividual variability of elimination, risk of residual NMB
Succinylcholine	Depolarizing muscle relaxant	–	↓↓↓	N/A	N/A	Rapid elimination after IOA	Contraindicated in MH and muscular dystrophies, pseudocholinesterase deficiency leads to long half-life

Arrows indicate an increase or decrease in the parameter. + mild effect, ++ moderate effect, +++ marked effect.

B:GC, Blood–gas partition coefficient (the higher the value, the more agent is dissolved in blood and the longer it takes for the volatile anesthetic to be eliminated); *$CMRO_2$*, cerebral metabolic rate for oxygen; *CNS*, central nervous system; *$CST_{1/2}$*, context-sensitive half-time (elimination half-life as a function of duration of infusion); *GABA*, γ-aminobutyric acid; *IOA*, induction of anesthesia; *MEPs*, motor evoked potentials; *MH*, malignant hyperthermia; *NDMR*, nondepolarizing muscle relaxant; *NMB*, neuromuscular blockade; *NMDA*, *N*-methyl-D-aspartate; *PONV*, postoperative nausea and vomiting; *SSEPs*, somatosensory evoked potentials.

From Rabai F, et al. Neurophysiological monitoring and spinal cord integrity. *Best Pract Res Clin Anaesthesiol.* 2016;30(1):53–68.

TABLE 2.7 Potencies of Volatile Anesthetics in Humans With and Without N_2O, Expressed as MAC Values

Anesthetic	MAC[a] (Expressed as % of 1 Atm)	MAC in 60%–70% N_2O
Nitrous oxide	104	—
Isoflurane	1.17	0.56
Desflurane	6	2.38
Sevoflurane	2	0.66

MAC, Minimum alveolar concentration; *N_2O,* nitrous oxide.
MAC-awake is the minimum alveolar concentration of anesthetic that inhibits responses to command in half of patients. It is approximately one-third of MAC. MAC-BAR is the minimum alveolar concentration of anesthetic that blunts the autonomic response to noxious stimuli. It is approximately 1.6 times higher than MAC.
[a]For patients aged 30–60 y.
From Elisha S, Heiner JS, Nagelhout JJ. *Nurse Anesthesia.* 7th ed. Elsevier; 2023.

TABLE 2.8 Cardiovascular Effects of Inhalation Anesthetics

	Cardiac Output	System Vascular Resistance	Mean Arterial Pressure	Heart Rate
Isoflurane	↓ Slight	↓	↓	↑
Desflurane	↔	↓	↓	↑
Sevoflurane	↔	↓	↓	↔
Nitrous oxide	↓	↑	↔	↑

Arrows indicate an increase, decrease, or no change in the parameter. All effects are dose dependent.
From Elisha S, Heiner JS, Nagelhout JJ. *Nurse Anesthesia.* 7th ed. Elsevier; 2023.

TABLE 2.9 Anesthetic Metabolism

Agent	Average Metabolism (%)
Sevoflurane	5–8
Nitrous oxide	<1
Isoflurane	<1
Desflurane	<0.1

From Elisha S, Heiner JS, Nagelhout JJ. *Nurse Anesthesia.* 7th ed. Elsevier; 2023.

irritation. Disadvantages include hepatic metabolism (5%–8%). Although there was some initial concern regarding renal toxicity due to liberation of compound A, it is now considered safe for patients with renal disorders.

- Desflurane is the most rapid acting of the modern anesthetics because it has the lowest blood gas solubility. It does not cause hepatic or renal toxicity. Disadvantages include respiratory irritation and cardiovascular stimulation (hypertension and tachycardia) when rapidly increasing the concentration. Because of its relative insolubility, it has gained popularity for patients having bariatric surgery. It significantly contributes to environmental contamination. Desflurane has a tropospheric life of 14 years, compared with sevoflurane at 1.1 years and isoflurane at 3.2 years. It also requires a specific heated vaporizer to administer as a gas.
- Isoflurane, which was introduced in the 1970s, is the oldest of the inhalation anesthetics. It exhibits the slowest onset and offset times, which limits its popularity. Like desflurane, isoflurane is irritating to the airway, and thus it is not suitable for mask inductions.
- A summary of the inhalation anesthetic pharmacokinetic concepts is provided in Table 2.14.

TABLE 2.10 Select Effects of the Inhalation Anesthetics

Variable	Isoflurane	Desflurane	Sevoflurane
Kinetics			
Alveolar equilibration	Moderate	Fast	Fast
Recovery	Moderate	Very fast	Fast
Liver			
Hepatotoxicity	No	No	No
Metabolism (%)	0.2	0.02	5–8
Musculoskeletal relaxation	Moderate	Moderate	Moderate
Respiratory System			
Respiratory irritation	Significant	Significant	No
Central Nervous System			
Seizure activity on EEG	No	No	Yes
Renal System			
Renal toxic metabolites	No	No	No

EEG, Electroencephalogram.
Modified from Aitkenhead AR, Thompson J, Rowbotham DJ, et al., eds. *Textbook of Anaesthesia*. 6th ed. Elsevier; 2013.

TABLE 2.11 Clinical Advantages and Disadvantages of Selected Inhalation Anesthetics

Anesthetic	Advantages	Disadvantages
Nitrous oxide	Analgesia Rapid uptake and elimination Little cardiac or respiratory depression Nonpungent Reduces MAC of the more potent agents Minimal biotransformation	Expansion of closed air spaces Requires high concentrations Amount of oxygen delivered is reduced. Diffusion hypoxia, increase in teratogenicity, PONV Supports combustion Immune suppression
Isoflurane	Moderate muscle relaxation Decreases cerebral metabolic rate Minimal biotransformation No significant systemic toxicity Inexpensive Possible neuroprotection and cardiac protection	Airway irritant Trigger for malignant hyperthermia Slower onset and offset
Desflurane	Rapid uptake and elimination Stable molecular structure, minimal biotransformation No significant systemic toxicity Possible neuroprotection and cardiac protection	Airway irritant Expensive compared with the other agents Needs special electrically heated vaporizer Rapid increases in inspired concentration can lead to reflex tachycardia and hypertension. Trigger for malignant hyperthermia
Sevoflurane	Rapid uptake and elimination Nonpungent Excellent for inhalation induction Cardiovascular effects broadly comparable to those of isoflurane Possible neuroprotection and cardiac protection	Reacts with soda lime Trigger for malignant hyperthermia Some hepatic biotransformation

MAC, Minimum alveolar concentration; *PONV,* postoperative nausea and vomiting.
From Elisha S, Heiner JS, Nagelhout JJ. *Nurse Anesthesia*. 7th ed. Elsevier; 2023.

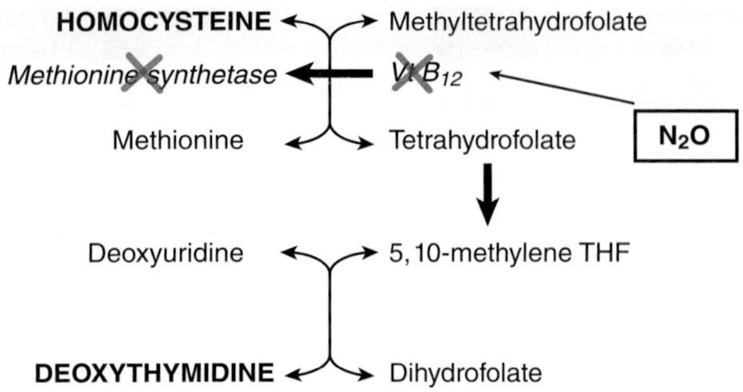

Fig. 2.1 Nitrous oxide (N_2O) oxidizes the cobalt atom on vitamin B_{12}, inhibiting methionine synthetase and causing accumulation of homocysteine and disruption of deoxythymidine synthesis. *THF,* Tetrahydrofolate. (From Fleisher LA. *Evidence-Based Practice of Anesthesiology*. 3rd ed. Elsevier; 2013.)

TABLE 2.12 Patients at Risk of Cobalamin Deficiency

Nutritional disorders	Elderly Vegans Alcoholics
Malabsorption disorders	Prolonged use of proton pump inhibitors or H_2 receptor antagonists Pernicious anemia Atrophic gastritis Postgastrectomy, Whipple procedure, ileal resection Crohn disease
Infection	Bacterial overgrowth, tapeworm

From Sanders RD, Weimann J, Maze M. Biologic effects of nitrous oxide: a mechanistic and toxicologic review. *Anesthesiology.* 2008;109(4):707–722.

TABLE 2.13 Recommended Contraindications to Administering Nitrous Oxide

Indications	Inhalational Analgesia/Sedation
Absolute contraindications	Known deficiency of enzyme or substrate in methionine synthase pathway Potential toxicity from expansion of gas-filled space (e.g., emphysema, pneumothorax, middle ear surgery, pneumocephalus, air embolus, bowel obstruction) Increased intracranial pressure
Relative contraindications	Pulmonary hypertension Prolonged anesthesia (>6 h) First trimester of pregnancy[a] High risk of postoperative nausea and vomiting

[a]Based on the theoretical (but unproven) detrimental effects.

From Sanders RD, Weimann J, Maze M. Biologic effects of nitrous oxide: a mechanistic and toxicologic review. *Anesthesiology.* 2008;109(4):707–722.

TABLE 2.14 Inhalation Anesthetic Pharmacokinetic Concepts

Concept	Comments
Minimum alveolar concentration (MAC)	The MAC required to achieve surgical anesthesia (immobility) in 50% of patients exposed to a noxious stimulus
Minimum alveolar concentration awake (MAC-awake)	The MAC suppressing appropriate response to commands in 50% of patients; memory is usually lost at MAC-awake; approximately 0.3–0.5 MAC.
Minimum alveolar concentration—block adrenergic responses (MAC-BAR)	The alveolar concentration of anesthetic that blunts the autonomic response to noxious stimuli; approximately 1.3–2.0 MAC
Ventilation effect	The greater the alveolar ventilation, the faster the patient achieves anesthesia.
Concentration effect	The higher the concentration of anesthetic delivered, the faster anesthesia is achieved; this is also referred to as *overpressuring;* as with any drug, the larger the initial dose administered, the faster the onset of action.

TABLE 2.14 Inhalation Anesthetic Pharmacokinetic Concepts—cont'd

Concept	Comments
Blood/gas solubility coefficient	The blood/gas solubility coefficient is the indicator of an anesthetic's speed of onset and emergence: The higher the coefficient, the slower the anesthetic; conversely, the lower the coefficient, the faster the anesthetic.
Oil/gas solubility coefficient	The oil/gas solubility coefficient is the indicator of an anesthetic's potency: The higher the coefficient, the more potent the agent.
Second-gas effect	The second-gas effect is a phenomenon in which two anesthetics of varying onset speeds are administered together: A high concentration of a fast anesthetic, such as nitrous oxide, is administered with a slower second anesthetic gas; the slower gas achieves anesthetic levels more quickly than if it had been given alone.
Diffusion hypoxia	Diffusion hypoxia occurs when high concentrations of nitrous oxide are administered; at the end of the procedure, when nitrous oxide is discontinued, it leaves the body very rapidly, causing a transient dilution of the oxygen and carbon dioxide in the lungs; hypocarbia and hypoxia may occur; administration of 100% oxygen for approximately 3–5 min when nitrous oxide is discontinued alleviates this problem.
Cardiac output effect	Increases in cardiac output decrease the speed of onset of all anesthetics; the more soluble anesthetics are affected to a much greater extent than the insoluble anesthetics.
Ventilation–perfusion abnormalities	Ventilation–perfusion abnormalities reduce the speed of onset of all anesthetics and affect the insoluble agents to a much greater degree than the soluble agents.
Pediatrics	Children achieve anesthesia more rapidly than adults because of a higher ventilatory rate and vessel-rich group blood flow; this occurs despite the fact that the required dose and cardiac output are higher in children.
Obesity	Obesity has minimal clinical effects on anesthetic induction; however, emergence may be slower because of deposition of anesthetics in fat.
Pregnancy	The kinetics of the inhalation anesthetics are similar in pregnant females and non-pregnant females; placental transfer is time dependent, as expected.

From Elisha S, Heiner JS, Nagelhout JJ. *Nurse Anesthesia*. 7th ed. Elsevier; 2023.

KNOWLEDGE CHECK

1. The blood/gas solubility coefficient of an inhalation agent indicates the
   a. potency.
   b. speed of induction and emergence.
   c. ability to vaporize an agent.
   d. efficacy.
   e. receptor affinity.
2. The minimum alveolar concentration value of an inhalation agent is defined as
   a. the potency of an inhalation agent.
   b. the speed of induction and emergence.
   c. the alveolar concentration at which 50% of patients do not respond to surgical stimuli.
   d. directly proportional to the blood/gas solubility coefficient.
3. Which inhalation agent will produce the slowest emergence from anesthesia?
   a. Desflurane
   b. Nitrous oxide
   c. Isoflurane
   d. Sevoflurane
4. Which is an absolute contraindication to the use of nitrous oxide? (*Select all that apply.*)
   a. Air embolism
   b. Bariatric surgery
   c. Pneumothorax
   d. Atrial fibrillation
5. The oil/gas solubility coefficient of an inhalation agent indicates the
   a. potency.
   b. speed of induction and emergence.

Continued

KNOWLEDGE CHECK—cont'd

c. ability to vaporize an agent.
d. receptor affinity.

6. Which agent undergoes the greatest amount of hepatic metabolism?
   a. Nitrous oxide
   b. Isoflurane
   c. Sevoflurane
   d. Desflurane
7. Which anesthetic medication exhibits analgesic properties as an NMDA agonist?
   a. Isoflurane
   b. Desflurane
   c. Sevoflurane
   d. Nitrous oxide
8. Which agent is relatively contraindicated during pregnancy?
   a. Nitrous oxide
   b. Isoflurane
   c. Desflurane
   d. Sevoflurane
9. MH is a contraindication to the use of
   a. sevoflurane.
   b. nitrous oxide.
   c. all inhalation anesthetics except nitrous oxide.
   d. all inhalation anesthetics.
10. Which anesthetic agent can produce significant dilution of alveolar oxygen and carbon dioxide (diffusion hypoxia)?
    a. Nitrous oxide
    b. Isoflurane
    c. Desflurane
    d. Sevoflurane
11. Which agent should be used with caution in patients with asthma?
    a. Nitrous oxide
    b. Isoflurane
    c. Desflurane
    d. Sevoflurane
12. Which inhalation agent can produce seizure activity on electroencephalography (EEG)?
    a. Isoflurane
    b. Nitrous oxide
    c. Sevoflurane
    d. Desflurane

Answers can be found in Appendix A.

ANESTHESIA INDUCTION MEDICATIONS

Anesthesia Implications

- The practice of using IV push boluses of sedatives to initiate anesthesia remains the standard because of the drugs' rapid onset of action.
- *Induction of general anesthesia* refers to the beginning of anesthesia when the patient is rendered unconscious and rapidly develops apnea. The IV induction agents allow loss of consciousness while also rapidly achieving surgical levels of anesthesia.
- Desirable properties of an induction agent include rapid onset and recovery, analgesia, minimal cardiac and respiratory depression, antiemetic actions, bronchodilation, lack of toxicity or histamine release, and advantageous pharmacokinetics and pharmacodynamic profile.
- Propofol is the most commonly used induction agent for inducing general anesthesia and IV sedation.
- Etomidate, dexmedetomidine, and ketamine are valuable agents for select anesthetics if propofol use is undesirable.
- Pharmaceutical preparations are noted in Tables 2.15–2.17.

Benzodiazepines

Anesthesia Implications

- Benzodiazepines act as an agonist on the γ-aminobutyric acid ($GABA_A$) receptor, which enhances the inhibitory effect of GABA. Flumazenil (Romazicon) is an antagonist at $GABA_A$ receptors and reverses the clinical effect of the agonists. Inverse agonists (not used clinically) are anxiogenic.
- Benzodiazepines cause the following:
  - Reduction of anxiety and aggression
  - Sedation, leading to decreased insomnia
  - Muscle relaxation and loss of motor coordination
  - Suppression of convulsions (antiepileptic effect)
  - Anterograde amnesia
- Differences in the pharmacological profile of different benzodiazepines are minor.
- Benzodiazepines are active orally and differ mainly in respect to their duration of action and half-lives. Some long-acting agents (e.g., diazepam and chlordiazepoxide) are converted to a long-lasting active metabolite, nordiazepam (Table 2.18).
- Benzodiazepines reduce the requirements (synergistic effect) for other anesthetic agents.

TABLE 2.15 Pharmaceutical Preparation of Intravenous Anesthetic Agents

Class	Drug Name	Available Solution	Pain on Injection[a]
Benzodiazepines	Diazepam (Valium)	0.5% in 40% propylene glycol and 10% alcohol	+++
	Lorazepam (Ativan)	0.4% in propylene glycol	+
	Midazolam (Versed)	0.5% Buffered aqueous solution (pH 3.5)	0
Imidazoles	Etomidate (Amidate)	Water-soluble at acidic pH, lipophilic at physiologic pH (pK_a 4.24); 0.2% solution in 30% propylene glycol (pH 5)	+++
	Dexmedetomidine (Precedex)	Dexmedetomidine HCl is freely soluble in water and has a pK_a of 7.1 with a pH of 4.5–7.0. The solution is preservative-free. Prepare by adding 2 mL of dexmedetomidine (100 mcg/mL) to 48 mL of 0.9% sodium chloride injection for a total of 50 mL. The final concentration is 4 mcg/mL.	0
Alkylphenol	Propofol (Diprivan)	1% Solution in an aqueous emulsion containing 10% soybean oil, 2.25% glycerol, and 1.2% egg phosphatide, EDTA (pK_a 11)	++
	Generic propofol	Generic formulations vary; may contain metabisulfite (use with caution in patients with allergies and asthma); formulations that contain benzyl alcohol pH 7–8.5 (benzyl alcohol should be avoided in infants)	++
Arylcyclohexylamines	Ketamine (Ketalar)	White crystalline salt 1% or 10% aqueous solution (pH 3.3–5.5; pK_a 7.5)	0

EDTA, Disodium ethylenediaminetetraacetic acid.
[a]0, None; +, mild; ++, moderate; +++, marked.
From Elisha S, Heiner JS, Nagelhout JJ. *Nurse Anesthesia.* 7th ed. Elsevier; 2023.

TABLE 2.16 Central Nervous System Effects of Intravenous Anesthetics

Agent	CBF	CPP	$CMRO_2$	ICP	IOP
Etomidate	↓↓	↓↓	↓↓	↓↓	↓
Propofol	↓↓	↓↓	↓↓	↓↓	↓↓
Ketamine	↑	↑	↑	↑	↑
Midazolam	↑↓	↓	↓	↓	↓
Dexmedetomidine	↓	↑↓	0	↓	↓

↓, Decreases; ↑, increases; 0, no effect.
CBF, Cerebral blood flow; *CPP,* cerebral perfusion pressure; *$CMRO_2$,* cerebral metabolic rate of oxygen consumption; *ICP,* intracranial pressure; *IOP,* intraocular pressure.
From Elisha S, Heiner JS, Nagelhout JJ. *Nurse Anesthesia.* 7th ed. Elsevier; 2023.

- Patients who are elderly or have hepatic and renal impairment have decreased clearance and dosage requirements.
- Benzodiazepines have been implicated in increasing the potential for postoperative cognitive dysfunction, especially in elderly patients.
- Zolpidem (Ambien, other brand names) is a short-acting drug that is not a benzodiazepine but acts similarly and is used as a hypnotic.
- Remimazolam is a benzodiazepine with an ester linkage that allows for rapid metabolism to inactive metabolites. It is administered by continuous infusion

TABLE 2.17 **Cardiac and Respiratory Effects of Intravenous Anesthetic Agents**

Drug Name	Mean Arterial Pressure	Heart Rate	Cardiac Output	Venous Dilation	Systemic Vascular Resistance	Respiratory Depression	Bronchodilation
Etomidate	0	0	0	0	0	0/−	0
Propofol	− −	−	−	++	− −	− −	0
Ketamine	++	++	+	0	+/−	0	+
Diazepam	0/−	−/+	0		−/0	0	0
Midazolam	0/−	−/+	0	+	−/0	0	0
Dexmedetomidine	−	− −	0/−	0	0	0	0

−, Mild decrease; − −, moderate decrease; +, mild increase; ++, moderate increase; 0, no effect.
From Elisha S, Heiner JS, Nagelhout JJ. *Nurse Anesthesia*. 7th ed. Elsevier; 2023.

TABLE 2.18 **Benzodiazepines Used Clinically in the United States**

Generic Name	Trade Name	Half-Life (h)	Clinical Application
Alprazolam	Xanax	12–15	Anxiolysis
Chlordiazepoxide	Librium	8–18	Treatment of alcohol withdrawal
Clonazepam	Klonopin	18.7–39	Treatment of epilepsy
Clorazepate	Tranxene	2.4	Treatment of epilepsy and alcohol withdrawal
Diazepam	Valium	36–50	Sedation; induction and maintenance of anesthesia
Estazolam	ProSom	14	Treatment of insomnia
Flurazepam	Dalmane	2–3	Treatment of insomnia
Lorazepam	Ativan	10–22	Anxiolysis and sedation
Midazolam	Versed	1.7–2.6	Sedation; induction and maintenance of anesthesia
Oxazepam	Serax	3–21	Anxiolysis
Quazepam	Doral	25–41	Treatment of insomnia
Temazepam	Restoril	10–21	Treatment of insomnia
Triazolam	Halcion	2–3	Treatment of insomnia
Flumazenil	Romazicon	0.7–1.3	Reversal of benzodiazepine agonists

From Elisha S, Heiner JS, Nagelhout JJ. Nurse Anesthesia. 7th ed. Elsevier; 2023.

and may prove useful as a fast-onset, short-duration induction drug.

Midazolam (Versed)

- Classification: benzodiazepine; hypnotic; sedative
- Indications: preoperative sedation; induction of anesthesia; long-term sedation in intensive care unit; sedation before short diagnostic and endoscopic procedures
- Dose: adults: preoperative sedation: intramuscular (IM): 0.07–0.08 mg/kg 30–60 minutes before surgery; usual dose: approximately 2–5 mg; IV: initial: 0.5–2 mg slowly over 2 minutes; usual total dose: 2–5 mg; decrease dose in elderly patients; reduce dose by 30% if other CNS depressants are administered concomitantly.
- Onset: IV: 1–5 minutes; IM: 15 minutes; oral/rectal: less than 10 minutes
- Duration: 2–6 hours
- Elimination half-life: 14 hours
- Adverse effects: tachycardia, hypotension, bronchospasm, laryngospasm, apnea, hypoventilation, vasovagal episodes, euphoria, prolonged emergence, agitation, hyperactivity, pruritus, rash
- Precautions and contraindications: intolerance to benzodiazepines and in those with acute narrow-angle glaucoma, shock, coma, or acute alcohol intoxication

- Anesthesia considerations: Use midazolam with caution in elderly patients and in patients with chronic obstructive pulmonary disease, chronic renal failure, or congestive heart failure (CHF).
- Reduce the dose in hypovolemia and with the concomitant use of other sedatives or narcotics.
- Hypotension and respiratory depression may occur when it is administered with opioids.

Flumazenil (Romazicon)

- GABA-A receptor antagonist
- Indications: reversal of benzodiazepine receptor agonist
- Dose: IV: 0.2–1 mg (4–20 mcg/kg); titrate to patient response; may repeat at 20-minute intervals (maximum single dose: 1 mg; maximum total dose: 3 mg in any 1 hour).
- Onset: IV 1–2 minutes
- Duration: 30–90 minutes
- Adverse effects: arrhythmia, tachycardia, bradycardia, hypertension, angina, flushing, reversal of sedation, seizures, agitation, emotional lability, nausea and vomiting, pain at injection site, thrombophlebitis
- Precautions and contraindications: Resedation may occur and is more common with large doses of long-acting benzodiazepines.
- Monitor for resedation.

KNOWLEDGE CHECK

1. Which physiologic effect is associated with benzodiazepine administration? (*Select all that apply.*)
   a. Muscle excitation
   b. Antiepileptic
   c. Anxiogenic
   d. Anterograde amnesia
   e. Antiemetic
2. Benzodiazepines are agonists at _______ receptors?
   a. mu
   b. muscarinic
   c. $GABA_A$
   d. NMDA
3. Flumazenil (Romazicon) administered IV begins to inhibit benzodiazepine-induced respiratory depression in
   a. 30 seconds.
   b. 2 minutes.
   c. 5 minutes.
   d. 10 minutes.

Answers can be found in Appendix A.

INDUCTION AGENTS

Dexmedetomidine

- Dexmedetomidine is a highly selective α_2-receptor agonist causing CNS sympatholysis.
- Dexmedetomidine does not interfere with neurologic monitoring and has minimal respiratory depressant effects.
- Hypotension and bradycardia are the most frequent cardiovascular adverse effects.
- Hypertension may occur upon starting an IV infusion as a result of peripheral α_2 receptor stimulation.
- It is useful for procedural sedation and as an analgesic.
- It reduces postoperative agitation and emergence reactions.

Propofol

- Propofol is the most commonly used IV anesthetic as an induction drug and for sedation.
- Respiratory effects include respiratory depression or apnea that is more pronounced as doses increase. Although not a bronchodilator, safe use in patients with asthma has been well established.
- Propofol exhibits mild antiemetic properties and has a short half-life (0.5–1.5 hours).
- Propofol has a rapid onset and provides for rapid emergence after bolus or shorter continuous infusions of the drug.
- Patients emerge with a mild euphoria followed by rapid dissipation of the sedative effects.
- Propofol reduces cerebral blood flow, cerebral metabolic rate of oxygen consumption ($CMRO_2$), and intracranial pressure (ICP).
- Propofol decreases blood pressure, cardiac output, and systemic vascular resistance (SVR) to a greater degree than etomidate at equipotent doses.
- The induction dose is 1–2 mg/kg, followed by a maintenance infusion of 100–200 mcg/kg/min.
- As a result of the formulation of propofol, severe burning occurs at the IV site if an induction dose is administered without first administering lidocaine.

Etomidate

- Etomidate is used when hemodynamic stability is critically important (i.e., massive hemorrhage resulting from trauma).
- The major advantage of etomidate is minimal cardiorespiratory depression.

- Etomidate reduces ICP, cerebral blood flow, and $CMRO_2$. Even though etomidate causes CNS depression, it can be associated with epileptogenic activity on EEG. For this reason, it may be prudent to use other induction agents for neurologic procedures or in patients with known seizure disorders.
- The mechanism of action of etomidate appears to be GABA-mimetic.
- Involuntary movements or myoclonus during IV bolus can occur.
- Etomidate frequently causes burning on injection, which is minimized by preemptively administering lidocaine.
- Etomidate inhibits the enzyme 11β-hydroxylase, which is essential in the production of both corticosteroids and mineralocorticoids from the adrenal cortex. Clinically significant reductions in steroid (cortisol and aldosterone) production may occur with single doses or prolonged infusions for up to 24 hours.
- Etomidate increases the incidence of PONV.
- The induction dose is 0.2–0.3 mg/kg.

Ketamine

- The site of action of ketamine appears to be the NMDA receptor, where it inhibits glutamate as a noncompetitive antagonist. Multiple mechanisms of action are likely.
- Ketamine produces an anesthetic state referred to as *dissociative anesthesia.*
- The onset of effect is relatively slow compared with other induction drugs (2–5 min).
- Ketamine produces a rise in cerebral perfusion pressure.
- Ketamine is a bronchodilator, preserves airway reflexes, and increases secretions.
- Emergence phenomena include vivid dreams, floating sensations, and delirium. They are more common in adults than in children and are reduced by benzodiazepine or other sedatives.
- Ketamine is an indirect sympathomimetic, releasing endogenous catecholamines. This action accounts for the cardiovascular stimulation and bronchodilation.
- Ketamine should be avoided in patients with catecholamine depletion because the drug may cause hypotension and myocardial depression.
- Ketamine is a moderate analgesic and can be used preoperatively as a component of preemptive analgesia.
- Clinical uses for ketamine are listed in Box 2.3.

BOX 2.3 Clinical Uses of Ketamine

Induction of Anesthesia in High-Risk Patients
- Shock or cardiovascular instability
- Hypovolemia
- Cardiomyopathy
- Trauma
- Bronchospasm

Obstetric Patients

Induction of General Anesthesia
- Severe hypovolemia/trauma
- Acute hemorrhage
- Acute bronchospasm

Low Dose for Analgesia
- To supplement regional anesthetic techniques
- As an additive to opioids in patient-controlled analgesia
- For use in therapy for chronic pain and depression

Adjunct to Local and Regional Anesthetic Techniques
- For sedation and analgesia during intravenous sedation or when a regional block is used
- To supplement an inadequate block

Outpatient Surgery
- For brief diagnostic and therapeutic procedures
- To supplement local and regional block techniques

Use Outside the Operating Room
- In burn units (e.g., debridement, dressing changes)
- In emergency rooms for minor procedures
- In intensive care units (e.g., sedation, painful procedures)
- During radiology procedures

From Elisha S, Heiner JS, Nagelhout JJ. *Nurse Anesthesia.* 7th ed. Elsevier; 2023.

Primary Clinical Characteristics and Effects of Ketamine

- Phencyclidine derivative sympathomimetic
- Causes unconsciousness; amnesia referred to as *dissociative anesthesia*, which can result in emergence delirium, nightmares, and hallucinations
- Increases blood pressure and heart rate
- Increases cerebral metabolic rate, cerebral blood flow, and intracranial and intraocular pressure
- Causes nystagmus
- Causes moderate analgesia via NMDA-receptor agonism
- Potent bronchodilator

- Maintains respirations and airway reflexes (NOTE: A period of initial apnea may occur, especially with high doses and rapid administration.)
- Increases salivation and respiratory secretions
- Increases muscle tone
- Should be used with caution in patients with hypertension, angina, CHF, increased ICP, increased intraocular pressure, and psychiatric dysfunction

Recommendation Doses of Ketamine

Premedication

- A benzodiazepine such as midazolam can be administered to decrease the potential for emergence delirium.
- An antisialagogue may also be given to decrease oral secretions.

Induction of anesthesia

- Ketamine 2–4 mg/kg IV or 4–6 mg/kg IM (oral dose is 10 mg/kg)

Maintenance of anesthesia

- Ketamine 15–45 mcg/kg/min (1–3 mg/min) by continuous IV infusion or 0.5–1.0 mg/kg supplemental IV doses as needed

Sedation and analgesia

- Ketamine 0.2–0.8 mg/kg IV (over 2–3 min) followed by a continuous ketamine infusion (5–120 mcg/kg/min); 10–20 mg IV may produce preemptive analgesia.

KNOWLEDGE CHECK

1. Which induction agent is associated with antiemetic properties?
   a. Propofol
   b. Dexmedetomidine
   c. Etomidate
   d. Ketamine
2. The term *dissociative anesthesia* is used to describe the anesthetic state produced by
   a. ketamine.
   b. propofol.
   c. isoflurane.
   d. midazolam.
3. Each physiologic effect contributes to hypotension after induction with propofol *except*
   a. direct myocardial depression.
   b. anticholinergic effect.
   c. CNS depression.
   d. vasodilation.
4. The induction agent of choice for a patient who is actively wheezing is
   a. dexmedetomidine.
   b. propofol.
   c. etomidate.
   d. ketamine.
5. A decrease in ICP, $CMRO_2$, cerebral blood flow, and cerebral perfusion pressure would be expected after the administration which agent? (*Select all that apply.*)
   a. Sevoflurane
   b. Ketamine
   c. Dexmedetomidine
   d. Propofol
6. Which physiologic effect is associated with etomidate? (*Select all that apply.*)
   a. Salivation
   b. Bronchodilation
   c. Myoclonus
   d. Tachycardia
   e. Adrenal cortical suppression
7. Emergence delirium associated with ketamine can be mitigated by administering
   a. fentanyl.
   b. lidocaine.
   c. dexmedetomidine.
   d. midazolam.

Answers can be found in Appendix A.

OPIATES

Anesthetic Implications

- Fentanyl and its analogs are most commonly used for their high potency and relatively short duration.
- Depending on their mechanism of action, opioids can be divided into four categories: agonists, partial agonists, agonists-antagonists, and antagonists.
- There are three main types of opioid receptors in the CNS: mu, delta, and kappa (Table 2.19).
- Mu-receptor stimulation produces supraspinal analgesia, euphoria, and a decrease in ventilation.
- Delta-receptor stimulation produces spinal analgesia, responds to enkephalins, and serves to modulate activity of the mu receptors.
- Kappa-receptor stimulation produces spinal analgesia, sedation, and miosis.

TABLE 2.19 Actions Produced at Each Opioid Receptor Subtype

Effects	Mu (μ) Receptor	Kappa (κ) Receptor	Delta (δ) Receptor
IUPHAR name	MOP	KOP	DOP
Analgesia	Supraspinal, spinal	Supraspinal, spinal	Supraspinal, spinal; modulates mu-receptor activity
Cardiovascular	Bradycardia		
Respiratory	Depression	Possible depression	Depression
Central nervous system	Euphoria, sedation, prolactin release, mild hypothermia, catalepsy, indifference to environmental stimulus	Sedation, dysphoria, psychomimetic reactions (hallucinations, delirium)	
Pupil	Miosis	Miosis	
Gastrointestinal	Inhibition of peristalsis, nausea, vomiting		
Genitourinary	Urinary retention	Diuresis (inhibition of vasopressin release)	Urinary retention
Pruritus	Yes		Yes
Physical dependence	Yes	Low abuse potential	Yes
Antishivering		Yes	

DOP, Delta opioid peptide; *IUPHAR*, International Union of Basic and Clinical Pharmacology; *KOP,* kappa opioid peptide; *MOP,* mu opioid peptide.

From Elisha S, Heiner JS, Nagelhout JJ. *Nurse Anesthesia*. 7th ed. Elsevier; 2023.

TABLE 2.20 Side Effects—Opioids and Related Frequency

Opioid Side Effect	Observed Frequency	Notes
Constipation	40%–95%	• Caused by opioid receptors in the gut • Does not resolve over time
Nausea	25%	• Direct stimulation of the chemotactic trigger zone, gastric distention, and increased vestibular sensitivity
Pruritus	10%	• Some histamine release, but more significantly, a direct stimulation of mu receptors
Sedation	60%	• Transient
Respiratory depression	Dose dependent	• Long-term opioid use may lead to sleep apnea
Endocrinologic	52%–74%	• Amenorrhea and low testosterone
Immunologic	?	• Inhibition of cellular immune response

From Elisha S, Heiner JS, Nagelhout JJ. *Nurse Anesthesia*. 7th ed. Elsevier; 2023.

Side Effects

- Some common side effects of opioids are listed in Table 2.20.

Clinical Effects

- See Table 2.21 for common clinical effects of opioid agonists.

Central Nervous System Effects: Analgesia, Sedation, and Euphoria

- Opiate analgesia results from actions in the CNS, spinal cord, and peripheral sites.
- Opioids are less effective in treating neuropathic pain that requires chronic multimodal therapy.

TABLE 2.21 Common Clinical Effects of Opioids

Acute	Chronic
Analgesia	Tolerance
Respiratory depression	Physical dependence
Sedation	Constipation
Euphoria	
Dysphoria	
Vasodilation	
Bradycardia	
Cough suppression	
Miosis	
Nausea and vomiting	
Skeletal muscle rigidity	
Smooth muscle spasm	
Constipation	
Urinary retention	
Biliary spasm	
Pruritus, rash	
Antishivering (meperidine only)	
Histamine release	
Hormonal effects	

From Elisha S, Heiner JS, Nagelhout JJ. *Nurse Anesthesia*. 7th ed. Elsevier; 2023.

- The analgesic effects of opioids come from their ability to do the following:
  1. Directly inhibit the ascending transmission of nociception information from the spinal cord dorsal horn
  2. Activate pain control pathways that descend from the midbrain via the rostral ventromedial medulla to the spinal cord dorsal horn
- The effect of opioids on electroencephalographic and evoked-potential activity is minimal; neurophysiologic monitoring can be conducted during opioid anesthetic techniques.
- The comparative potency of the opioid agonists that are used in anesthesia is as follows: sufentanil > fentanyl = remifentanil > hydromorphone (Dilaudid).
- Physical and psychological dependence occur with repeated administration, as evidenced by physical withdrawal with abstinence and drug-seeking behaviors.

Respiratory depression

- All opiate agonists produce a dose-dependent depression of respiration via effects on mu and delta receptors in the respiratory centers in the brainstem.
- Opiate agonists reduce the responsiveness of the respiratory centers to increasing carbon dioxide and decreasing oxygen.
- Respiratory rate is affected first, and a classically "narcotized" patient will take slow, deep breaths.
- Both analgesia and respiratory depression are mediated via the same receptors, and therefore reversal of respiratory depression with opiate receptor antagonists such as naloxone also reverses analgesia.

Nausea and vomiting

- Opioids cause nausea and vomiting by stimulating the chemoreceptor trigger zone in the area postrema of the medulla.
- Clinically, when opiates are used as part of the anesthetic plan, there may be an increased incidence of PONV.

Cardiac Effects

- Bradycardia may be caused by opioid administration and results from medullary vagal stimulation.
- All opioids induce dose-dependent peripheral vasodilation.
- Myocardial contractility, baroreceptor function, and autonomic responsiveness remain intact.
- The hypotension produced by morphine and codeine is attributed to histamine release, which is absent with fentanyl, sufentanil, alfentanil, and remifentanil.

Muscle rigidity

- A generalized skeletal muscle hypertonus can be produced by large IV bolus doses of most opioid agonists.
- Although morphine can produce skeletal muscle rigidity, it is most often associated with fentanyl, sufentanil, and remifentanil.
- The difficulty is caused in part by loss of chest wall compliance and by constriction of pharyngeal and laryngeal muscles, which can make manual ventilation difficult. This effect is referred to as *rigid chest* or *truncal rigidity*.
- Truncal rigidity most often occurs during anesthesia induction when high doses of potent opiates are administered rapidly IV.
- Opioid-induced muscle rigidity is thought to be mediated by central mu receptors interacting with dopamine and GABA pathways.
- This rigidity is easily eliminated by the administration of muscle relaxants or naloxone.

Pruritus

- Opiates may produce a rash, itching, and a feeling of warmth in the "blush" area of the face, upper chest, and arms.

- This occurs with both histamine-releasing and non–histamine-releasing narcotics. Pruritus is especially common with neuraxial administration of narcotics.
- Pruritus is common with the administration of neuraxial morphine and, to a lesser extent, with other opioids.
- Nalbuphine, droperidol, antihistamines, and ondansetron may be effective at decreasing opioid-induced pruritus.

Gastrointestinal Effects

- Opioids decrease gastric motility and intestinal propulsive activity, prolong gastric emptying time, and reduce secretory activity throughout the GI system, leading to opiate-induced constipation and postoperative ileus.
- Alvimopan (Pamora), methylnaltrexone (Relistor), and naloxegol (Movantik) are locally acting opiate receptor antagonists approved for use in treating GI hypomotility.
- These medications do not cross biological compartments, owing to solubility barriers, and therefore affect only the GI system. Thus they do not affect analgesia.
- Lubiprostone (Amitiza), a bicyclical fatty acid, activates intestinal chloride channel 2 in the small intestine and increases fluid secretion and gut motility.
- Opioids produce a dose-dependent increase in biliary duct pressure and sphincter of Oddi tone via opioid-receptor–mediated mechanisms.

Endocrinological Effects

- Opiates reduce the stress response to surgery and have an immunosuppressant effect.
- Endocrinologic effects of opioids include the release of vasopressin and inhibition of the stress-induced release of corticotropin-releasing hormone and adrenocorticotropic hormone from the hypothalamus and anterior pituitary, respectively.
- Opioids slightly decrease body temperature by resetting the equilibrium point of temperature regulation in the hypothalamus.
- Opioids produce an antidiuretic effect.

Opioids and Cancer

- Although controversial, inhalation anesthetic agents and opioid analgesia are independent risk factors for cancer recurrence.
- Conversely, regional anesthesia and propofol-based total IV anesthesia may have chemopreventive effects.
- Opioids may have a protumor action and may have negative effects on cancer survival. A definitive conclusion has not been reached.
- Opioid type and dose, as well as the underlying disease pathology and organs involved, are important factors.
- The effect of various anesthetic techniques on cancer recurrence is summarized in Table 2.22.

Neuraxial Effects

- Opioids are administered via epidural or subarachnoid routes.
- Opioids with a higher lipid solubility are rapidly absorbed into the spinal tissues after central administration, resulting in a faster onset of action.
- However, higher lipid solubility is associated with a small area of distribution of the drug along the length of the spinal cord and therefore a more limited area of analgesia.
- Higher lipid solubility is also associated with more rapid clearance of the drug out of the epidural and intrathecal spaces, resulting in a shorter duration of action and higher blood concentrations of the opioid.
- Spinal opioids are advantageous in selective analgesia, which occurs in the absence of motor and sympathetic blockade.
- Small portions of epidural opioids cross the dura, enter the cerebrospinal fluid (CSF), and penetrate spinal tissue in amounts proportional to their lipid solubility.
- The remaining drug is absorbed by the vasculature, producing plasma levels comparable to those after IM injections and providing supraspinal analgesia.
- Pain that is unresponsive to systemic opioids may respond to the same drugs given centrally, reducing some side effects while increasing the incidence of others.
- Intrathecal administration allows injection of the opioids directly into the CSF, a more efficient method of delivering the drug to the spinal cord opiate receptors.
- Side effects include those described previously with systemic administration. However, pruritus and urinary retention occur with much greater frequency.
- Respiratory depression is the most common serious complication associated with intrathecally and epidurally administered opioids.
- Less lipid-soluble agents such as morphine and hydromorphone produce a delayed ventilatory depression,

TABLE 2.22 Effect of Anesthetic Technique on Cancer Recurrence or Metastasis

Anesthetic Technique	Effect on Cancer Recurrence and Metastasis
Volatile anesthetic agents	Conflicting evidence; some in vitro studies suggest enhanced expression of tumorigenic markers, migration of cancer cells, angiogenesis, and metastasis in tumors. Insufficient evidence exists to avoid in cancer surgery.
Nitrous oxide	No impact on cancer recurrence
Local anesthetics	Reduced cancer recurrence and metastasis secondary to antiinflammatory actions and direct effects on the proliferation and migration of cancer cells
Neuraxial anesthesia	Conflicting results but generally thought to reduce cancer recurrence and metastasis by attenuating the immunosuppressive consequences of the stress response and possibly an opiate-sparing effect
Nonsteroidal antiinflammatory drugs	Acute or chronic use associated with tumor regression, presumably via cyclooxygenase 2 (COX-2) and prostaglandin inhibition in cancer cells. Beneficial choice as analgesics in patients with cancer.
Acetylsalicylic acid (ASA)	Reduces cancer metastasis
Opioids	Promote cancer progression and reduce long-term survival. Promote cancer cell growth, inhibit cellular immunity, enhance angiogenesis and tumor cell signaling pathways; inhibit natural killer cell function.
Supplemental oxygen	Patients given 80% oxygen postoperatively have a shorter cancer-free survival period; has an angiogenic effect on micrometastasis
Dexamethasone	No effect on cancer survival

Adapted from Byrne K, Levins KJ, Buggy DJ. Can anesthetic-analgesic technique during primary cancer surgery affect recurrence or metastasis? *Can J Anaesth.* 2016;63(2):184–192.

the result of migration of opioid via the CSF to the midbrain vestibular centers.

- Two phases of respiratory depression can occur after neuraxial morphine administration. An early phase observed soon after administration reflects rapid systemic absorption and is similar to parenteral dosing. A secondary, more insidious respiratory depression occurs over a period of 8–12 hours and has been related to rostral flow of CSF and delivery of morphine to the brainstem respiratory center.
- Awareness of delayed respiratory depression has resulted in increased monitoring of patients and dose reductions, thereby greatly reducing the incidence of serious respiratory depression and possible arrest.
- Urinary retention after spinal opioid analgesia administration is related to inhibition of sacral parasympathetic outflow, which results in relaxation of the bladder detrusor muscle and an inability to relax the sphincter.
- Preemptive analgesia is an antinociceptive treatment that prevents establishment of altered processing of afferent input, which amplifies postoperative pain. Three different definitions have been used as the basis for the concept. Preemptive analgesia has been defined as treatment that
  1. begins before surgery;
  2. prevents the establishment of central sensitization caused by incisional injury (covers only the period of surgery); and
  3. prevents the establishment of central sensitization caused by incisional and inflammatory injuries (covers the period of surgery and the initial postoperative period).
- Preemptive analgesia initiated before the surgical procedure to prevent pain in the early postoperative period has the potential to be more effective than a similar analgesic treatment initiated after surgery.
- Recently, there has been a concern over the judicious use of narcotics during anesthesia. Factors that have changed the opinions of anesthetists to provide opioid-sparing or opioid-free anesthesia include enhanced recovery after surgery (ERAS) protocols, the opioid epidemic, the potential for postoperative ileus, nausea and vomiting, sedation, cancer risk, and postoperative addiction.

- Preoperative multimodal analgesia, regional nerve blocks, and other techniques are gaining popularity.

Methadone

- Methadone is a synthetic opioid often used for the treatment of opioid misuse in detoxification or treatment programs.
- It is also used to treat severe acute and chronic cancer pain, as well as noncancer pain.
- Methadone is a viable option for chronic pain for patients who have developed tolerance (intolerable side effects or inadequate analgesia) to opioids.
- Because of its high degree of lipid solubility, it is well absorbed via the gastric mucosa, with peak analgesic effects in 30–60 minutes. When given IV, the drug has peak effects that are seen in 15–20 minutes. Methadone has a long half-life of approximately 15–60 hours.
- Metabolism of methadone is primarily via the CYP450 enzyme, specifically CYP3A4 and CYP2B6, into inactive metabolites that are excreted in the urine. Therefore, any medication that inhibits (e.g., phenytoin, carbamazepine) or induces CYP450 may alter methadone metabolism.
- Side effects associated with methadone are similar to those associated with other opioids, including respiratory depression and excessive sedation; respiratory depression peak effects occur later than the analgesic peak effects.
- A unique side effect of methadone is QT interval prolongation.
- Patients taking methadone on a continuous basis should be monitored with a cardiac evaluation.
- An electrocardiogram (ECG) should be obtained before treatment and periodically thereafter, depending on dose changes, baseline ECG findings, and other risk factors for QT interval prolongation.
- In complex surgical procedures, methadone administered intraoperatively decreases postoperative pain scores and reduces postoperative opioid requirements.
- Methadone's lack of active metabolites, long half-life, and low cost make it desirable for chronic nonmalignant pain management.
- Recommendations for management of the chronic opioid-dependent patient are listed in Table 2.23.

Opioid Antagonist

- Naloxone (Narcan) is a pure opioid antagonist that reverses the physiologic effects associated with narcotics, such as respiratory depression and analgesia.
- It provides competitive antagonism at mu, kappa, and delta receptors within the CNS.
- The clinical duration of action of naloxone (30–40 minutes) is less than that of most narcotics.
- If extreme narcosis is reversed, a second dose of naloxone may be necessary within 30 minutes of the initial dose.
- Because of the rapid reversal of the "narcotic effect" associated with naloxone, catecholamine output from the CNS greatly increases.
- This phenomenon can result in hypertension, neurogenic pulmonary edema, and/or ventricular dysrhythmias.

Partial Agonists/Antagonists Opiate Analgesics

Partial agonist

- The partial agonist buprenorphine is available in oral transmucosal (Belbuca) and parenteral formulations (Buprenex and generics) and in a transdermal patch (Butrans) for treatment of pain.
- Buprenorphine is approved by the US Food and Drug Administration (FDA) for maintenance treatment of opioid use disorder in oral transmucosal formulations (alone and in combination with the opioid antagonist naloxone), as a subdermal implant (Probuphine), and as a once-monthly injection (Sublocade); it is safer than methadone because it has a ceiling on its respiratory depressant effect and a lower abuse potential, and it is less likely to prolong the QT interval. (In high doses, buprenorphine can prolong the QT interval.) Nausea, headache, dizziness, and somnolence are common adverse effects of buprenorphine.

Mixed agonist/antagonists

- The mixed agonist/antagonists pentazocine (Talwin), butorphanol, and nalbuphine all have a ceiling on their analgesic effects and can precipitate withdrawal symptoms in patients physically dependent on full opioid agonists.
- All are less likely than full agonists to cause physical dependence.

Anesthetic implications

- The opiate partial agonists and mixed agonist/antagonist drugs have limited use in anesthesia. They have a ceiling effect to their analgesic action. As noted later, they can be used for chronic pain secondary to a lower likelihood of respiratory depression than the full agonists. Rarely, they are also used to treat pruritus because, unlike naloxone, they have some analgesic effects.

TABLE 2.23 Recommendations for Perioperative Management for Patients on Chronic Opioid Therapy

Preoperative	Intraoperative	Postoperative
Pain assessment	Continue baseline opioid (oral, transdermal, IV, intrathecal pump)	Multimodal analgesic techniques
Precise opioid use (dose/type)—continue DOS	Increases in intraoperative opioids because of tolerance—titrate or continuous infusion	Maintain baseline opioid
Adjuvant medications for CP—continue DOS	Consider opioid rotation	Titrate opioids aggressively to achieve adequate pain control
Reassurance and address fears/anxiety	Multimodal approach	PCA—primary or supplementary for epidural/regional
Multimodal pain plan—consider NSAIDs, acetaminophen, 1–2 h before surgery, anxiolytics	Consider regional, LA wound infiltration, PNB, CPNB, epidural/SAB	Continue applicable regional techniques
Consult with addiction specialist/clinic if indicated—continue methadone maintenance	Consider adjuvants—ketorolac, ketamine, clonidine, dexmedetomidine	Continue ketamine or low-dose ketamine infusion, if started in the OR
Plan for postoperative analgesia	Anticipate increases in inhalation agent	Monitor for respiratory depression
	Avoid opioid antagonists and mixed agonists	Continued assessment of analgesia
		Implement nontraditional comfort measures

CP, Chronic pain; *CPNB,* continuous peripheral nerve block; *DOS,* day of surgery; *LA,* local anesthetic; *NSAIDs,* nonsteroidal anti-inflammatory drugs; *OR,* operating room; *PCA,* patient-controlled analgesia; *PNB,* peripheral nerve block; *SAB,* subarachnoid blockade.

From Elisha S, Heiner JS, Nagelhout JJ. *Nurse Anesthesia.* 7th ed. Elsevier; 2023.

KNOWLEDGE CHECK

1. Which is the most potent narcotic?
   a. Alfentanil
   b. Fentanyl
   c. Sufentanil
   d. Remifentanil
2. Which narcotic produces histamine release?
   a. Morphine
   b. Alfentanil
   c. Remifentanil
   d. Sufentanil
3. Remifentanil metabolism is catalyzed by
   a. pseudocholinesterase.
   b. hepatic microsomal enzymes.
   c. monoamine oxidase.
   d. nonspecific esterases.
4. Narcotics are primarily metabolized
   a. in the gastrointestinal tract.
   b. in the kidneys.
   c. by pseudocholinesterase.
   d. in the liver.
5. Opiate-induced increases in biliary pressure are due to
   a. constriction of intestinal sphincters.
   b. increase in bile flow.
   c. increase in hepatic metabolic activity.
   d. decrease bile viscosity.
6. Which is a side effect associated with neuraxial opioid administration? (*Select all that apply.*)
   a. Direct myocardial depression
   b. Pruritus
   c. Respiratory depression/arrest
   d. GI hypermotility
   e. Urinary retention
   f. Tachycardia
7. When administered in the subarachnoid space, which narcotic can cause delayed onset respiratory depression?
   a. Morphine
   b. Fentanyl
   c. Alfentanil
   d. Sufentanil

Continued

KNOWLEDGE CHECK—cont'd

8. Which side effect is associated with methadone? (*Select all that apply.*)
   a. Direct myocardial depression
   b. QT interval prolongation
   c. Sedation
   d. Respiratory depression
9. Which opioid receptor subtype causes respiratory depression?
   a. Mu
   b. Delta
   c. Kappa
   d. Sigma
10. Which adverse physiologic reactions can be associated with Naloxone administration?
   a. Disseminated intravascular coagulation
   b. Pulmonary edema
   c. Ventricular tachycardia
   d. Respiratory arrest

Answers can be found in Appendix A.

NEUROMUSCULAR BLOCKING AGENTS

Depolarizing Muscle Relaxant: Succinylcholine Chloride

- Succinylcholine chloride (Anectine, Quelicin) use in clinical anesthesia has been the standard of care for a variety of situations. However, opinions regarding its use remain divided because of the side effects that can occur.
- The major advantages associated with succinylcholine include rapid onset and offset.
- The use of succinylcholine is contraindicated in patients who are MH-susceptible (Table 2.24).
- However, with the advent of sugammadex, more anesthetists may opt not to use succinylcholine in the future.

Nondepolarizing Muscle Relaxants

- The efficacy of the nondepolarizing muscle relaxants is similar, so the choice of one drug over another is largely made on the basis of other factors.
- Specific patient characteristics, type of surgical procedure, pharmacokinetics, and side-effect profile guide the selection of an individual relaxant for a given situation.
- The intermediate-duration nondepolarizing relaxants are almost exclusively used in current clinical practice.
- The nondepolarizing agents are divided into two chemical groups: aminosteroids and benzylisoquinolines:
  1. The aminosteroids are named with "-curonium" suffixes, such as rocuronium, vecuronium, and pancuronium. These drugs are metabolized by the liver and excreted by the kidneys.
  2. The benzylisoquinolines are named with "-curium" suffixes, such as atracurium, cisatracurium, and mivacurium. Atracurium is primarily metabolized by nonspecific esterases (~66%). The balance is degraded by Hofmann elimination. Mivacurium is metabolized by pseudocholinesterase only.

Characteristics of Neuromuscular Blockade (Box 2.4 and Table 2.25)

Depolarizing (Phase I) Block

- Muscle fasciculation precedes onset of neuromuscular blockade (NMB).
- Sustained response to tetanic stimulation
- Absence of posttetanic potentiation, stimulation, or facilitation
- Lack of fade to tetanus, train of four (TOF), or double-burst stimulation (DBS)
- Block antagonized by prior administration of nondepolarizing muscle relaxant as pretreatment (approximately 20% more succinylcholine required)
- Block potentiated by anticholinesterase drugs

Nondepolarizing (Phase II) Block

- Absence of muscle fasciculation
- Appearance of tetanic fade and posttetanic potentiation, stimulation, or facilitation
- TOF and double-burst fade
- Reversal with anticholinesterase drugs
- In rare cases, may be produced by an overdose and desensitization with succinylcholine at doses greater than 6 mg/kg (Boxes 2.5 and 2.6)

Commonly Used Terminology Related to Neuromuscular Blockade

- *Onset time:* Time from drug administration to maximum effect

TABLE 2.24 Side Effects Associated With Succinylcholine

Side Effect	Probable Cause
Hyperkalemia	Normally, serum K^+ is increased by up to 0.5 mEq/L secondary to potassium leaking from the depolarized muscle; in upregulated patients, levels may rise much higher.
Dysrhythmias	Tachycardia (usually mild) is the most common effect; bradycardia secondary to hyperkalemia, especially with repeat doses, can occur. (Wide electrocardiographic complexes leading to cardiac arrest have been seen in children with Duchenne muscular dystrophy and other muscular disorders.)
Myalgia	Secondary to fasciculation, even though some patients complain of muscle pain without having shown visible evidence of fasciculation
Myoglobinemia	Rare complication after extensive fasciculation or in malignant hyperthermia
Elevated intragastric pressure	Secondary to transient contraction of abdominal muscles during fasciculation; however, elevations of intragastric pressure seen after succinylcholine are not clinically relevant; less significant than occurs with CO_2 insufflation during laparoscopic procedures; barrier pressure is typically maintained due to increased lower esophageal sphincter (LES) tone.
Elevated intracranial pressure (ICP)	Postulated to be secondary to fasciculation, increased central venous pressure; associated with increased cerebral blood flow secondary to muscle-spindle afferent activity and actions on peripheral neuromuscular junctions; ICP effects can be blocked by pretreatment with a small dose of nondepolarizing relaxant and the usual initial administration of an induction agent; may safely be used in neurosurgical procedures.
Elevated intraocular pressure (IOP)	Increases IOP within 1 min and peaks at an increase of 9 mm Hg within 6 min after administration; increase is a vascular event, with choroidal vascular dilation or a decrease in drainage secondary to elevated central venous pressure temporarily inhibiting the flow of aqueous humor through the canal of Schlemm; generally considered safe in ocular emergencies.
Malignant hyperthermia	Associated with a genetic predisposition; mechanism by which succinylcholine triggers the syndrome is not understood.
Masseter spasm	Seen in anesthetic and emergency use; sometimes followed by malignant hyperthermia

CO_2, Carbon dioxide; *K^+*, potassium.

Modified from Kirby RR, Gravenstein N, Lobato EB, et al., eds. *Clinical Anesthesia Practice*. 2nd ed. Elsevier; 2002; Atlee JL. *Complications in Anesthesia*. 2nd ed. Elsevier; 2007.

BOX 2.4 Characteristics of Neuromuscular Blockade

Depolarizing (Phase I) Block

- Muscle fasciculation precedes onset of neuromuscular blockade
- Sustained response to tetanic stimulation
- Absence of posttetanic potentiation, stimulation, or facilitation
- Lack of fade to tetanus, train of four, or double-burst stimulation
- Block antagonized by prior administration of nondepolarizer as pretreatment (approximately 20% more succinylcholine required)
- Block potentiated by anticholinesterase drugs

Nondepolarizing (Phase II) Block

- Absence of muscle fasciculation
- Appearance of tetanic fade and posttetanic potentiation, stimulation, or facilitation
- Train of four and double-burst fade
- Reversal with anticholinesterase drugs and sugammadex (aminosteroid neuromuscular blocking drugs—rocuronium, vecuronium)
- In rare cases, a phase II may be produced by an overdose and desensitization with succinylcholine at doses greater than 6 mg/kg.

From Elisha S, Heiner JS, Nagelhout JJ. *Nurse Anesthesia*. 7th ed. Elsevier; 2023.

TABLE 2.25 A Comparison of Neuromuscular Monitoring Sites

Monitoring Site	Response	Comments
Ulnar nerve innervation of the adductor pollicis	Thumb adduction	Usually has easy access Best site to measure recovery
Facial nerves	Eyelid and eyebrow movement	Easily accessed when arm is not available Best site to measure onset Corrugator supercilii is more resistant to relaxants than the orbicularis oculi.

From Elisha S, Heiner JS, Nagelhout JJ. *Nurse Anesthesia.* 7th ed. Elsevier; 2023.

BOX 2.5 Pathologic Conditions With Potential for Succinylcholine-Induced Hyperkalemia

- Upper or lower motor neuron defect
- Spinal cord trauma
- Prolonged chemical denervation (e.g., muscle relaxants, magnesium, clostridial toxins)
- Direct muscle trauma, tumor, or inflammation
- Select muscular dystrophies and myopathies
- Thermal trauma
- Disuse atrophy
- Stroke
- Tetanus
- Severe infection

From Elisha S, Heiner JS, Nagelhout JJ. *Nurse Anesthesia.* 7th ed. Elsevier; 2023.

BOX 2.6 Contraindications to the Use of Succinylcholine

- Hyperkalemia
- Burn patients with injuries of over 35% total body surface area (TBSA), third-degree burn
- Severe muscle trauma
- Neurologic injury (e.g., paraplegia, quadriplegia)
- Hyperkalemia resulting from renal failure
- Severe sepsis (e.g., abdominal)
- Muscle wasting, prolonged immobilization, extensive muscle denervation
- Malignant hyperthermia
- Duchenne muscular dystrophy
- Selected muscle disorders
- Should be used in children under 8 years old only in emergency situations; not for routine intubation
- Genetic variants of pseudocholinesterase
- Allergy

From Elisha S, Heiner JS, Nagelhout JJ. *Nurse Anesthesia.* 7th ed. Elsevier; 2023.

- *Clinical duration:* Time from drug administration to 25% recovery of the twitch response
- *Total duration of action:* Time from drug administration to 90% recovery of twitch response
- *Recovery index:* Time from 25%–75% recovery of the twitch response
- *Train-of-four ratio:* Compares the fourth twitch of a TOF with the first twitch; when the fourth twitch is 90% of the first, recovery is indicated.

General Guidelines for Neuromuscular Monitoring

- Objective (quantitative) monitoring of neuromuscular function should be used when possible (Table 2.26).
- Peripheral nerve stimulator units should display the delivered current output, which should be at least 30 mA.
- During onset, paralysis begins with the eye muscles, followed by the extremities, trunk (from the neck muscles downward through the intercostals), abdominal muscles, and finally the diaphragm. Recovery returns in the opposite order (Table 2.27).
- Protective airway reflex muscles of the pharynx and upper esophagus recover later than the diaphragm, larynx, hands, or face.
- Monitoring of the facial nerve for determination of onset and readiness for intubation may be preferable to monitoring of the ulnar nerve.
- Monitoring of the offset and recovery from NMB is most reflective of the diaphragm at the ulnar nerve compared with the orbicularis oculi.
- Tactile evaluation of TOF (Fig. 2.2) and DBS fade reduces but does not eliminate the incidence of postoperative residual paralysis compared with the

TABLE 2.26 Common Neuromuscular Monitoring Tests

Monitoring Test	Definition	Comments	Stimulation Characteristics
Single twitch	A single supramaximal electrical stimulus ranging from 0.1 to 1.0 Hz	Requires baseline before drug administration; generally used as a qualitative rather than quantitative assessment	
Train of four (TOF)	A series of four twitches at 2 Hz every 0.5 s for 2 s	Reflects blockade from 70%–100%; useful during onset, maintenance, and emergence TOF ratio is determined by comparing T_1–T_4	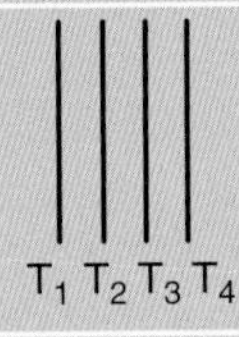
Double-burst simulation	Two short bursts of 50-Hz tetanus separated by 0.75 s	Similar to TOF; useful during onset, maintenance, and emergence; may be easier to detect fade than with TOF; tactile evaluation	
Tetanus	Generally consists of rapid delivery of a 30-, 50-, or 100-Hz stimulus for 5 s	Should be used sparingly for deep block assessment; painful	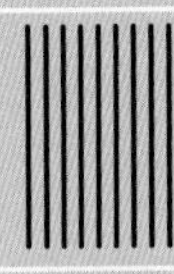
Posttetanic count	50-Hz tetanus for 5 s, a 3-s pause, then single twitches of 1 Hz	Used only when TOF and double-burst stimulation is absent; count of less than 8 indicates deep block, and prolonged recovery is likely	

From Elisha S, Heiner JS, Nagelhout JJ. *Nurse Anesthesia*. 7th ed. Elsevier; 2023.

TABLE 2.27 Key Points Related to Tests of Neuromuscular Transmission and Reversal

Test	Acceptable Clinical Result to Suggest Normal Function	Approximate Percentage of Receptors Occupied When Response Returns to Normal Value	Comments, Advantages, and Disadvantages
Tidal volume	At least 5 mL/kg	80%	Necessary but insensitive as an indicator of neuromuscular function
Single-twitch strength	Qualitatively as strong as baseline	75%–80%	Uncomfortable; need to know twitch strength before relaxant administration; insensitive as an indicator of recovery, but useful as a gauge of deep neuromuscular blockade
Train of four (TOF)	No palpable fade	70%–75%	Uncomfortable but more sensitive as indicator of recovery than single-twitch; used as a gauge of depth of block by counting the number of responses perceptible
Sustained tetanus at 50 Hz for 5 s	At least 20 mL/kg	70%	Very uncomfortable but a reliable indicator of adequate recovery

Continued

TABLE 2.27 Key Points Related to Tests of Neuromuscular Transmission and Reversal—cont'd

Test	Acceptable Clinical Result to Suggest Normal Function	Approximate Percentage of Receptors Occupied When Response Returns to Normal Value	Comments, Advantages, and Disadvantages
Vital capacity	At least 20 mL/kg	70%	Requires patient cooperation but is the goal for achievement of full clinical recovery
Double-burst stimulation	No palpable fade	60%–70%	Uncomfortable but more sensitive than TOF as an indicator of peripheral function; no perceptible fade indicates TOF of at least recovery of 60%
Inspiratory force	At least 40 cm H_2O	50%	Difficult to perform with endotracheal intubation, but a reliable gauge of normal diaphragmatic function
Head lift	Must be performed unaided with patient supine and sustained for 5 s	50%	Requires patient cooperation but remains the standard test of normal clinical function
Hand grip	Sustained at a level qualitatively similar to preinduction	50%	Sustained strong grip, although also requires patient cooperation; is another good gauge of normal function
Sustained bite	Sustained jaw clench on tongue blade	50%	Very reliable with patient cooperation; corresponds with TOF of 85%

Modified from Miller RD. Neuromuscular blocking drugs. In: Miller RD, Pardo M, eds. *Basics of Anesthesia.* 6th ed. Elsevier; 2011.

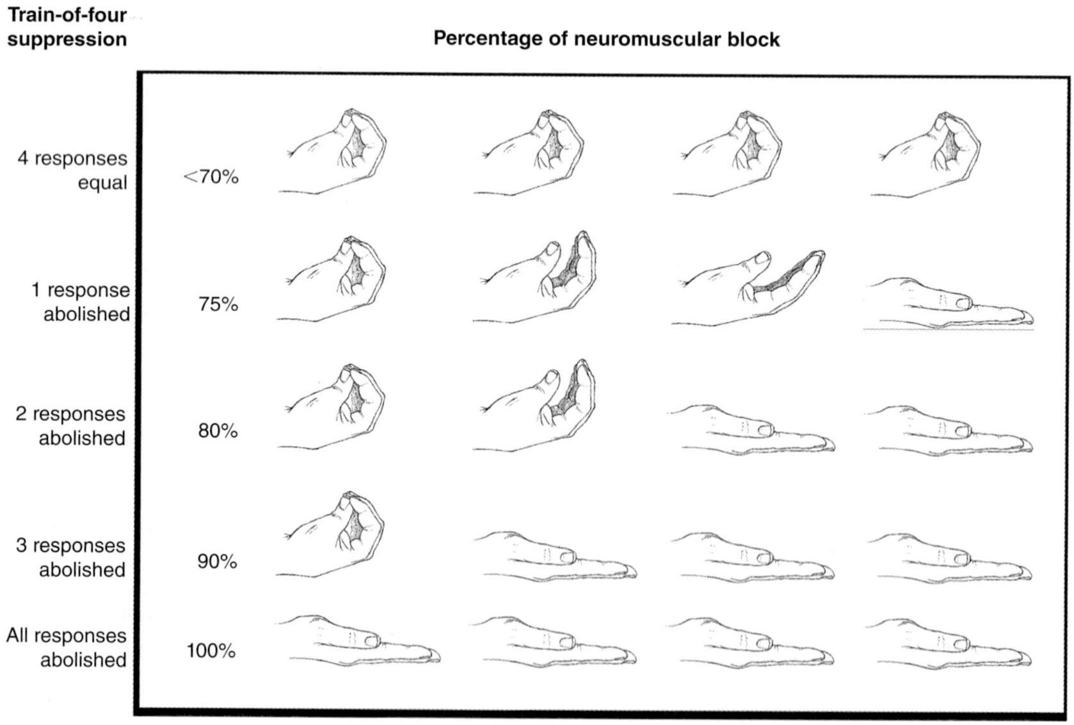

Fig. 2.2 Train-of-four test. (From Elisha S, Heiner JS, Nagelhout JJ. *Nurse Anesthesia.* 7th ed. Elsevier; 2023.)

TABLE 2.28 Select Inherited Variants of Plasma Cholinesterase

PChE Variant	Genetic Label	Frequency (%)	Population Incidence	Enzyme Activity	Duration of Succinylcholine
Usual	Homozygote U	96%	Normal	Normal	Normal; dibucaine number 70–80
—	Heterozygote U/A	3%	1 in 480	Decreased	Slightly prolonged; dibucaine number 50–69
Atypical	Homozygote A	0.3%	1 in 3200	Decreased by 70% or more	Significantly prolonged; dibucaine number 16–30
Fluoride	Homozygote F	0.03%	Extremely rare	Decreased by 60%	Moderately prolonged
Silent	Homozygote S	0.04%	Extremely rare	No activity	Significantly prolonged

PChE, Plasma cholinesterase.
From Elisha S, Heiner JS, Nagelhout JJ. *Nurse Anesthesia.* 7th ed. Elsevier; 2023.

use of clinical criteria to assess readiness for tracheal extubation.

- Adequate spontaneous recovery should be established before pharmacologic antagonism of a neuromuscular blocking drug (NMBD) block with anticholinesterases. This requirement does not apply to reversal with sugammadex.
- When there is only one response to TOF stimulation, successful reversal may take as long as 30 minutes with neostigmine.
- At a TOF count of two or three responses, recovery usually takes 4–15 minutes after intermediate-acting drugs.
- When the fourth response to TOF stimulation appears, adequate recovery can be achieved within 5 minutes of reversal with neostigmine or 2–3 minutes after use of edrophonium.
- When the fourth twitch of the TOF returns, the TOF ratio may be determined.
- The size of the fourth twitch (T_4) is compared with the size of the first twitch (T_1), using T_4:T_1 as a ratio.
- The timing of tracheal extubation should be guided by quantitative monitoring tests such as TOF greater than 0.9 or DBS_3 greater than 0.9.
- See Table 2.28 and Box 2.7.

BOX 2.7 Dibucaine Inhibition Test Outcomes

1. Low dibucaine number + slightly lower activity = atypical enzyme and prolonged apnea
2. Normal dibucaine number + low activity = normal enzyme with low levels present and prolonged apnea
3. Low dibucaine number + very low activity = possible rare variant–type enzyme with very low levels present and prolonged apnea
4. Normal dibucaine number + normal activity = normal enzyme and amount (Another reason for the prolonged apnea must be investigated.)

From Elisha S, Heiner JS, Nagelhout JJ. *Nurse Anesthesia.* 7th ed. Elsevier; 2023.

Histamine and Administration of Muscle Relaxants

- The effects of histamine release on histamine receptors are summarized in Table 2.29 and Box 2.8. The histamine-releasing potential of the relaxants is noted in Table 2.30.

TABLE 2.29 Effects of Stimulation of Histamine Receptors by Neuromuscular Blockers

H_1 Receptors	H_2 Receptors
Increased capillary permeability	Increased gastric acid production
Bronchoconstriction	Systemic and cerebral vasodilation
Intestinal contraction	Positive inotropic effects
Negative dromotropic effects	Positive chronotropic effects

H, Histamine.
Atracurium and mivacurium cause the release of histamine. Slight histamine release may occur with succinylcholine. The amount of histamine release is dependent on dose and speed of injection. With endogenous histamine release, all receptor responses are elicited.
Prophylaxis against histamine release requires administration of both H_1- and H_2-receptor blockers.
From Elisha S, Heiner JS, Nagelhout JJ. *Nurse Anesthesia.* 7th ed. Elsevier; 2023.

KNOWLEDGE CHECK

1. Which neuromuscular blocking medication is contraindicated for a patient with severe bronchial asthma? (*Select all that apply.*)
   a. Rocuronium
   b. Mivacurium
   c. Vecuronium
   d. Atracurium
2. Which anatomic site is most indicative of diaphragmatic recovery when used to assess adequacy of reversal of neuromuscular blockade?
   a. Ulnar nerve
   b. Orbicularis oculi muscle
   c. Corrugator supercilii muscle
   d. Superior laryngeal nerve
3. Which description represents a phase 2 block?
   a. Muscle fasciculation that precedes onset of neuromuscular blockade
   b. Absence of muscle fasciculation
   c. Sustained response to tetanic stimulation
   d. Absence of posttetanic potentiation, stimulation, or facilitation
4. Which is the definition of *clinical duration* in relation to neuromuscular blockade?
   a. Comparison of the size of the fourth twitch with the size of the first twitch
   b. Time from 25%–75% recovery of the twitch response
   c. Time from drug administration to 25% recovery of the twitch response
   d. TOF and double-burst fade
5. Which neuromuscular blocking medication is an aminosteroid compound?
   a. Succinylcholine
   b. Rocuronium
   c. Atracurium
   d. Mivacurium
6. Atracurium and cisatracurium are metabolized by
   a. hepatic extraction.
   b. plasma cholinesterase.
   c. Hoffman elimination.
   d. renal excretion.
7. Which neuromuscular blocking medication is contraindicated in a patient who is MH-susceptible?
   a. Succinylcholine
   b. Rocuronium
   c. Atracurium
   d. Mivacurium

Answers can be found in Appendix A.

BOX 2.8 Cardiac Effects of Neuromuscular Blocking Drugs

- Atracurium and mivacurium cause histamine release and may produce hypotension and tachycardia.
- Pancuronium is vagolytic and causes slight catecholamine release (indirect sympathomimetic), producing tachycardia.
- Repeat dosing in adults and any dose in children may produce sudden, abrupt bradycardia.

From Elisha S, Heiner JS, Nagelhout JJ. *Nurse Anesthesia*. 7th ed. Elsevier; 2023.

ANTICHOLINESTERASE AGENTS

Anesthetic Implications

- Anticholinesterase agents inhibit the effects of acetylcholinesterase, which is the enzyme that degrades acetylcholine. Increased concentrations of acetylcholine at the neuromuscular junction facilitate reversal of NMB. However, this mechanism causes cholinergic side effects in other organ systems (i.e., heart [bradycardia], lungs [bronchial constriction], and intestines [increased peristalsis]).
- The anticholinesterase agent neostigmine is the most commonly used nondepolarizing relaxant reversal agent because of its significant potency.
- It is coadministered with atropine or glycopyrrolate to minimize cholinergic side effects such as bradycardia, bronchoconstriction, increased oral secretions, and intestinal spasm.
- The onset of action of anticholinesterase agents is within several minutes, and bolus doses of an anticholinergic will cause tachycardia.

Neostigmine (Prostigmin)

- Reversal of NMB; myasthenia gravis
- Most commonly used anticholinesterase to reverse NMB because of its increased potency
- Reversal of NMB: slow IV: 0.05–0.07 mg/kg (maximum dose: 6 mg), with atropine (0.015 mg/kg) or glycopyrrolate (0.01 mg/kg). Myasthenia gravis: oral: 15–375 mg daily (three divided doses); IM/slow IV: 0.5–2 mg (dose must be individualized).
- Onset: reversal of NMB, onset 1 minute, peak effect 10 minutes, duration of action 30 minutes, dependent

TABLE 2.30 Summary of Select Properties of Neuromuscular Blocking Agents

Classification	ED95 (mg/kg)	Intubating Dose Usually 2–3 × ED95 (mg/kg)	Onset	Duration	Metabolism	ELIMINATION Kidney (%)	ELIMINATION Liver (%)	AUTOMATIC GANGLIA EFFECT (SNS and PNS)	CARDIAC MUSCARINIC EFFECT (Vagal Block)	Histamine Release	Resulting Cardiac Action
Ultrashort											
Succinylcholine (Anectine, Quelicin)	0.3	1–1.5	30–60 sec	5–10 min	Plasma cholinesterase	< 2%	0	Stimulates	Stimulates and/or blocks	0?	Usually tachycardia, bradycardia with repeat doses
Intermediate											
Atracurium (Tracrium)	0.15	0.5	2–4 min	30–60 min	Hofmann elimination, nonspecific esterase hydrolysis	10%–40% metabolites	0	0	0	Yes	Hypotension, tachycardia, flushing
Cisatracurium (Nimbex)	0.05	0.1	2–4 min	30–60 min	Hofmann elimination, nonspecific esterase hydrolysis	Up to 77% metabolites	0	0	0	0	0
Rocuronium (Zemuron)	0.3	1	1–3 min	30–60 min	Hepatic and renal	10%–30%	70%–90%	0	0	0	0
Vecuronium (Norcuron)	0.05	0.1	2–4 min	30–60 min	Hepatic and renal	40%–50%	50%–60%	0	0	0	0

PNS, Parasympathetic nervous system; *SNS*, sympathetic nervous system.
From Elisha S, Heiner JS, Nagelhout JJ. *Nurse Anesthesia*. 7th ed. Elsevier; 2023.

on dose and depth of blockade. Myasthenia gravis: IM: less than 20 minutes; oral: 45–75 minutes; duration of action 45–60 minutes.

- Adverse effects: bradycardia, tachycardia, atrioventricular (AV) block, nodal rhythm, hypotension, bronchospasm; respiratory depression; seizures; dysarthria; headaches; nausea, emesis, flatulence, increased peristalsis; urinary frequency; rash, urticaria, allergic reactions, anaphylaxis; increased oral, pharyngeal, and bronchial secretions
- Precautions and contraindications: caution in patients with bradycardia, asthma, epilepsy, cardiac arrhythmias, peptic ulcer, peritonitis, or mechanical obstruction of the intestines or urinary tract
- Excessive and or multiple doses of neostigmine may induce *cholinergic crisis*, characterized by nausea, vomiting, bradycardia or tachycardia, excessive salivation and sweating, bronchospasm, weakness, and paralysis; treatment includes discontinuation of neostigmine use and administration of atropine (10 mg/kg IV every 3–10 minutes until muscarinic symptoms disappear).
- Neostigmine may increase PONV.

Edrophonium (Tensilon)

- Indications: reversal of NMB; diagnostic assessment of myasthenia gravis
- Not recommended for reversal of profound NMB because of its lesser potency and shorter duration of action than neostigmine
- *Dose reversal of NMB:* IV: 0.5–1 mg/kg (maximum dose: 40 mg), with atropine (0.007–0.015 mg/kg), administered before the edrophonium because of rapid onset of action
- *Assessment of myasthenic/cholinergic crisis:* slow IV: 1 mg every 1–2 minutes until change in symptoms (maximum dose: 10 mg); IM: 10 mg
- *Onset:* IV: 30–60 seconds; IM: 2–10 minutes
- *Duration:* IV: 20 minutes; IM: 20–60 minutes
- Adverse effects: bradycardia, tachycardia, AV block, nodal rhythm, hypotension; increased oral, pharyngeal, bronchial secretions; bronchospasm; respiratory depression; seizures; miosis; visual changes; nausea/vomiting, increased peristalsis; rash, urticaria, allergic reactions, anaphylaxis.
- *Precautions and contraindications:* Edrophonium should be used with caution in patients with bradycardia, bronchial asthma, cardiac arrhythmias, peptic ulcer, peritonitis, or mechanical obstruction of the intestines or urinary tract.
- Excessive and/or repeated doses may induce a cholinergic crisis characterized by nausea, vomiting, bradycardia or tachycardia, excessive salivation and sweating, bronchospasm, weakness, and paralysis. Treatment involves discontinuation of edrophonium and administration of atropine, 10 mcg/kg IV every 10 minutes, until muscarinic symptoms disappear.
- Owing to the brief duration of action of edrophonium, neostigmine is generally preferred for reversal of the effects of nondepolarizing muscle relaxants.
- Administer with an anticholinergic to avoid cholinergic side effects (e.g., bronchoconstriction, bradycardia).
- Edrophonium is not recommended when deep block is present, owing to its short duration of action.

Physostigmine (Antilirium)

- *Indications:* reversal of prolonged somnolence and central anticholinergic syndrome
- Physostigmine is a tertiary amine compound (lipid soluble), and thus it is the only anticholinesterase agent that crosses the blood–brain barrier.
- *Dose:* IV/IM: 0.5–2 mg (10–20 mcg/kg) at rate of 1 mg/min; repeat dosing at intervals of 10–30 minutes.
- *Onset:* IV/IM: 3–8 minutes
- *Duration:* IV/IM: 30 minutes to 5 hours
- *Adverse effects:* bradycardia, bronchospasm, dyspnea, respiratory paralysis, seizures, salivation, nausea and vomiting, miosis
- *Precautions and contraindications:* High doses of physostigmine may cause tremors, ataxia, muscle fasciculations, and ultimately a depolarization block. Use it with caution in patients with epilepsy, parkinsonian syndrome, or bradycardia.
- Rapid IV administration may cause bradycardia and hypersalivation, leading to respiratory problems or possibly seizures.
- May cause cholinergic crises (increased acetylcholine within the brain has an excitatory effect), characterized by nausea, vomiting, bradycardia or tachycardia, excessive salivation and sweating, bronchospasm, weakness, and paralysis.
- Treatment of cholinergic crises includes mechanical ventilation and IV administration of atropine (anticholinergic), 10 mcg/kg every 10 minutes, until muscarinic symptoms decrease or until signs of atropine overdose (central anticholinergic syndrome) appear.

SELECTIVE MUSCLE RELAXANT BINDING AGENT

Selective Relaxant Binding Agents—Sugammadex

- Sugammadex (Bridion) is the first selective relaxant binding agent to be introduced as a reversal for clinical NMB.
- The name *sugammadex* is a combination of *sugar* and *gamma-cyclodextrin.*
- It is a modified gamma-cyclodextrin that works by encapsulating and forming very tight water-soluble complexes at a 1:1 ratio with steroidal neuromuscular blocking drugs. Once encapsulation occurs, it does not dissociate from the neuromuscular blocking compound, and the sugammadex-relaxant complex is excreted in the urine.
- Reversal occurs independent of the depth of neuromuscular blockade; therefore, even deep blockade can be reversed with the appropriate dose (Box 2.9).
- The concentration of free muscle relaxant falls rapidly, and muscle strength is rapidly reestablished (within 3 minutes).
- It is effective in reversing rocuronium, vecuronium, and pancuronium (aminosteroids), and it does not affect atracurium and cisatracurium (benzylisoquinolines).

BOX 2.9 Reversal of Neuromuscular Blockade: Considerations in Clinical Practice

Considerations When Return of Muscle Function Is Incomplete

- As with any reversal agent, the ability to counteract a nondepolarizing blocking agent depends on the amount of spontaneous recovery before the administration of a reversal drug.
- Has enough time been allowed for the anticholinesterase to antagonize the block (at least 15–30 min)?
- Is the neuromuscular blockade too intense to be antagonized?
- Even if recovery appears clinically adequate, a small dose of neostigmine may be prudent if the time since relaxant administration is less than 4 h.
- Has an adequate dose of antagonist been given?
- Are the other anesthetics and adjunctive agents contributing to patient weakness?
- Has metabolism or excretion of the relaxant been reduced by a possibly unrecognized process?
- Have acid–base and electrolyte status, temperature, age, drug interactions, and other factors that may prolong relaxant action been contemplated?
- The safest approach when any question about successful reversal remains is to provide proper sedation and controlled ventilation until adequate recovery is ensured.

From Elisha S, Heiner JS, Nagelhout JJ. *Nurse Anesthesia.* 7th ed. Elsevier; 2023.

Pharmacokinetics

- Sugammadex is biologically inactive and does not bind to plasma proteins or erythrocytes.
- The pharmacokinetics of sugammadex show a linear dose relationship in doses up to 8.0 mg/kg (Table 2.31).
- The elimination half-life is 2.3 hours.
- Up to 80% of an administered dose of sugammadex is eliminated in the urine within 24 hours.
- Because of the dependence on renal elimination, it should be used with caution in patients with renal disease and avoided in patients receiving dialysis.

Clinical Use

- The dosage range of sugammadex varies from 2 to 16 mg/kg according to the depth of blockade at the time of reversal.
- Monitoring for twitch responses to determine the timing and dose for sugammadex administration is essential.
- A dose of 2 mg/kg is recommended if spontaneous recovery has reached the reappearance of the second twitch in response to TOF stimulation.
- A dose of 4 mg/kg is recommended if spontaneous recovery of the twitch response has reached 1–2 posttetanic counts and there are no twitch responses to TOF stimulation.
- A dose of 16 mg/kg is recommended if there is a clinical need to reverse NMB soon (approximately 3 minutes) after administration of a single dose of 1.2 mg/kg of rocuronium.
- Suggested dosing strategy for reversal is given in Table 2.32.
- *Adverse reactions:* anaphylaxis (often occurring within 5 minutes after administration and is associated with the higher dosage ranges), bronchospasm, nausea/vomiting, hypertension, bleeding, and headache (Box 2.10)

TABLE 2.31 Commonly Used Anticholinesterase, Anticholinergic, and Select Relaxant Binding Agents

Agent	Dose Range	Onset (min)	Duration	Comments
Neostigmine	25–75 mcg/kg	5–15	45–90 min	Most commonly used reversal agent; may increase incidence of postoperative nausea and vomiting
Edrophonium	500–1000 mcg/kg	5–10	30–60 min	Not recommended for deep block; rapid onset, short duration
Atropine	15 mcg/kg	1–2	1–2 h	Should be combined with edrophonium because of more rapid onset
Glycopyrrolate	10–20 mcg/kg	2	2–4 h	Less initial tachycardia than atropine; no central nervous system effects; most frequently used
Sugammadex	2–16 mg/kg	1–2	2–16 h	Selective relaxant binding agent; up to 16 mg/kg has been safely used

From Elisha S, Heiner JS, Nagelhout JJ. *Nurse Anesthesia*. 7th ed. Elsevier; 2023.

TABLE 2.32 Strategies for Reversal of Neuromuscular Blockade

Type of Stimulus	Phase (Depth) of Neuromuscular Block	Reversal (Sugammadex Available)	Reversal (Sugammadex Unavailable)
Posttetanic count 50-Hz stimulus for 5 s followed by up to 20 single 1-Hz stimuli	Intense (count < 3) Deep (count > 3)	Sugammadex 4–16 mg/kg Sugammadex 4 mg/kg	Wait for train-of-four (TOF) count 4 Wait for TOF count 4
TOF count Four stimuli delivered every 0.5 s with 2-Hz frequency	Intermediate (TOF count 1–3) Recovery (TOF count 4) With fade Without fade	Sugammadex 2 mg/kg Neostigmine 50 mcg/kg Neostigmine 30 mcg/kg	Wait for TOF count 4 Neostigmine 50 mcg/kg Neostigmine 30 mcg/kg
TOF ratio Measurable using a quantitative monitor only, once the fourth twitch has returned on TOF stimulation	Recovery (TOF count 4) TOF ratio 0–0.8 TOF ratio > 0.9	Neostigmine 30–50 mcg/kg No reversal	Neostigmine 30–50 mcg/kg No reversal
Double-burst stimulus Two short-duration 50-Hz stimuli separated by 750-ms interval)	Recovery (TOF count 4) Fade (on second stimulus) No fade (on second stimulus)	Neostigmine 50 mcg/kg Neostigmine 30 mcg/kg	Neostigmine 50 mcg/kg Neostigmine 30 mcg/kg

- An increase in the coagulation parameters of activated partial thromboplastin time and prothrombin time/international normalized ratio (PT[INR]) of up to 25% for up to 1 hour following a 4-mg/kg dose has occurred.
- Patients using hormonal contraceptives must use an additional, nonhormonal method of contraception for the next 7 days after sugammadex administration because oral contraceptives are aminosteroid compounds that are also bound by sugammadex.

BOX 2.10 Adverse Effects of Residual Neuromuscular Block

Volunteer Studies

- Impairment of pharyngeal coordination and force of contraction
- Swallowing dysfunction/delayed initiation of the swallowing reflex
- Reductions in upper esophageal sphincter tone
- Increased risk of aspiration
- Impairment of upper airway dilator muscle function
- Decreased inspiratory airflow
- Upper airway obstruction
- Impaired hypoxic ventilatory drive
- Profound symptoms of muscle weakness (visual disturbances, severe facial weakness, difficulty speaking and drinking), generalized weakness

Clinical Studies in Surgical Patients

- Increased risk of postoperative hypoxemia
- Increased incidence of upper airway obstruction during transport to the postanesthesia care unit (PACU)
- Higher risk of critical respiratory events in the PACU
- Symptoms and signs of profound muscle weakness
- Delays in meeting PACU discharge criteria and achieving actual discharge
- Prolonged postoperative ventilatory weaning and increased intubation times (cardiac surgical patients)
- Increased risk of postoperative pulmonary complications (atelectasis or pneumonia)

From Murphy GS, Brull SJ. Residual neuromuscular block: lessons unlearned. Part I: definitions, incidence, and adverse physiologic effects of residual neuromuscular block. *Anesth Analg.* 2010;111(1):120–128; Brull SJ, Murphy GS. Residual neuromuscular block: lessons unlearned. Part II: methods to reduce the risk of residual weakness. *Anesth Analg.* 2010;111(1):129–140.

- If NMB needs to be reestablished after sugammadex administration, a benzylisoquinoline such as atracurium, mivacurium, or cisatracurium should be used.
- Succinylcholine is not affected by sugammadex.
- Recurarization is rare but has been reported.
- FDA approved for patients of all ages
- See Boxes 2.11 and 2.12 for common clinical signs of recovery and factors influencing the incidence of postoperative residual NMB.

KNOWLEDGE CHECK

1. Which is a side effect associated with anticholinesterase administration? (*Select all that apply.*)
   a. Bradycardia
   b. Cholinergic crises
   c. Bronchodilation
   d. Myocardial excitation
2. The mechanism of action associated with reversal of neuromuscular blockade with an anticholinesterase agent is
   a. decreased catecholamine secretion.
   b. increased acetylcholine at the neuromuscular junction.
   c. decreased muscarinic activity.
   d. increased release of serotonin.
3. Which anticholinesterase agent should *not* be used to reverse profound neuromuscular blockade?
   a. Neostigmine
   b. Sugammadex
   c. Edrophonium
   d. Physostigmine
4. Sugammadex antagonizes the effects of neuromuscular blockade from which agent? (*Select all that apply.*)
   a. Cisatracurium
   b. Vecuronium
   c. Succinylcholine
   d. Rocuronium
5. Patients should be counseled that sugammadex may reverse which prescription drug class?
   a. Statins
   b. Oral contraceptives
   c. Nonsteroidal antiinflammatory drugs
   d. Anticoagulants
6. Which is a side effect associated with sugammadex administration? (*Select all that apply.*)
   a. Anaphylaxis
   b. Hypertension
   c. Tachycardia
   d. Bronchospasm
   e. Bleeding

Answers can be found in Appendix A.

BOX 2.11 Common Clinical Signs of Recovery From Neuromuscular Blockers

- Adequate tidal volume and rate
- Respirations smooth and unlabored
- Opens eyes widely on command; no diplopia
- Sustained protrusion and purposeful movement of tongue
- Effective swallowing and sustained bite
- Able to sustain head or leg lift for at least 5 seconds (In small children, a strong knee-to-chest movement is equivalent.)
- Arm lift and touch the opposite shoulder
- Strong, constant hand grip
- Effective cough
- Adequate vital capacity of at least 15 mL/kg
- Adequate inspiratory force of at least 25–30 cm H_2O negative pressure
- Sustained tetanic response to 50 Hz for 5 seconds
- Train-of-four ratio greater than 0.9 without fade
- No fade to double-burst stimulation

From Elisha S, Heiner JS, Nagelhout JJ. *Nurse Anesthesia*. 7th ed. Elsevier; 2023.

BOX 2.12 Factors Influencing the Incidence of Postoperative Residual Neuromuscular Blockade

Definition of Residual Neuromuscular Blockade
- Objective train-of-four (TOF) measurements (TOF ratio less than 0.9)
- Clinical signs or symptoms of muscle weakness

Type and Dose of Neuromuscular Blocking Drug (NMBD) Administered Intraoperatively
- Intermediate-acting NMBD
- Long-acting NMBD
- Bolus versus infusion

Use of Neuromuscular Monitoring Intraoperatively
- Qualitative monitoring (TOF and double-burst stimulation studied)
- Quantitative monitoring (acceleromyography)

Degree of Neuromuscular Blockade Maintained Intraoperatively
- TOF count of 1–2
- TOF count of 2–3

Amount of Spontaneous Recovery at Time of Reversal
- The greater the extent of spontaneous recovery present, the more effective the reversal

Type of Anesthesia Used Intraoperatively
- Inhalation drugs
- Intravenous anesthesia (total intravenous anesthesia [TIVA])

Type and Dose of Reversal Drug
- Neostigmine 25–75 mcg/kg
- Edrophonium 500–1000 mcg/kg
- Sugammadex 2–16 mg/kg

Duration of Anesthesia

Time Interval Between Anticholinesterase Administration and Objective Monitoring
- TOF measurements

Patient Factors
- Metabolic derangements in the postanesthesia care unit (PACU; acidosis, hypercarbia, hypoxia, electrolyte imbalance, or hypothermia)
- Organ dysfunction, such as renal, hepatic, cardiac, or neuromuscular disease

Drug Therapy in PACU
- Aminoglycoside antibiotics
- Lithium
- Magnesium
- Local anesthetics

From Murphy GS, Brull SJ. Residual neuromuscular block: lessons unlearned. Part I: definitions, incidence, and adverse physiologic effects of residual neuromuscular block. *Anesth Analg.* 2010;111(1):120–128; Srivastava A, Hunter JM. Reversal of neuromuscular block. *Br J Anaesth.* 2009;103(1):115–129.

ANTICHOLINERGICS

Anesthetic Implications

- Glycopyrrolate is frequently the anticholinergic of choice during surgery and anesthesia because it does not pass the placental or blood–brain barrier.
- Anticholinergics are administered with neostigmine to prevent the muscarinic side effects (i.e., bradycardia, bronchial constriction).
- Anticholinergics that cross the blood–brain barrier, such as scopolamine, inhibit nausea and vomiting by inhibition of acetylcholine receptors in the

chemoreceptor trigger zone in the medulla and the vestibular apparatus.

Clinical Use

- Atropine, scopolamine, and glycopyrrolate are the three commonly used anticholinergics in anesthesia practice.
- These agents are competitive antagonists of acetylcholine at muscarinic receptors (Table 2.33).

Atropine

- Atropine, a belladonna alkaloid, is the prototype anticholinergic.
- Uses: antisialagogue, treatment of bradycardia, and concurrently administered with anticholinesterase agents in the reversal of muscle relaxants
- The typical adult IV dose for increasing heart rate during anesthesia is 0.4–0.6 mg.
- Atropine is a tertiary amine; this allows it to cross the blood–brain barrier freely, and it may result in transient bradycardia during onset when low doses are given.
- Hepatic metabolism accounts for approximately half of a dose of atropine, with the remainder being eliminated unchanged in the urine. The elimination half-life of atropine is approximately 4 hours.
- Atropine should be avoided in patients with narrow-angle glaucoma because it increases intraocular pressure.
- Atropine poisoning (central anticholinergic syndrome) or belladonna alkaloid toxicity manifests with extreme antimuscarinic effects, with potential progression to CNS depression and coma.
- The signs and symptoms associated with atropine poisoning include flushing (“red as a beet”), extreme mydriasis (“blind as a bat”), lack of secretions and dry mouth (“dry as a bone”), confusion (“mad as a hatter”), and hyperthermia (“hot as a hare”).
- Central anticholinergic syndrome (treatment: physostigmine, a.k.a. antilirium, 0.5–2 mg/kg)

Scopolamine

- Scopolamine (Isopto Hyoscine) is a tertiary amine resulting in sedation and amnesia.
- It produces greater sedation and amnesia and has greater antisialagogue and ocular effects than does atropine, with lesser effects on the heart, bronchial smooth muscle, and GI tract.
- Scopolamine is also used to diminish the incidence of PONV. A scopolamine patch (Transderm Scōp) containing a total dose of 1.5 mg is usually applied behind the ear. The patches have an onset of 4 hours and a duration of 3 days.
- For PONV, apply one patch at a minimum of 4 hours before surgery or 1 hour before cesarean section. Keep in place for 24 hours. Apply patch to hairless area behind the ear. Do not cut patch in half.
- Adverse effects: hallucinations, paradoxical bradycardia in low doses, mydriasis, blurred vision, tachycardia, drowsiness, restlessness, confusion, anaphylaxis, dry nose and mouth, constipation, urinary hesitancy, retention, increased intraocular pressure, decreased sweating
- Central anticholinergic syndrome (treatment: physostigmine, a.k.a. antilirium, 0.5–2 mg/kg)
- Children and elderly patients are more susceptible to adverse effects.

Glycopyrrolate

- Glycopyrrolate (Robinul) is a synthetic quaternary ammonium compound that prevents it from crossing

TABLE 2.33 Comparative Effects of Anticholinergic Drugs

Effect	Atropine	Scopolamine	Glycopyrrolate
Sedation	+	+++	0
Antisialagogue	+	+++	++
Increase heart rate	+++	+	++
Relax smooth muscle	++	+	++
Mydriasis, cycloplegia	+	+++	0
Prevent motion-induced nausea	+	+++	0
Decrease gastric hydrogen ion secretion	+	+	+

From Elisha S, Heiner JS, Nagelhout JJ. *Nurse Anesthesia.* 7th ed. Elsevier; 2023.

the blood–brain barrier to any significant degree; therefore, CNS effects are not seen.

- This property also makes it the agent of choice in obstetrics because it does not pass the placental barrier compared with atropine or scopolamine.
- Adult IV doses 0.1–0.2 mg for antisialagogue activity and for the treatment of bradycardia
- Onset of action is rapid, and the duration of action is up to 4 hours.
- Administered in combination with neostigmine for reversal of nondepolarizing NMB to minimize cholinergic effects

KNOWLEDGE CHECK

1. Which anticholinergic drug has the greatest antiemetic properties?
   a. Atropine
   b. Scopolamine
   c. Glycopyrrolate
   d. Tiotropium
2. Which anticholinergic drug does *not* have sedative properties?
   a. Atropine
   b. Scopolamine
   c. Glycopyrrolate
   d. Neostigmine
3. Which is a sign or symptom associated with central anticholinergic syndrome? (*Select all that apply.*)
   a. Mydriasis
   b. Excessive salivation
   c. Confusion
   d. Hyperthermia
   e. Bradycardia
4. The onset of action for a scopolamine patch used to prevent PONV is
   a. 1 hour.
   b. 2 hours.
   c. 3 hours.
   d. 4 hours.

Answers can be found in Appendix A.

AUTONOMIC NERVOUS SYSTEM—SYMPATHOMIMETIC AMINES

Anesthetic Implications

- The sympathomimetic amines include the three naturally occurring catecholamines epinephrine, norepinephrine, and dopamine and a number of synthetic agents, such as phenylephrine and dobutamine.
- These drugs are used for treating hypotension, bradycardia, anaphylaxis, shock, and heart failure and for cardiac resuscitation.
- The effects elicited by this pharmacologic class are the result of the stimulation of β-adrenergic, α-adrenergic, and dopamine adrenergic receptors.
- The innervation of the effector organs by the autonomic system is outlined in Table 2.34.
- The efficacy of sympathomimetic amines depends on their concentration at the receptor site, their affinity for specific receptors, and the population of receptors available for binding.
- The direct action of sympathomimetic amines occurs as a result of binding of the drug to an adrenergic receptor (e.g., phenylephrine).
- If a sympathomimetic amine has an indirect effect, the drug also stimulates the release of endogenous catecholamines (e.g., ephedrine).
- The effects of the common autonomic drugs are summarized in Table 2.35.

Epinephrine

- Epinephrine is a powerful agonist (stimulation) at α- and β-receptors (β_1- and β_2-receptors).
- The dominance of α or β effects is dose related.
- Epinephrine's stimulation of β_1 receptors produces marked positive inotropic (force of contraction), chronotropic (heart rate), and dromotropic (conduction velocity) actions.
- Left ventricular stroke work index, stroke volume, and cardiac output increase, causing myocardial oxygen consumption.
- Beneficial effects of β_2 stimulation include bronchodilation, vasodilation, and stabilization of mast cells, which decrease histamine release, especially during anaphylaxis. Thus epinephrine is the drug of choice to treat anaphylaxis.
- With low doses of epinephrine (10 mcg/min), the peripheral vasculature promotes the redistribution of blood flow to skeletal muscle, thereby producing a decrease in SVR.
- As the dose of epinephrine is increased, the α effect predominates, with resultant vasoconstriction and an increase in SVR.
- The increased α effect with greater doses of epinephrine also results in renal and splanchnic vasoconstriction.
- Beta 1 receptor stimulation leads to activation of the renin–angiotensin system (RAS)

TABLE 2.34 Typical Autonomic Influences on Peripheral Effector Organs

Organ System	Sympathetic Effect	Adrenergic Receptor Type	Parasympathetic Effect	Cholinergic Receptor Type
Eye				
Radial muscle, iris	Contraction (mydriasis)	α_1		
Sphincter muscle, iris			Contraction (miosis)	M_3, M_2
Ciliary muscle	Relaxation for far vision	β_2	Contraction for near vision (accommodation)	M_3, M_2
Heart				
Sinoatrial node	Increase in heart rate	β_1	Decrease in heart rate	M_2
Atria	Increase in contractility and conduction velocity	β_1	Decrease in contractility	M_2
Atrioventricular node	Increase in automaticity and conduction velocity	β_1	Decrease in conduction velocity; atrioventricular block	M_2
His-Purkinje system	Increase in automaticity and conduction velocity	β_1	Little effect	M_2
Ventricle	Increase in contractility, conduction velocity, automaticity	β_1	Slight decrease in contractility	M_2
Blood Vessels				
Arteries				
Coronary	Constriction; dilation	α; β_2	None	—
Skin and mucosa	Constriction	α_1; β_2	None	—
Skeletal muscle	Constriction; dilation	α_1; β_2	None	—
Cerebral	Constriction (slight)	α_1	None	—
Pulmonary	Constriction; dilation	α_1; β_2	None	—
Abdominal viscera	Constriction; dilation	α_1; β_2	None	—
Salivary glands	Constriction and reduced secretions	α_1; α_2	Dilation and increased secretions	M_3
Renal	Constriction; dilation	α_1, α_2; β_1, β_2	None	—
Veins	Constriction; dilation	α_1, α_2; β_2	None	—
Lung				
Tracheal and bronchial smooth muscle	Relaxation	β_2	Contraction	M_2, M_3
GI Tract				
Motility and tone	Decrease	α_1, α_2; β_1, β_2	Increase	M_2, M_3
Sphincters	Contraction	α_1	Relaxation	M_3, M_2
Secretion	Inhibition	α_2	Stimulation	M_3, M_2
Gallbladder and ducts	Relaxation	β_2	Contraction	M

Continued

TABLE 2.34 **Typical Autonomic Influences on Peripheral Effector Organs—cont'd**

Organ System	Sympathetic Effect	Adrenergic Receptor Type	Parasympathetic Effect	Cholinergic Receptor Type
Kidney				
Renin secretion	Increase	β_1	None	—
Urinary Bladder				
Detrusor	Relaxation	β_2, β_3	Contraction	M_3, M_2
Trigone and sphincter	Contraction	α_1	Relaxation	M_3, M_2
Uterus	Contraction (pregnant)	α_1	None	—
	Relaxation (pregnant and nonpregnant)	β_2		
Liver	Glycogenolysis and gluconeogenesis; increased blood sugar	α_1; β_2		
Pancreas				
Islets (β cells)	Decreased insulin secretion	α_2	None	—
	Increased insulin secretion	β_2	None	—
Adipocytes	Lipolysis	α_1; β_1, β_2, β_3	None	—

α, Alpha receptor; β, beta receptor; *GI*, gastrointestinal; *M*, muscarinic receptor.
From Elisha S, Heiner JS, Nagelhout JJ. *Nurse Anesthesia*. 7th ed. Elsevier; 2023.

- Increased beta 2 receptor stimulation results in lipolysis, glycogenolysis, and gluconeogenesis, which can result in ketone production and lactate release by skeletal muscle.
- Insulin secretion is inhibited by β_2 stimulation.
- Epinephrine-induced β_2 stimulation can also cause a transient hyperkalemia as potassium follows glucose out of hepatic cells.

Norepinephrine

- Norepinephrine is not as potent as epinephrine in stimulating α-receptors in equipotent doses, and it has minimal β_2 agonist activity at low doses.
- Increased SVR decreases peripheral perfusion; however, coronary artery perfusion may be increased as a result of diastolic pressure.
- Increased preload occurs because norepinephrine causes venoconstriction.
- Renal vascular resistance is increased, and urine output may decrease.
- Norepinephrine is often administered to patients with adequate cardiac output but low SVR.
- Intense norepinephrine-induced peripheral vasoconstriction decreases peripheral tissue perfusion/oxygenation even when adequate blood pressure has been achieved.

Dopamine

- Dopamine stimulates dopaminergic receptors, β-receptors, and α-receptors in a dose-dependent manner because of differing receptor affinities.
- Dopaminergic receptors are stimulated with low doses of less than 2 mcg/kg/min.
- At moderate doses of 2–10 mcg/kg/min, β effects are elicited, and α effects are seen with high infusion rates of greater than 10 mcg/kg/min.
- Dopamine also has an indirect sympathomimetic effect, eliciting the release of norepinephrine via β_1 stimulation.
- Dopamine inhibits aldosterone, resulting in increased sodium excretion and urine output.
- The monoamine oxidase enzymes metabolize dopamine; therefore, the effects of dopamine can be

TABLE 2.35 Effects of Autonomic Drugs

Organ Systems	α-Agonists	α-Blocker	β-Agonists	β-Blocker	Cholinergic Agonists	Anticholinergic
Eye	Mydriasis	Miosis (slight)	NCRE	↓ Intraocular pressure	Miosis, ↓ intraocular pressure	Mydriasis, cycloplegia, ↑ intraocular pressure
Heart						
Rate	Bradycardia (reflex)	Tachycardia (reflex)	Tachycardia	Bradycardia	Bradycardia	Tachycardia
Contractility	NCRE	Slight increase (reflex)	↑	↓	↓ (slight)	↑ (slight)
Conduction velocity	NCRE	NCRE	↑	↓	↓	↑
Blood (vessels)	Vasoconstriction	Vasodilation	Vasodilation	Vasoconstriction	NCRE	NCRE
Lungs	NCRE	NCRE	Bronchodilation	Bronchoconstriction	Bronchoconstriction	Bronchodilation (slight)
GI tract	↓ Motility and secretion	NCRE	↓ Motility and secretion	NCRE	↑ Motility and secretion	↓ Motility and secretion
Uterus	Contraction	NCRE	Relaxation	NCRE	NCRE	NCRE
Liver	↑ Blood sugar	NCRE	↑ Blood sugar	Hypoglycemia	NCRE	NCRE

↑, Increase; ↓, decrease; *GI,* gastrointestinal; *NCRE,* no clinically relevant effect.
From Elisha S, Heiner JS, Nagelhout JJ. *Nurse Anesthesia.* 7th ed. Elsevier; 2023.

prolonged in patients receiving a monoamine oxidase inhibitors (MAOIs). Tricyclic antidepressants (TCAs) may also augment the activity of sympathomimetic drugs.

Dobutamine

- Dobutamine's primary mechanism of action is as a β_1-agonist, and it has β_2-agonist effects.
- Dobutamine displays a strong inotropic response with minimal chronotropy.
- It produces a slight drop in SVR, owing to peripheral vasodilation from β_2 agonism.
- An increase in cardiac output compensates for the decrease in SVR, causing increased blood pressure.
- Pulmonary artery pressure decreases, and an increase in left ventricular stroke work index is observed.
- The positive inotropic effects, coupled with the reduced effects on chronotropy and maintenance of normal blood pressure, make dobutamine an option for treatment of cardiogenic and septic shock and in CHF.

Direct-Acting α-Agonist

Phenylephrine

- Phenylephrine has potent α-stimulating effects.
- An increase in blood pressure is produced as a result of a significant increase in peripheral vascular resistance secondary to the α_1 stimulation and venoconstriction that augments venous return.
- Reflex bradycardia occurs, caused by baroreceptor stimulation.
- The onset of action of IV phenylephrine resulting from a bolus dose of 50–100 mcg is within 30–60 seconds, and the duration of action ranges from 5 to 20 minutes.

Direct and Indirect α and β Agonists

Ephedrine

- Direct stimulation of α, β_1, and β_2 receptors results in increases in cardiac output, heart rate (β_1 effects), SVR = blood pressure (α_1 effects), and bronchodilation (β_2 effects).
- An indirect stimulatory effect causes the release of endogenous catecholamines, resulting in the same effects as described earlier. Tachyphylaxis may develop, and endogenous catecholamine stores become depleted.
- As a result of β_1 agonism, the increase in heart rate and myocardial oxygen consumption can be significant. As a result, ephedrine should be used with caution in patients who may have coronary artery disease.
- As a result of β_2 agonism, ephedrine causes bronchodilation and is indicated for patients who are hypotensive and exhibiting signs and symptoms associated with bronchospasm.
- The onset of action of IV ephedrine resulting from an IV bolus dose of 5–20 mg is 1–2 minutes, and the duration of action ranges from 15 minutes to 1.5 hours.

KNOWLEDGE CHECK

1. Which medication is most effective for the treatment of acute bronchospasm?
   a. Hydrocortisone
   b. Propofol
   c. Ephedrine
   d. Atropine
2. A 78-year-old patient is taking a preoperative β-blocker. Intraoperatively, his heart rate decreases from 58 to 52 beats/min, with blood pressure of 84/48 mm/Hg. Which vasopressor is relatively *contraindicated* in this patient?
   a. Epinephrine
   b. Vasopressin
   c. Isoproterenol
   d. Phenylephrine
3. Which adrenergic agonist would improve myocardial contractility without causing severe tachycardia?
   a. Norepinephrine
   b. Dobutamine
   c. Epinephrine
   d. Vasopressin
4. Which IV infusion dose of dopamine will primarily cause an increase in heart rate, impulse conduction velocity, and contractility?
   a. 1–2 mcg/kg/min
   b. 4–5 mcg/kg/min
   c. 10–11 mcg/kg/min
   d. 20–21 mcg/kg/min
5. Which describes the mechanism of action for indirect sympathomimetic activity?
   a. Directly stimulating adrenergic receptors
   b. Inducing endogenous catecholamine release
   c. Producing bronchoconstriction
   d. Inhibiting adrenergic receptors

Answers can be found in Appendix A.

Other Inotropic Agents

Vasopressin

- Arginine vasopressin, also known as *antidiuretic hormone*, is an endogenous hormone that is produced in the supraoptic nuclei within the hypothalamus.
- Its release is stimulated by an increased serum osmolality and hypovolemia.
- Vasopressin is a potent vasoconstrictor (agonist at V1 receptors); however, it selectively dilates renal afferent, pulmonary, and cerebral arterioles.
- Low-dose vasopressin infusion (0.03–0.04 units/min) increases blood pressure, urine output, and creatinine clearance and decreases the dosage of norepinephrine required to maintain blood pressure in patients with septic shock.
- Complications associated with vasopressin include GI ischemia, decreased cardiac output, skin or digital necrosis, and cardiac arrest (especially at doses greater than 0.04 units/min).
- See Tables 2.36 and 2.37 for vasopressor agents and doses of select drugs.

α-ADRENERGIC BLOCKING AGENTS

Anesthesia Implications

- Alpha-receptor antagonists have limited use in anesthesia.
- Phenoxybenzamine is used preoperatively in patients undergoing surgery for pheochromocytoma to control blood pressure.
- Patients may be receiving these agents preoperatively for benign prostatic hyperplasia (BPH) and hypertension.
- Patients with hypertension alone are rarely prescribed this class of drugs, owing to an unacceptable side-effect profile.
- Judicious use of fluids and induction agents can avoid hypotensive and tachycardic episodes during anesthesia induction.

α-Receptor Antagonists

- The α-receptor antagonists are used for treatment of hypertension, BPH, pheochromocytoma, Raynaud phenomenon, and ergot alkaloid toxicity.
- Common side effects include orthostatic hypotension and baroreceptor-mediated reflex tachycardia.

Phenoxybenzamine

- Phenoxybenzamine (Dibenzyline) has both α_1- and α_2-blocking activity.
- The α-receptors are noncompetitively, irreversibly bound by phenoxybenzamine, and its action is terminated only by metabolism of the drug and generation of new α-receptors.
- The preoperative course is started 1–3 weeks before surgery, with the oral dosage titrated up to 40–120 mg in two or three divided daily doses.
- Phenoxybenzamine also prevents the sympathomimetic response associated with phenylephrine administration.
- The primary side effect is orthostatic hypertension.
- The main clinical applicability related to phenoxybenzamine is preoperative blood pressure control for a patient with a pheochromocytoma.

Phentolamine

- Phentolamine is a competitive antagonist of α_1- and α_2-receptors.
- It has a rapid onset after IV administration and a much shorter duration of action than phenoxybenzamine.
- It can be used for the short-term control of hypertension in patients with pheochromocytoma.
- The recommended dose is 1–5 mg by slow IV push.
- Phentolamine has also been used in the treatment of inadvertent local infiltrations of vasoconstricting agents such as dopamine.
- Phentolamine (5–10 mg) can be mixed with 10 mL of normal saline and injected directly into the site of the infiltration.

Prazosin and Other α-Receptor Antagonists

- Prazosin (Minipress), doxazosin (Cardura), and terazosin (Hytrin) are selective α_1-antagonists used in the treatment of chronic hypertension.
- Their lack of α_2-blocking activity indicates that they have no effect on norepinephrine levels, and less norepinephrine-induced tachycardia results than when a nonselective α-antagonist is used.
- Prazosin induces vasodilation in both arterioles and veins and may cause orthostatic hypotension.
- Peripheral vascular resistance and cardiac preload and afterload are diminished.
- Tamsulosin (Flomax), alfuzosin (Uroxatral), and silodosin (Rapaflo) are α_1-selective antagonists that produce relaxation of the bladder neck and prostate and relieve obstructive urinary symptoms.

TABLE 2.36 Vasopressor Agents

		PERIPHERAL VASCULATURE		CARDIAC EFFECTS			
Agent	**Dose Range**	**Vasoconstriction**	**Vasodilation**	**Heart Rate**	**Contractility**	**Dysrhythmias**	**Typical Use**
Dopamine	1–4 mcg/kg per min	0	1+	1+	1+	1+	"Renal dose" does not improve renal function; may be used with bradycardia and hypotension
	5–10 mcg/kg per min	1–2+	1+	2+	2+	2+	
	11–20 mcg/kg per min	2–3+	1+	2+	2+	3+	Vasopressor range
Vasopressin	0.04–0.1 units/min	3–4+	0	0	0	1+	Septic shock, post–cardiopulmonary bypass shock state, no outcome benefit in sepsis
Phenylephrine	20–200 mcg/min	4+	0	Reflex bradycardia	0	1+	Vasodilatory shock, best for supraventricular tachycardia
Norepinephrine	1–20 mcg/min	4+	0	2+	2+	2+	First-line vasopressor for septic shock, vasodilatory shock
Epinephrine	1–20 mcg/min	4+	0	4+	4+	4+	Refractory shock, shock with bradycardia, anaphylactic shock
Dobutamine	1–20 mcg/kg/min	1+	2+	1–2+	3+	3+	Cardiogenic shock, septic shock
Milrinone	37.5–75 mcg/kg bolus followed by 0.375–0.75 mcg/min	0	2+	1+	3+	2+	Cardiogenic shock, right heart failure, dilates pulmonary artery; caution in renal failure

From Rivers EP. Approach to patient with shock. In Goldman L, Schafer AI. *Goldman's Cecil Medicine*. 25th ed. Elsevier; 2016.

TABLE 2.37 **Doses of Select Vasoactive Drugs**

Drug	Bolus Dose	Infusion Dose Rate	Comments
Calcium chloride ($CaCl_2$)	500–1000 mg (chloride) Slow IVP (over 5 minutes)		Onset: <1 min Peak effect: <1 min Duration: 10–20 min
Dobutamine (Dobutrex)	500–2000 mg	2–20 mcg/kg per min	Onset: 1–2 min Peak effect: 1–10 min Duration: 10 min
Dopamine		1–2 mcg/kg per min (renal doses) 2–10 mcg/kg per min (cardiac doses) 10–20 mcg/kg per min (vasopressor doses)	Onset: 2–4 min Peak effect: 2–10 min Duration: <10 min
Ephedrine	5- to 10-mg incremental doses		Dilute to 5 or 10 mg/mL Onset: <1 min Peak effect: 2–5 min Duration: 10–60 min
Epinephrine	10–100 mcg	0.01–0.03 mcg/kg/min (β doses) 0.03–0.15 mcg/kg per min (α and β doses) 0.15–0.3 mcg/kg per min (α doses)	Onset: <1 min Peak effect: 1–2 min Duration: 5–10 min
Fenoldopam		0.1–1.6 mg/kg per min	Onset: 4–5 min Peak effect: 7 min Duration: 15 min
Glucagon	1–5 mg over 2–5 min		
Isoproterenol (Isuprel)	1 mL over 1 min after diluting in 10 mL (= 0.02 mg/mL)	0.015–0.15 mcg/kg per min	Onset: <1 min Peak effect: 1 min Duration: 1–5 min
Milrinone (Primacor)	50 mcg/kg	0.375–0.75 mcg/kg per min	
Nesiritide (Natrecor)		0.01 mcg/kg per min	Onset: 15 min Peak effect: 1 h Duration: 60 min
Norepinephrine (Levophed)		0.01–0.2 mcg/kg per min	Onset: <1 min Peak effect: 1–2 min Duration: 2–10 min
Phentolamine	5 mg (50–100 mcg/kg); repeat as required	1–10 mcg/kg per min	Onset: 1–2 min Peak effect: 2 min Duration: 10–15 min
Phenylephrine (Neo-Synephrine)	40–100 mcg	0.15–0.75 mcg/kg per min	Onset: <1 min Peak effect: 1 min Duration: 15–20 min
Sodium nitroprusside (Nitropress)		0.1–10 mcg/kg per min	Onset: <1 min Peak effect: 1–2 min Duration: 1–10 min
Vasopressin (Pitressin)	10–20 units	0.1–1.0 units/min	Onset: 1–5 min Peak effect: 5 min Duration: 10–30 min

IVP, Intravenous push.
From Elisha S, Heiner JS, Nagelhout JJ. *Nurse Anesthesia*. 7th ed. Elsevier; 2023.

KNOWLEDGE CHECK

1. Which is the most common side effect associated with phenoxybenzamine?
   a. Orthostatic hypotension
   b. Laryngospasm
   c. Urinary retention
   d. Bronchospasm
2. Which medication can potentiate hypotension associated with general anesthesia?
   a. Vasopressin
   b. Milrinone
   c. Prazosin
   d. Calcium chloride

Answers can be found in Appendix A.

β-ADRENERGIC BLOCKING AGENTS

Anesthesia Implications

- Anesthesia implications can be found in Box 2.13.

Clinical Use

- Indications for the use of β-blockers include the treatment of angina pectoris, hypertension, post–myocardial infarction therapy, supraventricular tachycardia (i.e., Wolff-Parkinson-White syndrome, atrial fibrillation), increased sympathetic activity (e.g., as occurs with intubation), hypertrophic obstructive cardiomyopathies and CHF, and migraine headaches; preoperative preparation of patients with hyperthyroidism; and in digitalis-induced arrhythmias.
- Mechanism of action: competitive binding of β-receptors and preventing the actions of catecholamines and other β-agonists. β_1 blockade causes a decrease in myocardial oxygen demand and increased myocardial oxygen supply.
- β-Blockers are subdivided on the basis of their selectivity for cardiac β_1-receptors and other notable clinical differences, such as their ability to vasodilate by additional mechanisms or whether they have partial agonist activity.
- Table 2.38 lists the β-blockers according to subtype.
- Some of the β-blockers act as partial agonists and, as such, possess intrinsic sympathomimetic activity (ISA).
- A partial agonist does not stimulate β-receptors to the extent that a full agonist does, and in the presence of a full agonist, the partial agonist acts as a competitive antagonist.
- It follows that β-blockers with ISA competitively antagonize the effects of a full agonist (e.g., endogenous catecholamines released during times of maximal sympathetic tone).
- ISA minimizes the risk of bronchoconstriction in patients with reactive airway disease who require β-blockade.
- Pindolol, acebutolol, and penbutolol are β-adrenergic blocking agents that possess ISA.
- Side effects associated with β-blockers include bronchospasm, CHF, peripheral vasoconstriction, hyperkalemia, bradycardia, and hypotension, and they may mask signs of physiologic stress (i.e., absence of tachycardia associated with hypoglycemia).
- Selective β1 receptor blockers (i.e., esmolol) can induce β_2-receptor blockade, especially when administered as a bolus dose.
- Patients receiving β-blockers should continue their regimen throughout the perioperative period.
- β-Blockers should be instituted in patients with multiple cardiac risk factors, known ischemic heart disease, or myocardial ischemia.
- The American Heart Association/American College of Cardiology (ACC/AHA) guidelines recommend starting β-blocker therapy if indicated >7 days before surgery and anesthesia.

BOX 2.13 Anesthesia Implications of β-Adrenergic Blocking Agents

- β-Blockers should be continued in patients undergoing surgery who have been receiving β-blockers chronically.
- It is reasonable for the management of β-blockers after surgery to be guided by clinical circumstances, independent of when the agent was started.
- In patients with three or more revised cardiac risk index (RCRI) risk factors (e.g., diabetes, heart failure, coronary artery disease, renal insufficiency, cerebrovascular accident), it is necessary to begin β-blockers before surgery.
- β-Blocker therapy should not be started on the day of surgery.

Adapted from Thompson A. 2024 AHA/ACC/ACS/ASNC/HRS/SCA/SCCT/SCMR/SVM Guideline for Perioperative Cardiovascular Management for Noncardiac Surgery: a report of the American College of Cardiology/American Heart Association Joint Committee on Clinical Practice Guidelines. *J Am Coll Cardiol.* 2024;84(19):1869–1969.

TABLE 2.38 β-Adrenergic Drugs

Drug	Daily Adult Maintenance Dosage	Frequent or Severe Adverse Effects
β-Adrenergic Blocking Drugs		
Atenolol (Tenormin)	25–100 mg in one or two doses	Fatigue; depression; bradycardia; decreased exercise tolerance; congestive heart failure; aggravate peripheral arterial insufficiency; aggravate allergic reactions; bronchospasm; mask symptoms of and delay in recovery from hypoglycemia; Raynaud phenomenon; insomnia; vivid dreams or hallucinations; acute mental disorder; impotence; increased serum triglycerides
Betaxolol generic	5–40 mg in one dose	
Bisoprolol (Zebeta)	5–20 mg in one dose	
Metoprolol (Lopressor, Toprol-XL)	50–200 mg in one or two doses Extended release 25–400 mg once	
Nadolol (Corgard)	20–320 mg in one dose	
Propranolol (Inderal)	40–240 mg in two doses	
Timolol generic	10–60 mg in two doses	
β-Adrenergic Blocking Drugs With Intrinsic Sympathomimetic Activity		
Acebutolol (Sectral)	200–1200 mg in one or two doses	Similar to other β-adrenergic blocking drugs but with less resting bradycardia and fewer lipid changes; acebutolol has been associated with positive antinuclear antibody test and occasional drug-induced lupus
Penbutolol (Levatol)	10–80 mg in one dose	
Pindolol generic	10–60 mg in two doses	
α- and β-Blockers		
Carvedilol (Coreg)	12.5–50 mg in two doses	Similar to other β-adrenergic blocking drugs, but more orthostatic hypotension; no effect on serum lipids
Labetalol generic	200–1200 mg in two doses	
β-Blocker With Vasodilating Nitric Oxide–Mediated Activity		
Nebivolol (Bystolic)	5–40 mg once	Vasodilator due to nitric oxide–mediated action

From Drugs for hypertension. *Med Lett Drugs Ther.* 2017;59(1516):41–48.

Anesthetic Uses

Esmolol

- Rapid onset: 1 minute
- Short duration of action: elimination half-life of approximately 9 minutes
- Clinical duration of action: 10–15 minutes
- Recommended IV loading dose of esmolol is 500 mcg/kg.
- Infusion rate of 100–300 mcg/kg/min
- IV bolus doses of 10–20 mg may be given and titrated to patient response.
- Esmolol is metabolized by nonspecific plasma esterase found in red blood cells (RBCs).

Metoprolol

- Uses: post–myocardial infarction, angina, and hypertension
- Administration of 5-mg doses IV at 5-minute intervals to a maximum dose of 15 mg is recommended.

Labetalol

- Classified as a nonselective β-blocker that possesses an α-blocking component
- Labetalol provides β-blockade along with α-blockade in a ratio of 7:1.
- IV bolus dose of labetalol is 0.1–0.2 mg/kg, infusion rate 2 mg/min.

- In clinical practice, a bolus dose of labetalol (5–10 mg) is titrated and repeated on the basis of patient response.
- Duration of action is dose dependent, typically 2–6 hours.
- Because of its α-blocking effects, it is recommended for hypertensive episodes in obstetric patients. Uterine blood flow is unaffected.
- Labetalol undergoes hepatic metabolism and renal elimination.

KNOWLEDGE CHECK

1. Which β-blocker can decrease SVR?
   a. Esmolol
   b. Pindolol
   c. Labetalol
   d. Metoprolol
2. Which is a side effect associated with β-blockers? (*Select all that apply.*)
   a. Bronchospasm
   b. CHF
   c. Hyperkalemia
   d. Hyperglycemia
   e. Renal failure
3. Which is true regarding β-blocking medications? (*Select all that apply.*)
   a. Should be started the morning of surgery
   b. Must be continued perioperatively in patients on chronic therapy
   c. Should be administered only when the heart rate exceeds 90 beats/min
   d. Can induce a bronchospasm
4. Esmolol has a rapid elimination half-life as a result of
   a. hepatic degradation.
   b. pseudocholinesterase.
   c. hepatic elimination.
   d. RBC esterase.

Answers can be found in Appendix A.

BRONCHODILATORS

Anesthesia Implications

Selective β_2-Agonists

- Inhaled β_2-agonists include albuterol (Proventil, Ventolin, others), levalbuterol (Xopenex), pirbuterol (Maxair), and salmeterol (Serevent).
- These "selective" β_2-agonists are effective in treating obstructive airway diseases such as asthma, chronic obstructive pulmonary disease, and acute bronchospasm.
- Long-acting formulations include formoterol (Foradil) and salmeterol (Serevent).
- Because of their β_2 receptor selectivity, the result is bronchodilation and a lower incidence of tachycardia and arrhythmia from β_1-receptor agonism.
- None of these agents is completely β_2 selective.
- These agents are available in aerosol form, which is as effective as subcutaneous administration.
- Chronic use of these agents can result in tachyphylaxis secondary to receptor downregulation (i.e., diminished quantity).
- Some bronchodilation agents are listed in Table 2.39.

KNOWLEDGE CHECK

1. Tachycardia can occur from administration of inhaled albuterol as a result of ____ stimulation.
   a. β_1
   b. β_2
   c. α_1
   d. α_2
2. Tachyphylaxis can occur from the chronic use of β_2 agonists as a result of
   a. depletion of CNS catecholamine stores.
   b. adrenergic receptor downregulation.
   c. conjugation with glucuronic acid.
   d. decreased intracellular calcium.

Answers can be found in Appendix A.

CALCIUM CHANNEL BLOCKERS

Anesthetic Implications

- Calcium channel blockers (CCBs) are commonly prescribed for cardiovascular and cerebrovascular disorders.
- Side effects include hypotension, bradycardia, heart block, and reflexive tachycardia.

Clinical Uses

- The calcium channel antagonists/CCBs are used to treat angina, hypertension, arrhythmias, peripheral vascular disease, cerebral and coronary artery vasospasm, and esophageal spasm.
- There are three chemical classes of CCBs: 1,4-dihydropyridine derivatives, such as nifedipine (Adalat, Procardia); benzothiazepine derivatives, such as diltiazem (Cardizem), and phenylalkylamine derivatives, such as verapamil (Calan, Isoptin).

TABLE 2.39 FDA-Approved Drugs for COPD

Drug	Delivery Device	Usual Adult Dosage
Inhaled Short-Acting Anticholinergic		
Ipratropium		
Atrovent HFA (Boehringer Ingelheim)	HFA MDI (200 inhalations/unit)	2 inhalations qid PRN
Generic: single-dose vials	Nebulizer	500 mcg qid PRN
Inhaled Short-Acting β_2-Agonist/Short-Acting Anticholinergic Combination		
Albuterol/ipratropium		
Combivent (Boehringer Ingelheim)	CFC MDI (200 inhalations/unit)	2 inhalations qid PRN
Combivent respimat (Boehringer Ingelheim)	MDI (130 inhalations/unit)	1 inhalation qid PRN
DuoNeb(dey) generic	Nebulizer	2.5–9.5 mg qid PRN
Inhaled Long-Acting β_2-Agnoists		
Indacaterol—Arcapta Neohaler (Novartis)	DPI (30 inhalations/unit)	75 mcg qd
Salmeterol—Serevent Diskus (GSK)	DPI (60 inhalations/unit)	50 mcg bid
Formoterol—Foradil Aerolizer (Merk)	DPI (60 inhalations/unit)	12 mcg bid
Perforomist (Dey)	Nebulizer	20 mcg bid
Arformoterol—Brovana (Sunovion)	Nebulizer	15 mcg bid
Inhaled Long-Acting Anticholinergics		
Tiotropium—Spiriva HandiHaler (Boehringer Ingelheim)	DPI (60 inhalations/unit)	18 mcg qd
Aclidinium—Tudorza Pressair (Forest)	DPI (60 inhalations/unit)	400 mcg bid

CFC, Chlorofluorocarbon; *COPD*, chronic obstructive pulmonary disease; *DPI*, dry powder inhaler; *FDA*, US Food and Drug Administration; *MDI*, metered-dose inhaler.
From Elisha S, Heiner JS, Nagelhout JJ. *Nurse Anesthesia*. 7th ed. Elsevier; 2023.

Mechanism of Action

- Depolarization of the sinoatrial and AV nodes is dependent on the inward flux of calcium during the depolarization phases of the cardiac action potential. Calcium channel antagonists "block" these channels, diminishing the inward flux of calcium and prolonging phase 2, and in this way, they exert a negative chronotropic effect on the heart. Ventricular pacemaker foci are dependent on the inward flux of sodium, which is minimally affected by the calcium antagonists. Calcium antagonists are effective in patients with atrial tachyarrhythmias. This negative inotropic effect then leads to a decrease in myocardial oxygen consumption.
- Calcium channel antagonists produce relaxation of vascular smooth muscle, resulting in vasodilation. Systemic vasodilation of both arteries and veins results in a decreased preload and afterload, which contributes to an increase in cardiac output and a decrease in myocardial work and oxygen consumption.
- Varying degrees of AV block, myocardial depression, and hypotension are associated with the use of CCBs. An additive effect should be anticipated if the calcium channel antagonists are used with other cardiac depressant agents, such as anesthetics.
- All CCBs have negative inotropic and chronotropic actions. CCBs depress electrical impulses in the sinoatrial (SA) and AV nodes and produce coronary and systemic vasodilation.
- The CCBs help prevent angina resulting from spasm of the coronary arteries, such as Prinzmetal angina.
- Nimodipine is used to treat cerebral vasospasm associated with neurologic emergencies such as a ruptured cerebral aneurysm and neurosurgical procedures.

TABLE 2.40 **Calcium Channel Blocker Drugs**

Drug	Daily Adult Maintenance Dosage	Frequent or Severe Adverse Effects
Diltiazem (Cardizem CD)	120–360 mg in one dose	Dizziness; headache; edema; constipation (especially verapamil); AV block; bradycardia; heart failure; lupus-like rash
Diltiazem (Tiazac)	120–540 mg in one dose	
Verapamil (Calan)	120–480 mg in one or two doses	
Verapamil (Calan SR)	120–480 mg in one or two doses	
Verapamil (Isoptin SR)	120–480 mg in one or two doses	
Verapamil (Verelan)	120–480 mg in one dose	
Verapamil (Covera-HS)	180–540 mg in one dose	

AV, Atrioventricular.
From Drugs for hypertension. *Med Lett Drugs Ther.* 2017;59(1516):41–48.

KNOWLEDGE CHECK

1. Which are mechanisms by which CCBs exert their effect on the heart? (*Select all that apply.*)
   a. Inhibition of calcium entering myocytes
   b. Enhancement of potassium transport in exiting myocytes
   c. Enhancing phase 1 depolarization
   d. Inhibition of phase 2 depolarization
2. Clevidipine is rapidly metabolized by
   a. acetylcholinesterase.
   b. nonspecific esterases.
   c. combining to hepatocytes.
   d. oxidation.
3. Which cardiovascular effects are associated with CCBs? (*Select all that apply.*)
   a. Increased stroke volume
   b. Decreased rate of cardiac conduction
   c. Tachycardia
   d. Decreased SVR
4. CCBs are indicated to inhibit (*Select all that apply.*)
   a. cerebral artery vasospasm (nimodipine).
   b. atrial tachyarrhythmias.
   c. venous stasis.
   d. thromboembolism.

Answers can be found in Appendix A.

- Verapamil 2.5–10 mg IV (dose can be repeated every 30 minutes) can be given for the treatment of atrial tachyarrhythmias. The onset time is approximately 10 minutes, and the duration of action ranges from 2 to 4 hours. Verapamil is metabolized hepatically, has an elimination half-life of 4–7 hours, and is renally eliminated.
- Clevidipine (Cleviprex) is a dihydropyridine L-type CCB indicated as an IV antihypertensive. It is highly selective for vascular muscle and, unlike other CCBs, does not affect myocardial contractility or conduction. Its antihypertensive effect is largely due to arterial vasodilation. Clevidipine is rapidly metabolized by nonspecific esterases in the blood. The terminal half-life is approximately 15 minutes. It is formulated as a lipid emulsion, and aseptic technique for administration is essential. The starting dose is 1–2 mg/h, titrated up to 16 mg/h or less according to patient response. Time onset is 2–4 minutes, and duration is 5–15 minutes (Table 2.40).

ANTIHYPERTENSIVE AGENTS

Anesthetic Implications

- There is no clear evidence to support deferring surgery or for acute management of blood pressure in patients presenting with moderate hypertension without significant cardiac comorbidities (Table 2.41).
- Severe hypertension (>180/110 mm Hg) should be controlled before elective surgery.

Hypertension

- Hypertension is the most common condition seen in primary care, and it can lead to myocardial infarction, stroke, renal failure, and death if not detected early and treated appropriately.
- The main classes of drugs used to treat hypertension include diuretics, CCBs, angiotensin-converting enzyme inhibitors (ACEIs), angiotensin receptor blockers (ARBs), and β-receptor blockers.

TABLE 2.41 2018 High Blood Pressure Clinical Practice Guidelines

Categories of BP in Adults[a]	SBP		DBP
Normal	<120 mm Hg	and	<80 mm Hg
Elevated	120–129 mm Hg	and	<80 mm Hg
Hypertension			
Stage 1	130–139 mm Hg	or	80–89 mm Hg
Stage 2	≥140 mm Hg	or	≥90 mm Hg

BP, Blood pressure; *DBP,* diastolic blood pressure; *SBP,* systolic blood pressure.
[a]Individuals with SBP and DBP in two categories should be designated to the higher BP category. BP is based on an average of at least two careful readings obtained on two or more occasions.
From Jones D, Ferdinand KC, Taler SJ, et al. 2025 AHA/ACC/AANP/AAPA/ABC/ACCP/ACPM/AGS/AMA/ASPC/NMA/PCNA/SGIM guideline for the prevention, detection, evaluation and management of high blood pressure in adults: a report of the American College of Cardiology/American Heart Association. *J Circulation.* 2025;152:11.

- Hypertensive episodes during the perioperative period occur most often during emergence from anesthesia and may be associated with pain, airway stimulation, hypoxia-hypercarbia, hypothermia and shivering, bladder distention, withdrawal from preoperative medications, and intraoperative use of vasopressors.
- Drugs useful for the treatment of perioperative hypertension are listed in Table 2.42.

Centrally Acting α_2-Agonists

Clonidine

- Clonidine (Catapres) is a presynaptic α_2-agonist.
- It decreases blood pressure by acting as an agonist at peripheral presynaptic α_2-receptors and central α_2-receptors.
- Stimulation of the peripheral presynaptic α_2-receptors causes inhibition of catecholamine release, with subsequent vasodilation.
- Stimulation of the central α_2-receptors, which is considered the main antihypertensive mechanism of action, results in diminished sympathetic outflow and a resultant decrease in circulating catecholamines and renin activity.
- Continuing the medication throughout the perioperative period is essential.
- Clonidine is available in oral, transdermal, and epidural forms.
- Additional uses of clonidine include sedation, as an analgesic combined with opiates for epidural treatment of severe pain (Duraclon), and in suppression of alcohol withdrawal symptoms.

Dexmedetomidine (Precedex)

- Dexmedetomidine is a potent selective adrenergic α_2-agonist.
- Its specificity for α_2-receptors versus α_1-receptors is 1620:1, compared with clonidine's specificity of 220:1.
- Dexmedetomidine provides dose-dependent sedation, analgesia, sympatholysis, and anxiolysis without causing significant respiratory depression via central α_2-receptor agonism.
- Side effects include hypertension (increased incidence with initial and large doses), hypotension, bradycardia, excessive sedation, and delayed recovery.
- Elimination half-life is 2 hours, primarily via hepatic metabolism and renal excretion.

Angiotensin-Converting Enzyme Inhibitors

- ACEIs are widely prescribed for the treatment of hypertension, angina, diabetic neuropathy, and CHF and in the management of a myocardial infarction.
- These drugs exert their action by inhibiting angiotensin-converting enzyme (ACE).
- Renin, a proteolytic protein, is released from the juxtaglomerular apparatus in the kidney in response to diminished blood pressure.
- Renin is responsible for the conversion of precursor angiotensinogen, which is released from the liver, to angiotensin I. Angiotensin I is then converted to angiotensin II by the ACE.
- ACE is primarily located in the endothelial tissue of the lung.

TABLE 2.42 Parenteral Drugs for Treatment of Severe Hypertension

Drug	Class	Route and Dose	Onset	Duration	Comments
Fenoldopam (Corlopam)	Dopamine-1 receptor agonist	IV infusion pump: 0.1–1.6 mcg/kg per min	4–5 min	< 10 min	May cause reflex tachycardia; may increase intraocular pressure
Labetalol (Trandate Normodyne)	α- and β-Adrenergic blocker	IV: 20 mg initially, then 40–80 mg every 10 min (300 mg max)	5 min or less	3–6 h	Not for patients with bronchospasm, congestive heart failure, first-degree heart block, cardiogenic shock, or severe bradycardia
Nicardipine (Cardene IV)	Calcium channel blocker	IV: 5 mg/h, increased by 2.5 mg/h every 15 min up to 15 mg/h	1–5 min	3–6 h	May cause reflex tachycardia
Clevidipine (Cleviprex)	Calcium channel blocker	IV infusion: 1–2 mg/h initially; double the dose at 90-s intervals until desired results are achieved (16 mg/h max)	2–4 min	5–15 min	Rapidly degraded by tissue and blood esterases; contraindicated with allergy to soy or eggs; may cause reflex tachycardia
Nitroglycerin	Venous arteriolar vasodilator	IV infusion pump: 5–100 mcg/min	2–5 min	5–10 min	Headache, tachycardia can occur; tolerance may develop with prolonged use
Sodium nitroprusside	Arteriolar and venous vasodilator	IV infusion pump: 0.3–10 mcg/kg per min	Seconds	3–5 min	Thiocyanate or cyanide toxicity with prolonged or too rapid infusion
Esmolol	β-Blocker	IV: 500 mcg/kg per min for 1 min titrated to effect, usually 50 mcg/kg per min	1–2 min	5–10 min	Cardioselective; however, use with caution in patients with asthma
Labetalol	Combined α- and β-blocker	5–80-mg bolus titrated to effect; 2 mg/min infusion	1–2 min	3–6 min	Generally used in 5–10-mg incremental doses titrated to effect in the perioperative period

Adapted from Victor RG. Arterial hypertension. In: Goldman L, Schafer AI, eds. *Goldman's Cecil Medicine*. 25th ed. Elsevier; 2016; Victor RG, Libby P. Systemic hypertension: management. In: Mann DL, Zipes DP, Libby P, eds. *Braunwald's Heart Disease*. 10th ed. Elsevier; 2015; van den Born BJ, Beutler JJ, Gaillard CAJM, et al. Dutch guideline for the management of hypertensive crisis—2010 revision. *Neth J Med*. 2011;69(5):248–255.

- Angiotensin II is a potent vasopressor that also stimulates the release of endogenous norepinephrine and aldosterone. Higher aldosterone levels result in increased sodium and water reabsorption, with concomitant secretion of potassium.
- ACEIs block this action and produce vasodilation.
- ACEIs are renally excreted.
- Adverse effects include cough, angioedema, renal failure, hyperkalemia, neutropenia, and proteinuria.
- If an ACEI cannot be tolerated, an ARB is substituted.
- ACE is also responsible for the metabolism of bradykinin, which is blocked by these drugs. The resulting increase in bradykinin is felt to contribute to the cough.

Angiotensin 2 Receptor Antagonists

- ARBs are a class of drugs useful for the treatment of hypertension and CHF.
- Their pharmacologic actions are similar to those of the ACEIs, but their mechanism of action is competitive blockade of type 1 angiotensin II receptors.
- They are effective for lowering blood pressure without causing the side effects, such as cough and angioedema, that are associated with ACEIs.

Anesthesia Management of Patients Taking Angiotensin Axis Blockers

- Consider withholding ACEIs and ARBs the morning of surgery to minimize the potential for refractory hypotension.
- These medications should be restarted postoperatively unless hypotension exists.
- *Vasoplegic syndrome* (VS) is defined as unexpected refractory hypotension under general anesthesia with a mean arterial pressure < 50 mm Hg, a cardiac index > 2.5 L/min/m^2, and low SVR despite adrenergic vasopressor administration.
- The incidence of VS in cardiac surgery patients is 8%–10% but may increase to upwards of 50% of patients taking ACEIs/ARBs.
- The proposed mechanism involves selective depression of the three blood pressure support systems: the sympathetic nervous system, the renin–angiotensin system (RAS), and the vasopressin system.
- ACEIs and ARBs inhibit the RAS, leaving only vasopressin to maintain blood pressure.
- Other mechanisms for developing refractory hypotension include cytokine- and nitric oxide–mediated smooth muscle relaxation, catecholamine receptor downregulation, cell hyperpolarization, and endothelial injury.
- Treatment of VS includes decreasing the anesthetic agent, volume expansion, phenylephrine, ephedrine, glycopyrrolate, norepinephrine, epinephrine, and dopamine.
- Vasopressin, 0.5–1.0-unit bolus, may be given, followed by an infusion dose of 0.03 units/min for vasopressin.
- Methylene blue can be used as a bolus dose of 1–2 mg/kg over 10–20 minutes, followed by an infusion of 0.25 mg/kg/h for 48–72 hours, with a maximum dose of 7 mg/kg.
- Methylene blue interferes with the nitric oxide (NO)/cyclic guanosine monophosphate (cGMP) pathway, inhibiting the vasodilating effect on smooth muscle.

VASODILATORS

Nitrovasodilators

Sodium Nitroprusside

- Sodium nitroprusside is frequently used for the emergent control of hypertension, for inducing hypotension to decrease blood loss during surgical procedures, and for the treatment of acute cardiac disorders.
- Its rapid onset (within seconds) and its short duration of action (1–3 min) make it unique among agents for the rapid control of blood pressure.
- Sodium nitroprusside reduces both afterload and preload, which results in a decrease in cardiac filling pressures and an increase in stroke volume and cardiac output.
- The maximum recommended infusion rate is 10 mcg/kg/min.
- Sodium nitroprusside has the potential to cause cyanide toxicity; when more than 500 mcg/kg is administered faster than 2 mcg/kg/min, cyanide is generated faster than it can be eliminated.
- Signs of cyanide toxicity include metabolic acidosis, increased mixed venous oxygen content, tachycardia, and tachyphylaxis.
- Treatment of cyanide toxicity includes the following:
  - Discontinuing the sodium nitroprusside infusion
  - Administering oxygen
  - Treating metabolic acidosis
  - Methylene blue 1–2 mg/kg
  - Sodium nitrite 3%, 4–6 mg/kg, can be administered over 3–5 minutes.
  - Sodium thiosulfate, 150–200 mg/kg over 15 minutes, can be administered every 2 hours.
  - Vitamin B_{12} can also be administered.
  - Hydroxocobalamin administration

Nitroglycerin

- Nitroglycerin is used to treat angina pectoris and ischemia and can be used to lower blood pressure.
- Nitroglycerin causes venodilation, with an increase in venous capacitance and a resultant decrease in preload.
- This results in a lowering of cardiac filling pressures, a lessening of myocardial wall tension, and ultimately, a decrease in myocardial oxygen requirements.
- Nitroglycerin's primary mechanism of action in the relief of angina is a decrease in preload (myocardial oxygen demand factor).
- Use of sublingual nitroglycerin, up to a total of three tablets, is the most efficient treatment for acute angina.
- Relief is generally achieved in 1–2 minutes and lasts up to 30 minutes.
- IV nitroglycerin also has an onset time of 1–2 minutes and duration of action of up to 10 minutes.

- Nitroglycerin is extensively metabolized in the liver and has a half-life of only 3 minutes.
- IV nitroglycerin is used for "unloading" of the heart in CHF and myocardial infarction.

Hydralazine

- Hydralazine causes direct relaxation of arterial smooth muscle.
- It can be administered IV for the control of hypertension in doses ranging from 2.5 to 20 mg.
- Tachycardia frequently accompanies the decrease in blood pressure secondary to the baroreceptor response from a reduction in afterload.
- The onset of action can occur from 2 to 20 minutes after administration; therefore, adequate time should be allowed before the initiation of repeat dosing so that profound decreases in blood pressure can be prevented. However, there is a synergistic vasodilatory effect with concomitant administration of anesthetic agents. Thus, the hypotensive effects occur more rapidly, and the dose should be titrated incrementally to response to avoid hypotension.
- The elimination half-life in plasma is approximately 1 hour, but the duration of vasodilating action is 12 hours.
- Hydralazine is used to treat hypertensive episodes during pregnancy.

Inhaled Nitric Oxide

- Indications for use:
  - *Children:* Acute or chronic pulmonary hypertension associated with persistent pulmonary hypertension of newborn, meconium aspiration, and congenital diaphragmatic hernia
  - *Adults:* Acute or pulmonary hypertension associated with acute respiratory distress syndrome, pulmonary embolism, placement of a left ventricular assist device, and cardiac surgery
- Inhaled NO activates guanylate cyclase in lung vessels and airways and increases levels of cGMP, causing selective pulmonary vasodilation.
- Rapid onset and avid binding with RBCs
- Hemoglobin inactivates NO and thereby prevents systemic vasodilation.
- NO is metabolized to nitrate and excreted in urine.
- Inhaled NO is mixed with O_2-containing gas immediately before administration via intratracheal catheter, ventilator, mask, or nasal prongs.
- NO is a free radical with a short half-life in aqueous solutions (~17 seconds).
- The usual inhaled NO dose is 1–40 ppm by volume.
- Precautions:
  - Methemoglobinemia (especially breathing >80 ppm NO) monitoring is recommended.
  - Measure inhaled NO and nitrogen dioxide (NO_2) levels continuously.
  - Do not give if NO_2 levels are high (>2 ppm).
  - High inhaled NO levels may inhibit platelet aggregation.
  - Rebound pulmonary hypertension during acute NO withdrawal
  - Contraindicated in severe heart failure (e.g., pulmonary capillary wedge pressure [PCWP] > 25 mm Hg) or with pulmonary venous disease (e.g., pulmonary vein stenosis, pulmonary veno-occlusive disease).
- See Table 2.42 for parenteral drugs used to treat severe hypertension.

KNOWLEDGE CHECK

1. Which is the mechanism of action by which dexmedetomidine produces sedation?
   a. Central α_2-receptor agonism
   b. Peripheral α_2-receptor agonism
   c. Central α_2-receptor antagonism
   d. Peripheral α_1-receptor antagonism
2. Which side effect can occur with dexmedetomidine administration?
   a. Blurred vision
   b. Hypertension
   c. Tachycardia
   d. Hyponatremia
3. Which is a side effect associated with high-dose nitroprusside infusion?
   a. Porphyria
   b. Diffusion hypoxia
   c. Increased afterload
   d. Cyanide toxicity
4. Which is true regarding preoperative management of ACEIs and ARBs?
   a. Half of the usual dose should be taken 1 day before surgery.
   b. Hold the medication 24 hours before surgery.

KNOWLEDGE CHECK—cont'd

c. Continue the medication throughout the perioperative period.
d. Discontinue the medication and administer IV metoprolol preoperatively.

5. Which is an intervention used to treat VS? (*Select all that apply.*)
   a. Epinephrine
   b. Methylene blue
   c. Nitroglycerin
   d. Dobutamine
   e. Vasopressin
6. Which medication is used to treat cyanide toxicity? (*Select all that apply.*)
   a. Indigo carmine
   b. Methylene blue
   c. Sodium nitrite
   d. Sodium nitroprusside
   e. Sodium thiosulfate
7. The primary mechanism by which nitroglycerin decreases myocardial oxygen demand and angina is by decreasing
   a. afterload.
   b. cardiac contractility.
   c. preload.
   d. heart rate.
8. Which is true regarding the indication for the use of nitric oxide?
   a. Esophageal hiatus
   b. Left ventricular failure
   c. Potentiate the effects of inhalation agents
   d. Pulmonary hypertension
9. Hydralazine increases the heart rate via the
   a. chemoreceptor response.
   b. baroreceptor response.
   c. Cushing response.
   d. trigeminovagal response.
10. Which is the drug of choice for treatment of acute angina?
    a. Nitroglycerin
    b. β-blockers
    c. ACEIs
    d. ARBs
11. Which is a side effect associated with ACEIs?
    a. Hypertension
    b. Angina
    c. CHF
    d. Cough

Answers can be found in Appendix A.

ANTIARRHYTHMICS

Anesthetic Implications

- Patients receiving drug therapy for arrhythmias should have their medication continued throughout the perioperative period.
- Common antiarrhythmic drug side effects, such as heart block or prolonged ECG segment intervals, may be exacerbated by anesthetic agents.
- The goal of drug therapy for arrhythmias should be to treat immediate hemodynamic problems and prevent progression of serious arrhythmias.
- Treatment is similar to that in the nonoperative setting, with the caveat that most therapies should be carefully titrated to avoid unexpected proarrhythmic or excessive hypotensive outcomes.

Causes of Intraoperative Rhythm Disturbances

General Factors

- Advanced age
- Catecholamines release from physiologic stress
- Left atrial enlargement
- Heightened adrenergic state
- Drug toxicity (proarrhythmic)
- Hypoxia
- Hypovolemia
- Hemodynamic instability
- Reperfusion after cessation of bypass
- Hypertension
- Hypoglycemia or hyperglycemia
- Pulmonary disease
- β-Blocker withdrawal

Structural Heart Disease

- Coronary artery disease
- Myocardial infarction
- Valvular and congenital heart disease
- Cardiomyopathy
- Sick sinus or prolonged QT interval syndrome
- Wolff-Parkinson-White syndrome
- Heart disease secondary to systemic disease (e.g., uremia, diabetes)
- Sinus bradycardia
- Atrioventricular (AV) node heart block

TABLE 2.43 **Drugs Used to Treat Perioperative Arrhythmias**

Drug	Dosing	Indications	Side Effects
Adenosine	6 mg, then 12 mg rapid IVP	Paroxysmal SVT: diagnosis of wide or narrow QRS tachycardias	Transient heart block, flushing, chest pain
Atropine	0.4–1 mg IV	Bradycardia or AV block	Excessive tachycardia: myocardial ischemia
Diltiazem	10–20-mg IV bolus, then infusion at 5–15 mg/h	Heart rate control	Hypotension; CHF
Esmolol	0.5-mg/kg bolus and infusion at 0.05 mg/kg/h ↑ by 0.05 mg/kg/h q 5 min	Rapid heart rate control	Bronchospasm; hypotension, exacerbation of CHF
Metoprolol	5 mg IV q 5 min 3 ×	Heart rate control	Bronchospasm; hypotension, exacerbation of CHF
Ibutilide	1 mg IV over 10 min May repeat once	Conversion of AF	QT prolongation; torsades de pointes
Amiodarone	150 mg IV over 10 min, then 1 mg/min × 6 h, then 0.5 mg/min	Refractory VF or VT; rate control and conversion of AF	Occasional mild hypotension with bolus; heart block

AF, Atrial fibrillation; *CHF,* congestive heart failure; *SVT,* supraventricular tachycardia; *VF, ventricular fibrillation*; *VT,* ventricular tachycardia.
From Heintz KM, Hollenberg SM. Perioperative cardiac issues: postoperative arrhythmias. *Surg Clin North Am.* 2005;85(6):1103–1114.

Transient Imbalance

- Stress: electrolyte or metabolic imbalance
- Laryngoscopy, hypoxia, hypercarbia, superior/recurrent nerve stimulation
- Device malfunction, microshock
- Diagnostic or therapeutic intervention (pacemakers, cardioverter-defibrillators)
- Surgical stimulation
- Central vascular catheters
- Hypocarbia

Perioperative Management

- The incidence of serious arrhythmias during general anesthesia is low, possibly because of the myocardial depressant effects of anesthetic medications.
- New pharmacologic and nonpharmacologic management (e.g., implantable cardiac devices) and cardiac ablation therapy approaches for cardiac arrhythmias have emerged.
- The use of antiarrhythmic drugs in the United States is declining because of the increasing use of ablation therapy and implantable devices.
- Some cautionary statements should precede any discussion on the use of antiarrhythmic agents during anesthesia:
  - The cause of the arrhythmia should be explored before any treatment is instituted.
  - A cardiology consult should be obtained when necessary.
  - Adequacy of ventilation, depth of anesthesia, acid–base balance, and fluid and electrolyte balance must be verified before appropriate therapy can be formulated.
  - See Table 2.43 for a list of postoperative arrhythmic drugs.

DIGITALIS

Anesthetic Implications

- Digitalis is used for inotropic support in heart failure and to slow the rate in atrial tachyarrhythmias.
- Its use as both an antiarrhythmic and an inotrope has decreased significantly with the introduction of more efficacious and safer drugs.
- For patients taking digitalis preoperatively, it should be continued throughout the perioperative period.
- Cardiac arrhythmias (toxicity) can be precipitated by hypokalemia, hypomagnesemia, hypoxia, hypercalcemia, hypernatremia, and renal failure.
- AV block can occur with coadministration of β-adrenergic or calcium channel–blocking drugs.
- The dosing has a narrow therapeutic index (0.8–2 ng/mL or 1.2–2 nmol/L).

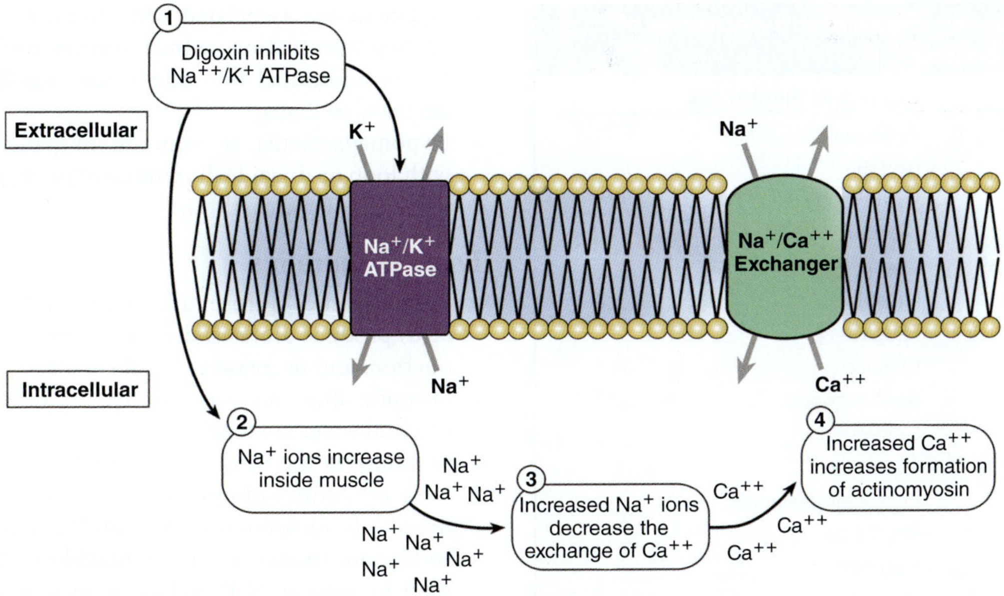

Fig. 2.3 The mechanism of action of digitalis. *(1)* The sodium-potassium ATPase is inhibited, resulting in increased intracellular sodium; *(2)* increased intracellular sodium produces a decrease in the exchange of sodium and calcium; *(3)* intracellular calcium increases; and *(4)* muscle contraction is enhanced. (From Elisha S, Heiner JS, Nagelhout JJ. *Nurse Anesthesia.* 7th ed. Elsevier; 2023.)

Mechanism of Action

- The primary inotropic effect of digitalis is achieved by binding to the α-subunit of the sodium-potassium adenosine triphosphatase (Na^+/K^+-ATPase) in cardiac cells. This results in an increase in the concentration of intracellular calcium during systole, which augments myocardial contractility. Normally, the Na^+/K^+-ATPase exchanges intracellular sodium for extracellular potassium against their concentration gradients. Inhibition of this exchange results in an increase in intracellular sodium that results in decreased calcium exchange and higher intracellular calcium.
- The mechanism of action of digitalis is shown in Fig. 2.3.
- The additional calcium enhances contraction. Digitalis produces an increase in both diastolic filling and ejection fraction.
- Enhanced vagal tone results in slowing of the heart rate and prolongation of AV conduction. Thus, digitalis is also used to control the ventricular response to atrial fibrillation and other atrial tachyarrhythmias.
- The digitalis-induced enhancement of vagal tone leads to slowing of impulse conduction through the AV node and prolongation of the effective refractory period of the AV node.
- Treatment for digitalis toxicity is symptomatic and includes discontinuing digoxin, obtaining laboratory tests for electrolytes and digitalis level, and treating the arrhythmias and GI symptoms as needed (Table 2.44).

KNOWLEDGE CHECK

1. Which electrolyte abnormality precipitates digoxin toxicity? (*Select all that apply.*)
   a. Hypokalemia
   b. Hypocalcemia
   c. Hyponatremia
   d. Hypomagnesemia
2. Which hemodynamic factor is directly increased by digitalis? (*Select all that apply.*)
   a. Ejection fraction
   b. Central venous pressure
   c. Diastolic filling
   d. Afterload
3. The mechanism of action of digitalis glycosides is inhibition of
   a. phosphodiesterase 3.
   b. cAMP release.
   c. cGMP release.
   d. Na^+/K^+-ATPase.

Answers can be found in Appendix A.

TABLE 2.44 Signs and Symptoms of Digitalis Toxicity

System	Signs and Symptoms
Gastrointestinal	Anorexia
	Nausea
	Vomiting
	Diarrhea
	Abdominal cramps
Neurologic	Headache
	Fatigue
	Malaise
	Restlessness
	Confusion
	Insomnia
	Personality changes
	Psychosis
	Neuralgia
	Convulsions
	Coma
Visual	Color-shaded vision (e.g., green, yellow, purple)
	Halo vision
	Flickering lights
	White borders on dark objects or dots
Cardiac	Every known cardiac arrhythmia has occurred secondary to digitalis toxicity, including bradycardia or tachycardia, premature ventricular contractions, bigeminy and trigeminy, paroxysmal atrial tachycardia with or without block, heart block (all types), atrial fibrillation, atrial flutter, ventricular tachycardia, ventricular fibrillation.

DIURETICS

Anesthetic Implications

- Diuretics are prescribed for patients with hypertension, heart failure, elevated ICP, edema, hemoglobinuria, low intraoperative urine output, hyperkalemia, volume overload, and rhabdomyolysis.
- Patients receiving diuretics during the preoperative period should be considered volume-depleted, and the degree of hypotension produced during anesthesia may be exaggerated.
- Hypokalemia associated with diuresis is worsened by hyperventilation, which further lowers serum K^+ an additional 0.5 mEq/L for each 10-mm Hg decrease in $Paco_2$.
- Hypomagnesemia is common in patients treated with loop or thiazide diuretics and predisposes them to ventricular arrhythmias.

Types of Diuretics

- Loop diuretics (furosemide, bumetanide, ethacrynic acid) produce diuresis, decrease the rate of CSF production, and decrease cerebral edema.
- Osmotic diuretics are effective in decreasing the cerebral water content.
- Mannitol is the most widely used osmotic diuretic for acute control of intracranial hypertension.
- Rapid administration of mannitol may produce vasodilation, an increase in cerebral blood flow, a transient increase in ICP, and an increase in circulating blood volume.
- The typically prescribed dose of mannitol is 0.25–1 g/kg.
- Decreases in ICP begin shortly after mannitol administration and may continue for up to 6 hours.
- Continued use of mannitol may produce volume depletion, causing hypotension, hyperosmolality, and electrolyte imbalance, which may be attenuated with concurrent administration of a loop diuretic.

Hypertension

- Thiazide-type diuretics are used for initial treatment of patients with hypertension (Table 2.45).
- Loop diuretics such as furosemide are used instead of thiazides to lower blood pressure in patients with moderate to severe renal impairment.
- Ethacrynic acid can be used for patients allergic to sulfonamides. (Thiazide and loop diuretics other than ethacrynic acid contain sulfonamide moieties.)
- Potassium-sparing diuretics (i.e., amiloride and triamterene) are used in conjunction with other diuretics to prevent or correct hypokalemia. These drugs cause hyperkalemia in patients with renal impairment and those taking ACEIs, ARBs, and β-blockers.
- Spironolactone, a mineralocorticoid receptor antagonist also used as a potassium-sparing diuretic, has been effective for patients with refractory hypertension.
- Both spironolactone and eplerenone have been shown to reduce the risk of death in patients with heart failure when added to standard therapy.

TABLE 2.45 **Diuretic Drugs**

Drug	Daily Adult Maintenance Dosage	Frequent or Severe Adverse Effects
Chlorothiazide (Diuril)	125–500 mg once	Hyperuricemia; hypokalemia; hypomagnesemia; hyperglycemia; hyponatremia; hypercholesterolemia; hypertriglyceridemia; pancreatitis; rashes and other allergic reactions; sexual dysfunction; photosensitivity reactions; may decrease excretion of lithium
Hydrochlorothiazide (Microzide)	12.5–50 mg once	
Chlorthalidone (Thalitone)	12.5–50 mg once	
Indapamide, generic	1.25–5 mg once	
Metolazone (Zaroxolyn)	1.25–5 mg once	
Loop Diuretics		
Bumetanide generic	0.5–2 mg in two doses	Dehydration; circulatory collapse; hypokalemia; hyponatremia; hypomagnesemia; hyperglycemia; metabolic alkalosis; hyperuricemia; blood dyscrasias; rashes; lipid changes as with thiazide-type diuretics
Ethacrynic acid (Edecrin)	25–100 mg in two or three doses	
Furosemide (Lasix)	20–320 mg in two doses	
Torsemide (Demadex)	5–20 mg in one or two doses	
Potassium-Sparing Diuretics		
Amiloride (Midamor)	5–10 mg in one or two doses	Hyperkalemia; GI disturbances; rash; headache
Triamterene (Dyrenium)	50–150 mg in one or two doses	Hyperkalemia; GI disturbances; nephrolithiasis
Aldosterone Antagonists		
Spironolactone (Aldactone)	12.5–100 mg in one or two doses	Hyperkalemia; hyponatremia; mastodynia; gynecomastia; menstrual abnormalities; GI disturbances; rash
Eplerenone (Inspra)	25–100 mg in one or two doses	Hyperkalemia; hypernatremia

GI, Gastrointestinal.
From Medical Letter Treatment Guidelines: Drugs for hypertension. *Treat Guidel Med Lett.* 2014;12(141):31–38.

KNOWLEDGE CHECK

1. Mannitol can transiently increase intracranial pressure by (*Select all that apply.*)
   a. increasing blood volume.
   b. increasing cardiac contractility.
   c. decreasing venous return.
   d. increasing cerebral blood flow.
2. Which abnormality is associated with most diuretic agents? (*Select all that apply.*)
   a. Hyperkalemia
   b. Hyponatremia
   c. Hyperglycemia
   d. Hypermagnesemia

Answers can be found in Appendix A.

NONSTEROIDAL ANTIINFLAMMATORY AGENTS

Anesthesia Implications

- Administered for their analgesic, antiinflammatory, and antipyretic properties (Fig. 2.4)
- A component of multimodal analgesia protocols
- Preoperative, intraoperative, and postoperative information, along with information on regional anesthesia, can be found in Box 2.14.
- The commonly used oral nonsteroidal antiinflammatory drugs (NSAIDs) are listed in Table 2.46.

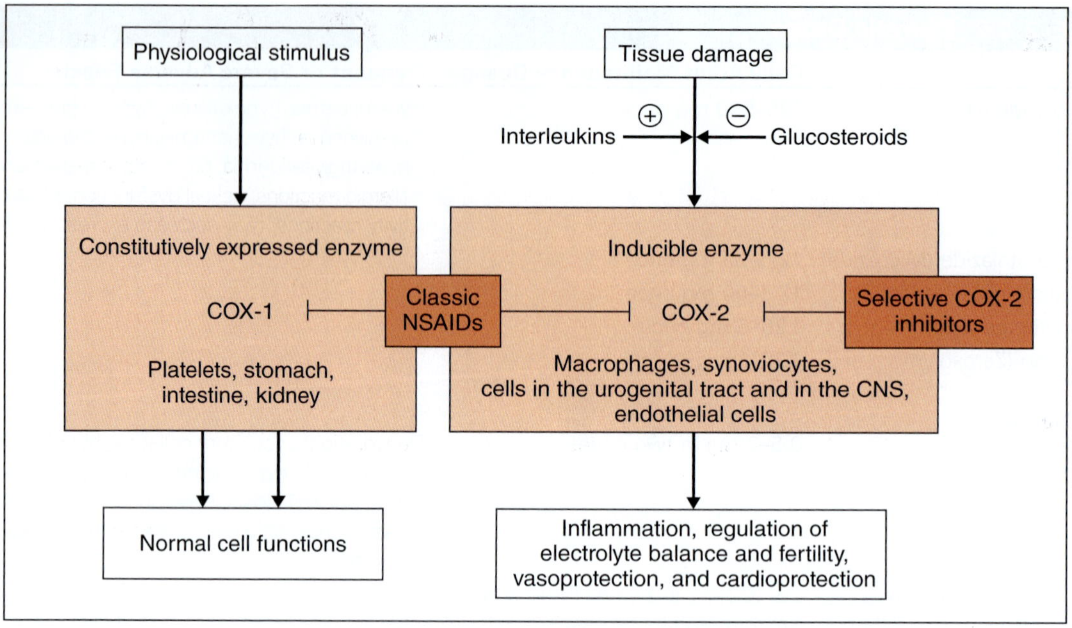

Fig. 2.4 Simplified description of the physiological and pathophysiological roles of cyclooxygenase (COX)-1 and COX-2. COX-1 is expressed constitutively in most tissues and fulfills housekeeping functions by producing prostaglandins. COX-2 is an inducible isoenzyme that is expressed in inflammatory cells (e.g., macrophages and synoviocytes) after exposure to proinflammatory cytokines and is downregulated by glucocorticoids. In the kidney (macula densa) and other areas of the urogenital tract and in the central nervous system (CNS), COX-2 is already significantly expressed even in the absence of inflammation. Induction of expression of COX-2 in peripheral and CNS tissues appears to be most prominent in connection with inflammatory painful reactions. Both enzymes are blocked by classic acidic antipyretic analgesics (nonsteroidal antiinflammatory drugs [NSAIDs]). (From McMahon S, et al. *Wall and Melzack's Textbook of Pain*. 6th ed. Elsevier; 2013.)

BOX 2.14 Perioperative Concerns Associated With NSAIDs

Preoperative Concerns

- Nonselective NSAID use has been associated with increased intraoperative blood loss due to platelet inhibition.
- NSAID platelet inhibition is reversible; common practice is to hold the NSAID for a period of five half-lives before surgery (e.g., ibuprofen 1 d, naproxen 5 d).
- Celecoxib, a COX-2-specific inhibitor, does not affect platelet function and therefore does not need to be held.

Regional Anesthesia

- According to the consensus guidelines of the American Society of Regional Anesthesia (ASRA), NSAIDs do not significantly increase the risk for spinal hematoma during neuraxial anesthesia.
- NSAIDs increase the risk of bleeding if combined with other anticoagulant/antiplatelet medications or if there is coexisting coagulopathy.
- Use of NSAIDs alone should not interfere with the performance of neuraxial blocks or the timing of neuraxial catheter removal.

Intraoperative Concerns

- May exacerbate asthma, especially in patients with a history of NSAID-induced bronchospasm, angioedema, chronic renal failure, urticaria, or rhinitis.

Postoperative Period

- The risk of adverse effects on renal function is the same for both nonselective NSAIDs and COX-2 inhibitors.

BOX 2.14 Perioperative Concerns Associated with NSAIDs—cont'd

- For patients with normal renal function, transient reduction in renal function with acute postoperative NSAID administration is usually clinically insignificant (normal function restored 2–7 d after stopping NSAID treatment).
- Caution when initiating therapy in patients with preexisting heart/kidney disease, use of loop diuretics, or loss of blood volume > 10%
- Both nonselective NSAIDs and celecoxib have been implicated in inhibition of bone healing.

COX-2, Cyclooxygenase-2; *NSAID,* nonsteroidal antiinflammatory drug.
Adapted from Fleisher LA, Roizen MF, Roizen J. *Essence of Anesthesia Practice.* 4th ed. Elsevier; 2018.

TABLE 2.46 Commonly Used Oral Nonsteroidal Antiinflammatory Drugs

Generic Name	Trade Name	Adult Dosage
Acetaminophen	Tylenol	500–1000 mg q 4 h
Acetylsalicylic acid	Aspirin	325–650 mg q 4 h
Celecoxib	Celebrex	200 mg q 12 h
Choline magnesium trisalicylate	Trilisate	500–750 mg q 8–12 h
Diclofenac sodium	Voltaren	25–75 mg q 8–12 h
Diflunisal	Dolobid	250–500 mg q 8–12 h
Etodolic acid	Lodine	200–400 mg q 6 h
Fenoprofen calcium	Nalfon	200 mg q 4–6 h
Flurbiprofen	Ansaid	100 mg q 8–12 h
Ibuprofen	Motrin	400–800 mg q 6–8 h
Indomethacin	Indocin	25–50 mg q 8–12 h
Ketoprofen	Orudis	25–75 mg q 6–8 h
Ketorolac	Toradol	10 mg q 6–8 h
Meclofenamate sodium	Meclomen	50 mg q 4–6 h
Meloxicam	Mobic	7.5–15 mg qd PRN
Naproxen	Naprosyn	275–500 mg q 8–12 h
Phenylbutazone	Butazolidin	100 mg q 6–8 h
Piroxicam	Feldene	10–20 mg once daily
Salsalate	Disalcid	500 mg q 4 h
Sulindac	Clinoril	150–200 mg q 12 h
Tolmetin	Tolectin	200–600 mg q 8 h

From Daroff RB, Jankovic J, Mazziotta JC, et al. *Bradley's Neurology in Clinical Practice.* 7th ed. Elsevier; 2016.

Clinical Uses

- NSAIDs and acetaminophen are used to decrease postoperative pain and have an opioid-sparing effect.
- Three NSAIDs are available in IV formulations and thus are used perioperatively. NSAIDs commonly used by anesthetists include ketorolac (Toradol), meloxicam (Mobic), and acetaminophen (Ofirmev).
- The mechanism of NSAIDs and acetaminophen is inhibition of the cyclooxygenase enzymes, which prevents the production of prostaglandins and thromboxane.
- Acetaminophen also possesses analgesic and antipyretic properties.

Ketorolac

- Ketorolac (Toradol) is an NSAID that can be administered via both IM and IV routes.
- The primary advantages are the low incidence of nausea and vomiting and lack of respiratory and CNS depression.
- Relative contraindications include asthma, renal or GI dysfunction, and bleeding disorders.

- It is effective at relieving shoulder tip pain associated with laparoscopic surgery.

Indications

- Short-term (less than 5 days) management of moderately severe acute pain that requires analgesia
- Ketorolac therapy should not exceed 5 days because of the potential for increased frequency and severity of adverse reactions (renal dysfunction, bleeding, inhibition of bone formation).
- Oral ketorolac is indicated only for continuation therapy after IV/IM ketorolac.

Dose

- IM: patients younger than 65 years: one dose of 60 mg; patients older than 65 years, renally impaired, and/or less than 50 kg: one dose of 30 mg
- IV: patients younger than 65 years: one dose of 30 mg; patients older than 65 years, renally impaired, and/or less than 50 kg: one dose of 15 mg
- Multiple-dose treatment (IV or subcutaneous): patients younger than 65 years: 30 mg every 6 hours, not to exceed 120 mg/d
- Patients older than 65 years, renally impaired, and/or less than 50 kg: 15 mg every 6 hours, not to exceed 60 mg/d
- Onset: IV/IM: 15–30 minutes. Peak effect: 1–2 hours
- Duration: 4–6 hours

Acetaminophen (Ofirmev)

- Acetaminophen (Ofirmev) is available as an IV analgesic and antipyretic drug for use in both adults and children over 2 years old.
- Acetaminophen does not exhibit the significant GI and cardiovascular side effects associated with NSAIDs.
- Hepatotoxicity is uncommon with doses less than 4000 mg/d.
- The recommended dose of Ofirmev for patients ≥12 years old weighing ≥50 kg is 1000 mg every 6 hours or 650 mg every 4 hours IV; the maximum daily dose of acetaminophen by any route is 4000 mg.
- For patients ≥2 years old weighing <50 kg, the recommended dose is 15 mg/kg every 6 hours or 12.5 mg/kg every 4 hours IV.
- Onset: 5–15 minutes; duration: 4–6 hours

Precautions and Contraindications

- Avoid acetaminophen in patients with liver disease.
- Overdose can cause serious or fatal hepatic injury, particularly in patients who are fasting.
- Hepatic toxicity after acetaminophen overdose can be treated with *N*-acetylcysteine.

Meloxicam (MOBIC)

- Used as a component part of preemptive analgesia
- Increased cyclooxygenase (COX)-2 selectivity, which inhibits inflammation and pain but preserves COX-1 prostaglandin functions (renal vascular tone, normal bronchial tone, and platelet function)
- Dose: 7.5 to 15 mg qd as needed
- Onset: 1–2 hours; duration: 10–24 hours

Precautions and Contraindications

- Use caution in asthma (bronchial), CHF, hypertension, fluid retention, renal impairment, stomatitis, and history of GI ulcers.
- Fluid retention and edema are observed in some patients treated with NSAIDs; use of meloxicam may blunt cardiovascular effects of several therapeutic agents used to treat these medical conditions (e.g., diuretics, ACEIs, or ARBs).
- Avoid use in patients with severe heart failure unless benefits are expected to outweigh risk of worsening heart failure; if meloxicam is used in patients with

KNOWLEDGE CHECK

1. Meloxicam should be used with caution in patients with (*Select all that apply.*)
   a. severe heart failure.
   b. autoimmune disease.
   c. renal dysfunction.
   d. acute myocardial ischemia.
2. Acetaminophen (Ofirmev) is contraindicated in patients with
   a. chronic obstructive pulmonary disease.
   b. hepatic disease.
   c. renal disease.
   d. coagulopathy.
3. Which condition is adversely affected by NSAID administration? (*Select all that apply.*)
   a. Bronchial asthma
   b. Bone healing
   c. Coagulopathy
   d. Hypertension
   e. Myasthenia gravis

Answers can be found in Appendix A.

severe heart failure, monitor patients for signs of worsening heart failure.

- Avoid the use of meloxicam in patients with recent myocardial infarction unless benefits outweigh risk of recurrent cardiovascular thrombotic events; if used in patients with recent myocardial infarction, monitor patients for signs of cardiac ischemia.
- The use of NSAIDs may compromise renal function.

MISCELLANEOUS ANALGESICS

Anesthetic Implications

- Patients frequently present for surgery having been treated for chronic pain syndromes (Table 2.47).
- They are also frequently induced by hepatic enzymes, and higher-dose requirements of many medications can be expected.

Chronic Pain Analgesics and Adjuncts

Anticonvulsants

- Anticonvulsants or antiepileptics are commonly used in certain neuropathic pain syndromes when treatment is refractory to traditional analgesics.
- First-generation anticonvulsants, such as carbamazepine and phenytoin, have been used for many years for neuropathic pain. The second-generation anticonvulsants gabapentin (Neurontin) and pregabalin (Lyrica) have become the most widely used.
- Anticonvulsants inhibit neuronal excitation and stabilize nerve membranes in an effort to decrease repetitive neural ectopic firing, which is common in neuropathic pain.
- Gabapentin and pregabalin are used for the management of postherpetic neuralgia, diabetic neuropathy, trigeminal neuralgia, and other neuropathic pain and chronic pain syndromes. Their mechanism of action is similar because it is believed that both block the alpha 2 delta ($\alpha 2\delta$) subunit of the presynaptic voltage-gated calcium channels in the CNS, thereby preventing excitatory neurotransmitter release. Pregabalin and gabapentin are structural analogs of GABA, which lack affinity for the GABA receptors. Both exhibit anticonvulsant, anxiolytic, and antihyperalgesic effects. Compared with gabapentin, pregabalin displays a pharmacokinetic profile that requires less frequent dosing with fewer side effects.

TABLE 2.47 Multimodal Treatment Options for Chronic Pain Management

Multimodal Treatment Modalities	Types
Medications	Antiinflammatory medications (NSAIDs, Tylenol), muscle relaxants, opioids, neuropathic medications (anticonvulsants, TCA, SNRI), SSRI, NMDA antagonist, α_2-agonist, topical medications
Rehabilitation	Physical therapy, occupational therapy, TENS, bracing
Psychology	Cognitive behavioral therapy, biofeedback, relaxation therapy, support groups
Interventional pain management	Epidural injections, facet joint injections, peripheral nerve block, major joint/bursa injections
Implantable therapies	Spinal cord stimulator therapy and intrathecal pumps
Complementary and alternative treatments	Acupuncture, chiropractic manipulation, massage, craniosacral therapy
Nutrition counseling	Weight loss, bone density
Vocational counseling	Return to work

NMDA, *N*-methyl-D-aspartate; *NSAIDs*, nonsteroidal antiinflammatory drugs; *SNRI*, selective norepinephrine reuptake inhibitor; *SSRI*, selective serotonin reuptake inhibitor; *TCA*, tricyclic antidepressant; *TENS*, transelectrical nerve stimulation.
From Dinakar P. Principles of pain management. In Daroff RB, Jankovic J, Mazziotta JC, et al., eds. *Bradley's Neurology in Clinical Practice*. 7th ed. Elsevier; 2016.

- Common side effects are dose dependent and include dizziness, somnolence, peripheral edema, and weight gain.
- Pregabalin and gabapentin are used as components in multimodal analgesia for acute postoperative pain management.
- Patients presenting for surgery who are routinely taking anticonvulsants as part of a chronic pain syndrome treatment regimen should continue taking their medication throughout the perioperative period because this will optimize their pain management.

Antidepressants

- In the presence of CNS sensitization, the descending inhibitory pathway, which uses inhibitory neurotransmitters (i.e., serotonin and norepinephrine), is altered. It is believed that antidepressants may exert their analgesic effects by blocking the reuptake of serotonin and norepinephrine in the CNS, thereby increasing their availability.
- Common antidepressants used to treat chronic pain include the TCAs, selective serotonin reuptake inhibitors (SSRIs), and selective norepinephrine and serotonin reuptake inhibitors (SNRIs) (Table 2.48).
- The analgesic dosage is much lower than the recommended antidepressant dose.
- The analgesic effects may not occur until 4–10 days after initiating treatment.
- Regardless of the type of antidepressant taken for chronic pain, the drug should be continued throughout the perioperative period.
- TCAs are commonly used for the treatment of postherpetic neuralgia, headaches, and fibromyalgia.
- TCAs (amitriptyline and nortriptyline) are associated with more side effects than the SSRIs and SNRIs because they antagonize other receptors, including muscarinic (e.g., dry mouth, blurred vision, and urinary retention), histaminergic (e.g., sedation, appetite stimulation with subsequent weight gain), and adrenergic (e.g., orthostatic hypotension, prolonged QT interval) receptors. They are contraindicated in patients with a history of a recent myocardial infarction, prolonged QT segment prolongation, cardiac dysrhythmias, or unstable CHF. Drug levels can be monitored to prevent unintentional overdose. The metabolism of all antidepressants is primarily hepatic.
- SNRIs (duloxetine, venlafaxine) lack affinity for the adrenergic, histaminergic, and cholinergic receptors. Therefore, they are preferred for those patients with cardiac disease. Both drugs (duloxetine and venlafaxine) have similar side effects: nausea, dry mouth, somnolence, headaches, and sexual dysfunction. Likewise, the concomitant use of SNRIs with SSRIs is not recommended because this may precipitate a serotonin syndrome.
- Serotonin syndrome is an acute toxicity of serotonin manifesting as anxiety, agitation, delirium, seizures, hyperthermia, diaphoresis, tachycardia, hypertension or hypotension, hyperreflexia, myoclonus, and muscle rigidity. Symptoms vary from mild to life threatening, and diagnosis is based on patient medication history, physical examination, and exclusion of other neurologic disorders.

TABLE 2.48 Common Antidepressants Used for Chronic Neuropathic Pain

Drug Class	Generic Name	Trade Name
TCAs	Amitriptyline	Elavil
	Nortriptyline	Pamelor
	Imipramine	Tofranil
SNRIs	Venlafaxine	Effexor
	Duloxetine	Cymbalta
	Milnacipran	Savella
SSRIs	Fluoxetine	Prozac
	Citalopram	Celexa

SNRI, Selective serotonin-norepinephrine reuptake inhibitors; *SSRI,* selective serotonin reuptake inhibitors; *TCA,* tricyclic antidepressant.
From Elisha S, Heiner JS, Nagelhout JJ. *Nurse Anesthesia.* 7th ed. Elsevier; 2023.

Corticosteroids

- Exogenous corticosteroids (glucocorticoids) are administered by a variety of routes (e.g., orally, IV, epidurally, caudally, and via intraarticular) as adjunct analgesics for multiple types of acute-onset and chronic pain syndromes.
- They exert multiple effects on the body, including autoimmune, antiinflammatory, antiedematous, and antiallergic effects.
- Typical disease processes and pain syndromes that are treated with corticosteroids include rheumatoid arthritis, osteoarthritis, herpetic neuralgia, chronic low back pain, and chronic neck pain. In the treatment of acute and chronic pain syndromes, corticosteroids exert their effects in several ways.
- They are primarily known for their antiinflammatory effect because they prevent the release of arachidonic acid by inhibiting phospholipase A2 on cell membranes. Through this mechanism, they decrease inflammatory cytokines (interleukin [IL]-6, IL-1, tumor necrosis factor alpha [TNF-α]) and prostaglandins.
- Side effects associated with corticosteroids include acute adrenal crises. Acute adrenal crises are a risk after discontinuation. This can occur if supraphysiologic doses of steroids, exceeding the rate of endogenous steroid production (approximately 20 mg/d) of hydrocortisone or its equivalent, are administered for more than 3 weeks within 1 year (Box 2.15).

BOX 2.15 Systemic Effects of Steroids

Endocrine
- Adrenal-pituitary insufficiency
- Hypercortisolism
- Hyperglycemia
- Cushing syndrome

Cardiovascular
- Hypertension
- CHF
- DVT
- Cardiomyopathy

Respiratory
- Asthma
- COPD

Musculoskeletal
- Muscle weakness
- Osteopenia/osteoporosis
- Avascular necrosis of bone
- Pathologic fractures
- Truncal obesity

Dermatologic
- Skin thinning
- Alopecia
- Petechiae
- Facial flushing
- Striae
- Hirsutism

Renal
- Sodium and water retention

Gastrointestinal
- Peptic ulceration
- Gastritis
- Hyperacidity

Neurologic/Psychological
- Headache
- Vertigo
- Euphoria
- Restlessness
- Insomnia
- Mood swings
- Depression

CHF, Congestive heart failure; *COPD,* chronic obstructive pulmonary disease; *DVT,* deep vein thrombosis.
Adapted from Baqai A, Bal R. The mechanism of action and side effects of epidural steroids. *Tech Reg Anesth Pain Manag.* 2009;13(4):205–211.

KNOWLEDGE CHECK

1. Which antidepressants are used to treat chronic pain syndromes? (*Select all that apply.*)
   a. Tricyclic antidepressants
   b. Benzodiazepines
   c. Monoamine oxidase inhibitors
   d. SSRIs
2. Gabapentin (Neurontin) and pregabalin (Lyrica) are anticonvulsants frequently used to treat
   a. restless leg syndrome.
   b. myasthenia gravis.
   c. Parkinson disease.
   d. neuropathic pain.
3. Corticosteroids exert their antiinflammatory effects by inhibiting (*Select all that apply.*)
   a. serotonin.
   b. aldosterone.
   c. prostaglandins.
   d. cytokines.
4. Which condition can selective serotonin and norepinephrine reuptake inhibitors precipitate?
   a. MH
   b. Pseudocholinesterase deficiency
   c. Acute renal failure
   d. Serotonin syndrome

Answers can be found in Appendix A.

LOCAL ANESTHETICS

Anesthesia Implications

- Local anesthetic (LA) medications attenuate action potential propagation along nerves by inhibiting depolarization.
- Thus, sensory, motor, and vascular sympathetic tone are inhibited.
- The brain, compared with the heart, is more sensitive to the effects of elevated plasma concentrations of LA. This explains why, as the LA concentration increases, manifestations associated with LA toxicity begin with

TABLE 2.49 Nerve Fiber Characteristics and Sensitivity to Local Anesthetics

Fiber Type	Function	Diameter (μm)	Myelination	Anesthetic Block Onset
Type A				
Alpha (Aα)	Proprioception, motor	6–22	Heavy	Last
Beta (Aβ)	Touch, pressure	6–22	Heavy	Intermediate
Gamma (Aγ)	Muscle tone	3–6	Heavy	Intermediate
Delta (Aδ)	Pain, cold temperature, touch	1–5	Heavy	Intermediate
Type B				
	Preganglionic autonomic vasomotor	< 3	Light	Early
Type C				
Sympathetic	Postganglionic vasomotor	0.3–1.3	None	Early
Dorsal root	Pain, warm and cold temperature, touch	0.4–1.2	None	Early

From Elisha S, Heiner JS, Nagelhout JJ. *Nurse Anesthesia*. 7th ed. Elsevier; 2023.

mild to moderate neurologic signs/symptoms, then progress to severe neurologic signs and, last, cardiotoxicity. However, if toxic doses of LA are injected directly into the central circulation, loss of consciousness caused by rapid onset of cardiovascular collapse can occur.

- Pharmacokinetics:
  - The greater the degree of lipid solubility, the greater the *potency.*
  - The greater the degree of protein binding, the greater the *duration of action.*
  - The closer the pK_a (acid dissociation constant at logarithmic scale) is to body pH, the *faster the onset of action.*
- Suspected causes of cardiotoxicity include LA blockade of cardiac sodium, potassium, and calcium channels, as well as cardiomyocyte mitochondrial inhibition.
- Because of its high potency, bupivacaine has most often been implicated in cases when cardiac arrest caused by LA toxicity occurs.
- LA toxicity is dependent on multiple factors, which include the following:
  - The specific LA medication (LA with greater potency will cause toxicity at lower plasma concentrations [i.e., bupivacaine])
  - The speed of absorption of LA into plasma
  - Total LA plasma concentration (mg/kg dose)
  - Addition of epinephrine to LA, which slows the systemic absorption caused by vasoconstriction
  - The individual's ability to metabolize and excrete the LA
- Amide LAs are metabolized by hepatic microsomal enzymes.
- Ester LAs are metabolized by plasma and tissue cholinesterase.
- Therefore, if a patient has severe liver disease or a pseudocholinesterase deficiency, the duration of metabolism will be increased.
- LAs are most often classified according to their chemical structure (Table 2.49).
- The differences between esters and amide-type LAs can be found in Table 2.50.

Clinical Effects Associated With Neuraxial Anesthesia

- The smaller the nerve fiber, the faster it is affected by an LA drug.
- A greater degree of nerve fiber myelination increases the effect of the LA.
- The degree of ionization of the LA plays an important role in its clinical actions.
- All LAs are basic, and their degree of lipid and water solubility is influenced by the pH of the solution in which they are placed (Box 2.16).

Side Effects Associated With Local Anesthetics

Methemoglobinemia

- Methemoglobinemia is a disorder characterized by high concentrations of methemoglobin (MetHb) in the blood, which can lead to tissue hypoxia.

TABLE 2.50 Clinical Differences Between Ester- and Amide-Type Local Anesthetics

Esters	Amides
Ester metabolism is catalyzed by plasma and tissue cholinesterase via hydrolysis; occurs throughout the body and is rapid.	Amides are metabolized in the liver by CYP1A2 and CYP3A4, and thus a significant blood level may develop with rapid absorption.
Although local anesthetic allergy is uncommon, esters have a higher allergy potential, and if patients exhibit an allergy to any ester drug, all other esters should be avoided.	Allergy to amides is extremely rare; there is no cross-allergy among the amide class or between the ester and amide agents.
Ester drugs tend to be shorter-acting due to their ready metabolism; tetracaine is the longest-acting ester.	Amides are longer-acting because they are more lipophilic and protein bound and require transport to the liver for metabolism.

From Elisha S, Heiner JS, Nagelhout JJ. *Nurse Anesthesia*. 7th ed. Elsevier; 2023.

BOX 2.16 Ion Trapping: Clinical Situations in Which Differences Between PK and pH May Affect Patient Response

- In the event of local anesthetic overdose, associated respiratory depression may occur, resulting in hypoxia and acidosis. The acidosis resulting from hypoxia increases the ionized fraction of local anesthetic (LA) within the cerebral circulation, thereby decreasing the ability of the anesthetic to cross the blood–brain barrier, leave the brain, and reenter the systemic circulation. This phenomenon may prolong and enhance the central nervous system toxicity of LAs.
- LA accumulation in the fetal circulation is enhanced by fetal pH being lower than maternal pH, which may result in high fetal levels of LAs.
- LAs injected into acidotic, infected tissues are rendered ineffective because of the loss of lipid solubility. The lipid solubility of LAs is diminished in an acidotic environment because of an increased concentration of the ionized, water-soluble form of the drug. The loss of lipid solubility prevents absorption into the nerve, thereby preventing access to the site of action.
- Carbonation of LAs speeds the onset and intensity of action of neural blockade. Carbon dioxide readily diffuses into the nerve, lowering the pH within the nerve. The lipid-soluble form of LA, after passing through the neuronal membrane, receives protons from the intraneuronal environment and ionizes. An increase in the ionized fraction within the neuron produces a higher concentration of the active form of the anesthetic available at the sodium channel, the site of action.
- Commercially available LAs are prepared in a slightly acidic formulation that improves the stability of the drug by increasing the concentration of the ionized, water-soluble form of the drug. Addition of sodium bicarbonate to the LA mixture increases the pH of the solution, thereby increasing the concentration of the un-ionized, lipid-soluble form of the drug. Improving the lipid solubility of the LA improves diffusion of the local anesthetic through the neuronal membrane, leading to a more rapid onset of action, especially with epidural and peripheral nerve blocks.

From Elisha S, Heiner JS, Nagelhout JJ. *Nurse Anesthesia*. 7th ed. Elsevier; 2023.

The ferrous form of hemoglobin (Fe^{2+}) is oxidized to the ferric form (Fe^{3+}). MetHb is an oxidized form of hemoglobin with reduced capacity to carry oxygen, which causes a leftward shift of the oxygen–hemoglobin dissociation curve. Normal MetHb levels are less than 1%.

- Signs and symptoms of developing methemoglobinemia are shown in Table 2.51. Decreasing oxygen saturation via pulse oximetry, which is unresponsive to oxygen supplementation, may occur.
- Methemoglobinemia can be diagnosed by CO oximetry or laboratory testing or can be implied by symptoms. Medications are the most common cause of MetHb in clinical practice, and of these, LAs (benzocaine and prilocaine), antibiotics (Dapsone), and nitrites (nitroglycerin/nitric oxide) are the most common (Box 2.17).

TABLE 2.51 Signs and Symptoms Associated With Methemoglobin Blood Concentrations

Methemoglobin Concentration	Percentage of Total Hemoglobin	Symptoms
<1.5 g/dL	<10	None
1.5–3.0 g/dL	10–20	Cyanotic skin discoloration
3.0–4.5 g/dL	20–30	Anxiety, lightheadedness, headache, tachycardia
4.5–7.5 g/dL	30–50	Fatigue, confusion, dizziness, tachypnea, increased tachycardia
7.5–10.5 g/dL	50–70	Coma, seizures, arrhythmias, acidosis
>10.5 g/dL	>70	Death

From Cortazzo JA, Lichtman AD. Methemoglobinemia: a review and recommendations for management. *J Cardiothorac Vasc Anesth.* 2014;28:1043–1047.

BOX 2.17 Clinical Clues to Diagnosis of Methemoglobinemia in the Anesthetized Patient

1. Hypoxia that does not improve with increased fraction of inspired oxygen (FIO_2)
2. Abnormal coloration of blood
3. Physiologically appropriate PaO_2 in blood gas sample with low pulse oximeter saturation ("saturation gap")
4. New-onset cyanosis and/or hypoxia after ingestion of an agent with oxidative properties

From Cortazzo JA1, Lichtman AD. Methemoglobinemia: a review and recommendations for management. *J Cardiothorac Vasc Anesth.* 2014;28(4):1043–1047.

- *Benzocaine:* The development of methemoglobinemia does not seem to be dose related. Symptoms appear from within minutes to up to 2 hours after benzocaine use. Benzocaine sprays are marketed under different brand names, such as Cetacaine, HurriCaine, Exactacain, and Topex. Benzocaine should not be used in children under 2 years old.
- *Prilocaine:* Prilocaine can produce methemoglobinemia because of one of its metabolites, *o*-toluidine, which oxidizes hemoglobin to methemoglobin. The tendency of prilocaine to produce MetHb is dose related. Current recommendations are that prilocaine should not be used in children younger than 6 months old, in pregnant females, or in patients taking other oxidizing drugs. The dose should be limited to 2.5 mg/kg. The treatment for elevated MetHb is methylene blue, which is initiated at a rate of 1–2 mg/kg IV over 3–10 minutes. If the MetHb level is greater than 50% or the clinical condition worsens, then the higher dose of methylene blue 2 mg/kg can be given initially. The dose can be repeated if symptoms fail to improve or high MetHb levels persist. A level of MetHb greater than 70% may require transfusion or dialysis. Recognition is critical because a delay in treatment can lead to cardiopulmonary compromise, neurologic sequelae, and death.

Allergic reactions

- Relatively uncommon
- Patients may describe palpitations associated with the injection of a local anesthetic that is combined with epinephrine, which is a possible side effect and not necessarily a symptom associated with an allergic reaction.
- Hypersensitivity
  - Amides are more likely to cause hypersensitivity reactions because of the metabolic product, para-aminobenzoic acid.
  - Esters can cause hypersensitivity reactions caused by the preservative methylparaben.

Local Tissue Toxicity

- Cauda equina syndrome (CES) manifests as bowel and bladder dysfunction with various degrees of bilateral lower extremity weakness and sensory impairment.
- Known risk factors for anesthetic-related CES are supernormal doses of intrathecal LA and/or the maldistribution of LA spread within the intrathecal space.
- Cases of CES have been associated with previously undiagnosed spinal stenosis.
- Increased pressure within the spinal canal may lead to pressure-induced spinal cord ischemia or limit normal LA distribution within the intrathecal sac,

BOX 2.18 American Society of Regional Anesthesia Recommendations for Minimizing Cauda Equina Syndrome

These recommendations are intended to encourage optimal patient care but cannot ensure the avoidance of adverse outcomes. As with any practice advisory recommendation, these are subject to revision as knowledge advances regarding specific complications.

- Inadequate initial dosing or redosing of subarachnoid local anesthetic, in addition to maldistribution (usually sacral) of local anesthetic spread, should be ruled out before redosing single-injection or continuous subarachnoid blocks (class I).
- The risks and benefits of neuraxial techniques should be considered in patients known to have moderate to severe spinal stenosis, especially if within the vertebral territory of the intended injection (class II).
- The incidence of transient neurologic symptoms after 40–50 mg of intrathecal 2-chloroprocaine seems to be remarkably low. The number of 2-chloropocaine spinal anesthetics reported in the literature is insufficient to determine the risk for cauda equina syndrome or other manifestations of neurotoxicity (class III).
- Physically and temporally separate disinfectant use from block trays and instruments during neuraxial procedures. Allow the solution to completely dry on skin before needle placement (2–3 min). Care should be taken to avoid needle or catheter contamination from chlorhexidine spraying or dripping, or from applicator device disposal, onto aseptic work surfaces (class II).

From Neal JM, Barrington MJ, Brull R, et al. The second ASRA practice advisory on neurologic complications associated with regional anesthesia and pain medicine: executive summary 2015. *Reg Anesth Pain Med.* 2015;40(5):401–430.

thereby exposing the cauda equina to high LA concentrations.

- Either of these conditions could promote LA neurotoxicity and could be exacerbated by additional compromise of the spinal canal, as may occur with surgical positioning.
- Controversy remains regarding whether transient neurologic syndrome (TNS) after spinal anesthesia is a form of LA neurotoxicity.
- See Box 2.18 for recommendations on minimizing CES.
- **Lidocaine** has been associated with CES when used for continuous spinal anesthesia, and as a result, it is no longer routinely used in this anesthetic technique in the United States. Single-dose spinal administration of lidocaine has also been implicated in TNS, which results in back and lower extremity pain for up to 5 days postoperatively. Symptoms include a burning, aching, cramping, and radiating pain in the anterior and posterior aspects of the thighs. Pain radiates to the lower extremities, and lower back pain is common. Other anesthetics have been implicated, but it is much more prevalent after spinal lidocaine. Surgical positioning may be a factor as well. The exact mechanism is unclear; however, CES is more likely to occur when patients are placed in the lithotomy position. Treatment for CES is supportive and should include NSAIDs.

Tumescent Anesthesia

- Tumescent local anesthesia (TLA) involves the use of lidocaine, sodium bicarbonate, and epinephrine diluted in normal saline to provide anesthesia for liposuction.
- The term *tumescent* refers to the physical appearance of tissues after the instillation of large volumes.
- Very low concentrations (0.05%–0.1%) of lidocaine mixed with epinephrine are used.
- Common preparations involve the dilution of 500–1000 mg to 1000 mL of normal saline.
- Epinephrine (0.5–1 mg) and sodium bicarbonate are added to the preparation. The volume of tumescent anesthesia solution used is determined by the achievement of palpable tumescence (uniform swelling) of the surgical field.
- The maximum dose of lidocaine in TLA can approach 35–55 mg/kg.
- Peak serum levels occur 12 hours after infiltration, and complete elimination is usually within 36 hours.

Sustained Release of LA

- A sustained-release formulation of the LA bupivacaine that does not require an indwelling catheter to achieve a long duration of action is available.
- Bupivacaine extended-release liposome injection, Exparel, consists of bupivacaine encapsulated in DepoFoam.
- It provides continuous and extended postsurgical analgesia for up to 72 hours.

- It is marketed as a 20-mL single-use vial, 1.3% (13.3 mg/mL).
- The maximum dosage should not exceed 266 mg (20 mL, 1.3% of undiluted drug).
- It is indicated for single-dose injection into the surgical site to produce postsurgical analgesia.

Local Anesthetic Systemic Toxicity

Prevention

Be prepared

- Establish a plan for managing local anesthetic systemic toxicity (LAST; i.e., crisis management checklist).
- Creating an LA toxicity kit and posting instructions for its use are encouraged.

Risk reduction

- Use the lowest dose of LA necessary to achieve the desired extent and duration of block.
- LA blood levels are influenced by site of injection and dose. Factors that can increase the likelihood of LAST include advanced age, heart failure, ischemic heart disease, conduction abnormalities, metabolic disease (e.g., mitochondrial disease), liver disease, low plasma protein concentration, metabolic or respiratory acidosis, and medications that inhibit sodium channels. Patients with severe cardiac dysfunction, particularly very low ejection fraction, are more sensitive to LAST and more prone to receive "stacked" injections (with resulting elevated LA tissue concentrations) because of slowed circulation time.
- Consider using a pharmacologic marker and/or test dose, for example, epinephrine 5 mcg/mL of LA.
- Use ultrasound guidance for LA injection.
- Aspirate before LA injection to check for blood and/or CSF.
- For epidural or regional anesthesia, inject LA in 3–5-mL increments.
- Add epinephrine to LA solutions for injection to assess for increased heart rate.
- Consistent verbal discussion with patient to assess level of consciousness and other signs and symptoms associated with neurologic LA toxicity
- Calculation of the toxic dose per patient's kilogram weight before LA administration or before additional LA infiltration by the surgeon

Detecting LAST

- Use standard American Society of Anesthesiologists (ASA) monitors.
- Monitor the patient during and after completing the injection because clinical toxicity can be delayed up to 30 minutes or longer after tumescent procedures.
- Consider LAST in any patient with new-onset altered mental status, neurologic symptoms, or cardiovascular instability after regional anesthesia.
- CNS signs/symptoms most often begin first (may be subtle):
  1. Nonspecific (metallic taste, circumoral numbness, diplopia, tinnitus, dizziness)
  2. Excitation (agitation, confusion, muscle twitching, seizure)
  3. Depression (drowsiness, obtundation, coma, apnea)
- Cardiovascular signs (often the only manifestation of severe LAST). If a large amount of local anesthesia is injected directly into a vein, the ensuing dramatic increase in plasma concentration can result in rapid bradycardia and asystole.
- For severe bradycardia/asystole associated with LAST, immediate administration of intralipids is critical (Box 2.19).
- Initially may be hyperdynamic (hypertension, tachycardia, ventricular arrhythmias), then:
  1. Progressive hypotension
  2. Conduction block, bradycardia, or asystole
  3. Ventricular arrhythmia (ventricular tachycardia, torsades de pointes, ventricular fibrillation)
- Sedative-hypnotic drugs reduce seizure risk, but even light sedation may abolish the patient's ability to recognize or report symptoms of rising LA concentrations.
- Epinephrine can impair resuscitation from LAST and reduce the efficacy of lipid rescue. Therefore, it is recommended to use smaller doses, such as 1 mcg/kg, for treating hypotension.
- Avoid vasopressin, CCBs, β-blockers, propofol, and LAs.
- Alert the nearest facility with cardiopulmonary bypass capability.
- See Box 2.19 for addressing mild to severe LA toxicity.
- Post LAST events at www.lipidrescue.org and report use of lipid to www.lipidregistry.org.

BOX 2.19 Actions for Mild, Moderate, and Severe Local Anesthetic Toxicity

If mild to moderate signs and symptoms of local anesthetic (LA) toxicity occur:

- Stop LA injection.
- Administer 100% oxygen.
- Assess airway, breathing, and circulation.
- Administer anticonvulsant drugs to increase seizure threshold.

  Administer:
  1. Benzodiazepine

If severe LA toxicity occurs and/or patient condition deteriorates:

- Call for help.
- Stop LA injection.
- Airway/breathing:
  1. Endotracheal intubation
  2. Adequate ventilation to prevent hypoxia, acidosis, and ion trapping
- Circulation:
  a. Perform cardiac resuscitation per American Heart Association protocol.
  b. Administer intralipids:
    1. Administer intravenous (IV) fluid bolus.
    2. Administer neuromuscular blockade for persistent tonic-clonic seizure activity.
    3. For hypotension, administer vasopressors and/or inotropic medications.
    4. For severe/sustained bradycardia, administer atropine 0.5–1 mg.
    5. Cardiac arrest caused by LA toxicity:
      1. Patients >70 kg, administer intralipid 20%, 100 mL IV bolus then 0.25 mL/kg/min infusion
      2. Patients <70 kg, intralipid 20%, 1.5 mL/kg IV bolus then 0.25 mL/kg/min infusion
      3. Repeat intralipid 20% IV bolus dose every 5 minutes (max-3 bolus doses)
      4. Maximum intralipid 20% IV dose is 12 ml/kg

KNOWLEDGE CHECK

1. The metabolism of the amide LAs is catalyzed by
   a. ALA synthetase.
   b. cholinesterase.
   c. hepatic microsomal oxidases.
   d. 11β-hydroxylase.
2. Which is the mechanism of action of LA drugs?
   a. Pressure reversal of the nerve membrane
   b. Blockade of sodium channels
   c. Blockade of adrenergic receptors
   d. Blockade of potassium and calcium receptors
3. Allergies to ester-type LA agents are caused by
   a. methylparaben.
   b. pseudocholinesterase metabolism.
   c. para-aminobenzoic acid.
   d. mitochondrial disease.
4. Which is an initial sign associated with LAST? (*Select all that apply.*)
   a. Circumoral numbness
   b. Supraventricular tachycardia
   c. Metallic taste
   d. Diplopia
   e. Seizures
   f. Hypotension
5. The greater the degree of protein binding of an LA, the
   a. longer the duration of action.
   b. shorter the duration of action.
   c. shorter the onset of action.
   d. longer the onset of action.
6. The closer the pK_a is to body pH, the
   a. longer the duration of action.
   b. shorter the duration of action.
   c. shorter the onset of action.
   d. longer the onset of action.
7. The metabolism of the ester local anesthetics is catalyzed by
   a. ALA synthetase.
   b. pseudocholinesterase.
   c. 11β-hydroxylase.
   d. monoamine oxidase.
8. Which effect will acidosis have on local anesthetic accumulation in the fetus?
   a. Enhance
   b. Reduce
   c. Varies with different drugs
   d. No effect
9. Which intervention is the curative treatment for LAST-induced cardiac arrest?
   a. Epinephrine 1 mcg/kg
   b. Intralipid bolus 1.5 mg/kg
   c. Midazolam 2 mg
   d. Propofol 1 mg/kg
10. Which is a method to prevent LAST during administration of epidural and regional anesthesia?
    a. Administration of hydrocortisone 100 mg
    b. Injection of LA in 3- to 5-mL increments
    c. Use of transesophageal echocardiography
    d. IV fluid bolus of 20 mL/kg

Answers can be found in Appendix A.

ORAL ANTACIDS

Anesthesia Implications

- Antacids are not commonly administered before anesthesia, except in the patient who may be considered "full stomach."
- Nonparticulate antacids are preferred to prevent damaging lung aspiration if vomiting does occur.

Antacids

- Antacids neutralize (remove hydrogen ions from) gastric contents or decrease the secretion of hydrogen chloride into the stomach.
- The oral antacids used most often are salts of aluminum, calcium, and magnesium.
- Hydrogen ions in stomach acid react with the base, forming a stable compound.
- Increasing gastric pH relieves the symptoms of gastritis, but if the pH of the stomach is too high, digestion of food is inhibited because an acidic pH is necessary for the breakdown of many foods.
- $NaHCO_3$ results in a prompt and rapid action, increasing the pH to the point that the stomach's pH is neutral, which can lead to acid rebound.
- Occasional failure of particulate antacids to increase gastric fluid pH may reflect inadequate mixing with stomach contents or an unusually large volume of gastric fluid such that the standard dose of antacid is inadequate to neutralize gastric hydrogen ions.

Types of Antacids

- **Magnesium hydroxide** (Milk of Magnesia) also produces prompt neutralization of gastric acid but is not associated with significant acid rebound.
- Systemic absorption of magnesium may be sufficient to cause neurologic, neuromuscular, and cardiovascular impairment in patients with renal dysfunction.
- **Calcium carbonate** can also produce metabolic alkalosis with chronic therapy.
- The plasma concentration of calcium is increased transiently.
- The administration of calcium carbonate–containing antacids may result in hypophosphatemia. Even small amounts of calcium carbonate–containing antacids evoke hypersecretion of hydrogen ions (acid rebound).
- **Aluminum hydroxide** is a mixture of aluminum hydroxide, aluminum oxide, and some fixed CO_2 as carbonate.
- Systemic absorption of aluminum is minimal, but in patients with renal disease, the plasma and tissue concentrations of aluminum may become excessive.
- **Sodium citrate**, a nonparticulate (clear) antacid, is less likely to cause a foreign body reaction if aspirated.
- Mixing with gastric fluid is more complete than with particulate antacids.
- The onset of effect is more rapid with sodium citrate than with particulate antacids that require a longer time for adequate mixing with gastric fluid.
- Sodium citrate, 15–30 mL, administered 15–30 minutes before the induction of anesthesia, is effective in reliably increasing gastric fluid pH in pregnant and nonpregnant patients.

Complications Associated With Antacid Therapy

- Chronic alkalinization of gastric fluid has been associated with bacterial overgrowth in the duodenum and small intestine.
- Alkalization of the urine may predispose to urinary tract infections.
- Increased urine pH may persist for >24 hours after administration of an antacid, leading to changes in the renal elimination of drugs.
- Acid rebound
- Milk-alkali syndrome is characterized by hypercalcemia, increased blood urea nitrogen and plasma creatinine concentrations, and systemic alkalosis, as reflected by an above-normal plasma pH. This syndrome is most commonly associated with ingestion of large amounts of calcium carbonate along with >1 L of milk every day.
- Phosphorus depletion can occur in patients who ingest large doses of aluminum salts.

Drug Interactions

- Gastric alkalinization increases gastric emptying, resulting in a faster delivery of orally administered drugs into the small intestine. This may facilitate absorption of drugs that are poorly absorbed, or it may shorten the time available for absorption.
- Antacids containing aluminum and, to a lesser extent, calcium or magnesium interfere with the absorption of tetracyclines and possibly digoxin from the GI tract.

KNOWLEDGE CHECK

1. Which antacid is likely to cause acid rebound? (*Select all that apply*).
   a. Magnesium hydroxide
   b. Aluminum hydroxide
   c. Calcium bicarbonate
   d. Sodium bicarbonate
2. Which antacid is nonparticulate?
   a. Magnesium hydroxide
   b. Sodium citrate
   c. Calcium bicarbonate
   d. Aluminum hydroxide

Answers can be found in Appendix A.

ANTIPARKINSONIAN DRUGS

Anesthetic Implications

- The motor symptoms associated with Parkinson disease (PD) are caused primarily by degeneration of dopaminergic neurons in the substantia nigra. The nonmotor symptoms of the disease are thought to be caused by degeneration of other neurotransmitter systems.
- Patients may be prone to hemodynamic instability, hypotension, arrhythmias, gastric aspiration, laryngospasm, postoperative cognitive dysfunction, and upper airway obstruction.
- Avoid administering drugs that exacerbate parkinsonism, such as the phenothiazines, butyrophenones, metoclopramide, and MAOIs.
- Continue PD medications the morning of surgery.

General Anesthesia

- Exquisitely sensitive to the cardiovascular and respiratory depressant effects of anesthetic agents
- Exaggerated vasodilation and cardiodepressant effects with volatile anesthetics, resulting in hypotension
- Possible enhanced opioid-induced muscle rigidity after fentanyl administration
- Increased risk of neostigmine-induced bronchoconstriction
- Drugs for PD can be found in Box 2.20 and Table 2.52.

BOX 2.20 Recommendations for Treatment of Parkinson Disease

- The combination of levodopa and carbidopa is the most effective treatment for the motor symptoms of Parkinson disease (PD), but its long-term use leads to motor fluctuations and dyskinesia.
- Dopamine agonists are less effective than levodopa; they can be used as monotherapy before the introduction of levodopa or as an adjunct to levodopa in patients with motor fluctuations.
- Addition of a peripherally acting catechol-O-methyltransferase (COMT) inhibitor or a monoamine oxidase B (MAO-B) inhibitor to levodopa can reduce motor fluctuations in patients with advanced disease.
- Amantadine can be used as monotherapy in early PD and as an adjunct in later stages; it may modestly improve PD symptoms and can decrease levodopa-induced dyskinesia.
- Anticholinergics can help control tremor and drooling but are rarely used because of their adverse effects.
- Deep brain stimulation is an option for patients with levodopa-induced motor complications and relatively intact cognition.
- Combining pharmacologic therapy with exercise therapy can improve physical function and quality of life.

ANTIBIOTICS

Anesthetic Implications

- Administration of the correct dose and timing of perioperative antibiotics has been a special focus for several years.
- Allergy to antibiotics remains a challenge throughout medicine; however, the use of cephalosporins has lessened unwanted side effects.

KNOWLEDGE CHECK

1. Which medication is contraindicated in patients with PD?
   a. Metoclopramide
   b. Ranitidine
   c. Zestril
   d. Decadron
2. PD is characterized by an increasing deficiency in
   a. acetylcholine.
   b. norepinephrine.
   c. dopamine.
   d. glutamate.
3. Which is an anesthetic implication for patients with PD? (*Select all that apply.*)
   a. Exaggerated vasodilation and cardiodepression
   b. Potential for opioid-induced muscle rigidity
   c. Increased incidence of supraventricular tachycardia
   d. Increased risk of neostigmine-induced bronchoconstriction

Answers can be found in Appendix A.

TABLE 2.52 Medications Used to Treat Parkinson Disease

Drug	Some Available Formulations	Usual Dosage[a]	Cost[b] ($)
Carbidopa/Levodopa			
Immediate release—generic	10/100-, 25/100-, 25/250-mg tabs	300–1500 mg levo/d, divided	6.70–18.30
Sinemet (Merck)			117.90–298.00
Orally disintegrating—generic	10/100-, 25/100-, 25/250-mg ODTs	300–1500 mg levo/d, divided	79.00–201.30
Sustained release—generic	25/100-, 50/200-mg tabs	400–1600 mg levo/d, divided	75.90–303.60
Sinemet CR (Merck)			168.00–672.00
Extended release—*Rytary* (Impax)	23.75/95-, 36.25/145-, 48.75/195-, 61.25/245-mg ER caps[c]	285–1170 mg levo/d, divided[d]	232.60–465.10
Intrajejunal infusion—*Duopa* (Abbvie)	100-mL single-use cassettes (4.63 mg/20 mg/mL)	2000 mg levo/d (1 cassette)[e]	6055.20
Dopamine Agonists			
Oral			
Pramipexole—generic	0.125-, 0.25-, 0.5-, 0.75-, 1-mg tabs	0.5–1.5 mg tid	13.30
Mirapex (Boehringer Ingelheim)	1.5-mg tabs		552.00
Extended release—generic	0.375-, 0.75-, 1.5, 2.25-, 3-mg tabs	1.5–4.5 mg once/d	295.00
Mirapex ER	3.75-, 4.5-mg ER tabs		522.20
Ropinirole—generic	0.25-, 0.5-, 1-, 2-, 3-, 4-, 5-mg tabs	3–8 mg tid	31.50
Requip (GSK)			499.60
Extended release—generic	2-, 4-, 6-, 8-, 12-mg ER tabs	8–24 mg once/d	132.00
Requip XL			422.00
Transdermal			
Rotigotine—*Neupro* (UCB)	1-, 2-, 3-, 4-, 6-, 8-mg/24-hr patches[f]	4–8 mg/24 hr[g]	621.80
Subcutaneous			
Apomorphine—*Apokyn* (US Worldmeds)	30-mg/3-mL cartridges	2–6 mg subcut 3–5x/d prn[h]	1008.00[i]
COMT Inhibitors			
Entacapone—generic	200-mg tabs	200 mg tid or qid[j]	450.00
Comtan (Novartis)			661.60
Tolcapone—generic	100-mg tabs	100 mg tid[k]	8319.20
Tasmar (Valeant)			10,668.50
Carbidopa/Levodopa/Entacapone			
Generic	12.5/50/200-, 18.75/75/200-mg tabs	300–1500 mg levo/d, divided	180.00–900.20
Stalevo (Orion)	25/100/200-, 31.25/125/200-, 37.5/150/200-, 50/200/200-mg tabs		437.40–2186.80
MAO-B Inhibitors			
Rasagiline—generic	0.5-, 1-mg tabs	0.5–1 mg once/d[l]	428.80
Azilect (Teva)			694.40

TABLE 2.52 **Medications Used to Treat Parkinson's Disease—cont'd**

Drug	Some Available Formulations	Usual Dosage[a]	Cost[b] ($)
Safinamide—*Xadago* (US Worldmeds)	50-, 100-mg tabs	50–100 mg once/d	669.90
Selegiline—generic	5-mg tabs, caps	5 mg once/d with breakfast	54.00
Eldepryl (Somerset)	5-mg caps		99.90
Orally disintegrating			
Zelapar (Valeant)	1.25-mg ODTs	1.25–2.5 mg once/d in the morning	2034.90
Other Drugs			
Amantadine—generic	100-mg caps, tabs	200–400 mg/d, divided	130.10
	50-mg/5-mL syrup		38.80
Extended release—*Gocovri* (Adamas)	68.5-, 137-mg ER caps	274 mg once/d at bedtime[m]	2375.00
Carbidopa—generic	25-mg tabs[n]	25 mg tid or qid[o]	1117.80
Lodosyn (Aton)			2369.70

COMT, Catechol-O-methyltransferase inhibitor; *ER,* extended release; *levo,* levodopa; *ODTs,* orally disintegrating tabs.
[a]Dosage adjustment may be needed for renal or hepatic impairment.
[b]Approximate WAC for 30 days' treatment with the lowest to highest dose of levodopa or the lowest usual dosage. WAC = wholesaler acquisition cost or manufacturer's published price to wholesalers. WAC represents a published catalog or list price and may not represent an actual transactional price. Source: AnalySource Monthly. November 5, 2017. Reprinted with permission by First Databank, Inc. All rights reserved. Copyright 2017. www.dbhealth.com/policies/drug-pricing-policy.
[c]Capsules may be opened and the contents sprinkled on 1–2 tablespoons of applesauce and taken immediately.
[d]Dosages of Rytary are not interchangeable with those of other carbidopa/levodopa products.
[e]Daily dosage is individualized based on clinical response and tolerability. Maximum recommended daily dose is 2000 mg of levodopa. Administered as a 16-hour infusion through a nasojejunal (NJ) or percutaneous endoscopic gastrostomy with jejunal (PEC-J) tube with the CADD-Legacy 1400 portable infusion pump.
[f]The 1-mg/24-hr formulation is not approved by the US Food and Drug Administration for Parkinson disease.
[g]Usual dose is 4–6 mg/day for early-stage disease and 6–8 mg/day for advanced-stage disease.
[h]Should be administered with the antiemetic trimethobenzamide.
[i]Cost of one 3-mL cartridge.
[j]With each dose of carbidopa/levodopa (max 8 tabs/day).
[k]Tolcapone does not need to be taken at the same time as carbidopa/levodopa. Discontinue within 3 weeks if no clinical benefit.
[l]Dose is 1 mg as monotherapy and 0.5–1 mg when given with carbidopa/levodopa.
[m]Equivalent to 340 mg of amantadine HCl. Capsules may be opened and the contents sprinkled over soft food such as applesauce and taken immediately.
[n]Tablets are scored.
[o]Starting dosage for patients who require individual titration of levodopa and carbidopa. Dosage for patients who need additional carbidopa is 25 mg given with the first dose of carbidopa/levodopa each day; additional doses of 12.5 or 25 mg may be needed.

Clinical Uses

- A surgical site infection (SSI) is an infection that occurs somewhere in the operative field after surgery (Box 2.21).
- SSIs are the most common perioperative infection and the most frequent cause of hospital readmission after surgery, accounting for nearly 20% of unplanned readmissions.
- The mortality rate associated with SSIs is 3%.
- Antimicrobial prophylaxis should be directed against the most likely organism without covering all possible pathogens to decrease drug resistance (Table 2.53).
- A drug for surgical prophylaxis should (1) prevent SSI, (2) prevent SSI-related morbidity and mortality, (3) reduce the duration and cost of healthcare, (4) produce no adverse effects, and (5) have no adverse consequences for the microbial flora of the patient or the hospital (Table 2.54).

BOX 2.21 Risk Factors for Surgical Site Infections

Patient-Related
- Age
- Nutritional status
- Diabetes
- Smoking
- Obesity
- Coexistent infections at a remote body site
- Colonization with microorganisms
- Altered immune response
- Length of preoperative stay
- Hypothermia

Operation
- Duration of surgical scrub
- Skin antisepsis
- Preoperative shaving
- Duration of operation
- Antimicrobial prophylaxis
- Operating room ventilation
- Inadequate sterilization of instruments
- Foreign material in the surgical site
- Surgical drains
- Surgical technique
- Poor hemostasis
- Failure to obliterate dead space
- Tissue trauma

Adapted from Young PY, Khadaroo RG. Surgical site infections. *Surg Clin North Am.* 2014;94(6):1245–1264.

TABLE 2.53 Antimicrobial Prophylaxis for Surgery

Nature of Operation	Common Pathogens	Recommended Antimicrobials	Usual Adult Dosage[a]
Cardiac			
	Staphylococcus aureus, Staphylococcus epidermidis	Cefazolin OR cefuroxime OR vancomycin[d]	1–2 g IV[b,c] 1.5 g IV[c] 1 g IV
Gastrointestinal			
Esophageal, gastroduodenal	Enteric gram-negative bacilli, gram-positive cocci	High-risk[e] only: cefazolin[f]	1–2 g IV[2]
Biliary tract	Enteric gram-negative bacilli, enterococci, clostridia	High-risk[g] only: cefazolin[f,h]	1–2 g IV[2]
Colorectal	Enteric gram-negative bacilli, anaerobes, enterococci	*Oral:* neomycin + erythromycin base[i] or metronidazole[i]	See footnote 9
		Parenteral:	
		cefoxitin[f] or cefotetan[f]	1–2 g IV
		OR cefazolin[f]	1–2 g IV[2]
		+ metronidazole	0.5 g IV
		OR ampicillin/sulbactam[f,j]	3 g IV
Appendectomy, nonpertorated[k]	Same as for colorectal	Cefoxitin[f] or cefotetan[f] OR cefazolin[f] + metronidazole	1–2 g IV 1–2 g IV[2] 0.5 g IV
Genitourinary			
Cystoscopy alone	Enteric gram-negative bacilli, enterococci	High-risk[l] only: ciprofloxacin[j]	500 mg PO or 400 mg IV 1 DS tablet
		OR trimethoprim/sulfamethoxazole	

TABLE 2.53 Antimicrobial Prophylaxis for Surgery—cont'd

Nature of Operation	Common Pathogens	Recommended Antimicrobials	Usual Adult Dosage[a]
Cystoscopy with manipulation or upper tract instrumentation[m]	Enteric gram-negative bacilli, enterococci	Ciprofloxacin[j]	500 mg PO or 400 mg IV
		OR trimethoprim/sulfamethoxazole	1 DS tablet
Open or laparoscopic surgery[n]	Enteric gram-negative bacilli, enterococci	Cefazolin[f]	1–2 g IV[2]
Gynecologic and Obstetric			
Vaginal, abdominal or laparoscopic hysterectomy	Enteric gram-negative bacilli, anaerobes, Gp B strep, enterococci	Cefazolin,[f] cefoxitin[f] or cefotetan[f] OR ampicillin/sulbactam[f,j]	1–2 g IV[2] 3 g IV
Cesarean section	same as for hysterectomy	Cefazolin[f]	1–2 g IV[2]
Abortion, surgical	same as for hysterectomy	Doxycycline	300 mg PO[o]
Head and Neck Surgery			
Incisions through oral or pharyngeal mucosa	Anaerobes, enteric gram-negative bacilli, *S. aureus*	Clindamycin OR cefazolin + metronidazole OR ampicillin/sulbactam[j]	600–900 mg IV 1–2 g IV[2] 0.5 g IV 3g IV
Neurosurgery			
	S. aureus, S. epidermidis	Cefazolin	1–2 g IV[2]
		OR vancomycin[d]	1 g IV
Ophthalmic			
	S. epidermidis, S. aureus, streptococci, enteric gram-negative bacilli, *Pseudomonas* spp.	Gentamicin, tobramycin, ciprofloxacin, gatifloxacin levofloxacin, moxifloxacin Ofloxacin or neomycin-gramicidin-polymyxin B	multiple drops topically over 2–24 hours
		OR cefazolin	100 mg subconjunctivally
Orthopedic			
	S. aureus, S. epidermidis,	Cefazolin[f] OR vancomycin[d,p]	1–2 g IV[2] 1 g IV
Thoracic (Noncardiac)			
	S. aureus, S. epidermidis, streptococci, enteric gram-negative bacilli	Cefazolin OR ampicillin/sulbactam[j] OR vancomycin[d]	1–2 g IV[2] 3g IV 1 g IV
Vascular			
Arterial surgery involving a prosthesis, the abdominal aorta, or a groin incision	*S. aureus, S. epidermidis,* enteric gram-negative bacilli	Cefazolin OR vancomycin[d]	1–2 g IV[2] 1 g IV

Continued

TABLE 2.53 Antimicrobial Prophylaxis for Surgery—cont'd

Nature of Operation	Common Pathogens	Recommended Antimicrobials	Usual Adult Dosage[a]
Lower extremity amputation or ischemia	*S. aureus, S. epidermidis,* enteric gram-negative bacilli, Clostridia	Cefazolin OR vancomycin[d]	1–2 g IV[2] 1 g IV

Gp B strep, Group B *Streptococcus; IV,* intravenous.

[a]Parenteral prophylactic antimicrobials can be given as a single IV dose begun within 60 minutes before the procedure. For prolonged procedures (>3 hours) or those with major blood loss, or in patients with extensive bums, additional intraoperative doses should be given at intervals 1–2 times the half-life of the drug (ampicillin/sulbactam q2 hours, cefazolin q4 hours, cefuroxime q4 hours, cefoxitin q2 hours, clindamycin q6 hours, vancomycin q12 hours) for the duration of the procedure in patients with normal renal function. If vancomycin or a fluoroquinolone is used, the infusion should be started within 60–120 minutes before the initial incision to have adequate tissue levels at the time of incision and to minimize the possibility of an infusion reaction close to the time of induction of anesthesia.

[b]The recommended close of cefazolin is 1 g for patients who weigh <80 kg and 2 g for those ≥80 kg. Morbidly obese patients may need higher doses.

[c]Some experts recommend an additional dose when patients are removed from bypass during open-heart surgery.

[d]Vancomycin can be used in hospitals in which methicillin-resistant *S. aureus* and *S. epidermidis* are a frequent cause of postoperative wound infection in patients previously colonized with methicillin-resistant *S. aureus* (MRSA) or for those who are allergic to penicillins or cephalosporins. Rapid IV administration may cause hypotension, which could be especially dangerous during induction of anesthesia. Even when the drug is given over 60 minutes, hypotension may occur; treatment with diphenhydramine (Benadryl, and others) and further slowing of the infusion rate may be helpful. Some experts would give 15 mg/kg of vancomycin to patients weighing more than 75 kg, up to a maximum of 1.5 g, with a slower infusion rate (90 minutes for 1.5 g). For procedures in which enteric gram-negative bacilli are common pathogens, many experts would add another drug, such as an aminoglycoside (gentamicin, tobramycin, or amikacin), aztreonam, or a fluoroquinolone.

[e]Morbid obesity, gastrointestinal (GI) obstruction, decreased gastric acidity or GI motility, gastric bleeding, malignancy or perforation, or immunosuppression.

[f]For patients allergic to penicillins and cephalosporins, clindamycin or vancomycin with either gentamicin, ciprofloxacin, levofloxacin, or aztreonam is a reasonable alternative. Fluoroquinolones should not be used for prophylaxis in cesarean section.

[g]Age >70 years, acute cholecystitis, nonfunctioning gall bladder, obstructive jaundice, or common bile duct stones.

[h]Cefotetan, cefoxitin, and ampicillin-sulbactam are reasonable alternatives.

[i]In addition to mechanical bowel preparation, 1 g of neomycin plus 1 g of erythromycin at 1 PM, 2 PM, and 11 PM or 2 g of neomycin plus 2 g of metronidazole at 7 PM and 11 PM the day before an 8 AM operation.

[j]Because of increasing resistance of *Escherichia coli* to fluoroquinolones and ampicillin/sulbactam, local sensitivity profiles should be reviewed before use.

[k]For a ruptured viscus, therapy is often continued for about 5 days.

[l]Urine culture positive or unavailable, preoperative catheter, transrectal prostatic biopsy, or placement of prosthetic material.

[m]Shock-wave lithotripsy, ureteroscopy.

[n]Including percutaneous renal surgery, procedures with entry into the urinary tract, and those involving implantation of a prosthesis. If manipulation of bowel is involved, prophylaxis is given according to colorectal guidelines.

[o]Divided into 100 mg before the procedure and 200 mg after.

[p]If a tourniquet is to be used in the procedure, the entire dose of antibiotic must be infused before its inflation.

- To achieve these goals, an antimicrobial agent should be (1) active against the pathogens most likely to contaminate the surgical site; (2) given in an appropriate dosage and at a time that ensures adequate serum and tissue concentrations during the period of potential contamination; (3) safe; and (4) administered for the shortest effective period to minimize adverse effects, the development of resistance, and costs.
- The Surgical Care Improvement Project (SCIP) is a national quality partnership of organizations interested in improving surgical care by significantly reducing surgical complications.
- SCIP guidelines include preoperative screening; decolonization; and targeted prophylaxis, such as preoperative removal of hair, rational antibiotic prophylaxis, avoidance of perioperative hypothermia, management of perioperative blood glucose, and effective preoperative bathing and skin preparation.
- Anesthesia providers should consider implementation of measures designed to target attenuation of

TABLE 2.54 **Select Antibiotic Classes and General Mechanisms**

Target and Group	Drugs	Mechanisms
Cell Wall		
β-Lactams	Penicillins, cephalosporins, carbapenems, monobactams	Inhibition of transpeptidases responsible for peptidoglycan cross-linking → loss of structural integrity
Glycopeptides	Vancomycin	Inhibition of peptidoglycan cross-linking by steric inhibition → loss of structural integrity
Cell Membrane		
Polymyxins	Colistin, polymyxin B	Disruption of outer cell membrane of gram-negative bacteria → altered cell membrane permeability
Ribosome		
Aminoglycosides	Gentamicin, tobramycin, amikacin, streptomycin	Binding to 30S ribosomal subunit → inhibition of protein synthesis, production of mistranslated proteins
Macrolides	Azithromycin, clarithromycin, erythromycin	Binding to 50S ribosomal subunit → inhibition of protein synthesis
Tetracyclines and glycylcyclines	Doxycycline, tigecycline	Binding to 30S ribosomal subunit → inhibition of protein synthesis
Lincosamides	Clindamycin	Binding to 50S ribosomal subunit → inhibition of protein synthesis
DNA Synthesis and Structure		
Fluoroquinolones	Ciprofloxacin, levofloxacin, moxifloxacin	Inhibition of bacterial topoisomerases, preventing DNA uncoiling → DNA strand breakage
Antifolates	Trimethoprim/sulfamethoxazole	Sequential inhibition of nucleotide precursors → interruption of DNA synthesis
Nitroimidazoles	Metronidazole	Generation of free radicals → DNA destabilization and strand breakage

Adapted from MacDougall C, Guglielmo BJ, Wiener-Kronish J. Antimicrobial therapy. In: Evers AS, Maze M, Kharasch ED, eds. *Anesthetic Pharmacology: Basic Principles and Clinical Practice*. 2nd ed. Cambridge University Press; 2011:59; Bryan CS. Infectious diseases. In: Rakel RE, Rakel DP. *Textbook of Family Medicine*. 9th ed. Elsevier; 2016, 183–236; Bratzler DW, Dellinger EP, Olsen KM, et al. Clinical practice guidelines for antimicrobial prophylaxis in surgery. *Am J Health Syst Pharm*. 2013;70(3):195–283.

bacterial transmission occurring during routine anesthesia administration.

- A multimodal approach including double-gloving during airway instrumentation, intraoperative hand hygiene, patient screening and decolonization, and environmental equipment decontamination, as well as improvements in intravascular handling and design, may reduce the risk of postoperative infections (Table 2.55).

Drug Administration

- The SCIP recommends that administration of the first dose of the prophylactic antibiotic should be 60 minutes before the initial surgical incision to ensure adequate serum and tissue levels.
- If vancomycin or a fluoroquinolone is used, the infusion should begin within 60–120 minutes before the incision because of the prolonged infusion times required for these drugs.
- Redosing of antibiotics is recommended at approximately 2 half-lives of the drug. For cefazolin (Ancef), for example, with an elimination half-life of 1.4–2.0 hours, that would be approximately 4 hours.
- The duration of antimicrobial prophylaxis should be <24 hours for most procedures.

TABLE 2.55 Surgical Wound Classification

Class	Type	Description
I	Clean	An uninfected operative wound in which no inflammation is encountered and the respiratory, alimentary, genital, or uninfected urinary tract is not entered. In addition, clean wounds are primarily closed and, if necessary, drained with closed drainage. Operative incisional wounds that follow nonpenetrating (blunt) trauma should be included in this category if they meet the criteria.
II	Clean—contaminated	An operative wound in which the respiratory, alimentary, genital, or urinary tract is entered under controlled conditions and without unusual contamination. Specifically, operations involving the biliary tract, appendix, vagina, and oropharynx are included in this category, provided no evidence of infection or major break in technique is encountered.
III	Contaminated	Open, fresh, accidental wounds. In addition, operations with major breaks in sterile technique (e.g., open cardiac massage) or gross spillage from the gastrointestinal tract and incisions in which acute, nonpurulent inflammation is encountered are included in this category.
IV	Dirty—infected	Old traumatic wounds with retained devitalized tissue and those that involve existing clinical infection or perforated viscera. This definition suggests that the organisms causing postoperative infection were present in the operative field before the operation.

Young PY, Khadaroo RD. Surgical site infections. *Surg Clin North Am.* 2014;94(6):1245–1264.

Antibiotic Allergy

- Antibiotics account for approximately 15% of anesthesia-related anaphylactic reactions, with penicillins and cephalosporins being responsible for 70% of these (Box 2.22).
- Penicillin allergy is the most commonly reported drug allergy in the United States. The prevalence of reported penicillin allergy is 10% in the general population.
- The rate of cephalosporin allergy is approximately 1%, although reports claim no cross-reactivity between these two classes of antibiotics.
- Immediate reactions occurring within 1 hour of exposure are almost always either immunoglobulin E (IgE)-mediated reactions or due to direct stimulation of mast cells.
- Reactions occurring later than 1 hour probably have multiple mechanisms, including IgE-mediated reactions, or involve cell-mediated reactions.

Antibiotic–Anesthetic Drug Interactions

- Aminoglycosides, polymyxins, lincomycin, clindamycin, and tetracycline antibiotics can potentiate NMB.
- If prolonged NMB occurs, ventilation should be controlled until muscle strength spontaneously returns.

BOX 2.22 Treatment of Anaphylaxis

- Discontinue suspected causative agent(s).
- Maintain patent airway and adequate ventilation.
- Monitor for the presence of rapidly developing airway edema and obstruction.
- Administer 100% FiO_2.
- Discontinue inhalation anesthetics.
- Administer fluid bolus.
- Epinephrine IV, 10–100-mcg bolus
- Antihistamine (H_1 blocker): diphenhydramine IV 0.5–1 mg/kg
  (H_2 blocker): famotidine 20 mg
- Bronchodilators: albuterol/terbutaline for persistent bronchospasm
- Corticosteroids: hydrocortisone IV, 100 mg
- Sodium bicarbonate IV, 0.5–1 mEq/kg for persistent hypotension or acidosis
- Vasopressin 1–2 units for refractory hypotension
  a. Epinephrine 2–10 mcg/min
  b. Norepinephrine 4–8 mcg/min
  c. Isoproterenol 0.5–1 mcg/min
     1. Vasopressor and inotropic medications as needed
- Invasive monitoring as indicated
- Check tryptase level.
- Follow advanced cardiac life support (ACLS) and pediatric advanced life support (PALS) guidelines as currently indicated.

- Calcium should not be given to reverse the interaction because the antagonism it produces is not sustained and it may diminish the antibacterial effect of the antibiotics.
- Direct-acting NMB reversal with sugammadex may be indicated.

KNOWLEDGE CHECK

1. Which medication is the initial treatment for anaphylaxis?
   a. Epinephrine
   b. Famotidine
   c. Diphenhydramine
   d. Hydrocortisone
2. Antibiotics should be readministered after
   a. 1 half-life.
   b. 2 half-lives.
   c. 3 half-lives.
   d. 4 half-lives.
3. According to SCIP, most antibiotic administration should be complete for ______ hour(s) at the time of surgical incision.
   a. 1
   b. 2
   c. 3
   d. 4
4. Which class of antibiotics potentiates neuromuscular blockade? (*Select all that apply.*)
   a. Aminoglycoside
   b. Penicillin
   c. Cephalosporin
   d. Tetracycline

Answers can be found in Appendix A.

ANTICOAGULANTS

Anesthetic Implications

- Anticoagulants are the drugs of choice for treatment and prevention of deep venous thrombosis and pulmonary embolism, collectively referred to as *venous thromboembolism* (VTE).
- Consultation with a hematologist is recommended for patients with complicated disease processes or major surgery.
- The advent of new antithrombotic medications has garnered increasing interest regarding the perioperative management of these medications.
- Antithrombotic medications can be categorized on the basis of their respective method of altering the normal physiologic process of hemostasis: antiplatelet, anticoagulant, and fibrinolytic medications.
- See Table 2.56 for common antithrombotic medications.
- Selection, dosing, and monitoring of antithrombotic therapy should be adjusted on the basis of the patient's primary diagnosis, comorbidities, type of therapy (e.g., treatment or prophylaxis), and renal impairment.
- Classification of antiplatelet drugs is noted in Box 2.23.
- The preoperative management of antithrombotic therapy is a pivotal topic in that the risk of perioperative bleeding must be weighed against the risk of disease exacerbation.
- Table 2.57 outlines guidelines for neuraxial anesthesia in patients receiving antithrombotic therapy.
- Uninterrupted administration of anticoagulant therapy, specifically warfarin, for low-risk procedures such as minor ophthalmic, dental, dermatologic, GI, orthopedic, and podiatric procedures is thought to be safe (Box 2.24).

Antiplatelet Drugs and Noncardiac Surgery: Patients With Coronary Stents

- Coronary stents are placed to improve coronary artery flow in patients with stable but symptomatic coronary artery disease or acute coronary syndromes, including unstable angina, non–Q-wave myocardial infarction, and ST-elevation acute myocardial infarction.
- The clinical efficacy of intracoronary stents is highly dependent on long-term antiplatelet therapy.
- As a result, anesthesia providers routinely manage patients with coronary artery disease who have had coronary stents placed and are typically receiving dual-antiplatelet therapy (DAPT) with aspirin and thienopyridines (e.g., clopidogrel) for 12 months.
- There are two distinct complications associated with stent placement: acute stent thrombosis and in-stent restenosis, which can lead to myocardial infarction.
- Stent thrombosis can occur anytime after stent implantation and anytime antiplatelet therapy is abruptly discontinued.
- Abrupt discontinuation of antiplatelet therapy can lead to a rebound effect, characterized by an inflammatory prothrombotic state.
- The AHA/ACC released their guidelines for management of patients with drug-eluting stents (Box 2.25).

TABLE 2.56 Pharmacologic Properties of Common Antithrombotic Medications

	Type	Mechanism	Half-Life	Reversal Available	General Anesthesia Recommendations	Laboratory Monitoring
ASA	Antiplatelet	COX-1 inhibitor (irreversible)	20 min	Platelets	Stop 7 d	None
NSAIDs	Antiplatelet	COX-1 inhibitor (reversible)	2–10 h	Platelets	Stop 24–48 h	None
Clopidogrel	Antiplatelet	ADP receptor antagonist	7 h	Platelets	Stop 5–7 d	None
Ticlopidine	Antiplatelet	ADP receptor antagonist	4 d	Platelets	Stop 7–10 d	None
Prasugrel	Antiplatelet	ADP receptor antagonist	7 h	Platelets	Stop 7–10 d	None
Abciximab	Antiplatelet	Glycoprotein IIb/IIIa receptor antagonist	30 min	Platelets	Stop 48–72 h	None
Eptifibatide	Antiplatelet	Glycoprotein IIb/IIIa receptor antagonist	2.5 h	Platelets	Stop 8–24 h	None
Tirofiban	Antiplatelet	Glycoprotein IIb/IIIa receptor antagonist	2 h	Platelets	Stop 8–24 h	None
Fondaparinux	Anticoagulant	Factor Xa antagonist (indirect[a])	14–17 h	None	Stop 2–4 d	Antifactor Xa assay
LMWH	Anticoagulant	Factors IIa and Xa antagonist (indirect[a])	4.5 h	Protamine (partial reversal)	Stop 12–24 h	Antifactor Xa assay
Heparin	Anticoagulant	Factors IIa and Xa antagonist (indirect[a])	1.5 h	Protamine	Stop 6 h	PTT
Warfarin	Anticoagulant	Vitamin K epoxide reductase antagonist	2–4 d	Vitamin K, FFP, recombinant factor VII	Stop 4–5 d	PT
Rivaroxaban	Anticoagulant	Factor Xa antagonist (direct)	7–11 h	Andexanet alfa	Stop 2–4 d	Antifactor Xa assay
Apixaban	Anticoagulant	Factor Xa antagonist (direct)	8–15 h	Andexanet alfa	Stop 1–2 d	Antifactor Xa assay
Dabigatran	Anticoagulant	Factor IIa antagonist (direct)	14–17 h	Idarucizumab	Stop 2–4 d	PTT
tPA	Fibrinolytic	Plasminogen activator	5 min	Antifibrinolytic	Stop 1 h	PT/PTT
Streptokinase	Fibrinolytic	Plasminogen activator	23 min	Antifibrinolytic	Stop 3 h	PT/PTT

ADP, Adenosine diphosphate; *ASA*, acetylsalicylic acid; *COX*, cyclooxygenase; *FFP*, fresh frozen plasma; *LMWH*, low-molecular-weight heparin, *NSAIDs*, nonsteroidal antiinflammatory drugs; *PT*, prothrombin time; *PTT*, partial thromboplastin time; *tPA*, tissue plasminogen activator.

[a]Antithrombin cofactor.

Adapted from Elisha S, Heiner J, Nagelhout J, et al. Venous thromboembolism: new concepts in perioperative management. *AANA J.* 2015;83(3):211–221.

BOX 2.23 Classification of Antiplatelet Drugs

Arachidonic Acid Inhibitors

1. COX inhibitors: aspirin, indobufen, triflusal, nonsteroidal antiinflammatory agents, sulfinpyrazone
2. Non-COX inhibition of arachidonic acid; phosphodiesterase inhibitors: dipyridamole, pentoxifylline, cilostazol, trapidil
3. Other: omega-3 fatty acids, eicosanoids (prostacyclin, prostaglandin analogs)

$P2Y_{12}$ ADP Receptor Inhibitors

1. Thienopyridines (ADP antagonists): ticlopidine, clopidogrel, prasugrel
2. ATP derivatives: cangrelor
3. CPTPs: ticagrelor

Thrombin Protease-Activated Receptor 1 Inhibitors

1. Vorapaxar, E-5555

Platelet Glycoprotein IIb/IIIa Receptor Blockers

1. Intravenous: abciximab, tirofiban, eptifibatide

Drugs With Secondary Antiplatelet Activity

1. Direct thrombin inhibitors, heparin, nitrates, fibrates, calcium channel antagonists, others

ADP, Adenosine diphosphate; *ATP,* adenosine triphosphate; *COX,* cyclooxygenase; *CPTPs,* cyclopentyltriazolopyrimidines.

From Wiviott SD, Giugliano RP. Non–ST-segment elevation acute coronary syndromes. In: Antman EM, Sabatine MS, eds. *Cardiovascular Therapeutics: A Companion to Braunwald's Heart Disease.* 4th ed. Elsevier; 2013:153–177.

TABLE 2.57 Neuraxial Anesthesia in Patients Receiving Antithrombotic Therapy

Drug	Contraindications and Comments
Antiplatelet medications	• NSAIDs: no contraindication • Discontinue ticlopidine 14 d, clopidogrel 7 d, GP IIB/IIIa inhibitors 8–48 h in advance • Ticagrelor 5–7 d; prasugrel 7–10 d • Epidural catheter removal: 6- to 24-h delay until restarting ticagrelor, prasugrel, or clopidogrel
Unfractionated heparin, subcutaneous	• No contraindication with twice-daily dosing and total daily dose < 10,000 units • Consider delaying heparin until after block if technical difficulty anticipated • The safety of neuraxial blockade in patients receiving doses > 10,000 units/d of UFH or more than twice-daily dosing of UFH has not been established.
Unfractionated heparin, intravenous	• Heparinize 1 h after neuraxial technique • Remove catheter 2–4 h after last heparin dose • No mandatory delay if traumatic insertion
LMWH	• Twice-daily dosing: LMWH 24 h after surgery, regardless of technique • Remove epidural catheter 2 h before first dose of LMWH
Warfarin	• Normal INR (before neuraxial technique) • Remove catheter when INR ≤ 1.5 (initiation of therapy)
Fondaparinux	• Single injection, atraumatic needle placement, or alternate thromboprophylaxis • Avoid indwelling catheters
Direct thrombin inhibitors	• ASRAPM: insufficient information; suggest avoiding neuraxial techniques • The Society for Anesthesia and Resuscitation of Belgium and the German Society of Anaesthesiology and Intensive Care Medicine: needle placement 8–10 h after dose; delay subsequent doses 2–6 h after needle placement
Thrombolytics	Absolute contraindication
Herbal therapy	• No evidence for mandatory discontinuation before placement neuraxial technique • Be aware of potential drug interactions with the "3 Gs": *Ginkgo biloba,* garlic, and ginseng

Continued

TABLE 2.57 Neuraxial Anesthesia in Patients Receiving Antithrombotic Therapy—cont'd

Drug	Contraindications and Comments
Factor Xa inhibitors: rivaroxaban, apixaban	• Time between epidural anesthetic technique and next anticoagulant dose: rivaroxaban, 4–6 h; apixaban, 6 h • Time before last anticoagulant dose and epidural catheter removal: rivaroxaban, 22–26 h; apixaban, 26–30 h • Time between removal of epidural catheter and next anticoagulant dose: rivaroxaban and apixaban, 4–6 h

For patients undergoing deep plexus or peripheral blocks, use these same recommendations.
ASRAPM, American Society of Regional Anesthesia and Pain Management; *GP*, glycoprotein; *INR*, international normalized ratio; *LMWH*, low-molecular-weight heparin; *NSAIDs*, nonsteroidal antiinflammatory drugs; *UFH*, unfractionated heparin.
Adapted from Elisha S, Heiner J, Nagelhout J, et al. Venous thromboembolism: new concepts in perioperative management. *AANA J.* 2015;83(3):211–221.

BOX 2.24 Procedures That May Be Performed Without Discontinuing Warfarin

Ophthalmic
- Cataract extractions
- Trabeculectomies

Dental
- Restorations
- Endodontics
- Prosthetics
- Uncomplicated extractions
- Dental hygiene treatment

Dermatologic
- Mohs micrographic surgery
- Simple excisions

Gastrointestinal
- Upper endoscopy and colonoscopy with or without biopsy
- Endoscopic retrograde cholangiopancreatography (ERCP) without sphincterotomy
- Biliary stent insertion without sphincterotomy
- Endosonography without fine-needle aspiration
- Push enteroscopy

Orthopedic or Podiatric
- Joint and soft tissue aspirations and injections
- Nail avulsions
- Phenol matrixectomies

From Elisha S, Heiner JS, Nagelhout JJ. *Nurse Anesthesia*. 7th ed. Elsevier; 2023.

Thromboembolism

- Most patients with acute VTE have traditionally been treated initially (5–10 days) with a parenteral anticoagulant such as low-molecular-weight heparin (LMWH), fondaparinux (Arixtra and generics), or unfractionated heparin (UFH), with an vitamin potassium antagonist such as warfarin (Coumadin and others) started at the same time (Box 2.26 and Table 2.58).
- After the parenteral anticoagulant is discontinued, warfarin is continued for at least 3 months and sometimes indefinitely.
- Two direct oral anticoagulants, apixaban (Eliquis) and rivaroxaban (Xarelto), have recently been approved as monotherapy for initial treatment of VTE, and two others, dabigatran (Pradaxa) and edoxaban (Savaysa), have been approved for use after initial treatment with a parenteral anticoagulant (Table 2.59).
- For primary prevention of VTE, LMWH has generally been recommended for orthopedic and nonorthopedic surgery patients for whom postoperative prophylaxis is indicated.
- Rivaroxaban and apixaban are FDA approved for prevention of VTE after knee or hip replacement surgery. Dabigatran is approved after hip replacement surgery (Table 2.60).

Antifibrinolytics

Tranexamic Acid (Lysteda)

Tranexamic acid (TXA) and ε-aminocaproic acid are used for antifibrinolytic therapy in major procedures such as

BOX 2.25 Perioperative Considerations for Patients With Coronary Stents

Stents

- Type of stent(s) (e.g., bare metal stent [BMS], drug-eluting stent [DES])
- When were stent(s) placed?
- Complications during the revascularization, such as malposition, longer length, overlapping

Antiplatelet Therapy

- What is antiplatelet regimen?
- What is the recommended duration of antiplatelet therapy?
- Consult patient cardiologist regarding antiplatelet management.

Elective Noncardiac Surgery

1. Elective noncardiac surgery should be delayed 30 days after BMS implantation and optimally 6 months after DES implantation.
2. In patients treated with dual-antiplatelet therapy (DAPT) after coronary stent implantation who must undergo surgical procedures that mandate the discontinuation of P2Y12 inhibitor therapy (clopidogrel or ticagrelor), it is recommended that aspirin be continued if possible and the P2Y12 platelet receptor inhibitor be restarted as soon as possible after surgery.
3. When noncardiac surgery is required in patients currently taking a P2Y12 inhibitor, a consensus decision among treating clinicians regarding the relative risks of surgery and discontinuation or continuation of antiplatelet therapy can be useful.
4. Elective noncardiac surgery after DES implantation in patients for whom P2Y12 inhibitor therapy will need to be discontinued may be considered after 3 months if the risk of further delay of surgery is greater than the expected risks of stent thrombosis.
5. Elective noncardiac surgery should not be performed within 30 days after BMS implantation or within 3 months after DES implantation in patients in whom DAPT will need to be discontinued perioperatively.

Nonelective Surgery

1. *Determine risk for surgical bleeding:* If not at high risk, continue DAPT. Discontinuation of DAPT in patients with incomplete stent endothelialization markedly increases the risk of stent thrombosis, myocardial infarction, and death.
2. *High risk for bleeding:* Risk primarily associated with closed-space surgeries (i.e., medullary canal spine surgery, intracranial surgery, posterior chamber eye surgery, and possibly prostate surgery) where increased tissue pressure would be deleterious. If DAPT must be interrupted, aspirin should be continued when possible. An evolving treatment option involves "bridging therapy" anticoagulation in which drugs of short duration (glycoprotein inhibitor, e.g., tirofiban, eptifibatide; direct thrombin inhibitor, e.g., bivalirudin; unfractionated heparin; low-molecular-weight heparin; nonsteroidal antiinflammatory drugs, e.g., flurbiprofen; cyclooxygenase-1 [COX-1] inhibitors) are administered for up to 6 hours during the surgery, with the goal of preventing stent thrombosis while DAPT is interrupted. Restart DAPT as soon as possible after the surgery.
3. Surgery should be performed in an institution where higher-acuity care and an interventional cardiologist are available when possible. Consult before surgery to determine procedural complexities and determine optimal antiplatelet therapy and requisite patient management.

Adapted from Fleisher LA, Roizen MF, Roizen J, et al. *Essence of Anesthesia Practice*. 4th ed. Elsevier; 2018.

cardiac surgery. The medication is also conventionally used to reduce bleeding in patients with hemophilia and von Willebrand disease. Both drugs prevent plasminogen from binding to fibrin by occupying the plasminogen lysine-binding site. Plasmin activation and subsequent fibrin degradation are inhibited because tissue plasminogen activator and plasminogen can no longer colocalize on the surface of fibrin.

Dose

- In cardiac surgery with cardiopulmonary bypass, the typical loading dose of IV TXA is 10–15 mg/kg after systemic anticoagulation. Continuous infusion of TXA is commonly used at 7.5 mg/kg/h for TXA until the end of surgery.
- Although there is a wide range in dosage and application, another suggested protocol for TXA is administration of an initial loading dose after heparin administration of 10 mg/kg with a maintenance dose of 1 mg/kg/h, or alternatively, a repetition dose of 5 mg/kg every 2 hours until chest closure after coronary artery bypass grafting.
- *Onset and duration:* IV onset is rapid, with peak action at approximately 1 hour and a dose-dependent duration of 6 hours.

BOX 2.26 VTE Recommendations

Treatment of Acute VTE

- LMWH or fondaparinux, with or without warfarin, has generally been recommended for initial treatment (5–10 days) of acute deep venous thrombosis (DVT) or pulmonary embolism (PE).
- Apixaban and rivaroxaban are oral alternatives for initial use as monotherapy in patients without active cancer.
- If a parenteral anticoagulant (UFH, LMWH, or fondaparinux) is used for initial treatment, warfarin or a DOAC (apixaban, rivaroxaban, dabigatran, or edoxaban) can be used for long-term treatment. A DOAC is preferred over warfarin.
- LMWH is recommended for initial and long-term treatment of patients with active cancer.
- Warfarin or UFH is recommended for treatment of patients with CrCl < 30 mL/min.
- LMWH is recommended for use during pregnancy.

Duration of Anticoagulation

- Patients with VTE should be treated for a minimum of 3 months.
- Patients with an unprovoked VTE and those with active cancer have the highest risk of recurrence; they should generally be treated for > 3 months.

Extended Treatment

- After 6–12 months of anticoagulation therapy, extended treatment for 1 year with low doses of apixaban or rivaroxaban can prevent symptomatic recurrences of VTE.
- After stopping an anticoagulant, aspirin therapy can reduce the risk of recurrence.

Primary Prevention of VTE

- LMWH is recommended for prevention of VTE in most orthopedic and nonorthopedic surgical patients for whom postoperative prophylaxis is indicated.
- Apixaban, rivaroxaban, and dabigatran are oral alternatives for prevention of VTE in patients undergoing knee or hip replacement surgery.
- The DOAC betrixaban is an oral alternative to parenteral treatment in patients hospitalized for an acute medical illness who are at increased risk of thrombosis.

DOAC, Direct oral anticoagulant; *LMWH,* low-molecular-weight heparin; *UFH,* unfractionated heparin; *VTE,* venous thromboembolism.
From Elisha S, Heiner JS, Nagelhout JJ. *Nurse Anesthesia.* 7th ed. Elsevier; 2023.

Precautions and contraindications

- Not approved for pediatric hemorrhage
- Subarachnoid hemorrhage
- Disseminated intravascular coagulation
- Concurrent thrombosis management
- Concurrent seizure activity
- Severe renal impairment
- Concurrent factor concentrate (cryoprecipitate) administration

KNOWLEDGE CHECK

1. DAPT is generally continued for how long after placement of a drug-eluting coronary stent?
   a. 1 month
   b. 6 months
   c. 12 months
   d. 24 months
2. Tranexamic acid should be used with caution or is contraindicated in patients with *(Select all that apply.)*
   a. disseminated intravascular coagulation.
   b. hepatic disease.
   c. subarachnoid hemorrhage.
   d. asthma.
   e. sepsis.

Answers can be found in Appendix A.

ANTIEMETICS

Anesthetic Implications

- Postanesthesia care unit (PACU) discharge may be delayed with PONV, or hospital readmission may be necessary for postdischarge nausea and vomiting (PDNV).

Risk Factors

- Several nonpharmacologic strategies to reduce the risk of PONV include the use of regional rather than general anesthesia when feasible.
- Preferential use of propofol infusions and avoidance of volatile anesthetics and nitrous oxide
- Reducing or avoiding the use of intraoperative and postoperative opioids and administering nonopioid analgesics if appropriate
- Adequate hydration is also helpful, especially in children (Box 2.27).

Multimodal Antiemetic Therapy

- Because the causes of nausea and vomiting are multifactorial, a multimodal approach using multiple drugs with different mechanisms is the most effective prophylaxis and therapy (Box 2.28).

TABLE 2.58 Some Parenteral Anticoagulants Used to Prevent VTE

Drug	Usual Adult Treatment Dosage	Usual Adult Prophylaxis Dosage[a]	Cost[b] ($)
Unfractionated Heparin (UFH)			
Generic	80 units/kg IV bolus, then 18 units/kg/h IV[c] or 333 units/kg subcut initially, followed by 250 units/kg subcut q12h[c]	5000 units subcut q8–12h	651.00
Low-Molecular-Weight Heparins (LMWHs)			
Dalteparin—Fragmin (Pfizer)	200 international units/kg subcut once/d[c,d,e]	2500–5000 international units subcut once/d[d]	3527.40
Enoxaparin—generic Lovenox (Sanofi)	1 mg/kg subcut bid or 1.5 mg/kg subcut once/d[c,d]	30 mg subcut bid or 40 mg subcut once/d[d]	630.00 3473.40
Direct Thrombin Inhibitor			
Desirudin—Iprivask (Valeant)	Not an FDA-approved indication	15 mg subcut q12h[d,f]	5400.00[g]
Factor Xa Inhibitor			
Fondaparinux—generic Arixtra (Mylan)	5–10 mg subcut once/d[c,d,h,i]	2.5 mg subcut once/d[d,i,j]	1755.00 3926.10

FDA, US Food and Drug Administration; *IV*, intravenous; *VTE*, venous thromboembolism.
[a]Prophylaxis is recommended for ≥10 to 14 days and for up to 35 days after major orthopedic surgery (Falck-Ytter Y, Francis CW, Johanson NA, et al. *Chest.* 2012;141:e278S).
[b]Approximate WAC for 30 days' treatment of a 70-kg patient at the lowest usual adult dosage for treatment. WAC = wholesaler acquisition cost or manufacturer's published price to wholesalers. WAC represents a published catalog or list price and may not represent an actual transactional price. Source: Analy-Source Monthly. February 5, 2018. Reprinted with permission by First Databank, Inc. All rights reserved. Copyright 2018. www.fdbhealth.com/policies/drug-pricing-policy.
[c]Warfarin is generally started at the same time. The parenteral anticoagulant can be stopped after a minimum of 5 days when INR is ≥2 for at least 24 hours (Smythe MA, Priziola J, Dobesh PP, et al. *J Thromb Thrombolysis.* 2016;41:165).
[d]Dosage adjustments may be needed for renal impairment.
[e]For extended VTE treatment in patients with cancer, the dose is 200 IU/kg subcut once/d for 30 days, followed by 150 IU/kg subcut once/d × 5 months (max 18,000 IU/day).
[f]Has only been studied for up to 12 days' use.
[g]Cost for 12 days' prophylaxis.
[h]Dose is 5 mg if patient weighs <50 kg, 7.5 mg if 50–100 kg, 10 mg if >100 kg.
[i]Contraindicated in patients with creatinine clearance (CrCl) 30 mL/min.
[j]Dosage for adults weighing >50 kg. Contraindicated in patients weighing <50 kg.

Glucocorticoids

- Decadron 4 mg IV administered within 1 hour before the induction of anesthesia is recommended.
- The efficacy of dexamethasone 4 mg IV is similar to that of ondansetron 8 mg IV.
- The mechanism of action is unclear, although several theories have been proposed. Glucocorticoids may act via the following mechanisms: (1) an antiinflammatory effect; (2) direct central action at the solitary tract nucleus; (3) interaction with the neurotransmitter serotonin, receptor proteins tachykinin NK1 and NK2, alpha-adrenaline, and prostaglandins; (4) maintaining the normal physiologic functions of organs and systems; (5) regulation of the hypothalamic–pituitary–adrenal axis (HPA); and (6) reducing pain and the concomitant use of opioids, which in turn reduces opioid-related nausea and vomiting.
- The effect on wound healing and infection after a single dose of dexamethasone is minimal.
- An increase in blood glucose may occur 6–12 hours postoperatively in patients with impaired glucose tolerance, type 2 diabetes, or obesity.

5-HT_3 Receptor Antagonists

- Ondansetron is the most widely used antiemetic and the gold standard for comparison of other agents.
- The standard dose is 4 mg, and it is commonly administered prior to extubation.

TABLE 2.59 Some Oral Anticoagulants Used to Prevent VTE

Drug	Usual Adult Treatment Dosage	Usual Adult Prophylaxis Dosage[a]	Cost[b] ($)
Vitamin K Antagonist			
Warfarin—generic	2–10 mg once/d[c,d]	2–10 mg once/d[c]	7.80
Coumadin (BMS)			64.50
Jantoven (USL)			10.80
Direct Thrombin Inhibitor			
Dabigatran etexilate—Pradaxa (Boehringer Ingelheim)	150 mg bid[e-h]	110 mg once, then 220 mg once/d[e-g]	400.60
Factor Xa Inhibitors			
Apixaban—Eliquis (BMS)	10 mg bid × 7 days, then 5 mg bid[i,j]	2.5 mg bid[i]	419.00
Betrixaban—Bevyxxa (Portola)	Not an FDA-approved indication	160 mg once, then 80 mg once/d for a total of 35–42 d[e,k,l]	450.00
Edoxaban—Savaysa (Daiichi-Sankyo)	60 mg once/d[e,h,m]	Not an FDA-approved indication	336.50
Rivaroxaban—Xarelto (Janssen)	15 mg bid × 3 weeks, then 20 mg once/d[e,g,n,o]	10 mg once/d[e,g]	333.30

FDA, US Food and Drug Administration; *VTE*, venous thromboembolism.

[a]Prophylaxis is recommended for a minimum of 10–14 days and for up to 35 days after major orthopedic surgery (Falck-Ytter Y, Francis CW, Johanson NA, et al. *Chest.* 2012; 141:e278S).

[b]Approximate WAC for 30 days' treatment at the lowest usual adult dosage for treatment. Cost of betrixaban is based on dosage for prophylaxis. WAC = wholesaler acquisition cost or manufacturer's published price to wholesalers. WAC represents a published catalog or list price and may not represent an actual transactional price. Source: AnalySource Monthly. February 5, 2018. Reprinted with permission by First Databank, Inc. All rights reserved. Copyright 2018. www.fdbhealth.com/policies/drug-pricing-policy.

[c]Monitor daily and adjust dose until international normalized ratio (INR) is in therapeutic range (INR 2–3).

[d]Requires overlap with low-molecular-weight heparin (LMWH), fondaparinux, or unfractionated heparin (UFH) for ≥5 days and until INR is ≥2 for at least 24 hours.

[e]Dosage adjustments may be needed for renal impairment.

[f]Avoid coadministration with P-glycoprotein (P-gp) inhibitors in patients with creatinine clearance (CrCl) <50 mL/min.

[g]Should not be used in patients with CrCl <30 mL/min.

[h]FDA approved for treatment of VTE after 5–10 days of initial therapy with a parenteral anticoagulant.

[i]When coadministered with dual strong CYP3A4/P-gp inhibitors, reduce dose by 50%; patients taking 2.5 mg bid should not take dual strong CYP3A4/P-gp inhibitors.

[j]For extended treatment after at least 6 months of treatment for deep vein thrombosis (DVT) or pulmonary embolism (PE), the dosage for reduction in risk of recurrence of VTE is 2.5 mg bid.

[k]Should not be used in patients with CrCl <15 mL/min.

[l]Dosage in patients taking a P-gp inhibitor concurrently is 80 mg once, then 40 mg once/d.

[m]Dosage is 30 mg once/d in patients taking a P-gp inhibitor concurrently or who weigh 40 kg.

[n]Avoid coadministration with dual P-gp/strong CYP3A4 inhibitors or inducers. Avoid coadministration in patients with CrCl 15<80 mL/min taking dual P-gp/moderate CYP3A4 inhibitors.

[o]For extended treatment after at least 6 months of treatment for DVT or PE. The dosage for reduction in risk of recurrence of VTE is 10 mg once/d.

TABLE 2.60 FDA-Approved Indications of Anticoagulants for VTE

Heparin	
Unfractionated Heparin	• Prophylaxis of DVT and PE • Treatment of DVT and PE
Low Molecular-Weight Heparins (LMWHs)	
Enoxaparin (Lovenox, and generics)	• Prophylaxis of DVT after abdominal surgery or hip or knee replacement surgery • Prophylaxis of DVT in medical patients with severely restricted mobility during acute illness • Treatment of acute DVT (without PE in outpatients and with or without PE in inpatients)
Dalteparin (Fragmin)	• Prophylaxis of DVT after abdominal surgery or hip replacement surgery • Prophylaxis of DVT in medical patients with severely restricted mobility during acute illness • Reduction in the risk of recurrent symptomatic VTE in cancer patients (extended treatment for 6 months)
Parenteral Direct Thrombin Inhibitor	
Desirudin (Iprivask)	• Prophylaxis of DVT after hip replacement surgery
Parenteral Factor Xa Inhibitor	
Fondaparinux (Arixtra, and generics)	• Prophylaxis of DVT after hip fracture surgery, hip or knee replacement surgery, or abdominal surgery • Treatment of acute DVT or PE in combination with warfarin
Vitamin K Antagonist	
Warfarin (Coumadin, and others)	• Prophylaxis of DVT and PE • Treatment of DVT and PE
Direct Oral Anticoagulants (DOACs)	
Apixaban (Eliquis)	• Prophylaxis of DVT after hip or knee replacement surgery • Treatment of DVT and PE • Reduction in the risk of recurrent DVT and PE after initial treatment lasting at least 6 months
Betrixaban (Bevyxxa)	• Prophylaxis of VTE in patients hospitalized for an acute medical illness who are at risk for thromboembolic complications due to moderate or severe restricted mobility and other risk factors for VTE
Dabigatran etexilate (Pradaxa)	• Prophylaxis of DVT and PE after hip replacement surgery • Treatment of DVT and PE after 5–10 days of initial therapy with a parenteral anticoagulant • Reduction in the risk of recurrent DVT and PE after initial therapy
Edoxaban (Savaysa)	• Treatment of DVT and PE after 5–10 days of initial therapy with a parenteral anticoagulant
Rivaroxaban (Xarelto)	• Prophylaxis of DVT after hip or knee replacement surgery • Treatment of DVT and PE • Reduction in the risk of recurrent DVT and/or PE after initial treatment lasting at least 6 months

DVT, Deep vein thrombosis; *FDA*, US Food and Drug Administration; *PE*, pulmonary embolism; *VTE*, venous thromboembolism.

BOX 2.27 Risk Factors for Nausea and Vomiting

Postoperative Nausea and Vomiting
- Female sex
- Age <50 y
- History of PONV
- High doses of intraoperative or postoperative opioids
- Duration of surgery more than 1 h
- Laparoscopic procedures

Postoperative Discharge Nausea and Vomiting
- Female sex
- Age <50 y
- History of PONV
- PONV in PACU

PACU, Postanesthesia care unit; *PONV*, postoperative nausea and vomiting.
From Gan TJ, Diemunsch P, Habib AS, et al. Consensus guidelines for the management of postoperative nausea and vomiting. *Anesth Analg*. 2014;118(1):85–113; Apfel CC, Philip BK, Cakmakkaya OS, et al. Who is at risk for postdischarge nausea and vomiting after ambulatory surgery? *Anesthesiology*. 2012;117(3):475–486; Apfel CC, Heidrich FM, Jukar-Rao S, et al. Evidence-based analysis of risk factors for postoperative nausea and vomiting. *Br J Anaesth*. 2012;109(5):742–753.

- At higher doses, QT interval prolongation and torsades de pointes can occur.
- The relatively short duration of action of 4–6 hours makes it unlikely to be effective for PDNV.
- The efficacy of the 5-HT antagonists increases when combined with dexamethasone (Box 2.29).

Neurokinin 1 Receptor Antagonists

- Aprepitant (Emend) and its IV prodrug fosaprepitant (Emend), netupitant/palonosetron (Akynzeo), and rolapitant (Varubi) are substance P/neurokinin-1 (NK-1) receptor antagonists.
- Rolapitant is characterized by a long half-life of 180 hours and an active metabolite with a half-life of 158 hours.

Transdermal Scopolamine

- A scopolamine patch is an effective antiemetic when applied the evening before surgery.
- It has an onset of action of 2–4 hours and a minimum duration of 24 hours.
- Common side effects: sedation, blurred vision, dizziness, and dry mouth

BOX 2.28 Current Antiemetic Medications by Drug Classes

Corticosteroids
Dexamethasone, methylprednisolone

Phenothiazines
Chlorpromazine, prochlorperazine

Butyrophenones
Droperidol, haloperidol

Benzamides
Metoclopramide

Anticholinergics
Scopolamine

Antihistamines
Hydroxyzine, dimenhydrinate, meclizine

5-HT$_3$ Antagonists
Ondansetron, dolasetron, granisetron, tropisetron, palonosetron, ramosetron

NK-1 Antagonists
Aprepitant, vestipitant, fosaprepitant, netupitant, rolapitant, casopitant

Benzodiazepines
Midazolam, lorazepam

5-HT3, 5-Hydroxytryptamine-3; *NK-1*, neurokinin-1.
From Elisha S, Heiner JS, Nagelhout JJ. *Nurse Anesthesia*. 7th ed. Elsevier; 2023.

BOX 2.29 Medical Conditions at Risk for Development of Pronged QT Syndrome

- Congestive heart failure
- Bradycardia
- Hypertension
- Heart block
- Cardiac hypertrophy
- Cardiomyopathy
- Hypomagnesemia
- Medications
  - Diuretics
  - Antihypotensives
  - Antidepressants
  - Antiarrhythmics

Adapted from Kovac AL. Update on the management of postoperative nausea and vomiting. *Drugs*. 2013;73(14):1525–1547.

Metoclopramide

- Metoclopramide exerts a mild dopamine-receptor-blocking effect.
- Minimal effects occur with doses of less than 20 mg.
- Half-life: 30–45 minutes
- Dyskinesia or extrapyramidal effects can be seen with higher doses.
- Use is contraindicated in patients with PD and bowel obstruction.

Anesthetic Implications

- Metoclopramide is a dopaminergic (D_2) and serotonergic ($5\text{-}HT_3$, peripheral $5\text{-}HT_4$ at higher doses) antagonist with gastric prokinetic properties to enhance gastric emptying.
- Its use is contraindicated in PD and other motion disorders because of extrapyramidal symptoms (EPSs). It is also contraindicated for patients with bowel obstruction because the gastrokinetic effects can result in intestinal rupture.
- Parkinson-like symptoms are produced by central dopamine receptor blockade.
- Mild antiemetic properties in doses of 20 mg or higher

Gastric Acid Secretions

- The ASA recommends the "timely administration of oral nonparticulate antacids, IV (IV) H_2-receptor antagonists, and/or metoclopramide for aspiration prophylaxis" before the induction of anesthesia in pregnant patients.
- Metoclopramide IV significantly decreases gastric volume in as little as 15 minutes, but it does not affect gastric pH.
- Gastric hypomotility associated with prior opioid administration reduces the effectiveness of metoclopramide.
- Dyskinesia or EPSs can be seen with higher doses ($\geq$20 mg).
- EPSs are caused by the drug's antidopaminergic effects, especially if administered as a rapid IV bolus.
- Symptoms associated with EPSs include the following:
  - Dystonia (continuous muscle contractions and spasm)
  - Akathisia (motor dysfunction)
  - Parkinsonism (rigidity)
  - Bradykinesia (slowed movements)
  - Tardive dyskinesia (tremors or jerky movements)
- Treatment of EPSs:
  - Diphenhydramine 25–50 mg IV, benztropine 1–2 mg IM

Clinical Use of Antiemetics

- Multimodal PONV and PDNV prophylaxis should be instituted for patients at moderate to high risk for PONV.
- All prophylaxis in children at moderate or high risk for PONV should include combination therapy using a $5\text{-}HT_3$ antagonist and a second drug.
- The effects of interventions from different drug classes are additive, and combining interventions has an additive effect in risk reduction.
- When rescue therapy is required, the antiemetic should be chosen from a different therapeutic class than the drugs used initially.
- If PONV occurs within 6 hours postoperatively, patients should not receive a repeat dose of the prophylactic antiemetic (Table 2.61).

KNOWLEDGE CHECK

1. Which medication can produce QT interval prolongation?
   a. Ondansetron
   b. Dexamethasone
   c. Aprepitant
   d. Metoclopramide
2. Which is the mechanism of action by which metoclopramide produces antiemetic effects?
   a. Gastric prokinetic effect
   b. Lowering intragastric pressure
   c. Antihistamine effect
   d. Dopamine-blocking effect
3. Which antiemetic medication can cause hyperglycemia?
   a. Scopolamine
   b. Decadron
   c. Metoclopramide
   d. Ondansetron
4. The antiemetic effects associated with ondansetron are caused by
   a. serotonin receptor antagonism.
   b. dopamine receptor blockade.
   c. antihistamine.
   d. neurokinin antagonist.
5. Which condition is a contraindication to metoclopramide administration? (*Select all that apply.*)
   a. Asthma
   b. Gastric ulcers
   c. Parkinson's disease
   d. Bowel obstruction

Answers can be found in Appendix A.

TABLE 2.61 Drugs for Postoperative and Postdischarge Nausea and Vomiting

Drug	Usual Adult Dose	Comment
$5\text{-}HT_3$ Antagonists		
Ondansetron (Zofran)	Adult 4–8 mg IV Child 50–100 mcg/kg (max 4 mg)	Effective for prevention of both nausea and vomiting; more effective for PONV than PDNV. Administer at the end of the procedure.
Granisetron (Kytril)	Adult 1 mg IV Child 40 mcg/kg up to 0.6 mg	Administer at the end of the procedure.
Palonosetron (Aloxi)	0.075 mg IV	Long duration makes it effective for PDNV.
Dopamine Antagonists		
Droperidol (Inapsine)	0.625–1.25 mg IV	See text for discussion of black-box warning.
Haloperidol (Haldol)	1–2 mg IV	Sedation, extrapyramidal symptoms, and QT prolongation may occur.
Metoclopramide (Reglan)	10–20 mg IV	Contraindicated in patients with gastric obstruction because of prokinetic effects. Also contraindicated in patients with Parkinson disease.
Prochlorperazine (Compazine)	10 mg IV	Sedation prominent
Antihistamines		
Hydroxyzine (Atarax)	12.5–25 mg IV	Sedation prominent
Promethazine (Phenergan)	12.5–25 mg IV	Sedation prominent
Diphenhydramine (Benadryl)	25 mg IV or IM	Sedation prominent
Glucocorticoid		
Dexamethasone (Decadron)	Adult 4–8 mg IV Child 150 mcg/kg up to 8 mg	May produce hyperglycemia postoperatively in diabetics
Anticholinergic		
Scopolamine transdermal (Transderm-Scōp)	2.5-cm^2 patch contains 1.5 mg of scopolamine	Long duration may make it effective for PDNV.
Neurokinin 1 Antagonist		
Aprepitant (Emend)	40 mg PO	Long duration may make it effective for PDNV.
Rolapitant (Varubi)	90 mg PO	Approved for chemotherapy-induced nausea and vomiting. Should not be taken more than once every 2 wk.

$5\text{-}HT_3$, Serotonin; *PDNV*, postdischarge nausea and vomiting; *PONV*, postoperative nausea and vomiting.
From Elisha S, Heiner JS, Nagelhout JJ. *Nurse Anesthesia*. 7th ed. Elsevier; 2023.

HISTAMINE RECEPTOR ANTAGONISTS

- Histamines are released from mast cells, basophils, and neurons within the CNS. Histamine causes contraction of smooth muscles in the airways; increases the secretion of acid in the stomach; and stimulates the release of neurotransmitters in the CNS through stimulation of three primary receptor subtypes, H_1, H_2, and H_3. A fourth H_4 receptor has been identified but not completely characterized.
- Histamine receptor antagonists do not inhibit release of histamine but rather bind to receptors and prevent responses mediated by histamine.
- H_3- and H_4-receptor modulators do not currently play a role in anesthetic practice.

- The H_4 receptor is expressed on mast cells, dendritic cells, basophils, and T lymphocytes. Activation of the H_4 receptor induces chemotaxis of immune cells.
- Activation of H_3 receptors inhibits the synthesis and release of histamine from neurons in the CNS, acting as presynaptic autoreceptors.
- In patients with chronic urticaria, H_1-receptor antagonists relieve pruritus and decrease the number, size, and duration of urticarial lesions.
- The second-generation H_1-receptor antagonists (cetirizine, fexofenadine, loratadine, desloratadine, azelastine) are supplanting first-generation drugs (diphenhydramine, chlorpheniramine, cyproheptadine) in the treatment of allergic rhinoconjunctivitis and chronic urticaria.
- Cimetidine, ranitidine, famotidine, and nizatidine are H_2-receptor antagonists that produce selective and reversible inhibition of H_2-receptor–mediated secretion of hydrogen ions by parietal cells in the stomach. The relationship between gastric hypersecretion of fluid containing high concentrations of hydrogen ions and peptic ulcer disease emphasizes the potential value of a drug that selectively blocks this response. Despite the presence of H_2 receptors throughout the body, inhibition of histamine binding to the receptors on gastric parietal cells is the beneficial effect of H_2-receptor antagonists.
- The relative potencies of the four H_2-receptor antagonists for inhibition of secretion of gastric hydrogen ions vary from 20- to 50-fold, with cimetidine being the least potent and famotidine the most potent.
- The onset of action to reliably increase gastric pH is 60–90 minutes.
- The duration of inhibition ranges from approximately 6 hours for cimetidine to 10 hours for ranitidine, famotidine, and nizatidine.
- Discontinuation of chronic H_2-receptor antagonist therapy is followed by rebound hypersecretion of gastric acid (Table 2.62).

Anesthetic Implications

- Uses: Increase gastric pH in patients considered "full stomach"; mild antiemetic properties, antipruritic, allergic rhinitis, treatment for anaphylaxis

TABLE 2.62 Antihistamines

Antihistamine Group	Generic Name	Average Oral Adult Doses
First-Generation H_1-Type Antihistamines		
Alkylamine	Brompheniramine (Dimetapp)	4 mg q4–6h
	Chlorpheniramine (Chlor-Trimeton)	4 mg q4–6h (short acting); 8–12 mg q8–12h (long acting)
Amino alkyl ether (ethanolamine)	Clemastine fumarate	1.34 mg bid or 2.68 mg qd–tid
	Diphenhydramine (Benadryl)	25–50 mg q4–6h
Ethylenediamine	Pyrilamine (Triaminic)	30 mg bid
Phenothiazine	Promethazine (Phenergan)	10–12.5 mg qid
	Trimeprazine (Temaril)	2.5 mg q6h
Piperidine	Azatadine	1–2 mg q8–12h
	Cyproheptadine	4 mg q8h
	Diphenylpyraline	2 mg tid–qid
Piperazine	Hydroxyzine (Atarax)	25–100 mg tid–qid
Second-Generation H_1-Type Antihistamines		
Alkylamine	Acrivastine (combined with pseudoephedrine in allergy medication)	8 mg qid
Piperidine	Astemizole (Hismanal)	10 mg qd
	Loratadine (Claritin)	10 mg qd
	Fexofenadine (Allegra)	60 mg bid or 180 mg qd
Piperazine	Cetirizine (Zyrtec)	5–10 mg/d

Continued

TABLE 2.62 Antihistamines—cont'd

Antihistamine Group	Generic Name	Average Oral Adult Doses
H_2-Type Antihistamines		
	Cimetidine (Tagamet)	400 mg bid
	Ranitidine (Zantac)	150 mg bid
	Famotidine	10 mg bid
	Nizatidine	300 mg at bedtime
H_1- and H_2-Type Antihistamines	Doxepin (Sinequan)	10–25 mg at bedtime

Adapted from Rakel RE, Rakel DP. *Textbook of Family Medicine*. 9th ed. Elsevier; 2016.

- Administration of the H_2 blockers alone may cause a histamine reaction as a result of stimulation of presynaptic histamine receptor release and a lack of H_1 blockade.

Clinical Uses

- All nonspecific histamine receptor antagonists have sedative side effects that may delay recovery when administered immediately before the end of anesthesia.
- Diphenhydramine (Benadryl) and dimenhydrinate (an aminophylline salt of diphenhydramine) are histamine (H_1)-receptor antagonists known for their effectiveness in preventing or minimizing motion sickness and their relatively weak anticholinergic (antimuscarinic) activity.
- Cyclizine (Marezine) and promethazine (Atosil, Phenergan) have equivalent antihistaminic and anticholinergic properties.
- Diphenhydramine, cyclizine, and promethazine are effective for the prevention of PONV.
- Side effects: drowsiness, urinary retention, dry mouth, blurred vision, and EPSs.

KNOWLEDGE CHECK

1. Which histamine antagonist blocks histamine 1 receptors?
   a. Diphenhydramine
   b. Ranitidine
   c. Nizatidine
   d. Famotidine
2. In which time period do IV histamine receptor blockers reliably increase gastric pH?
   a. 10–30 minutes
   b. 60–90 minutes
   c. 100–130 minutes
   d. 140–170 minutes
3. Which is a side effect associated with antihistamines? (*Select all that apply.*)
   a. Urinary retention dry
   b. Blurred vision
   c. Serotonin syndrome
   d. Antiemetic effects
   e. Extrapyramidal reaction

Answers can be found in Appendix A.

ANTIEPILEPTIC DRUGS

Anesthetic Implications

- Valproate is the most widely prescribed drug used in the treatment of epilepsy (Table 2.63). It is also widely used for acute mania, bipolar disease, impulse-control disorders, migraine headaches, and neuropathic pain.
- It may affect platelet function and other coagulation factors; thus, laboratory coagulation tests (coagulation factors, fibrin formation, fibrinogen, platelet count, bleeding time, prothrombin time (PT), partial thromboplastin time (PTT), von Willebrand factor level, thromboelastography (TEG), and liver function tests (LFTs) should be obtained when considerable blood loss is anticipated.
- Valproate should be continued perioperatively if possible and should resume immediately postoperatively to decrease the risk of seizure.
- Increased sedation in elderly patients with alcohol and/or benzodiazepine use and delayed emergence after general anesthesia is possible.

TABLE 2.63 Treatment of Epilepsy[a]

Partial, Including Secondarily Generalized Seizures[b]

Drugs of Choice:	Some Alternatives:
Carbamazepine	Brivaracetam
Lamotrigine	Clobazam
Levetiracetam	Eslicarbazepine
Oxcarbazepine	Gabapentin Lacosamide Perampanel Phenytoin Pregabalin Topiramate Valproate Zonisamide

Primary Generalized Tonic-Clonic Seizures[b]

Drugs of Choice:	Some Alternatives:
Lamotrigine	Perampanel
Levetiracetam	Topiramate
Valproate	Zonisamide

Absence Seizures

Drugs of Choice:	Some Alternatives:
Ethosuximide	Clonazepam
Valproate	Lamotrigine Levetiracetam Zonisamide

Atypical Absence, Myoclonic, and Atonic Seizures

Drugs of Choice:	Some Alternatives:
Lamotrigine	Clobazam
Levetiracelam	Clonazepam
Valproate	Felbamate Rufinamide Topiramate Zonisamide

[a]Some of the drugs listed here have not been approved by the US Food and Drug Administration for such use. Approved indications can be found in the text.
[b]In the revised International League Against Epilepsy (ILAE) classification of seizure types, "partial" is replaced with "local" and "primary generalized" with "bilateral tonic-clonic" (Fisher, Cross JH, French JA, et al. Operational classification of seizure types by the International League Against Epilepsy: Position Paper of the ILAE Commission for Classification and Terminology. *Epilepsia*. 2017; 58(4):522–531.
From Drugs for epilepsy. *Med Lett Drugs Ther.* 2017;59(1526): 121–130.

Anticonvulsants

- Anticonvulsants or antiepileptics are commonly used in certain neuropathic pain syndromes when treatment is refractory to traditional analgesics.
- Anticonvulsants inhibit neuronal excitation and stabilize nerve membranes to decrease repetitive neural ectopic firing, which is common in neuropathic pain.
- Second-generation anticonvulsants such as gabapentin (Neurontin) and pregabalin (Lyrica) are the most widely used.
- Gabapentin and pregabalin are used for the management of postherpetic neuralgia, diabetic neuropathy, trigeminal neuralgia, and other neuropathic pain and chronic pain syndromes.
- Pregabalin and gabapentin exhibit anticonvulsant, anxiolytic, and antihyperalgesic effects.
- Common side effects are dose dependent and include dizziness, somnolence, peripheral edema, and weight gain.
- Pregabalin and gabapentin are also used as components in multimodal analgesia for acute postoperative pain management.
- Patients taking anticonvulsants as part of a chronic pain syndrome treatment regimen should continue taking their medication throughout the perioperative period.

KNOWLEDGE CHECK

1. Which laboratory result may be affected by the use of valproic acid? (*Select all that apply*)
   a. Fibrinogen
   b. Hemoglobin
   c. White blood cell count
   d. LFTs
2. Which is *not* a physiologic effect associated with gabapentin and pregabalin?
   a. Antiemetic
   b. Anxiolysis
   c. Anticonvulsant
   d. Antihyperalgesia

Answers can be found in Appendix A.

DANTROLENE

Anesthesia Implications

- Definitive pharmacologic treatment for MH
- Enhanced patient monitoring, earlier diagnosis and treatment, and the introduction of dantrolene

are responsible for the dramatic decrease in mortality from nearly 80% 30 years ago to less than 5% today.

- Mechanism of action: Dantrolene is a unique muscle relaxant that does not work at the neuromuscular junction as do standard neuromuscular blocking drugs. It binds to the ryanodine calcium channel (Ryanodine receptor type 1) and reduces calcium efflux from the sarcoplasmic reticulum, counteracting the abnormal intracellular calcium levels accompanying MH.
- Dantrolene may cause significant muscle weakness and respiratory insufficiency, especially in patients with preexisting muscle disease.
- Dantrolene may be efficacious in treating neuroleptic malignant syndrome.
- CCBs should not be administered with dantrolene because they may induce life-threatening myocardial depression and hyperkalemia.
- There are three preparations of dantrolene available: Dantrium, Revonto, and Ryanodex.
- The dose (mg/kg) should be calculated on the basis of actual body weight.
- The initial bolus does of dantrolene is 2.5 mg/kg to be repeated up to 10 mg/kg.
- The typical total dose used to treat an episode of MH is 6 mg/kg.
- If the cause of the hypermetabolism is indeed MH, the onset of action is approximately 6 minutes.
- Dantrium and Revonto are packaged as a 20-mg vial that must be reconstituted with 60 mL of *sterile water* for injection. There are 3 g of mannitol in each 20-mg vial of Dantrium/Revonto, which acts as an osmotic diuretic. With this preparation, the initial dantrolene dose (2.5 mg/kg) equates to 8–10 vials of Dantrium/Revonto for an average-weight adult patient. Thus, it is time-consuming to mix and administer the requisite doses during an MH emergency.
- Ryanodex is easier to reconstitute than Dantrium and Revonto. It is available as 250 mg per vial and only requires 5 mL of sterile water diluent. Therefore with Ryanodex, the initial dantrolene treatment can be administered more rapidly, and an initial loading dose for an average-weight adult patient is contained within one 250-mg vial. The provider should note that there is only 0.125 g of mannitol in each 250-mg vial of Ryanodex.

KNOWLEDGE CHECK

1. Which is the primary mechanism of action of dantrolene?
   a. Promoting calcium elimination in the kidneys and liver
   b. Inhibition of the temperature-regulating centers in the brain
   c. Inhibition of intracellular calcium release
   d. Muscle relaxation via an antimuscarinic effect
2. Which is the initial loading dose required for dantrolene?
   a. 1.0 mg/kg
   b. 1.5 mg/kg
   c. 2.0 mg/kg
   d. 2.5 mg/kg
3. In addition to dantrolene administration, which is a condition that contraindicates the use of CCBs during MH? (*Select all that apply.*)
   a. Hypertension
   b. Myocardial depression
   c. Dysrhythmias
   d. Hyperkalemia

Answers can be found in Appendix A.

HERBAL SUPPLEMENTS

Anesthesia Implications

- During the preoperative evaluation, patients should be queried regarding their use of nonprescription herbal medications to determine the herb's name, the duration of herbal therapy, and the dose taken.
- Certain herbal products are known to influence blood clotting, affect blood glucose levels, produce CNS stimulation or depression, or interact with psychotropic drugs (Table 2.64).
- Discontinuation of dietary supplements should be encouraged for a minimum of 2 weeks before anesthesia and surgery.

Dietary Supplements

- Dietary supplements (vitamins, minerals, herbs, amino acids, enzymes) are products ingested orally and intended to supplement the diet with nutrients thought to improve health. Herbs include flowering plants, shrubs, seaweed, and algae.
- It is estimated that 25% of patients use alternative therapies characterized as dietary supplements or herbal remedies.

TABLE 2.64 Clinically Important Effects and Perioperative Concerns of Selected Herbal Medicines and Recommendations for Discontinuation of Use Before Surgery

Herb: Common Name(s)	Relevant Pharmacologic Effects	Perioperative Concerns	Preoperative Discontinuation
Echinacea: purple coneflower root	Activation of cell-mediated immunity	Allergic reactions; decreased effectiveness of immunosuppressive actions of corticosteroids and cyclosporine; potential for immunosuppression with long-term use; inhibition of hepatic microsomal enzymes may precipitate toxicity of drugs metabolized by the liver (e.g., phenytoin, rifampin, phenobarbital)	No data
Ephedra: ma huang	Increased heart rate and blood pressure through direct and indirect sympathomimetic effects	Risk of myocardial ischemia and stroke from tachycardia and hypertension; ventricular arrhythmias with halothane; long-term use depletes endogenous catecholamines and may cause intraoperative hemodynamic instability (control hypotension with direct vasoconstrictor, e.g., phenylephrine); life-threatening interaction with monoamine oxidase inhibitors	At least 24 h before surgery
Garlic: *Allium sativum*	Inhibition of platelet aggregation (may be irreversible); increased fibrinolysis; equivocal antihypertensive activity	Potential to increase risk of bleeding, especially when combined with other medications that inhibit platelet aggregation	At least 7 d before surgery
Ginkgo: duck foot tree, maidenhair tree, silver apricot	Inhibition of platelet-activating factor	Potential to increase risk of bleeding, especially when combined with other medications that inhibit platelet aggregation	At least 36 h before surgery
Ginseng: American ginseng, Asian ginseng, Chinese ginseng, Korean ginseng	Lowers blood glucose; inhibition of platelet aggregation (may be irreversible); increased PT-PTT in animals; many other diverse effects	Hypoglycemia; potential to increase risk of bleeding; potential to decrease anticoagulation effect of warfarin	At least 7 d before surgery
Kava: awa, intoxicating pepper, kawa	Sedation, anxiolysis	Potential to increase sedative effect of anesthetics; potential for addiction, tolerance, and withdrawal after abstinence unstudied	At least 24 h before surgery
St. John's wort: amber, goatweed, hardhay, *Hypericum*, Klamath weed	Inhibition of neurotransmitter reuptake, monoamine oxidase inhibition is unlikely	Induction of cytochrome P450 enzymes, affecting cyclosporine, warfarin, steroids, protease inhibitors, and possibly benzodiazepines, calcium channel blockers, and many other drugs; decreased serum digoxin levels	At least 5 d before surgery
Valerian: all-heal, garden heliotrope, vandal root	Sedation	Potential to increase sedative effect of anesthetics; benzodiazepine-like acute withdrawal; potential to increase anesthetic requirements with long-term use	No data

PT-PTT, Prothrombin time–partial thromboplastin time.

Modified from Ang-Lee MK, Moss J, Yuan CS. Herbal medicines and perioperative care. *JAMA.* 2001;286:208-216; Kaye AD, Kucera I, Sabar R. Perioperative anesthesia clinical considerations of alternative medicines. *Anesthesiol Clin N Am.* 2004;22: 125–139; Hogg LA, Foo L. Management of patients taking herbal medicines in the perioperative period: a survey of practice and policies within anaesthetic departments in the United Kingdom. *Eur J Anaesthesiol.* 2010;27(1):11–15.

- These products are not subject to FDA approval because they are considered nutrients.
- The FDA has no control over the herbal industry in terms of safety guidelines that would regulate the purity and consistency of therapeutic medications.

Adverse Effects and Drug Interactions

- Individuals who take dietary supplements and/or herbal remedies in combination with prescription drugs may be at risk for experiencing adverse interactions.
- The most serious side effects include cardiovascular instability; bleeding tendency, particularly in conjunction with other anticoagulants such as warfarin; and delayed awakening from anesthesia.
- Ephedra (ma huang) is a common ingredient in herbal weight-loss products, stimulants, decongestants, and bronchodilators. The active moiety in ephedra is ephedrine, a sympathomimetic amine structurally related to amphetamines. Serious adverse reactions, including hypertension, cardiac arrhythmias, prolonged QTc interval on the ECG, myocardial infarction, stroke, and death, have been described in patients taking ephedra. Although tachycardia and vasoconstriction can occur in healthy patients, those with heart disease or systemic hypertension or who engage in strenuous physical exercise are at greatest risk for ephedra's sympathomimetic-related effects.
- Ginseng may cause tachycardia or systemic hypertension, particularly in combination with other cardiac stimulant drugs. Ginseng may decrease the anticoagulant effects of warfarin.
- *Ginkgo biloba* has been suggested to possess antiplatelet effects, and spontaneous hemorrhage has been reported. Warfarin may also be potentiated by concomitant use of garlic, *Ginkgo biloba*, and ginger.
- St. John's wort, which is taken for its potential natural antidepressant effects, has been shown to inhibit serotonin, dopamine, and norepinephrine reuptake. Thus the possibility of interactions with MAOIs and other serotonergic drugs exists. Valerian, kava kava, and possibly St. John's wort may delay awakening from anesthesia by prolonging the sedative effects of anesthetic drugs.
- Herbal medications that may affect hemostasis and thus pose some concern are noted in Table 2.65.

TABLE 2.65 Herbal Medications Affecting Hemostasis[a]

Herb	Important Effects	Perioperative Concerns	Time to Normal Hemostasis After Discontinuation
Garlic	Inhibition of platelet aggregation (may be irreversible) Increased fibrinolysis Equivocal antihypertensive activity	Potential to increase bleeding, especially when combined with other medications that inhibit platelet aggregation	7 d
Ginkgo	Inhibition of platelet-activating factor	Potential to increase bleeding, especially when combined with other medications that inhibit platelet aggregation	36 h
Ginseng	Lowers blood glucose Increased prothrombin (PT) and activated partial PTs in animals Other diverse effects	Hypoglycemia Potential to increase risk of bleeding Potential to decrease anticoagulant effect of warfarin	7 d

[a]At this time, it is not deemed necessary to discontinue herbal medications and allow resolution of their effects on hemostasis before surgery or anesthesia.

Adapted from Horlocker TT. Regional anaesthesia in the patient receiving antithrombotic and antiplatelet therapy. *Br J Anaesth.* 2011;107(suppl 1):i96–i106.

KNOWLEDGE CHECK

1. Which side effect is associated with *Gingko biloba*?
   a. Jaundice
   b. Increased bleeding
   c. Hirsutism
   d. Angioedema
2. It is recommended that patients stop taking all herbal supplements ________ before anesthesia and surgery.
   a. 2 days
   b. 2 weeks
   c. 3 weeks
   d. 4 weeks
3. Which is a side effect associated with the use of ephedra? (*Select all that apply.*)
   a. QT interval prolongation
   b. Dysrhythmias
   c. Delayed emergence
   d. Hypertension
   e. Bleeding

Answers can be found in Appendix A.

INSULIN

Anesthetic Implications

Preoperative Concerns

- Poor preoperative glycemic control (Hb $A_{1c} > 8.5\%$) may warrant referral to a diabetes specialist.
- Traditionally, long-acting insulin is discontinued 2–3 days before surgery; glucose levels are then stabilized with a combination of intermediate- and short-acting insulin.
- Prandial insulin should be withheld while fasting, and blood glucose is measured before surgery in all patients with diabetes.
- If capillary blood ketones are >300 mol/L or urinary ketones are >3+, cancel surgery, follow diabetic ketoacidosis (DKA) therapeutic guidelines, and contact a diabetes specialist.
- Symptomatic hyperglycemia > 400 mg/dL may also justify delay of surgery.
- In patients with type 1 diabetes, rapid-acting analog insulin may be given subcutaneously, assuming that 1 unit decreases blood glucose by 54 mg/dL.

Intraoperative Concerns

- Surgical trauma reduces tissue insulin sensitivity, resulting in hyperglycemia in both patients with diabetes and those without it.
- Acute insulin resistance is aggravated in the presence of physiologic stress, such as cardiopulmonary bypass, use of catecholamines, and hypothermia, and after long periods of preoperative fasting.
- Even moderate hyperglycemia contributes to morbidity and mortality after major surgery.
- Although the ideal level of glycemia regarding surgical outcomes is unknown, most professional associations recommend a blood glucose level < 200 mg/dL.
- From a metabolic perspective, anesthetic techniques that seem preferable allow early return to normal diet, mobilization, and usual pharmacologic diabetes management.
- Neuraxial blockade (spinal and or epidural anesthesia) has been demonstrated to attenuate the hyperglycemic response to surgery and facilitate recovery.
- Glycemia in anesthetized, unconscious patients must be monitored and hypoglycemia avoided.
- If hypoglycemia occurs, administer D50W 10–25 g (20–50-mL 50% solution)

Postoperative Period

- Blood sugar levels should be checked and assessed before discharge.

Insulin

- Insulin is synthesized within the β cells of the pancreas, and it is packaged and stored in membrane-lined vesicles within the β-cell cytoplasm.
- About 200 units of insulin are stored in the pancreas in this form.
- With stimulation, insulin is released via exocytosis from the β cell to the surrounding capillaries, where it enters the portal circulation.
- During the first pass through the hepatic circulation, the liver removes about 50% of the circulating insulin.
- Total daily insulin secretion is estimated to be about 60 units, but the total daily peripheral delivery is about 30 units.
- The circulating half-life of insulin is about 7 minutes, and it is mainly cleared from the circulation in 10–15 minutes.
- Both adrenergic and cholinergic fibers of the autonomic nervous system innervate the islets.
- Parasympathetic vagal activity and sympathetic β-receptor stimulation increase insulin release.
- Sympathetic nervous system predominance has a suppressive effect on insulin release (via α_2-adrenergic receptor activation).

- Pancreatic insulin secretion, however, does not require intact autonomic innervation; appropriate secretion responses occur in the transplanted pancreas as well.
- Almost all tissues in the body can metabolize insulin, but the major site of hormone degradation is the liver, with the kidney also metabolizing insulin but to a lesser degree.
- As a result, patients with liver dysfunction or kidney disease may have prolonged effects of insulin with increased risk of hypoglycemia.

Effects of Insulin

- Intimately involved in the regulation of carbohydrate, fat, and protein metabolism
- Insulin promotes the storage of carbohydrate, fat, and protein for future use when substrate supply is low.
- Most cells in the body have insulin receptors, but the major targets of insulin action are the liver, muscle, and adipose tissue.
- Insulin is the body's key hormone controlling glucose removal from the plasma. It facilitates rapid uptake, as well as storage and use of glucose in all cells, but especially liver, muscle, and adipose cells.
- The brain is one of the few tissues in the body that does not require insulin for glucose transport into its cells.
- In the liver, and to a lesser extent in muscle cells, insulin promotes the efficient storage of excess glucose in the form of glycogen (glycogenesis).
- Between meals, when blood glucose levels decrease, insulin secretion decreases, and glucose can be released back into the blood (glycogenolysis).
- Glycogen content in the liver is limited and is largely depleted after an overnight fast. Therefore gluconeogenesis becomes the predominant source of glucose after prolonged fasting.
- Insulin also conserves amino acids in existing proteins by inhibiting the breakdown of protein stores.
- Potassium, phosphate, and magnesium uptake into cells is mediated by an insulin mechanism, leading to decreased serum levels. Thus the administration of insulin is used to treat hyperkalemia.
- Hypokalemia secondary to vigorous insulin treatment can occur.
- Insulin promotes glucose transfer into cells and fosters glucose use for energy.
- When energy needs are met, insulin promotes glucose storage.
- The greatest risk with all forms of insulin administered is hypoglycemia.

Insulin Preparations

- Insulin preparations are created using DNA recombinant technology, mimicking the amino acid sequence of human insulin.
- Most insulin formulations in the United States are prepared as U-100 (100 IU/mL).
- A current exception is the concentrated form of insulin glargine (Toujeo), which contains 300 IU/mL, instead of insulin glargine (Lantus) at 100 IU/mL.
- Protamine is added to some insulins to prolong their effect. Protamine-containing insulins (e.g., neutral protamine Hagedorn, protaminated insulin aspart) may cause sensitization by stimulating antibodies against protamine sulfate. In patients taking protamine-containing insulins, particular care must be exercised (slow and titrated doses) to monitor for anaphylaxis when administering protamine sulfate to reverse the coagulant effects of heparin.
- The available insulins can be divided on a pharmacokinetic basis into three broad categories: rapid-acting, intermediate-acting, and long-acting insulins (Table 2.66).

Timing of Insulin Effects

- It is imperative to know the surgical patient's normal insulin dosage regimen and their treatment compliance.
- Many patients with diabetes mellitus (DM) are on a regimen of long-acting insulin at bedtime and rapid-acting insulin analogs given with meals ("basal bolus regimen").
- Rapid-acting insulins, such as lispro, aspart, and glulisine, have an onset of action of 1 hour or less and are used to reduce glycemia that occurs after meal ingestion.
- Long-acting insulins, including glargine, detemir, and degludec, have delayed absorption from subcutaneous tissue and prolonged effects. They are titrated to produce a steady, basal insulin level throughout the night.
- Continuous subcutaneous insulin infusion is increasingly used to produce an optimal physiologic regimen.
- These infusion pumps administer rapid-acting insulin through a catheter that is inserted into the subcutaneous tissues of the anterior abdominal wall.

TABLE 2.66 Pharmacokinetic Properties of Insulin Preparations

Insulin Type	Onset	Peak	Duration
Rapid Acting			
Aspart (Novolog)	15 min	1 h	3–4 h
Lispro (Humalog)	15 min	1 h	3–4 h
Glulisine (Apidra)	15 min	1 h	3–4 h
Regular (Humulin R, Novolin R)	30–60 min	2–4 h	6–8 h
Intermediate Acting			
NPH	1–3 h	6–8 h	12–16 h
Long Acting			
Detemir (Levemir)	1 h	3–9 h	6–24 h
Glargine (Lantus) U-100	1 h	No peak	29 h
Glargine (Toujeo) U-300	1 h	12–16	32–34 h

Time course is based on subcutaneous administration.
Adapted from Atkinson MA. Type 1 diabetes mellitus. In: Melmed S, Polonsky KS, Larsen PR, et al., eds. *Williams Textbook of Endocrinology*. 13th ed. Elsevier; 2016:1451–1483.

- The pump delivers a basal insulin infusion (usually about 0.5–1 unit/h) and can be programmed to increase and decrease at predetermined times of the day.

Type 1 Diabetes Mellitus

- About 5% of diabetic patients have type 1 DM.
- Individuals with type 1 DM have an absolute deficiency or lack of insulin secretion and are therefore entirely dependent on exogenous insulin therapy.
- In the absence of sufficient exogenous insulin, the disease course may be complicated by periods of ketosis and acidosis.
- Type 1 DM may be caused by an unusually vigorous autoimmune destruction of the β cells of the pancreatic islets.
- Environmental factors such as infection or exposure to specific antigenic proteins are cited as possible initiators of the immune assault.
- Patients with type 1 DM are also more likely to have other autoimmune diseases, such as Graves disease, Hashimoto thyroiditis, myasthenia gravis, and Addison disease.
- A genetic predisposition for development of the disease is also involved.
- Type 1 DM usually develops before age 30 years, but it can develop at any age.
- The lack of insulin has three major sequelae: (1) increased blood glucose levels, (2) increased use of fat for energy, and (3) depletion of the body's protein stores.

KNOWLEDGE CHECK

1. The intraoperative blood sugar in patients with type 1 diabetes should be maintained at
   a. <100 mg/dL.
   b. <200 mg/dL.
   c. <300 mg/dL.
   d. the patient's preoperative blood glucose value.
2. Which medication may cause anaphylaxis in a patient with type 1 diabetes?
   a. Fentanyl
   b. Heparin
   c. Rocuronium
   d. Protamine

Answers can be found in Appendix A.

ORAL HYPOGLYCEMICS

Anesthetic Implications

- Anesthetic concerns with patients with DM taking oral hypoglycemics:
  - Hypoglycemia (sulfonylureas and meglitinides)
  - Ketoacidosis (sodium/glucose cotransporter 2 [SGLT2] inhibitors)
  - Metformin-associated lactic acidosis
  - Delayed gastric emptying and potential for aspiration (glucagon-like peptide 1 [GLP-1] analogs and dipeptidyl peptidase IV [DPP-IV] inhibitors)
- Patients on glucose-lowering drugs must be assessed preoperatively to determine suitability for continuation of drugs.
- Oral hypoglycemics are most often discontinued during the perioperative period.
- Blood sugar should be monitored intraoperatively to determine whether normoglycemia is maintained.
- Renal function must be monitored.
- If omitted preoperatively, these agents should be reintroduced only once normal diet has been resumed and adequate renal function is ensured.

Types of Oral Hypoglycemic Agents

- Oral glucose-lowering agents (Table 2.67) and insulin are used as adjuncts to diet therapy and exercise for treating type 2 DM.
- Most patients with type 2 DM require multiple drugs to achieve glycemic control.
- There are currently eight different classes of noninsulin glucose-lowering drugs that can be used to treat hyperglycemia caused by diabetes:
  1. Biguanides
  2. Sulfonylureas
  3. Meglitinides
  4. Thiazolidinediones
  5. GLP-1 agonists
  6. Dipeptidyl peptidase 4 (DPP-4) inhibitors
  7. α-Glucosidase inhibitors
  8. SGLT2 inhibitors
- *Metformin,* a biguanide, decreases hepatic glucose production and increases peripheral insulin uptake. Metformin is generally preferred as the first-line oral hypoglycemic agent and is available in fixed-dose combinations with many other glucose-lowering drugs. Lactic acidosis has been reported in surgical patients taking metformin, and some recommend that metformin be discontinued 24 hours or more before surgery. Impaired renal function, liver failure, major surgery, heart failure, and alcoholism may increase the risk of lactic acidosis. Alternatively, perioperative administration of metformin has been reported without increased risk of adverse outcomes, including increasing the risk of lactic acidosis compared with other antihyperglycemic treatments.
- *Sulfonylurea agents* increase the secretion of insulin from the pancreas and thus require the presence of functioning β cells. Persistent and severe hypoglycemia is a possible adverse effect of sulfonylureas.
- *Meglitinides* or *nonsulfonylurea secretagogues* increase insulin production by pancreatic β cells similarly to the sulfonylureas. Multiple daily doses are required. Hypoglycemia is a possible adverse effect of meglitinides.
- *Thiazolidinedione derivatives* lower blood glucose levels in patients with type 2 DM by decreasing hepatic glucose production and by increasing the insulin sensitivity of adipose tissue, skeletal muscle, and the liver. Thiazolidinediones may be associated with myocardial infarction and liver failure.
- *GLP-1 receptor agonists* are approved for treatment of patients with type 2 DM and are only available via subcutaneous injection. This class of drugs, called *incretin mimetics*, potentiates insulin release, lowers serum glucagon levels, slows gastric emptying, and promotes satiety. The GLP-1 receptor agonists dulaglutide, exenatide, and albiglutide are approved as once-weekly treatment for type 2 DM. This class of medications should be held for a minimum of 7 days before surgery and anesthesia to decrease gastroparesis and the potential for aspiration.
- *DPP-4 inhibitors* are oral agents that inhibit the destruction of incretin mimetics by blocking the DPP-4 enzyme responsible for GLP-1 degradation. The long-term safety of inhibiting DPP-4, which degrades not only incretin hormones but also cytokines and other peptides, is unknown. Both GLP-1 receptor agonists and DPP-4 inhibitors have been linked to acute pancreatitis.
- *α-Glucosidase inhibitors* block the intestinal enzymes that digest starches into absorbable monosaccharides, resulting in a slower and lower rise in postprandial plasma glucose.
- *SGLT2 inhibitors* block the transport of glucose from the proximal renal tubule, decreasing renal glucose reabsorption and increasing glucose excretion. Because of their diuretic effect, these agents may lead to dehydration, hypovolemia, and hypotension, particularly in the elderly patient with renal dysfunction. The use of SGLT2 inhibitors may cause ketoacidosis.
- *Pramlintide (Symlin)* is an injected antihyperglycemic medication for use in patients with type 2 or type 1 DM who use insulin. It is a synthetic analog of human amylin, a naturally occurring hormone synthesized from pancreatic β cells and normally cosecreted with insulin. Amylin, similar to insulin, is absent or deficient in patients with DM, and its administration contributes to glucose control during the postprandial period.

KNOWLEDGE CHECK

1. Which is the most serious adverse side effect associated with metformin?
   a. Diarrhea
   b. Renal dysfunction
   c. Lactic acidosis
   d. Peripheral neuropathy
2. Which class of oral hypoglycemic agents is associated with ketoacidosis?
   a. Biguanide
   b. SGLT2 inhibitor
   c. α-glucosidase inhibitor
   d. Sulfonylurea

Answers can be found in Appendix A.

TABLE 2.67 Oral Drugs Used to Manage Type 2 Diabetes Mellitus

Drug Class	Mechanism	Adverse Effects
Biguanide Metformin (glucophage) Metformin extended release	Decreases hepatic glucose production and increases peripheral insulin sensitivity	Vitamin B_{12} deficiency; gastrointestinal effects; rare lactic acidosis
Sulfonylurea Glimepiride (Amaryl) Glipizide (Glucotrol), Glyburide (DiaBeta, Micronase)	Increases insulin production and secretion by pancreatic β-cells and increases peripheral insulin sensitivity	Hypoglycemia; weight gain; possible aggravation of myocardial ischemia
Meglitinide Nateglinide (Starlix) Repaglinide (Prandin)	Increases insulin production and secretion by pancreatic β-cells	Hypoglycemia; weight gain; must be taken before each meal
Thiazolidinedione Pioglitazone (Actos), Rosiglitazone (Avandia)	Decreases hepatic glucose production and increases insulin sensitivity of adipose, muscle, and liver cells	Increased risk of heart failure (contraindicated in NYHA class III or IV heart failure), weight gain, decrease bone mineral density and fractures, hepatotoxicity, bladder cancer
GLP-1 Receptor Agonists ("Incretin mimetics") Exenatide (Byetta, Bydureon) Liraglutide (Victoza) Albiglutide (Tanzeum) Dulaglutide (Trulicity) Lixisenatide (Lyxumia)	Potentiates insulin release, lowers serum glucagon levels, slows gastric emptying, and promotes satiety	Only available via subcutaneous injection; nausea; vomiting; acute renal failure; acute pancreatitis; should not be used in patients with gastroparesis; medullary thyroid C-cell cancer in animals
DPP-4 Inhibitors Sitagliptin (Januvia) Saxagliptin (Onglyza) Linagliptin (Tradjenta) Alogliptin (Nesina)	Inhibits metabolism of endogenously released incretin hormones. Potentiates insulin release, lowers serum glucagon levels, slows gastric emptying, and promotes satiety	Hypersensitivity reactions (urticarial, angioedema, anaphylaxis, Stevens-Johnson syndrome, vasculitis); acute pancreatitis; fatal hepatic failure; long-term safety unknown
Alpha-Glucosidase Inhibitor Acarbose, Miglitol	Blocks the intestinal enzymes that digest starches into absorbable monosaccharides, resulting in slower and lower rise in postprandial plasma glucose	Abdominal pain; diarrhea; flatulence; contraindicated in patients with intestinal disease
SGLT2 Inhibitor Canagliflozin (Invokana) Dapagliflozin (Farxiga) Empagliflozin (Jardiance)	Blocks the transport of glucose from the proximal renal tubule, decreasing renal glucose reabsorption and increasing glucose excretion	Ketoacidosis, genital mycotic infections; recurrent urinary tract infections; volume depletion; hypotension; hyperkalemia; hypomagnesemia; hyperphosphatemia; fractures; cardiovascular and long-term safety unknown

DPP-4, Dipeptidyl peptidase-4; *GLP-1,* glucagon-like peptide; *NYHA,* New York Heart Association; *SGLT2,* sodium/glucose cotransporter 2.
Modified from Drugs for type 2 diabetes. *Med Lett Drugs Ther.* 2017;59(1512):9–18.

INTRAVENOUS DYES

Anesthetic Implications

- Intravenous contrast medium (ICM) can cause an allergic reaction in some patients, varying from itching with hives to anaphylactoid and anaphylactic reactions (Box 2.30).
- Adverse reactions to ICM are more likely to develop in patients with asthma or a history of allergy or in patients with multiple morbidities.
- Fatal reactions are rare.
- Contrast media–induced renal impairment can be reduced with the use of low-osmolality contrast media and extracellular volume expansion.
- ICM can also cause local tissue sloughing and necrosis if the ICM extravasates from the vein.
- The radiologist should use the smallest amount of contrast agent necessary.

BOX 2.30 Considerations and Treatment Protocols for Preventing Intravenous Contrast Medium Extravasation

Considerations

- Avoid use of the same vein if the first attempt at intravenous catheterization was not achieved.
- Ensure the intravenous catheter is patent and free-flowing.

Treatments

- Attempt to aspirate as much ICM as possible.
- Elevate the affected limb.
- Apply ice packs for 20–60 min until swelling resolves.
- A heating pad may be necessary in place of ice for swelling.
- Observe the patient for possible tissue damage related to continual contact with ice or heat.
- Observe the patient for 2–4 h before discharge; consider medical/surgical consultation if necessary.
- Follow up with patient, assessing for residual pain, increased or decreased temperature, hardness, change in sensation, redness, or blistering.

ICM, Intravenous contrast medium.
Modified from American College of Radiology. Extravasation of contrast media. In: *ACR Manual on Contrast Media,* version 10.1, 2015. Accessed May 15, 2016, https://www.acr.org/Clinical-Resources/Clinical-Tools-and-Reference/Contrast-Manual; Reynolds PM, MacLaren R, Mueller SW, et al. Management of extravasation injuries: a focused evaluation of noncytotoxic medications. *Pharmacotherapy.* 2014;34(6):617–632.

- To safeguard against the possibility of renal failure, the patient should be adequately hydrated beginning 1 hour before the procedure and continuing for another 24 hours.
- Patients who are at risk for possible nonimmunologic anaphylactic reactions should be pretreated with corticosteroids, such as methylprednisolone or prednisone, administered by mouth or IV.
- In cases of moderate or severe previous ICM reactions, a histamine-1 (H_1) blocker such as diphenhydramine and an H_2-blocker such as famotidine should be given together, either IV or by mouth.

Clinical Use

- ICM is typically a water-soluble, iodine-containing solution of two available types: media that can dissociate into ions in solution and media that will remain in a neutral state in solution.
- ICM is also formulated as high-osmolar contrast media (HOCM), which contain few dissolved particles and iodine atoms, and low-osmolar contrast media (LOCM), which contain greater numbers of dissolved particles with iodine.
- An HOCM solution causes fluid shift from the cell to the vein with the ICM, whereas an LOCM solution is closely iso-osmolar, inducing less fluid shift from the cell.
- Reactions are possible with either type of ICM solution, although fewer reactions occur with LOCM. Some reactions may present anywhere from half an hour to 1 week after the administration of the ICM.
- Reactions to ICM are theorized to be caused by the ICM molecule's serving as an antigen and affixing itself to either mast cells or basophils. This causes release of mediators such as histamine and tryptase, which can inhibit coagulation, dilate blood vessels, release complement, or even stimulate an IgE-modulated immune reaction.
- A new ICM using gold nanoparticles is available and undergoing tests before use in humans. It has many advantages over iodinated ICM, such as higher radiation absorption, yielding better images with lower x-ray dose, low allergenic response, and longer imaging times because of its nanoparticle size.

KNOWLEDGE CHECK

1. Which IV contrast medium is associated with the fewest allergic reactions?
   a. High osmolar
   b. Low osmolar
   c. Lipid soluble
   d. Iodine based
2. Which complication is associated with IV contrast medium? (*Select all that apply.*)
   a. Hepatic failure
   b. Gastrointestinal bleeding
   c. Renal failure
   d. Extravasation and tissue necrosis

Answers can be found in Appendix A.

LIPID-LOWERING AGENTS

Anesthetic Implications

- Statins have been associated with improved postoperative outcomes by decreasing cardiac morbidity and mortality.
- Statins should be continued throughout the perioperative period when possible or started as soon as feasible postoperatively (Table 2.68).

Statins

- Statins have documented benefits for primary and secondary prevention of cardiovascular disease and are thought to improve perioperative outcomes in patients undergoing surgery.
- Compliance with statin therapy in vascular surgical patients was associated with significantly improved long-term survival.

Nonstatin Lipid-Lowering Agents

- Several agents have a long history of use as hyperlipidemic agents. These include niacin, fibrates, bile acid sequestrants, and ezetimibe. Some perioperative considerations are described in the subsections that follow.

Preoperative Concerns

- Ezetimibe should be discontinued before surgery; the perioperative safety is not clear.
- Stop niacin or niacinamide at least 2 weeks before surgery because of the potential for hypotension and hyperglycemia.
- Fibrates should be withheld on the day of surgery.
- Bile sequestrants interfere with bowel absorption of multiple medications that may be required perioperatively and should be withheld on the day of surgery.

Intraoperative Concerns

- Niacin and niacinamide may exacerbate allergies by increasing histamine, increasing bleeding, and accentuating the effects of anticoagulants.

TABLE 2.68 HMG-CoA Reductase Inhibitors ("Statins")

Drug	Initial Dosage	Maximum Dosage	Comments
Atorvastatin (Lipitor)	10 mg daily	80 mg daily	Statins are generally tolerated better than other lipid-lowering drugs. Mild transient gastrointestinal disturbances, muscle pain, rash, and headache have occurred. Some patients have reported sleep disturbances. An increase in liver enzymes and creatine phosphokinase may occur with significant myalgia and muscle weakness.
Fluvastatin (Lescol)	20 mg daily	40 mg bid	
Lovastatin (Mevacor)	20 mg daily	80 mg daily	
Pitavastatin (Livalo)	2 mg daily	4 mg daily	
Pravastatin (Pravachol)	40 mg daily	80 mg daily	
Rosuvastatin (Crestor)	10 mg daily	40 mg daily	
Simvastatin (Zocor)	20 mg daily	80 mg daily	

HMG-CoA, 3-Hydroxy-3-methylglutaryl-coenzyme A.
Adapted from Drugs for lipids. *Treat Guidel Med Lett.* 2014;12(137):1–6.

- Statins do not increase bleeding associated with regional anesthesia. They may exacerbate the effects of antihypertensive drugs. Cardiac arrhythmias have been reported. Use of nicotine patches may worsen or increase the risk of flushing.
- Niacin and fibrates can cause myopathy and rhabdomyolysis, which may be exacerbated by surgery. Risk is higher when these agents are used in combination with statins.
- Lipid-lowering agents should be restarted in the postoperative period.

KNOWLEDGE CHECK

1. Statin medications should be
   a. continued throughout the perioperative period.
   b. discontinued 1 week before surgery.
   c. discontinued 2 days before surgery.
   d. restarted 1 week postoperatively.
2. Which preoperative recommendation is associated with niacin and niacinamide?
   a. Continued throughout the perioperative period
   b. Continued until the day before surgery
   c. Discontinued at least 2 weeks before surgery
   d. Discontinued permanently

Answers can be found in Appendix A.

PHOSPHODIESTERASE INHIBITORS

Anesthetic Implications

- Milrinone improves heart contractility while causing pulmonary artery and systemic vasodilation (inotrope and vasodilator).
- It may be used during cardiac surgery to supplement other inotropes, such as dobutamine, and to lower pulmonary artery pressures in cor pulmonale.
- Milrinone improves weaning of high-risk patients from cardiopulmonary bypass.

Milrinone

- The phosphodiesterase 3 (PDE3) inhibitors, also known as *nonglycoside noncatecholamines*, include milrinone (Primacor).
- Phosphodiesterases (PDEs) are a group of enzymes that play a role in a variety of physiologic actions. They break down the second messengers, cyclic adenosine monophosphate (cAMP) or cGMP, in various cells. The PDE3 inhibitors, such as milrinone, prevent the breakdown of cAMP and thus enhance its action.
- Milrinone substantially improves left ventricular function in association with an acceleration of calcium uptake by the sarcoplasmic reticulum. This allows for the buildup of cAMP and a subsequent increase in the uptake of intracellular calcium. Because adrenergic receptors are responsible for this inotropic effect, it follows that these drugs retain their inotropic effect even in the presence of β-blocking agents or the phenomenon of β-receptor downregulation, situations frequently encountered in patients with heart failure. Therefore PDE3 inhibitors may be used to augment the effect of direct-acting β-agonists such as dobutamine or dopamine. Milrinone acts to enhance diastolic function, increase cardiac output, and decrease PCWP.
- In the smooth muscle, milrinone prevents the breakdown of cAMP, causing an efflux of calcium and relaxation of the smooth muscle and vasodilation. The clinical result is a decrease in both preload and afterload. This effect, along with the absence of an associated increase in heart rate, probably contributes to the absence of an increase in myocardial oxygen consumption.
- Sildenafil (Viagra, Revatio) is a PDE5 inhibitor that produces vasodilation and is used to treat pulmonary arterial hypertension. Pulmonary vasodilation reduces the workload of the right ventricle and improves symptoms of right-sided heart failure. The medication is also used to treat erectile dysfunction (ED). Severe and refractory hypotension can occur in patients who receive anesthesia and are taking PDE5 inhibitors. It is recommended that patients withhold PGE5 inhibitors used to treat ED for 7 days before anesthesia.

Side effects and elimination

- Side effects include supraventricular arrhythmias, ventricular arrhythmias, torsades de pointes, anaphylaxis, hypotension, bronchospasm, hyperthermia, and thrombocytopenia.
- Elimination is via the kidney; therefore milrinone should be used with caution in patients in renal failure because of the potential for life-threatening arrhythmias.

Indications

- Therapy for CHF, cardiac bypass procedures, and heart transplants

Dose

- IV: loading dose: 50 mcg/kg over 10 minutes; maintenance dose: 0.375 mcg/kg/min, 0.5 mcg/kg/min, or 0.75 mcg/kg/min. Rapid IV bolus can result in hypotension.

Onset and duration

- Onset: IV: 2 minutes; oral: 1–1.5 hours. Duration of action: 2 hours

Precautions and contraindications

- Use with caution in patients with renal insufficiency and in those with aortic or pulmonary valvular disease.
- Milrinone is contraindicated in patients with hypersensitivity to milrinone or amrinone (see Table 2.36).

KNOWLEDGE CHECK

1. Which is a cardiovascular effect associated with milrinone? (*Select all that apply.*)
   a. Increased preload
   b. Increased contractility
   c. Decreased afterload
   d. Decreased myocardial oxygen consumption
2. Which is a side effect associated with milrinone? (*Select all that apply.*)
   a. Hypertension
   b. Polycythemia
   c. Bronchospasm
   d. Anaphylaxis
3. When sildenafil is used to treat ED, it is recommended that the medication be discontinued a minimum of _____ days preoperatively to avoid refractory hypotension.
   a. 2
   b. 5
   c. 7
   d. 9

Answers can be found in Appendix A.

PSYCHOPHARMACOLOGY

Anesthesia Implications

- Most psychiatric drug therapy should be continued throughout the preoperative period.
- Continuation of antidepressants, anxiolytics, antipsychotics, and other psychotropic agents will ensure the patient's disease is better controlled during the postoperative period.

Antidepressants

- Depression is treated with antidepressant medications, psychotherapy, electroconvulsive therapy, or a combination of these approaches.
- Several drug classes are useful for the treatment of depression; they are listed in Table 2.69.
- The goal of antidepressant treatment is complete remission of symptoms because partial response is associated with an increased risk of relapse.

Selective Serotonin Reuptake Inhibitors

- SSRIs are the first-line therapy for major depression and the most widely prescribed class of antidepressants.
- Unless a patient-specific concern develops, SSRIs should be continued throughout the perioperative period.
- Common side effects include restlessness, insomnia, nausea, diarrhea, headache, dizziness, fatigue, and sexual dysfunction.
- SSRIs can cause hyponatremia, particularly in elderly patients, and increase the risk of bleeding by inhibiting serotonin uptake by platelets.
- When SSRIs are stopped abruptly, discontinuation may cause nervousness, anxiety, irritability, paresthesia, dizziness, insomnia, confusion, and nausea and vomiting.
- Withdrawal effects are most severe with paroxetine because of its short half-life and are least likely to occur with fluoxetine because of its long half-life.
- SSRIs have an inhibitory effect on CYP450 isoenzymes and may interact with other drugs that rely on hepatic metabolism, including β-blockers, benzodiazepines, and antiarrhythmics.
- Interactions with other serotonergic drugs may lead to serotonin syndrome.

Serotonin syndrome

- Serotonin syndrome is a rare but potentially life-threatening condition associated with increased serotonergic activity in the central and peripheral nervous systems.
- It can be caused by individual drugs, an overdose, or most commonly, a drug interaction.
- The syndrome is characterized by mental status changes, autonomic instability, neuromuscular hyperactivity, and hyperthermia.
- Drugs that are associated with serotonin syndrome are listed in Tables 2.70 and 2.71.
- Symptoms may appear within minutes or up to 24 hours after the initial use of medication, a change in dose, or the addition of a new serotonergic drug.
- Mortality may result from rhabdomyolysis with renal failure, hyperkalemia, disseminated intravascular coagulation, and/or acute respiratory distress syndrome.

TABLE 2.69 Antidepressant Drugs

Drug Class	Generic Name	Trade Name	Comment
SSRIs	Fluoxetine	Prozac	First-line treatment for depression. May increase the risk of bleeding due to inhibition of serotonin uptake by platelets. Significant effects on CYP450 isoenzymes may lead to various drug interactions. Abrupt discontinuation may lead to discontinuation syndrome. May lead to serotonin syndrome when combined with other serotonergic drugs.
	Paroxetine	Paxil	
	Sertraline	Zoloft	
	Fluvoxamine	Luvox	
	Citalopram	Celexa	
	Escitalopram	Lexapro	
SNRIs	Desvenlafaxine	Pristiq	May produce dose-dependent increase in blood pressure. Can precipitate serotonin syndrome or neuroleptic malignant syndrome. Abrupt withdrawal may lead to severe discontinuation syndrome. Used for analgesic effect in diabetic neuropathy.
	Duloxetine	Cymbalta	
	Venlafaxine	Effexor	
TCAs	Amitriptyline	Elavil	Anticholinergic side effects such as urinary retention, dry mouth, blurred vision, and confusion are common. Orthostatic hypotension and cardiac conduction abnormalities may occur. A preoperative ECG should be obtained to rule out conduction changes. Direct-acting vasopressors such as phenylephrine are preferred over indirect drugs such as ephedrine.
	Desipramine	Norpramin	
	Imipramine	Tofranil	
	Nortriptyline	Pamelor	
	Protriptyline	Vivactil	
	Doxepin	Sinequan	
MAOIs	Isocarboxazid	Marplan	Enzyme-inhibiting effects can persist for up to 2 wk after discontinuation. Interaction with serotonergic drugs, bupropion, and sympathomimetics can lead to serotonin syndrome. Avoid meperidine due to severe excitatory drug interaction.
	Selegiline	Ensam	
	Phenelzine	Nardil	
	Tranylcypromine	Parnate	
Atypical	Bupropion	Wellbutrin	Bupropion produces dose-related seizures. It is prescribed for smoking cessation. Blocks reuptake of both norepinephrine and dopamine.
	Mirtazapine	Remeron	
	Trazodone	Desyrel	
	Nefazodone	Serzone	
	Vilazodone	Vibryd	

ECG, Electrocardiogram; *MAOIs*, monoamine oxidase inhibitors; *SNRIs*, selective norepinephrine reuptake inhibitors; *SSRIs*, selective serotonin reuptake inhibitors; *TCAs*, tricyclic antidepressants.
From Elisha S, Heiner JS, Nagelhout JJ. *Nurse Anesthesia*. 7th ed. Elsevier; 2023.

TABLE 2.70 Drugs Implicated in Serotonin Syndrome

Drug Class	Agents
Monoamine oxidase inhibitors	Phenelzine, moclobemide, isocarboxazid, selegiline, tranylcypromine
SSRIs	Sertraline, fluoxetine, fluvoxamine, paroxetine, citalopram, escitalopram
SNRIs	Duloxetine, venlafaxine, desvenlafaxine
Tricyclic antidepressants	Amitriptyline, doxepin, clomipramine, nortriptyline, imipramine, desipramine
Antibiotics	Linezolid
Opiate analgesics and pain medications	Meperidine, fentanyl, tramadol, pentazocine
OTC cough/cold medications	Dextromethorphan
Antimigraine agents	Almotriptan, sumatriptan
Drugs of abuse	Amphetamine, cocaine, methylenedioxymethamphetamine (MDMA or ecstasy), lysergic acid diethylamide (LSD)
Antiemetics	Metoclopramide, ondansetron
Anticonvulsants	Carbamazepine, valproic acid
Herbal products	Ginseng, nutmeg, St. John's wort
Other	Lithium, methylene blue, buspirone, tryptophan

OTC, Over the counter; *SNRIs,* selective norepinephrine reuptake inhibitors; *SSRIs,* selective serotonin reuptake inhibitors.
From Elisha S, Heiner JS, Nagelhout JJ. *Nurse Anesthesia*. 7th ed. Elsevier; 2023.

TABLE 2.71 Triad of Neuromuscular, Autonomic, and Mental Status Effects Seen in Serotonin Syndrome

Neuromuscular Effects	Autonomic Effects	Mental Status Effects
• Hyperreflexia	• Hyperthermia	• Anxiety
• Tremor	• Tachycardia	• Agitation
• Myoclonus	• Tachypnea	• Confusion
• Ocular clonus	• Abdominal pain	• Hallucinations
• Hypertonia	• Diarrhea	• Delirium
• Rigidity	• Diaphoresis	• Hyperreactivity
	• Flushing	• Disorientation
	• Mydriasis	
	• Hyper- or hypotension	

From Elisha S, Heiner JS, Nagelhout JJ. *Nurse Anesthesia*. 7th ed. Elsevier; 2023.

- Benzodiazepines may be used to treat agitation and tremor.
- Although rare, hospitalization is required for patients with moderate or severe serotonin syndrome.
- Critically ill patients may require neuromuscular paralysis, sedation, and intubation.

Tricyclic Antidepressants

- TCAs are valuable alternatives to the SSRIs and SNRIs for patients with moderate to severe treatment-resistant depression.
- TCAs are commonly used adjunct analgesics in the management of both neuropathic and somatic chronic pain.
- Amitriptyline is the prototype antidepressant used in this context. In general, pain relief may be expected in 7–14 days. It should be avoided in patients with a history of heart disease (conduction disorders, arrhythmias, or heart failure) and closed-angle glaucoma.
- TCAs cause anticholinergic effects (urinary retention, constipation, dry mouth, blurred vision, and confusion), orthostatic hypotension, weight gain,

sedation, sexual dysfunction, and cardiac conduction delay.
- Patients treated with TCAs may have altered responses to anesthesia-related drugs.
- An increase in CNS catecholamine levels may increase the minimum alveolar concentration (MAC) of the inhalation anesthetics.
- Increased peripheral catecholamines may produce exaggerated responses to indirect-acting vasopressors, such as ephedrine; thus a direct-acting vasopressor, such as phenylephrine, is preferred.

Monoamine Oxidase Inhibitors

- MAOIs were widely used as antidepressants before the introduction of SSRIs, which have an improved safety profile.
- They are now used only when other first-line treatments are ineffective because of the risk of drug and food interactions eliciting a hypertensive crisis and difficulty with proper dosing.
- Inhibition of monoamine oxidase (MAO) leads to central and peripheral increases in norepinephrine, serotonin, and dopamine, producing a sympathomimetic action in nerve terminals. MAO has two subtypes, MAO-A and MAO-B. MAO-A preferentially metabolizes serotonin, norepinephrine, and epinephrine. MAO-B preferentially metabolizes phenylethylamine.
- About 60% of human brain MAO activity is of the A subtype.
- Because of the risk of serotonin syndrome, serotonergic drugs and MAOIs should not be used together or within 2 weeks of each other.
- Because an exaggerated hypertensive response may occur with administration of an indirect-acting vasopressor, such as ephedrine, the use of a direct-acting agent, such as phenylephrine, is preferred.
- The use of meperidine in a patient treated with MAOIs may result in agitation, headache, skeletal muscle rigidity, hyperpyrexia, hypertension, and death.
- An increase in serotonin activity in the brain is presumed to be responsible for excitatory reactions evoked by meperidine.
- Derivatives of meperidine (fentanyl, sufentanil, alfentanil) have been associated with adverse reactions in patients treated with MAOIs.
- Morphine does not inhibit uptake of serotonin, but its opioid effects may be potentiated in the presence of MAOIs.

Serotonin and Norepinephrine Reuptake Inhibitors

- The SNRIs are indicated to treat major depression, anxiety, mood disorders, and chronic neuropathic pain, particularly pain associated with diabetic peripheral neuropathy.
- SNRIs are mediated via increases in levels of serotonin and norepinephrine in the brain.
- Side effects include increased sweating, tachycardia, and urinary retention.
- Symptoms can recur when these drugs are abruptly stopped, especially with venlafaxine and desvenlafaxine because of their short half-lives.
- SNRIs can cause a dose-dependent increase in blood pressure.

Antipsychotics

- Patients with chronic schizophrenia should continue their antipsychotic medications preoperatively.
- Anesthesia management consists of avoiding hypotension during induction because of the additive depressive effects of the anesthetic drugs, assessing QT interval prolongation, and observing for abnormal temperature regulation.
- Antipsychotics include two major classes: dopamine receptor antagonists and serotonin-dopamine antagonists.
- The first-generation drugs are also referred to as *typical antipsychotics* and include the phenothiazines, thioxanthenes, and butyrophenones. They block dopamine receptors in the basal ganglia and limbic portions of the forebrain.
- Dopamine receptor antagonists, such as haloperidol and fluphenazine, tend to cause EPSs or parkinsonian syndrome.
- All first-generation antipsychotic drugs have been associated with sexual dysfunction, hyperprolactinemia, neuroleptic malignant syndrome, and tardive dyskinesia.
- Second-generation antipsychotics have a relatively low risk of EPSs and are less likely than first-generation antipsychotics to cause tardive dyskinesia and neuroleptic malignant syndrome.
- Some second-generation drugs, particularly clozapine, olanzapine, and quetiapine, cause weight gain and hyperglycemia.
- Clozapine is the most effective antipsychotic drug, but it should be reserved for refractory disease because of its potential for serious hematologic toxicity and strict monitoring requirements.

KNOWLEDGE CHECK

1. Which is a physiologic effect associated with serotonin syndrome? (*Select all that apply.*)
   a. Hyperthermia
   b. Hypokalemia
   c. Bradycardia
   d. Autonomic instability
2. Which medication should be used to treat hypotension in a patient taking an MAOI?
   a. Ephedrine
   b. Phenylephrine
   c. Epinephrine
   d. Dobutamine

Answers can be found in Appendix A.

CORTICOSTEROIDS

Anesthesia Implications

Perioperative Steroid Replacement

- The stress response associated with surgery and the suppression of the HPA axis with supraphysiologic doses of corticosteroids has led to administering perioperative glucocorticoids to patients who have taken steroids in the preoperative period.
- Synthesis and secretion of cortisol can increase 5- to 10-fold under conditions of severe stress, such as surgery, trauma, or infection.
- In adult patients who have received supraphysiologic doses of glucocorticoids (oral, topical, or inhaled), it may take up to 12 months from the time of discontinuation of steroids for the HPA axis to function adequately.
- A single dose of etomidate induces decreased cortisol output for up to 24 hours by inhibiting 11β hydroxylase.
- Acute adrenal crisis is life threatening, and even though there is a small risk of adrenal insufficiency, steroid supplementation is warranted.
- Preoperative steroid supplementation should occur in the following scenarios:
  1. The patient has taken oral pharmacologic doses of prednisone greater than 20 mg/d or its equivalent (16 mg/d methylprednisolone, 80 mg/d of hydrocortisone, 3 mg/d of dexamethasone).
  2. The period of treatment was for 3 weeks or longer.
  3. The treatment occurred during the 12 months immediately before surgery.
- A common perioperative protocol for steroid supplementation is included in Table 2.72.
- Signs and symptoms associated with acute adrenal crises:
  - Neurologic
    1. Altered level of consciousness
    2. Loss of consciousness
  - Respiratory
    1. Respiratory distress/arrest
  - Cardiovascular
    1. Hypotension that is unresponsive/minimally responsive to vasopressor therapy
  - Endocrine
    1. Hypoglycemia
    2. Hypovolemia
    3. Hyponatremia, hyperkalemia
    4. Metabolic acidosis
- Treatment for acute adrenal crises can be found in Box 2.31.
- Therapeutic uses of corticosteroids can be found in Tables 2.72–2.74.

TABLE 2.72 Guidelines for Perioperative Adrenal Supplementation Therapy

Type of Surgery-Related Stress	Additional Hydrocortisone Dose
Superficial Surgery Dental biopsies	None
Minor Surgery Inguinal hernia Colonoscopy	25 mg IV before induction of anesthesia
Moderate Surgery Colon resection Total abdominal hysterectomy Total joint replacement	50–75 mg IV before induction of anesthesia; taper by 50%/d over 1–2 d
Major Surgery Cardiovascular Thoracic Liver	100–150 mg IV before induction of anesthesia; taper by 50%/d over 1–2 d

Modified from Wall RT III. Endocrine disease. In: Hines RL, Marschall KE, eds. *Stoelting's Anesthesia and Co-existing Disease*. 6th ed. Elsevier; 2012:376–406.

BOX 2.31 Treatment for Acute Adrenal Crises

- Endotracheal intubation and controlled ventilation for respiratory arrest
- Intravascular volume expansion with isotonic crystalloid (e.g., Ringer lactate or normal saline)
- Hydrocortisone 100 mg IV bolus, followed by hydrocortisone 50–100 mg every 6 h for 24 h (total 300 mg/d)
- Administer D50W bolus if hypoglycemia is present.
- Administer vasopressors or positive inotropes to treat hypotension.
- Invasive monitoring (e.g., arterial line or central venous line) as necessary
- Monitor laboratory values (i.e., electrolytes, cortisol, ACTH, and glucose).
- Perform cardiac resuscitation per American Heart Association ACLS/PALS protocol as necessary.

ACLS/PALS, Advanced cardiac life support/pediatric advanced life support; *ACTH,* adrenocorticotropic hormone; *D50W,* 50% dextrose in water.

KNOWLEDGE CHECK

1. Which medication is administered to treat acute adrenal crises?
   a. Cortisol
   b. Dexamethasone
   c. Prednisone
   d. Hydrocortisone
2. Which medication decreases the synthesis of cortisol by inhibition of 11β hydroxylase?
   a. Propofol
   b. Etomidate
   c. Dexmedetomidine
   d. Ketamine
3. Which metabolic abnormality is associated with acute adrenal crises? (*Select all that apply.*)
   a. Metabolic acidosis
   b. Metabolic alkalosis
   c. Hyperkalemia
   d. Hypokalemia
4. Which is a criterion for providing preoperative steroid coverage? (*Select all that apply.*)
   a. Prednisone greater than 20 mg/d or its equivalent
   b. Hydrocortisone greater than 20 mg/d or its equivalent
   c. Period of treatment of 3 weeks or longer
   d. Treatment occurring during the 12 months immediately before surgery

Answers can be found in Appendix A.

TABLE 2.73 Clinical Features of Primary Adrenal Insufficiency

Feature	Frequency (%)
Symptoms	
Weakness, tiredness, fatigue	100
Anorexia	100
Gastrointestinal symptoms	92
Nausea	86
Vomiting	75
Constipation	33
Abdominal pain	31
Diarrhea	16
Salt craving	16
Postural dizziness	12
Muscular or joint pain	13
Signs	
Weight loss	100
Hyperpigmentation	94
Hypotension (<110 mm Hg systolic)	88–94
Vitiligo	10–20
Auricular calcification	5
Laboratory Findings	
Electrolyte disturbances	92
Hyponatremia	88
Hyperkalemia	64
Hypercalcemia	6
Azotemia	55
Anemia	40
Eosinophilia	17

From Melmed S, Polonsky KS, Larsen, PR, et al., eds. *Williams Textbook of Endocrinology*. 13th ed. Elsevier; 2016.

UTEROTONICS

Anesthesia Implications

- Oxytocic drugs are used for several indications in obstetric anesthesia:
  1. Induction and management of labor
  2. Treatment of uterine atony and postpartum hemorrhage
- After vaginal delivery, there can be increased uterine atony in the setting of retained products, a long labor, high parity, macrosomia, polyhydramnios,

TABLE 2.74 Steroid Preparation

Steroid	Glucocorticoid Potency[a]	Mineralocorticoid Potency (Salt Retention)	Approximate Equivalent Dose
Cortisol (Hydrocortisone)	1.0	1.0	20 mg
Prednisone	4.0	0.25	5 mg
Prednisolone	4.0	0.25	5 mg
Methylprednisolone	5.0	0	4 mg
Dexamethasone	30	0	0.75 mg
Fludrocortisone	12	125	

[a]Glucocorticoid and mineralocorticoid potencies are relative to cortisol, with cortisol being 1.0. Prednisone, prednisolone, methylprednisolone, and dexamethasone have less mineralocorticoid effect than hydrocortisone.
From Elisha S, Heiner JS, Nagelhout JJ. *Nurse Anesthesia*. 7th ed. Elsevier; 2023.

excessive oxytocin augmentation during labor, and chorioamnionitis.

- In these settings, bimanual uterine massage is first attempted before administration of an oxytocic agent. Oxytocic drugs are also given routinely after cesarean section and delivery of the neonate to prevent the development of uterine atony.
- The uterus has α and β receptors, with α-receptor stimulation resulting in contraction and β_2-receptor stimulation resulting in uterine relaxation.
- **Oxytocin (Pitocin)** is the first-line agent used to increase uterine tone and is administered as a dilute solution of 20–40 units/L after delivery. The hemodynamic effects include tachycardia, vasodilation, and hypotension.
- **Methylergonovine (Methergine)** (0.2 mg IM) can also be given to improve uterine tone. It causes intense and prolonged contractions and therefore is only given after delivery as a single IM injection. Its use is contraindicated in patients with preeclampsia and cardiovascular disease because it can cause severe hypertension.
- **Carboprost (Hemabate)**, a synthetic analog of prostaglandin E2 (0.25 mg IM), is another alternative to stimulate uterine contractions. It is also administered IM and should be avoided in patients with asthma because of its association with bronchospasm. Side effects include the following:
  - Nausea, vomiting, and diarrhea
  - Mild fever, chills
  - Flushing (warmth, redness, or tingly feeling)
  - Cough, hiccups
  - Headache
  - Mild pelvic pain or menstrual-type cramps

KNOWLEDGE CHECK

1. Which physiologic effect can be associated with methergine administration?
   a. Hypertension
   b. Bradycardia
   c. Supraventricular tachycardia
   d. Premature ventricular contractions
2. Which uterotonic should be avoided in patients with asthma?
   a. Methergine
   b. Pitocin
   c. Hemabate
   d. Terbutaline

Answers can be found in Appendix A.

3

Human Physiology, Pathophysiology, and Anesthesia Case Management

CARDIOVASCULAR SYSTEM

Physiologic Principles

The human heart is one of the most amazing organs in the body. Its compensatory ability to constantly regulate blood flow to tissues during various physiologic periods (e.g., exercise vs. sleep) is a major reason for the high rate of myocardial oxygen consumption. Assuming that the average adult heart rate is 72 beats/min (BPM), this translates into 100,000 beats/d and 2.5 billion beats/lifetime. The heart, which approximates the size of your fist, pumps approximately 2000 gallons of blood through 60,000 miles of blood vessels each day. Thus rapid and constant synthesis of cellular energy in the form of adenosine triphosphate (ATP) is necessary. Oxygen is a necessary component of maximizing ATP creation during glycolysis.

As a result of rapid hemodynamic changes that occur during anesthesia and surgery, the anesthetist should predicate management decisions based on myocardial oxygen supply and demand factors (Table 3.1).

Myocardial Oxygen Supply

- *Coronary artery patency:* Vascular occlusion decreases the ability of the coronary arteries to deliver blood to the myocardium. When oxygen demand is increased, the coronary arteries dilate to allow more oxygenated blood to perfuse the heart. In areas where blood flow is decreased because of plaque formation, maximal vasodilation is constant, and if myocardial oxygen demand is increased, myocardial ischemia and infarction are possible.
- *Coronary artery autoregulation:* Under normal physiologic conditions, the coronary circulation exhibits *autoregulation*, which is the ability to maintain coronary blood flow across a range of mean arterial pressures (MAPs) by dilating or constricting. Because of the high oxygen extraction ratio by the heart, which is nearly 70%, greater oxygenation during periods of increased demand occurs by vasodilation, resulting in increased coronary artery blood flow and myocardial perfusion. Coronary blood flow is maintained at a constant flow rate across a range of MAPs between 60 and 140 mm Hg. When arterial blood pressure (ABP) is less than or exceeds these pressure limits, coronary blood flow becomes pressure dependent (Fig. 3.1). In patients with chronic and untreated hypertension and or neurologic/coronary artery atherosclerosis, the autoregulation curve is shifted to the right of the normal curve. In this example, a MAP of 60 mm Hg, which is the lower limit of normal physiologic autoregulation, may be too low for adequate myocardial perfusion. Current critical care practice is to maintain a MAP of ≥65 mm Hg.
- *Diastolic time (heart rate):* The majority of coronary artery perfusion to the left ventricle (LV) occurs during diastole. Therefore a slow heart rate (50–60 BPM) increases diastolic time and maximizes left ventricular perfusion (Fig. 3.2).
- *Hemoglobin*
  - *Oxygen saturation:* Avoiding periods of hypoxemia allows hemoglobin to release an adequate amount of oxygen to tissues.
  - *Concentration:* Periods of acute blood loss can cause decreased oxygen-carrying capacity despite normal blood pressure (BP) and adequate oxygenation. There is no absolute hemoglobin value that is a trigger to administer packed red blood cells (RBCs). At hemoglobin values <5 g/dL, oxygenation of the myocardium may be inadequate to sustain cardiac function. It is prudent to maintain higher hemoglobin values in patients

TABLE 3.1 **Determinants of Myocardial Oxygen Supply and Demand**

Supply	Demand
Coronary artery anatomy and patency	Heart rate
Coronary artery autoregulation (DBP)	Preload
Diastolic time (heart rate)	Afterload
Hemoglobin concentration	Contractility

DBP, Diastolic blood pressure.

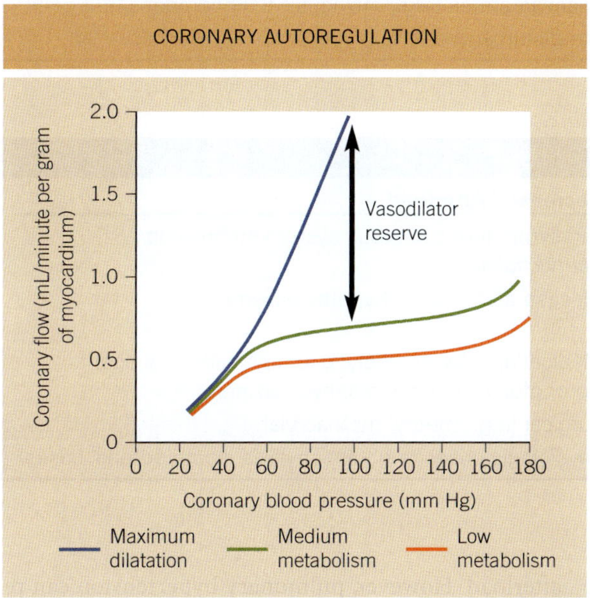

Fig. 3.1 Coronary autoregulation. Note that coronary blood flow is reasonably constant despite changes in coronary artery pressure. Below the autoregulatory range (approximately 60 mm Hg), flow is strongly pressure dependent. Vasodilator reserve is the increase in flow between the prevailing flow and a specified "maximum" vasodilator stimulus. Below the autoregulatory range, vasodilator reserve is exhausted. (From Crawford MH, DiMarco JP, Paulus WJ. *Cardiology*. 3rd ed. Elsevier; 2010.)

with known coronary artery disease. Signs of inadequate myocardial blood flow include but are not limited to hypotension that is minimally or unresponsive to vasopressor administration, new-onset dysrhythmias, and evidence of myocardial ischemia/infarction on an electrocardiogram (ECG) and decreased cardiac contractility (wall function abnormalities) on a transesophageal echocardiogram (TEE).

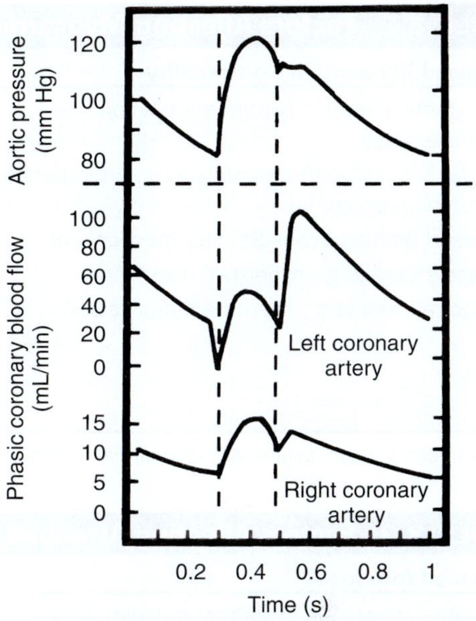

Fig. 3.2 Blood flow in the left and right coronary arteries. The right ventricle is perfused throughout the cardiac cycle. Flow to the left ventricle is largely confined to diastole. (From Kaplan JA, Reich DL, Savino JS, eds. *Kaplan's Cardiac Anesthesia: The Echo Era*. 6th ed. Elsevier; 2011.)

Myocardial Oxygen Demand

The hemodynamic factors that affect myocardial oxygen demand in order from greatest to least are as follows:

Heart rate > Contractility > Afterload > Preload

- *Heart rate:* Increasing heart rate not only increases demand but also decreases the diastolic perfusion time period of the LV. An increased heart rate is the most important factor that negatively affects MVO_2. Doubling the heart rate doubles myocardial oxygen demand. This phenomenon most dramatically affects patients with coronary artery disease because coronary blood supply is compromised; increasing demand without increasing supply can result in myocardial ischemia/infarction. By slowing heart rate and decreasing contractility, β-blocking medications increase supply and decrease demand, protecting the heart from ischemia. Conversely, medications that increase heart rate (e.g., ephedrine) increase myocardial oxygen demand.
- *Contractility:* The efficiency of cardiac contraction is measured as a ratio of work output and total energy expenditure. The inhalation anesthetic agents are

TABLE 3.2 Factors Affecting Myocardial Contractility

Increased Myocardial Contractility	Decreased Myocardial Contractility
Sympathetic nervous system stimulation *Catecholamines*	Parasympathetic nervous system stimulation *Acetylcholine*
Medications: Sympathomimetic (e.g., amiodarone, ketamine, ephedrine)	Medications: Sympatholytic (e.g., inhalational agents, propofol, β-blockers)
Increased preload (Frank-Starling mechanism)	Hypoxia/hypercarbia/acidosis
Disease states (e.g., hyperthyroidism)	Disease states (e.g., hypothyroidism)
Cardiac reflexes (e.g., chemoreceptor reflex)	Cardiac reflexes (e.g., baroreceptor reflex, celiac reflex, oculocardiac reflex)
	Cardiac disease states (e.g., previous MI, uncompensated CHF)
	Electrolyte disturbances (e.g., hyperkalemia, hypocalcemia)

CHF, Congestive heart failure; *MI*, myocardial infarction.

TABLE 3.3 Factors Affecting Afterload

Increased Afterload	Decreased Afterload
Sympathetic nervous system stimulation *Catecholamines*	Parasympathetic nervous system stimulation *Acetylcholine*
Disease states (e.g., pheochromocytoma, coarctation of the aorta)	Disease states (e.g., hypothyroidism)
Medications: Sympathomimetic (e.g., phenylephrine/ ephedrine, ketamine)	Medications: Sympatholytic (e.g., inhalational agents, propofol, ACE inhibitors, hydralazine)
Surgical (e.g., aortic cross-clamping)	Surgical (e.g., methyl methacrylate)
Hypoxia/hypercarbia/acidosis	Physiologic crises (e.g., anaphylaxis, acute adrenal crises)

ACE, Angiotensin-converting enzyme.

known to inhibit myocardial contractility in a dose-dependent manner. If contractility is inhibited such that severe hypotension occurs, neurologic and cardiac ischemia/infarction are possible. However, if MAP is adequate, inhibition of contractility can be desirable because it decreases myocardial oxygen demand. Factors that affect myocardial contractility are listed in Table 3.2.

- *Afterload:* When the pressure in the LV exceeds the pressure in the aorta, the aortic valve opens, and left ventricular systole or ejection occurs. Afterload encompasses the period spanning from closure of the mitral valve to increased LV muscle fiber shortening, aortic valve opening, LV ejection, and finally aortic valve closure. Afterload is dependent on systemic vascular resistance (SVR). Because the highest pressures and thus greatest increases in myocardial oxygen consumption are associated with left ventricular contraction, it is assumed that *afterload* refers to LV afterload. However, pulmonary hypertension can result in increased right ventricular afterload. Factors that affect afterload are presented in Table 3.3.
- *Preload* begins when the mitral valve opens and LV filling begins, and it concludes after closure of the mitral valve after atrial systole. The volume of blood contained within the LV at the end of atrial systole is known as *end-diastolic volume.* The Frank-Starling mechanism theorizes that increased blood volume increases the "stretch" on cardiac muscle fibers, which increases the force of LV contraction. Thus stroke volume (SV; volume of blood ejected from the LV after each heartbeat) increases as preload increases. However, this compensatory mechanism that minimizes the potential for volume overload has a limit. If LV preload is excessive, myocardial performance decreases, which can lead to congestive heart failure (CHF). Factors that affect preload are presented in Table 3.4.

TABLE 3.4 Factors Affecting Preload

Increased Preload	Decreased Preload
Sympathetic nervous system stimulation *Catecholamines*	Parasympathetic nervous system stimulation *Acetylcholine*
Disease states (e.g., Cushing syndrome)	Disease states (e.g., all forms of shock)
Medications: Sympathomimetic (e.g., phenylephrine/ephedrine, ketamine)	Medications: Sympatholytic (e.g., inhalation agents, propofol, ACE inhibitors, hydralazine)
Hypervolemia	Hypovolemia
Hypoxia/hypercarbia/acidosis	Physiologic crises (e.g., anaphylaxis, acute adrenal crises)

ACE, Angiotensin-converting enzyme.

KNOWLEDGE CHECK

1. Which best describes coronary artery autoregulation?
   a. Intrinsic ability of the coronary arteries to dilate and constrict to maintain constant myocardial blood flow
   b. Coronary artery blood flow is decreased at a MAP of 96 mm Hg.
   c. Most coronary artery blood flow to the LV occurs during systole.
   d. During periods of increased MVO_2, vasodilation occurs, resulting in increased coronary artery blood flow.
2. Which are factors that contribute to myocardial oxygen supply? *(Select all that apply.)*
   a. Hemoglobin
   b. Systolic time
   c. Heart rate
   d. Contractility
3. When increased, which factor increases myocardial oxygen consumption to the greatest degree?
   a. Afterload
   b. Heart rate
   c. Contractility
   d. Preload
4. Which factor increases afterload? *(Select all that apply.)*
   a. Parasympathetic nervous system predominance
   b. Septic shock
   c. Ketamine
   d. Acidosis
5. Which factor is representative of LV preload? *(Select all that apply.)*
   a. IV fluid, which increases LV preload
   b. Labetalol, which increases LV preload
   c. End-systolic volume
   d. Increased LV volume, which increases SV

Answers can be found in Appendix A.

Hypertension

Hypertension is the leading cause of cardiovascular disease, affecting one-third of adults in the United States. The incidence is expected to increase as a result of an increasing elderly population and the prevalence of obesity. The rate of hypertension is similar between males and females. There is a genetic predisposition associated with hypertension, which affects non-Hispanic Black adults to the greatest degree. There is scientific evidence showing the relationship between hypertension and cardiovascular disease.

Essential hypertension, which is also known as *primary* or *idiopathic hypertension*, has no identifiable causes and accounts for 95% of all cases. It is subjectively defined as systolic/diastolic blood pressure (SBP/DBP) > 160/90 mm Hg. The most current BP targets stated by the Joint National Committee on Prevention, Detection, Evaluation, and Treatment of High Blood Pressure are as follows:

- Patients ≥60 years old, BP goal ≤ 150/90 mm Hg
- Patients <60 years old with chronic kidney disease or diabetes mellitus, BP goal ≤ 140/90 mm Hg

Decreased vascular compliance is a part of the normal aging process because decreased elastin within the vascular endothelium causes arterial hardening (e.g., atherosclerosis). Secondary causes of hypertension include renal artery stenosis, endocrine disorders (e.g., Cushing disease, pheochromocytoma), drug-induced hypertension, and coarctation of the aorta. Hypertension accelerates and exacerbates the onset of atherosclerotic changes in the arterial vessels of the target organs. It is a primary risk factor for the development of coronary artery disease. Hypertension is a significant cause of CHF and cardiomyopathy because it causes increased afterload as a result of chronic vasoconstriction. Hypertension increases the likelihood of the development of atherosclerosis, and thus chronic untreated hypertension increases the incidence of myocardial infarction (MI), stroke, and chronic kidney injury.

The result of long-standing untreated hypertension is end-organ damage (Box 3.1). Preventive medical management consists of identifying a definitive cause, lifestyle changes (e.g., smoking cessation), and pharmacologic therapy. Antihypertensive treatment of chronic hypertension can include the use of one or a combination of the following medications: Thiazide diuretics, vasodilators (e.g., angiotensin-converting enzyme inhibitors [ACEIs] or angiotensin receptor blockers [ARBs]), and adrenergic antagonists (e.g., β-blockers and/or calcium blockers).

BOX 3.1 End-Organ Damage Caused by Hypertension

Vasculopathy
- Endothelial dysfunction
- Remodeling
- Generalized atherosclerosis
- Arteriosclerotic stenosis
- Aortic aneurysm

Cerebrovascular Damage
- Acute hypertensive encephalopathy
- Stroke
- Intracerebral hemorrhage
- Lacunar infarction
- Vascular dementia
- Retinopathy

Heart Disease
- Left ventricular hypertrophy
- Atrial fibrillation
- Coronary microangiopathy
- Coronary heart disease, myocardial infarction
- Heart failure

Nephropathy
- Albuminuria
- Proteinuria
- Chronic renal insufficiency
- Renal failure

From Hines RL, Jones RL. *Stoelting's Anesthesia and Co-Existing Disease*. 8th ed. Elsevier; 2022.

Anesthesia Case Management

- There is an increased possibility of significant hemodynamic variability during intraoperative anesthetic management as a result of the following:
  - Autonomic nervous system (ANS) dysfunction
  - Baroreceptor desensitization
  - Intravascular volume depletion

Preoperative

- There is no definitive degree of systolic hypertension that has been proven to increase physiologic complications in patients without cardiovascular disease during the perioperative period. Anecdotally, an SBP <180 mm Hg is desirable.
- A DBP >110 mm Hg is associated with increased perioperative cardiovascular complications and should be treated before anesthesia.
- ACEIs or ARBs can cause severe or refractory hypotension. It is reasonable to hold ACEIs or ARBs for 24 hours after the surgical procedure. Restarting ACEIs/ARBs postoperatively is indicated unless hypotension exists.
- Reinstitution of ACEIs and ARBs within 2 weeks postoperatively is associated with decreased 30-day mortality.
- Cardiac history (Box 3.2)
  - Dyspnea on exertion
  - Decreased functional capacity (metabolic equivalents [METs])
  - Angina
  - Dysrhythmias
  - MI
  - Atherosclerosis
  - CHF
  - Percutaneous coronary intervention (PCI)
  - Coronary artery bypass graft (CABG)
- Physical examination
  - *Auscultation heart sounds:* S1, S2, rate 60–90 BPM, regular; *abnormal:* extra heart sounds (snaps, clicks, friction rub, murmurs); excessively high or low rate, irregularity
  - *Auscultation breath sounds:* Equal, bilateral, clear apex to base; *abnormal:* Rales, rhonchi, wheezing, pleural friction rub

BOX 3.2 Revised Cardiac Risk Index

Risk Categories

- High-risk surgery (aortic, major vascular, peripheral vascular)
- Ischemic heart disease (previous myocardial infarction, previous positive result on stress test, use of nitroglycerin, typical angina, ECG Q waves, previous PCI or CABG)
- History of compensated previous congestive heart failure (history of heart failure, previous pulmonary edema, third heart sound, bilateral rales, evidence of heart failure on chest radiograph)
- History of cerebrovascular disease (previous TIA, previous stroke)
- Diabetes mellitus (with or without preoperative insulin)
- Renal insufficiency (creatinine >2.0 mg/dL)

Estimated Rates for Postoperative Major Adverse Cardiac Events per Number of Risks

- 0 risk factors: 0.4%
- 1 risk factor: 0.9%
- 2 risk factors: 7%
- 3 risk factors or more: 11%

CABG, Coronary artery bypass grafting; *ECG*, electrocardiogram; *PCI*, percutaneous coronary intervention; *TIA*, transient ischemic attack.
From Lee TH, Marcantonio ER, Mangione CM, et al. Derivation and prospective validation of a simple index for prediction of cardiac risk of major noncardiac surgery. *Circulation.* 1999;100:1043–1049; Freeman WK, Gibbons RJ. Perioperative cardiovascular assessment of patients undergoing noncardiac surgery. *Mayo Clin Proc.* 2009;84:79–90.

- Preoperative cardiac test results should be obtained on the basis of the patient's history, physical examination, and other coexisting diseases.
  - ECG
  - Echocardiography, chest x-ray (CXR)
  - Angiography

Intraoperative Goals

- No single anesthetic technique has been scientifically proven to be superior at decreasing an acute MI or cerebrovascular accident (CVA).
- Minimizing extreme hemodynamic variability is desirable to maintain a steady state of blood flow to the heart and the brain.
- Maintain MAP within 20% of preoperative MAP.

General anesthesia

- Because of the myocardial depression, vasodilation, and central nervous system (CNS) inhibition that occur with most anesthetic medications, profound and sustained hypotension may occur during induction.
- IV fluid loading preinduction, vasopressor support, incremental administration of medications, and use of higher doses of opiates instead of greater concentrations of inhalational agents may help minimize hypotension.

Neuraxial anesthesia

- The degree of hypotension is likely increased as the sensory block egresses toward higher dermatome levels (e.g., T10 [umbilicus] vs. T4 [nipple line]).
- The onset of hypotension is frequently slower with epidural administration, especially if incremental dosing is performed.
- Rapidly occurring nausea and vomiting several minutes after local anesthetic administration are frequently associated with severe hypotension caused by medullary hypoxia.
- To minimize the degree of hypotension with neuraxial anesthesia, administer an IV fluid bolus before administration of neuraxial anesthesia.
- Vasopressor support may be necessary. Caution should be used when administering phenylephrine for hypotension because it may worsen the bradycardia associated with cardioaccelerator nerve fiber blockade (T1–T4 distribution) if a high spinal block occurs.
- In the setting of severely elevated BP that is sustained despite a significant anesthetic depth and treatment with antihypertensive medications, the anesthetist should consider hypermetabolic syndromes (malignant hyperthermia [MH], pheochromocytoma, thyroid storm).

Treatment of Hypotension

- Assess noninvasive BP (recheck measurement).
- Assess invasive BP (assess level of transducer).
- Administer fraction of inspired oxygen (Fio_2) to keep saturation >90%.
- Decrease/discontinue administration of anesthetic agents.
- Identify and treat the cause of severe hypotension.
- Expand intravascular volume.
  - Crystalloids, colloids, packed RBCs if significant anemia is present
- Administer vasoactive medications (drug and dose are dependent on the degree of hypotension and the patient's condition).
  - Ephedrine
  - Phenylephrine

- Epinephrine
- Vasopressin
- Methylene blue
- Elevate lower extremities/mild Trendelenburg positioning.
- Minimize peak inspiratory pressure and/or positive end-expiratory pressure (PEEP)
- Consider other causes:
  - All shock states (see later discussion)
  - Medication error
  - Acute adrenal crises

KNOWLEDGE CHECK

1. Which hemodynamic value is associated with increased cardiovascular complications?
   a. SBP >180 mm Hg
   b. BP 170/96 mm Hg
   c. DBP >110 mm Hg
   d. MAP 100 mm Hg
2. Which interventions may decrease the degree of hypotension during the induction period?
   a. Administer 200 mg propofol.
   b. Preload with 500 mL lactated Ringer's solution IV.
   c. Ventilate with PEEP 10 cm H_2O.
   d. Deliver sevoflurane concentration of 3%.
3. Severe hypotension may be caused by *(Select all that apply.)*
   a. acute MI.
   b. inadvertent administration of hydralazine.
   c. dermatome level C8 sensory blockade from neuraxial anesthesia.
   d. acute adrenal crises.
   e. pheochromocytoma.

Answers can be found in Appendix A.

Valvular Heart Disease

The cardiac valves are membranous leaflets that separate the chambers of the heart. The atrioventricular (AV) valves include the following:

- Tricuspid valve between the right atrium (RA) and right ventricle
- Biscuspid or mitral valve between the left atrium (LA) and LV

The semilunar valves include the following:

- Pulmonic valve between the right ventricle and pulmonary artery (PA)
- Aortic valve between the LV and aorta

When open, cardiac valves allow blood flow between the chambers and great vessels, and when closed, they prevent regurgitant blood flow between the chambers or backflow from the great vessels. A valvular orifice of normal size presents a small degree of flow obstruction and thereby creates a hemodynamically insignificant gradient. Primary dysfunction of the mitral and aortic valves represents the most common, and causes the most severe, hemodynamic abnormalities. Acquired primary dysfunction of the tricuspid or pulmonic valves is rare.

Valvular heart disease is classified according to the type of lesion that exists: Stenosis, insufficiency, or mixed lesions. Valvular stenosis is a narrowing of the valvular orifice that restricts flow through the orifice when the valve is open. This situation creates an increase in flow resistance and increases turbulent blood flow. Valvular insufficiency results in regurgitation secondary to incomplete or partial valve closure, which allows for regurgitant blood flow into the atria.

Mitral Stenosis

Pathophysiology

- *Causes:* Annulus calcification, rheumatic heart disease, congenital, endocarditis
- *Signs and symptoms:* Fatigue, dyspnea, basilar crackles, hemoptysis, hoarseness, CHF, palpitations, atrial fibrillation (AF)
- An enlarged LA can impinge on the left recurrent laryngeal nerve, causing hoarseness.
- Normal mitral valve orifice is 4–6 cm^2; symptoms begin with mitral valve orifice narrowing of <1.5 cm^2.
- AF/atrial flutter can cause blood clot formation in LA, leading to hypotension and possibly systemic embolization.
- Decreased blood flow from LA to LV causes LA pressure overload.
- Pulmonary hypertension is likely to occur if pulmonary capillary wedge pressure (PCWP) exceeds 25 mm Hg (Fig. 3.3).

Medical/surgical therapy

- Diuretics are prescribed to decrease overall fluid volume, decreasing LA volume and thus LA pressure.
- AF occurs in one-third of patients with significant mitral stenosis (MS). Medical treatment includes β-blockers, calcium channel blockers, and/or digoxin.
- The incidence of embolic stroke with AF associated with MS is approximately 10%; thus anticoagulation is necessary.

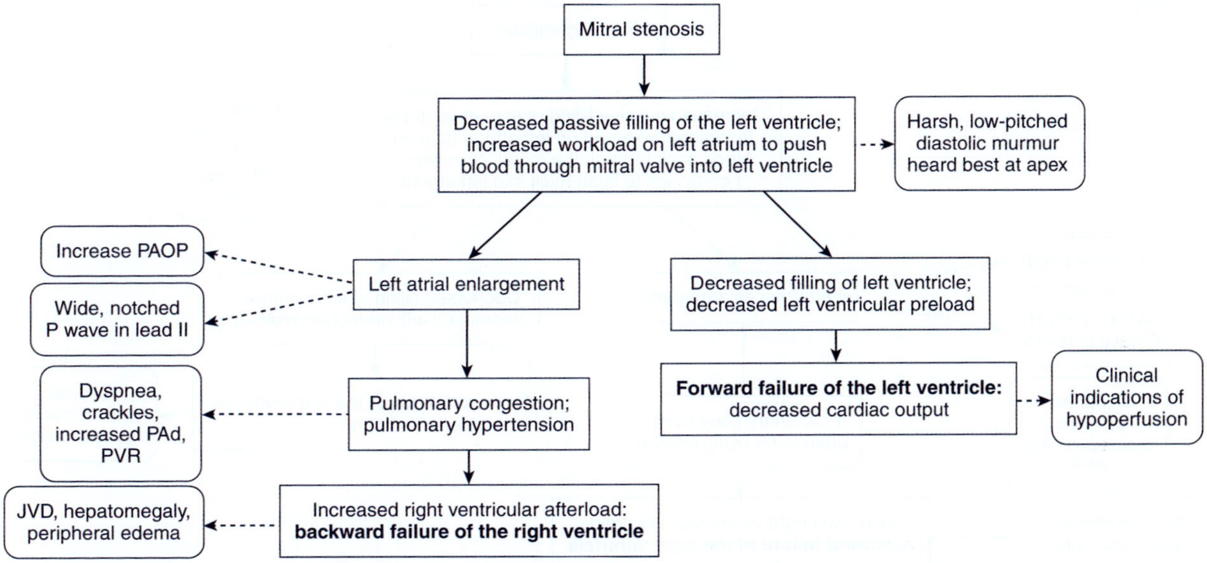

Fig. 3.3 Pathophysiology of mitral stenosis. *Dotted lines* connect pathology to the clinical presentation. *JVD*, Jugular venous distention; *PAd*, pulmonary artery diastolic pressure; *PAOP*, pulmonary artery occlusive pressure; *PVR*, pulmonary vascular resistance. (From Dennison RD. *Pass CCRN [Adult]*. 6th ed. Elsevier; 2024.)

- Surgical correction for MS includes percutaneous balloon valvotomy or direct valvular replacement.

Diagnostic testing/intraoperative monitoring

- *Auscultation:* Increased intensity of S1; early in diastole, a snap followed by a low-pitched murmur is heard best over the apex of the heart.
- CXR shows LA enlargement, right ventricular hypertrophy (RVH), pulmonary congestion, and mitral valve calcification.
- ECG shows notched P waves suggestive of LA enlargement, RVH, and dysrhythmias (e.g., AF).
- TEE reveals degree of mitral valve calcification and incompetence, atrial/ventricular dilation/wall motion abnormalities, and transmitral valve gradient.
- Intraoperative: Intraarterial monitoring.
- PCWP is an indirect measure of left-sided heart pressures in a normal heart. Therefore it is assumed that left-sided heart pressures increase as a result of increased left-sided heart volume.
- In patients with significant MS, PCWP *overestimates* left ventricular end-diastolic volume (LVEDV) or LV preload (e.g., PCWP 21 mm Hg and actual left ventricular end-diastolic pressure [LVEDP] = 12 mm Hg, decreased LVEDV or LV preload).
- Clinical significance: If PCWP = 21 mm Hg, the anesthetist may administer vasodilators/diuretics to decrease the elevated PCWP. Because PCWP overestimates LVEDV, this intervention causes significant hypotension.
- PCWP waveform associated with MS: Prominent *a* wave, decreased *y* descent.

Intraoperative hemodynamic considerations

- Maintain normal sinus rhythm (NSR): Loss of atrial kick further decreases LV preload.
- Minimize tachycardia: Ideal heart rate is between 60 and 70 BPM; rapid heart rate decreases LV diastolic filling time. Significant afterload reduction caused by vasodilation in patients who are not receiving β-blocking medication will result in increased heart rate.
- Significant increases in preload (e.g., fluid, blood, vasopressors) and/or myocardial depression can precipitate CHF.
- Phenylephrine: Vasopressor of choice for hypotension

Anesthetic considerations

- Neuraxial anesthesia is permissible. Either subarachnoid block (SAB) or epidural blockade is acceptable. An advantage associated with epidural anesthesia is incremental dosing and more gradual effects associated with hemodynamic manipulation. The lowest dermatome level possible minimizes significant decreases in afterload.

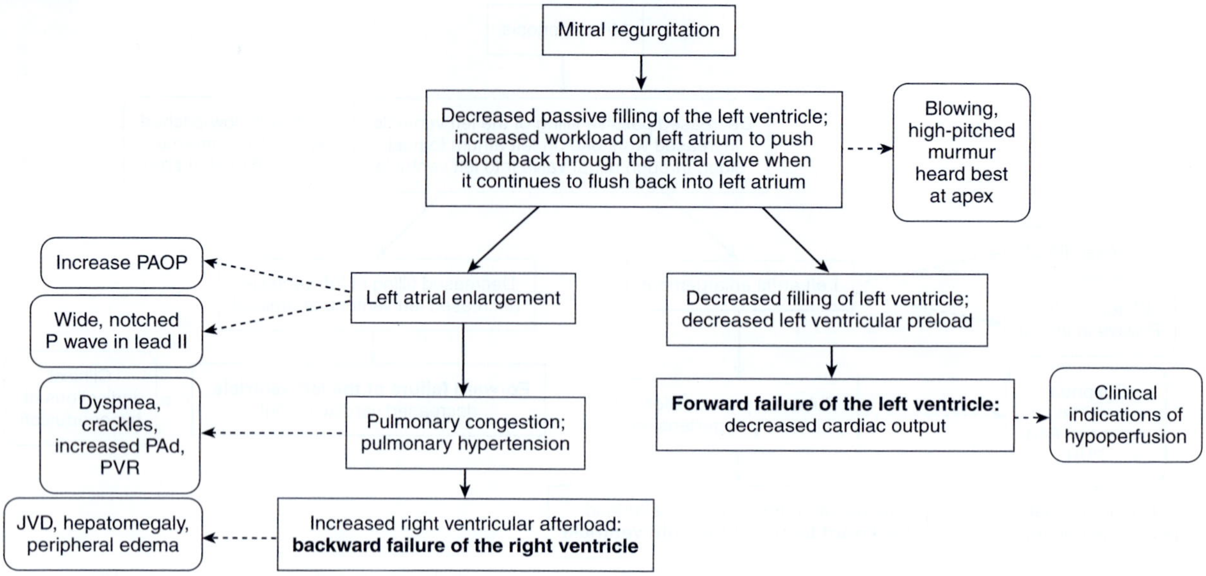

Fig. 3.4 Pathophysiology of mitral regurgitation. *Dotted lines* connect pathology to the clinical presentation. *JVD*, Jugular venous distention; *PAd*, pulmonary artery diastolic pressure; *PAOP*, pulmonary artery occlusive pressure; *PVR*, pulmonary vascular resistance. (From Dennison RD. *Pass CCRN [Adult]*. 6th ed. Elsevier; 2024.)

- Avoid tachycardia (ketamine, anticholinergics, ephedrine, adequate depth of anesthesia) and rapidly ensuing hypotension.
- Acute-onset AF with rapid ventricular response/supraventricular tachycardia (SVT) can be treated with synchronized cardioversion, amiodarone, calcium channel blockers, or β-blockers.
- Avoid large/rapid increases in central blood volume, which can cause CHF.
- If hypotension requiring vasopressor therapy occurs, incremental doses of phenylephrine increase SVR without causing tachycardia.

Mitral Regurgitation

Pathophysiology

- Mitral regurgitation (MR) can result as part of acute dysfunction (e.g., papillary muscle rupture) or chronic disease (e.g., cardiomyopathy).
- *Acute MR* can result in rapidly ensuing decreased SV, LA volume overload, pulmonary edema, and cardiovascular collapse. The signs and symptoms are dependent on the severity and rapidity of onset.
- *Chronic MR* causes compensatory LV dilation over time and preserves SV. As MR becomes more severe, a decrease in SV and pulmonary edema occurs.
- Moderate symptoms occur with regurgitant fraction of 30%–60%. Severe symptoms occur with regurgitant fraction $> 60\%$ (Fig. 3.4).

Medical/surgical therapy

- Pharmacologic medical therapy: Vasodilators (e.g., ACEIs/ARBs), positive inotropic effect (e.g., digoxin, amrinone), diuretics, anticoagulants
- Ventricular pacing
- Open or percutaneous mitral valve repair

Diagnostic testing/intraoperative monitoring

- CXR with moderate to severe MR consistent with cardiomegaly
- Auscultation; holosystolic apical murmur
- Echocardiography shows the presence of wall motion abnormalities, atrial and ventricular chamber size, severity of MR, and estimate of LV function.
- ABP/central venous pressure (CVP) monitoring is indicated for significant MR and/or surgical procedures associated with extensive hemodynamic variability.
- PCWP is indicated for severe MR with history of CHF. A large V wave is associated with MR.
- Similar to MS, PCWP may not accurately reflect LVEDP/LVEDV because of a loss of LV compliance from remodeling associated with chronic volume overload.

Intraoperative hemodynamic considerations

- Maintain NSR: Loss of atrial kick further decreases LV preload. New-onset AF can occur.
- The phrase *fast, full, and forward* can be used to conceptualize general hemodynamic goals for patients with MR.
  - Avoiding bradycardia and maintaining a more rapid heart rate ≥80 BPM decreases regurgitant blood flow and maximizes SV.
  - Avoiding rapid increases in intravascular volume can result in LA and LV overload. Maintaining adequate preload is necessary for adequate LV preload and SV.
  - Rapid and significant increases in SVR (afterload) can decrease SV and lead to LA/LV overload and pulmonary edema.
- Preserve myocardial contractility.
- Ephedrine: Vasopressor of choice for hypotension

Anesthetic considerations

- For moderate to severe MR, consider higher doses of narcotics in relation to inhalational agents to minimize myocardial depression.
- Neuraxial anesthesia is permissible. Either SAB or epidural blockade is acceptable. An advantage associated with epidural anesthesia is incremental dosing and more gradual effects associated with hemodynamic manipulation. The lowest dermatome level possible minimizes significant decreases in afterload. If the patient is receiving anticoagulants, the anesthetist should abide by the most current American Society of Regional Anesthesia and Pain Medicine (ASRA) guidelines before performing neuraxial anesthesia.
- If hypotension that requires vasopressor therapy occurs, incremental doses of ephedrine increase SVR without causing bradycardia.
- Avoid large tidal volume (V_t) breaths and PEEP if possible during mechanical ventilation to maximize venous return.

Aortic Stenosis

Pathophysiology

- *Causes:* Congenital defect (e.g., bicuspid aortic valve, coarctation), rheumatic heart disease, calcification
- Normal aortic valve orifice (AVO) = 2.5–3.5 cm^2, mild to moderate aortic stenosis (AS) AVO = 1.0–1.5 cm^2, critical AS AVO < 1.0 cm^2.
- If hypotension occurs, sympathetic nervous system (SNS) predominance causes a compensatory increase in SV to improve peripheral perfusion. As aortic valve narrowing progresses, the amount of blood that can be ejected from the LV is fixed despite an increase in heart rate, contractility, and cardiac conduction velocity.
- LV pressure overload results in compensatory LV hypertrophy, which increases the MVO_2.
- Increased LV ejection time decreases LV diastolic perfusion.
- LV ischemia and infarction can cause pulmonary edema and cardiogenic shock.
- The signs and symptoms associated with moderate to severe AS are also dependent on the adequacy of ejection fraction, dyspnea on exertion, angina, orthostatic hypotension, and exertional syncope.
- Critical AS produces a triad of symptoms: Angina (even in the absence of significant coronary artery disease), syncope, and CHF (Fig. 3.5).

Medical/surgical therapy

- Pharmacologic medical therapy: Inotropes (e.g., digoxin, amrinone), diuretics, ACEIs/ARBs
- Surgical options: Aortic valve replacement, balloon valvuloplasty, transcatheter aortic valve replacement

Diagnostic testing/intraoperative monitoring

- Auscultation: Systolic ejection murmur over the second intercostal space, right sternal border
- Preoperative ECG: LA/LV hypertrophy, dysrhythmia (e.g., AF), left bundle branch block
- Preoperative CXR: Cardiomegaly, left ventricular hypertrophy (LVH), RVH, pulmonary congestion
- Preoperative echocardiography: Aortic valve thickening, calcification of aortic valve annulus, aortic valve area, LVH, transvalvular pressure gradient
- ABP/CVP monitoring is indicated for moderate to critical AS and/or surgical procedures associated with extensive hemodynamic variability; a narrowed pulse pressure is consistent with AS.
- PCWP monitoring is indicated for severe AS with history of CHF.

Intraoperative hemodynamic considerations

- Maintenance of NSR to achieve adequate LVEDV; acute-onset AF may result in severe hypotension, rapid-onset pulmonary edema, and cardiovascular collapse.
- Avoid acute and extreme decreases in SVR.
- Avoid bradycardia (LV overload → decreased SV, left-sided heart failure).
- Avoid tachycardia (increased MVO_2 and decreased oxygen supply → LV ischemia) (tachycardia → decreased systolic ejection time → decreased SV).

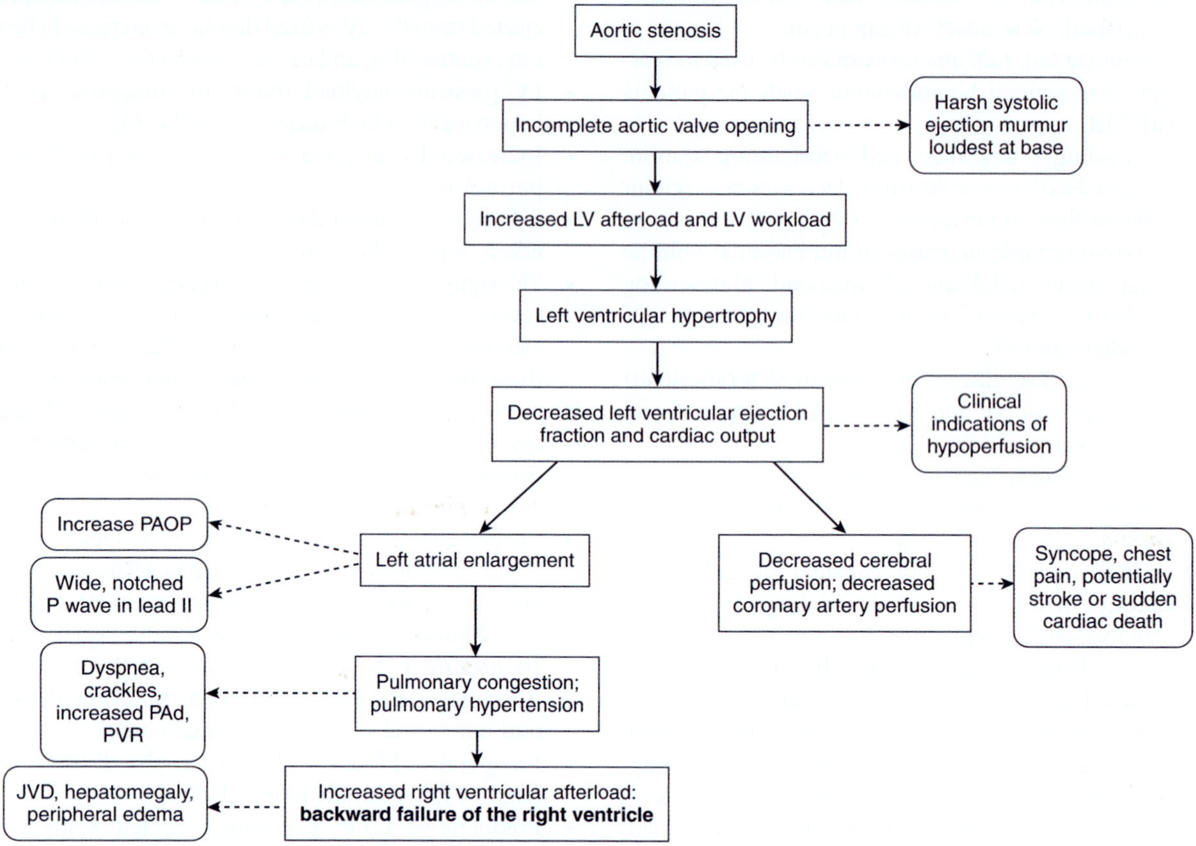

Fig. 3.5 Pathophysiology of aortic stenosis. *Dotted lines* connect pathology to the clinical presentation. *JVD*, Jugular venous distention; *LV*, left ventricular; *PAd*, pulmonary artery diastolic pressure; *PAOP*, pulmonary artery occlusive pressure; *PVR*, pulmonary vascular resistance. (From Dennison RD. *Pass CCRN [Adult]*. 6th ed. Elsevier; 2024.)

- Maintain normovolemia (adequate preload) necessary for LVEDV.
- Preserve myocardial contractility, especially if LV ejection fraction (EF) is compromised.
- Phenylephrine: Vasopressor of choice for hypotension

Anesthetic considerations

- Consider higher-dose narcotics in relation to inhalation agent to minimize myocardial depression.
- *Extreme caution* must be used if neuraxial anesthesia is administered. The use of neuraxial anesthesia for patients with AS is controversial. An advantage associated with epidural anesthesia compared with spinal anesthesia is incremental dosing and more gradual effects associated with hemodynamic manipulation. The lowest dermatome level possible minimizes significant decreases in afterload. If the patient is receiving anticoagulants, the anesthetist should abide by the current ASRA guidelines before performing neuraxial anesthesia. For patients with critical AS, neuraxial anesthesia is contraindicated.
- If hypotension that requires vasopressor therapy occurs, incremental doses of phenylephrine increase SVR without causing tachycardia.
- In the event of cardiac arrest associated with ventricular tachycardia (VT), early defibrillation is essential because external cardiac compressions will not create adequate SV.

Aortic Regurgitation

Pathophysiology

- Aortic regurgitation (AR) can be caused by acute dysfunction (e.g., papillary muscle rupture) or chronic disease (e.g., cardiomyopathy).
- *Acute AR* can result in rapidly ensuing decreased SV, LA volume overload, pulmonary edema, and cardiovascular collapse. The signs and symptoms are dependent on the severity and rapidity of onset. Causes include trauma, aortic dissection, and endocarditis.
- *Chronic AR* causes compensatory LV dilation over time and preserves SV. As AR becomes more severe, a decrease in SV, LV overload, and pulmonary edema occurs. Causes include rheumatic heart disease, Marfan syndrome, and connective tissue diseases (systemic lupus erythematosus).
- Symptoms: Mild = regurgitant volume < 40% SV; severe = regurgitant volume > 60% SV, exertional chest pain, syncope, palpitations, consistent with LV failure (dyspnea, orthopnea, fatigue)
- Signs: Widening pulse pressure, pulmonary congestion, and decreased DBP (Fig. 3.6)

Medical treatment

- Pharmacologic medical therapy: Inotropes (e.g., digoxin, amrinone), diuretics, ACEIs/ARBs, calcium channel blockers
- Surgical option: Aortic valve replacement

Diagnostic testing/intraoperative monitoring

- Auscultation: High-pitched diastolic murmur loudest at base; also possible, middiastolic low-pitched murmur
- Preoperative ECG: LVH, dysrhythmias

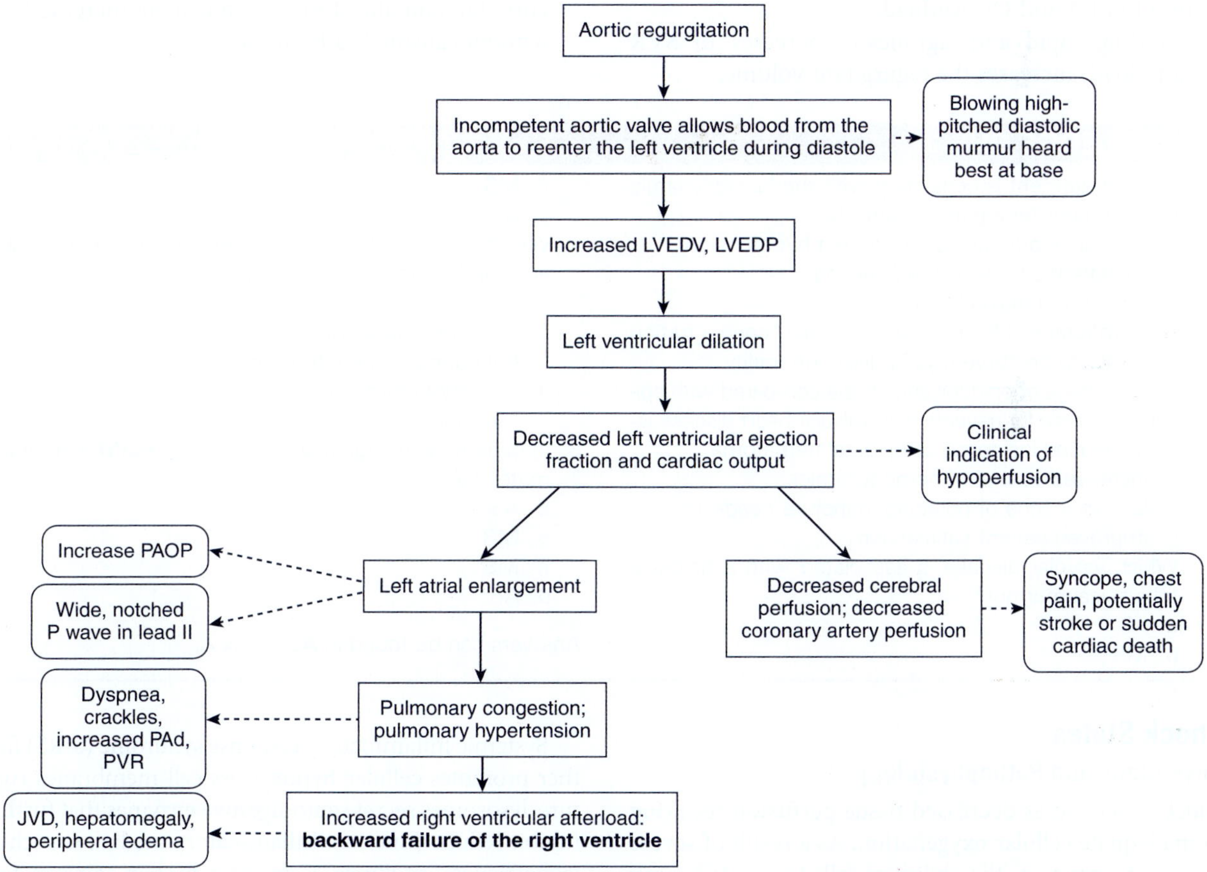

Fig. 3.6 Pathophysiology of aortic regurgitation. Dotted lines connect pathology to the clinical presentation. *JVD*, Jugular venous distention; *LVEDP*, left ventricular end-diastolic pressure; *LVEDV*, left ventricular end-diastolic volume; *PAd*, pulmonary artery diastolic pressure; *PAOP*, pulmonary artery occlusive pressure; *PVR*, pulmonary vascular resistance. (From Dennison RD. *Pass CCRN [Adult]*. 6th ed. Elsevier; 2024.)

- Preoperative CXR: LVH, LA enlargement, pulmonary congestion
- Preoperative echocardiography: Aortic valve thickening, LVH, EF, regurgitant fraction
- ABP/CVP monitoring is indicated for moderate to severe AR and/or surgical procedures associated with extensive hemodynamic variability; a widened pulse pressure is consistent with AR.
- PCWP measurement indicated for severe AR with history of CHF; large V wave present

Intraoperative hemodynamic considerations

- The phrase *fast and forward* can be used to conceptualize general hemodynamic goals for patients with AR.
- Avoiding bradycardia and maintaining a more rapid heart rate ≥80 BPM decreases regurgitant blood flow by shortening diastolic time and the regurgitant volume.
- Avoiding rapid increases in intravascular volume can result in LA and LV overload.
- Avoiding rapid and significant increases in SVR (afterload) increases the regurgitant volume.
- Preserve myocardial contractility.
- Ephedrine: Vasopressor of choice for hypotension

Anesthetic considerations

- For moderate to severe AR, consider higher doses of narcotics in relation to inhalational agent to minimize myocardial depression. Titration of narcotics is vital to avoid bradycardia.
- Neuraxial anesthesia is permissible. Either SAB or epidural blockade is acceptable. An advantage associated with epidural anesthesia is incremental dosing and more gradual effects associated with hemodynamic manipulation. The lowest dermatome level possible minimizes significant decreases in afterload. If the patient is receiving anticoagulants, the anesthetist should abide by the current ASRA guidelines before performing neuraxial anesthesia.
- If hypotension that requires vasopressor therapy occurs, incremental doses of ephedrine increase SVR without causing bradycardia.

KNOWLEDGE CHECK

1. Which treatment is consistent with the hemodynamic management for a patient with AS?
   a. Ephedrine administration to treat hypotension
   b. Hydralazine to decrease afterload
   c. Albumin to maximize SV
   d. Sevoflurane 1.5 minimum alveolar concentration (MAC) to preserve myocardial contractility
2. An advantage of epidural anesthesia compared with spinal anesthesia for patients with valvular heart disease is
   a. decreased incidence of epidural hematoma.
   b. increased control of hemodynamics.
   c. less incidence of postdural puncture headache
   d. improved patient satisfaction.
3. Which valvular disease is associated with a holosystolic apical murmur?
   a. AS
   b. MR
   c. MS
   d. AR
4. Which are desirable hemodynamic goals for both AR and MR? *(Select all that apply.)*
   a. NSR
   b. Heart rate 60 BPM
   c. Ephedrine for hypotension
   d. BP 150/98 mm Hg
   e. Maximize preload
5. In patients with significant ________, PCWP overestimates LVEDV.
   a. AS
   b. MR
   c. MS
   d. AR

Answers can be found in Appendix A.

Shock States

Physiology and Pathophysiology

Shock is defined as decreased tissue perfusion resulting in inadequate cellular oxygenation. As a result of severe oxygen deprivation, the ability of cells to create energy in the form of ATP is severely diminished. Cellular acidosis ensues as pyruvic acid (byproduct of anaerobic metabolism) is converted to lactic acid.

Systemic inflammatory response syndrome (SIRS) further promotes cellular hypoxia. As cell membranes rupture, lysosomes secrete autodigestive enzymes that further inhibit cellular function. Inflammatory mediators such as leukotrienes, cytokines, C-reactive protein, oxygen free radicals, and prostaglandins are liberated and further decrease physiologic adaptation by promoting capillary vasodilation, cellular edema, and metabolic acidosis.

If cellular hypoxia and acidosis are inadequately treated, progression of the shock state can result in multiple organ dysfunction syndrome (MODS). When two or more organ systems are adversely affected, MODS can occur. A continuum from the initial shock state to the development of MODS includes cellular hypoxia → SIRS → progression of the shock state → MODS. The development of MODS dramatically increases the mortality rate. Respiratory failure, gastrointestinal bleeding, hepatic failure, and renal failure are frequently associated with MODS.

This pathologic process occurs over a continuum and is divided into the three stages of shock: (1) compensatory (physiologic adaptation), (2) progressive (progressive failure of physiologic adaptation), and (3) irreversible (refractory; the physiologic state is refractory to resuscitative efforts). The physiologic insults are systemic, extreme, and not able to be overcome. The more rapidly the shock state is treated and cellular hypoxia is reversed, the greater the chance of survival. The specific shock states, signs, symptoms, and treatments are presented in Table 3.5.

Classification of Shock

- Fig. 3.7 is a visual reference that categorizes shock states.
- Hypodynamic shock is associated with low cardiac output and vasoconstriction (e.g., hypovolemic, cardiogenic, obstructive [cardiac compressive]).
- Hyperdynamic shock is associated with high cardiac output and vasodilation (e.g., distributive shock [anaphylactic, septic]).

Intravascular volume—"the tank"

- *Hypovolemic shock:* Inadequate intravascular volume; the degree of intravascular volume depletion determines the severity of the signs and symptoms that occur.

Heart—"the pump"

- *Cardiogenic shock:* Inadequate SV; 40% is caused by MI.
- *Obstructive shock (cardiac compressive shock):* External cardiac compression, outflow tract obstruction, and/or decreased ventricular compliance impair SV (e.g., cardiac tamponade).

Arterial and venous vasculature—"the pipes"

The "pipes" distribute blood from the heart to peripheral tissues. Regardless of the definitive cause, distributive shock causes severe vasodilation and hypotension.

- *Anaphylactic shock:* An allergen (e.g., medication, blood transfusion, latex) causes immunoglobulin E (IgE) antibody production. A type 1 hypersensitivity reaction results from degranulation of mast cells, releasing histamine, tryptase, kinins, leukotrienes, and other chemical mediators that cause severe vasodilation and hypotension. Histamine is responsible for many of the adverse effects, including bronchoconstriction, vasodilation, urticaria, pruritus, and increased mucus production. It is also involved in complement system activation.

TABLE 3.5 Severity of Hemorrhagic Shock

Indicator	Class I	Class II	Class III	Class IV
Blood loss (% of blood volume)	Less than 15%	15%–30%	30%–40%	Greater than 40%
Blood loss (mL)	Less than 750 mL	750–1500 mL	1500–2000 mL	Greater than 2000 mL
Heart rate, beats/min	Less than 100	Greater than 100	Greater than 120	140 or greater
Blood pressure	Normal	Normal	Decreased	Decreased
Pulse pressure	Widened or normal	Narrowed	Narrowed	Narrowed
Capillary refill	Normal	Delayed	Delayed	Delayed or absent
Ventilatory rate/min	14–20	20–30	30–40	Greater than 35
Urine output (mL/h)	30 or greater	20–30	Less than 20	Negligible
Skin appearance	Cool, pink	Cool, pale	Cold, moist, pale	Cold, clammy, cyanotic
Neurologic status	Slightly anxious	Mildly anxious	Anxious, confused	Confused, lethargic

Modified from American College of Surgeons. *ATLS: Advanced Trauma Life Support for Doctors.* 8th ed. American College of Surgeons; 2008.

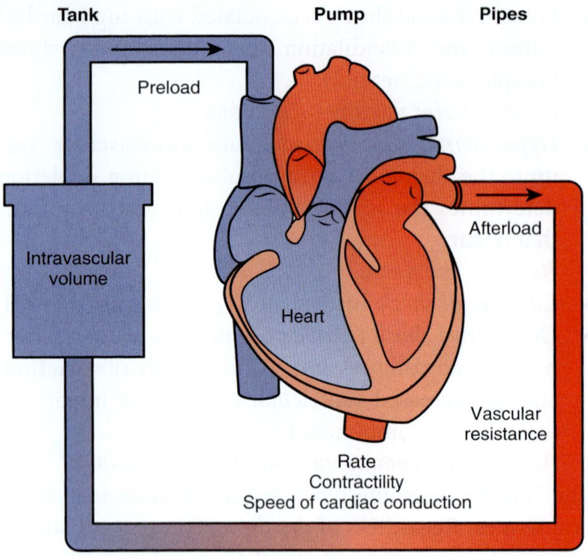

Fig. 3.7 Cardiovascular components affected by shock states.

- *Septic shock:* The Society of Critical Care Medicine and the European Society of Intensive Care Medicine decided to collaborate to attempt to reduce the morbidity and mortality of sepsis and septic shock. The Surviving Sepsis Campaign is a collection of the most effective evidence-based treatment strategies. The coalition publishes updated guidelines on a periodic basis.
  - *Sepsis*: Life-threatening organ dysfunction caused by systemic infection resulting in a loss of physiologic autoregulation. It is associated with hypotension, cellular hypoxia, inflammatory mediator release, SIRS, oliguria, and elevated lactate.
  - *Septic shock*: Worsening progression of sepsis that is minimally responsive/refractory to treatment. It is associated with a high risk of mortality.
- *Neurogenic shock*: A loss of SNS influence on SVR resulting in severe vasodilation and hypotension. If neurogenic shock is caused by a spinal cord injury (SCI), the higher the disruption, the greater the degree of hypotension. Signs include the following:
  - *C3–C5 distribution:* Absence of motor innervation to the diaphragm via the phrenic nerve causes apnea.
  - *T1–T4 distribution:* SNS stimulation via the cardioaccelerator fibers that innervate the heart. Parasympathetic nervous system predominance occurs and causes bradycardia.

Treatment

General intraoperative treatment strategy for acute shock before determining a definitive cause (Table 3.6):

- Administer 100% oxygen.
- Evaluate adequacy of breathing: Endotracheal intubation as needed.
- Administer IV fluids (e.g., crystalloids/colloids/blood/blood products).
- Maintain appropriate BP (MAP ≥65 mm Hg).
  - Decreased anesthetic depth
  - Pharmacologic treatment (vasopressors/positive inotropic medications)
- Place at least two large-bore peripheral IV lines.
- Invasive line placement (e.g., arterial line, central line).
- Consider IV scopolamine/ketamine for sedation if severe hypotension is present.
- Obtain diagnostic tests (e.g., ECG, arterial blood gas [ABG], CXR, echocardiography).
- Monitor complete blood count, coagulation status, renal function, and electrolyte status.
- Monitor acid–base status and manage acidosis appropriately.
- Monitor urine output (≥0.5 mL/kg/h).
- Perform cardiac resuscitation per American Heart Association (AHA) advanced cardiac life support/pediatric advanced life support (ACLS/PALS) protocol.

Cardiac Conduction System: Dysrhythmias

During the course of a normal cardiac cycle, the conduction pathways and structural components of the heart work in coordination. This synchrony is vital to venous oxygenation and ultimately oxygen delivery (DO_2) to peripheral and central tissues. Cardiac dysrhythmias represent conduction and/or structural aberrancies of the cardiac cycle. The severity of a particular cardiac dysrhythmia is dependent on its (1) etiology, (2) onset and duration (e.g., acute or chronic presentation), (3) effect on venous oxygenation and DO_2, and (4) adequacy of preoperative medical management. Medical management includes antidysrhythmic medication, antithrombotic medication, use of external or insertion of internal pacemaker, and automatic implantable cardioverter-defibrillator efficacy.

The cardiac dysrhythmias to be discussed are (1) sinus bradycardia and AV heart block, (2) sinus tachycardia, (3) atrial tachyarrhythmias (e.g., AF, atrial flutter, and SVT), (4) ventricular tachyarrhythmias (e.g., VT,

KNOWLEDGE CHECK

1. Which shock state is associated with hypotension associated with decreased afterload? *(Select all that apply.)*
   a. Cardiogenic
   b. Anaphylactic
   c. Neurogenic
   d. Obstructive
   e. Hypovolemic
   f. Septic
2. Which sign is associated with cardiac tamponade? (*Select all that apply.*)
   a. Hypotension, jugular venous distention, and muffled heart sounds
   b. Tachycardia, hypertension, and angioedema
   c. Hyperthermia, bradycardia, and widened pulse pressure
   d. Unilateral breath sounds, tachycardia, and increased CVP
3. Which medication should be administered as an initial treatment for anaphylactic shock?
   a. Hydrocortisone
   b. Ranitidine
   c. Epinephrine
   d. Diphenhydramine
4. During the initial treatment of shock, which value represents a major goal of hemodynamic management?
   a. CVP 5 mm Hg
   b. Heart rate <110 beats per minute
   c. Urine output >1 mL/kg/h
   d. MAP ≥65 mm Hg
5. According to the Surviving Sepsis Campaign, which is a major recommendation to improve survivability?
   a. Titrating dobutamine to maintain MAPs >60 mm Hg
   b. Administering broad-spectrum antibiotics within 1 hour after diagnosis
   c. Maintaining blood glucose <200 mg/dL
   d. Maintaining oxygen venous saturation ≥60%

Answers can be found in Appendix A.

TABLE 3.6 Signs, Symptoms, and Treatments of Various Shock States

Shock States	Cause(s)	Signs and Symptoms	Treatment
Hypovolemic	• Major vascular disruption and exsanguination • Excessive fluid loss (e.g., vomiting, diarrhea) • Inadequate fluid intake • Major burns	• Tachycardia • Initial hypertension followed by hypotension • Oliguria • Cool, clammy skin • Anxiety and/or confusion • Decreased CVP	• Identify cause and stop blood loss • Replace volume • Administer blood products • For massive blood transfusion, consider replacement ratio of 1 PRBC/1 FFP/1 Platelet • Provide vasopressor and inotropic support as needed
Cardiogenic	• Damage to cardiac tissue causing myocardial dysfunction from ischemia, contusion, drugs, or toxins	• Hypotension • Decreased pulse pressure (e.g., <25 mm Hg) • Tachycardia • Increased CVP/PCWP • Tachypnea • Pulmonary edema • Oliguria • Cool, clammy skin • Anxiety and/or confusion	• Decrease the workload of heart (e.g., nitrates, morphine) • Provide inotropic and vasopressor support as needed • Aspirin therapy • Obtain serum cardiac markers (e.g., CK-MB, troponin I and II) and an ECG • Consider transesophageal echocardiogram to evaluate cardiac function • Consider pulmonary artery catheter monitoring • Consider intraaortic balloon pump or ventricular assist device • Consider thrombolytic therapy, cardiac stent placement, or coronary artery bypass surgery

Continued

TABLE 3.6 Signs, Symptoms, and Treatments of Various Shock States—cont'd

Shock States	Cause(s)	Signs and Symptoms	Treatment

Obstructive (cardiac compressive)	• Cardiac tamponade
	• Tension pneumothorax with mediastinal compression
	• Constrictive pericarditis
	• Massive pulmonary embolus
		• Hypotension
		• Tachycardia
		• Tachypnea
		• Anxiety and/or confusion
		• Increased CVP/PCWP
		• Cardiac tamponade
		  • Beck's triad (hypotension, JVD, muffled heart sounds)
		  • Narrowed pulse pressure (e.g., <25 mm Hg)
		  • Tachypnea
		• Tension pneumothorax
		  • Decreased breath sounds
		  • Unilateral breath sounds
		  • Tracheal deviation
		  • Cyanosis
		  • Tachypnea
		  • Respiratory compromise
			• Identify and correct cause
			• Pericardiocentesis
			• Needle decompression in affected lung
			• Chest tube placement in affected lung
			• Provide inotropic and vasopressor support as needed

Septic	• Infection by a microorganism in the body causing a systemic inflammatory response (gram-negative or gram-positive bacteria are most common pathogens) • Severe burns • Bowel perforation • Major trauma • Indwelling devices (e.g., Foley catheters, central lines) • IV drug use	• Hyperthermia • Tachycardia • Hypotension • Wide pulse pressure • Decreased CVP • Tachypnea • Mental status changes • Conjunctival petechiae • Oliguria • Liver dysfunction • Coagulopathy • DIC	• Broad-spectrum IV antibiotic therapy within 1 hour of diagnosis • Provide IV crystalloid 30 mL/kg within 3 hours of diagnosis • Provide inotropic and vasopressor support as needed (norepinephrine is first-line therapy) • Repair perforated bowel and clean peritoneum • Remove and culture indwelling devices • Obtain urine, blood, and/or CSF cultures • Obtain CBC, electrolyte panel, renal function, coagulation studies, D-dimer, ABG analysis, LFTs, and urinalysis Goals: • MAP ≥μ65 mm Hg • Urine output ≥0.5 mL/kg/h • CVP 8–12 mm Hg • $Scvo_2$ ≥70% • Blood glucose ≤180 mg/dL
Neurogenic	• Central nervous system damage (brain and/or spinal cord)	• Hypotension (from loss of sympathetic tone) • Decreased CVP • Bradycardia • Neurologic dysfunction (e.g., paresthesias, paralysis) • Warm, dry skin • Hypothermia	• Provide adequate volume • Provide inotropic and vasopressor support as needed • Atropine as necessary • Careful airway management (avoid movement of head and neck) • Cautious succinylcholine administration (K^+ release)

TABLE 3.6 Signs, Symptoms, and Treatments of Various Shock States—cont'd

Shock States	Cause(s)	Signs and Symptoms	Treatment
Anaphylactic	• Antigen–antibody reaction (immunologic hypersensitivity reaction) • Nonimmunologic hypersensitivity reaction • Delayed hypersensitivity reaction	• Pruritus • Urticaria • Angioedema • Tachycardia • Hypotension • Decreased CVP • Tachypnea • Respiratory compromise (i.e., stridor, wheezing, arrest) • Cardiac arrest	• Identify offending agent and discontinue use • Administer 1. Epinephrine 10–100 mcg Epinephrine infusion 1–10 mcg/min 2. H_1 receptor blockade Diphenhydramine 50 mg 3. H_2 receptor blockade Famotidine 20 mg or Ranitidine 50 mg or Cimetidine 300 mg 4. Hydrocortisone 100 mg • Provide adequate volume • Provide inotropic and vasopressor support as needed

ABG, Arterial blood pressure; *CBC*, complete blood count; *CK-MB*, creatine kinase-MB; *CSF*, cerebrospinal fluid; *CVP*, central venous pressure; *DIC*, disseminated intravascular coagulation; *ECG*, electrocardiogram; FFP, fresh frozen plasma; H_2, histamine; *IV*, intravenous; *JVD*, jugular venous distention; *LFT*, liver function test; *MAP*, mean arterial pressure; *PCWP*, pulmonary capillary wedge pressure; *PRBC*, packed red blood cell; $Scvo_2$, central venous oxygen saturation.

ventricular fibrillation [VF], and torsade de pointes), and (5) pulseless electrical activity (PEA) and asystole. Differential diagnosis and treatment of cardiac dysrhythmias should be based on treating the underlying pathologic state and carrying out ACLS/PALS protocols.

Cardiac Conduction Pathway (Fig. 3.8 and Table 3.7)

Sinoatrial node

- Located along the epicardial surface at the junction between the superior vena cava and RA
- Intrinsic cardiac impulse origination begins at the sinoatrial (SA) node at a rate of between 60 and 100 times per minute.

Internodal pathways

- The anterior (Bachmann bundle), middle (Wenckebach bundle), and posterior internodal tracts are located within the RA and conduct impulses to the AV node.

Atrioventricular node

- Located beneath the endocardium on the right atrial septum
- Responsible for a delay in cardiac conduction
- Slowed cardiac conduction at the AV node allows for atrial depolarization and contraction to occur.

Atrioventricular bundle (bundle of his)

- Located on the posterior aspect of the RA and tricuspid valve
- Only electrical connection between the atria and ventricles
- The intrinsic pacemaker cells in the AV bundle depolarize at a rate of 40–60 times per minute.

Left and right bundle branches

- Transmission of impulse from AV bundle to Purkinje fibers
- Left branches: Left anterior and posterior fascicles
- Right branch: Terminates near the right venticular apex
- Both left and right bundle branches intertwined with the Purkinje fibers

Purkinje fibers

- Distal position of the cardiac conduction system: Rapid rate of conduction
- Impulse conduction to right and left ventricular walls
- The intrinsic pacemaker cells in the AV bundle depolarize at a rate of 20–40 times per minute (see Table 3.7).

Relationship of Cardiac Conduction to ECG Wave Morphology (Fig. 3.9)

- *P wave*: Initiated by SA node, completed after impulse conduction and atrial depolarization via right and left bundle branches

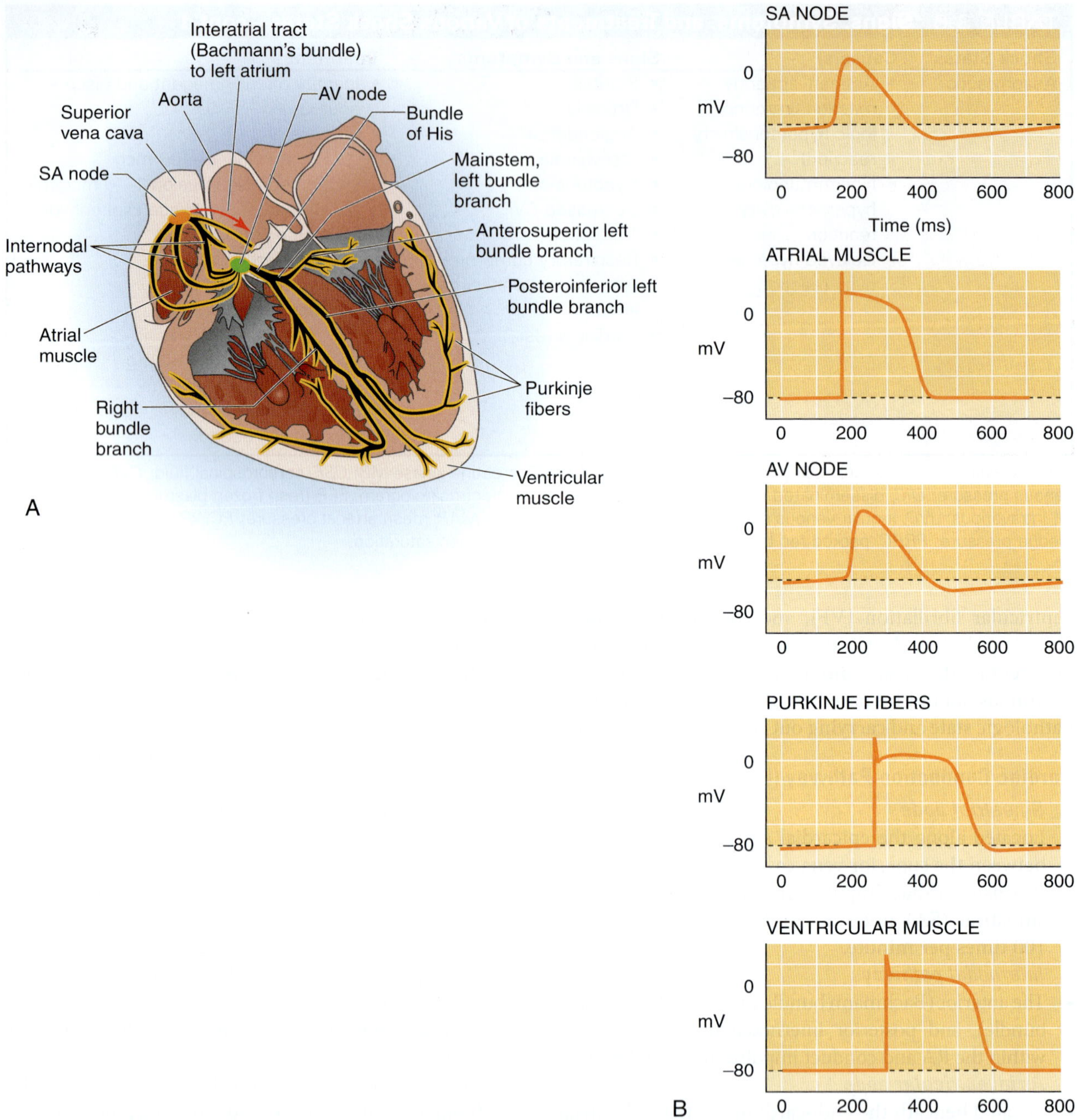

Fig. 3.8 Electrical activity in heart tissue. (A) Conduction pathways through the heart. A section through the long axis of the heart is shown. (B) Cardiac action potentials. The distinctive shapes of action potentials at five sites along the spread of excitation are shown. *AV,* Atrioventricular; *SA,* sinoatrial. (From Boron WF, Boulpaep EL. *Medical Physiology*. 3rd ed. Elsevier; 2017.)

TABLE 3.7 Conduction Speed in Cardiac Tissue

Tissue	Conduction Rate (m/s)
SA node	0.05
Atrial internodal pathways	1
AV node	0.05
Bundle of His	1
Purkinje system	4
Ventricular system	1

AV, Atrioventricular; *SA*, sinoatrial.

- *QRS complex*: Impulse conduction through the Purkinje fibers results in ventricular depolarization.
- *T wave*: Ventricular repolarization
- *ST segment*: Segment that begins at the end of the QRS complex and extends to the beginning of the T wave. Ventricular depolarization ends, and repolarization begins. ST-segment elevation or depression may be one sign of myocardial ischemia or infarction, respectively.
- *QT interval*: Segment that includes QRS complex, ST segment, and T wave, specifically from the beginning of the Q wave to the end of the T wave, and represents ventricular depolarization to the end of ventricular repolarization. QT interval prolongation can occur for a variety of reasons, including electrolyte abnormalities and medications. Prolongation can be a precursor to dysrhythmias, including torsade de pointes.
- The electrical component on the ECG waveform ***precedes*** the physical cardiac event (contraction/relaxation).

Refractory Period (Fig. 3.10)

- The extended duration of the action potential of the myocardial cell protects it against premature excitation. This period of quiescence is known as the *refractory period* and can be divided into effective or absolute and relative refractory periods.
- *Absolute refractory period:* The electrical time segment during the cardiac action potential in which a second conducted action potential may not be evoked, even if an active response is elicited by a supramaximal stimulus.
- *Relative refractory period:* The electrical time segment during the cardiac action potential when a second stimulus can result in an action potential with decreased amplitude, upstroke velocity, and conduction velocity.
- *Clinical application:* This information can be related to synchronized cardioversion. When in a synchronized mode, a shock will not be delivered during the T wave on the ECG, which represents ventricular repolarization. The relative refractory period occurs during the T wave, and electricity delivered during this time can cause electrical disorganization in cardiac cells, resulting in VT or VF (Table 3.8).

KNOWLEDGE CHECK

1. Cardiac impulse conduction is slowed when traveling through the
   a. Purkinje fibers.
   b. left anterior fascicle.
   c. atrial internodal pathways.
   d. atrioventricular node.
2. Ventricular depolarization is synonymous with which electrical event on the ECG?
   a. QRS complex
   b. SA node
   c. P wave
   d. T wave
3. During unstable AF, synchronized cardioversion is employed to ensure that the shock does not occur during the
   a. supramaximal stimulus.
   b. absolute refractory period.
   c. QRS complex.
   d. T wave.

Answers can be found in Appendix A.

Arrhythmia Identification and Treatment Review

Heart rate

- Is the rhythm associated with bradycardia (<60 BPM), normal (60–100 BPM), or tachycardia (>100 BPM)?

Regular or irregular rhythm?

- Is the R-to-R interval regular or irregular?
- Is the rhythm regularly irregular (same pattern of recurring irregularity)? Example: A premature ventricular contraction regularly replaces every third QRS complex.
- Is the rhythm irregularly irregular (variable patterns of consistent irregularity)? Example: P waves and QRS complexes consistently vary with AF.

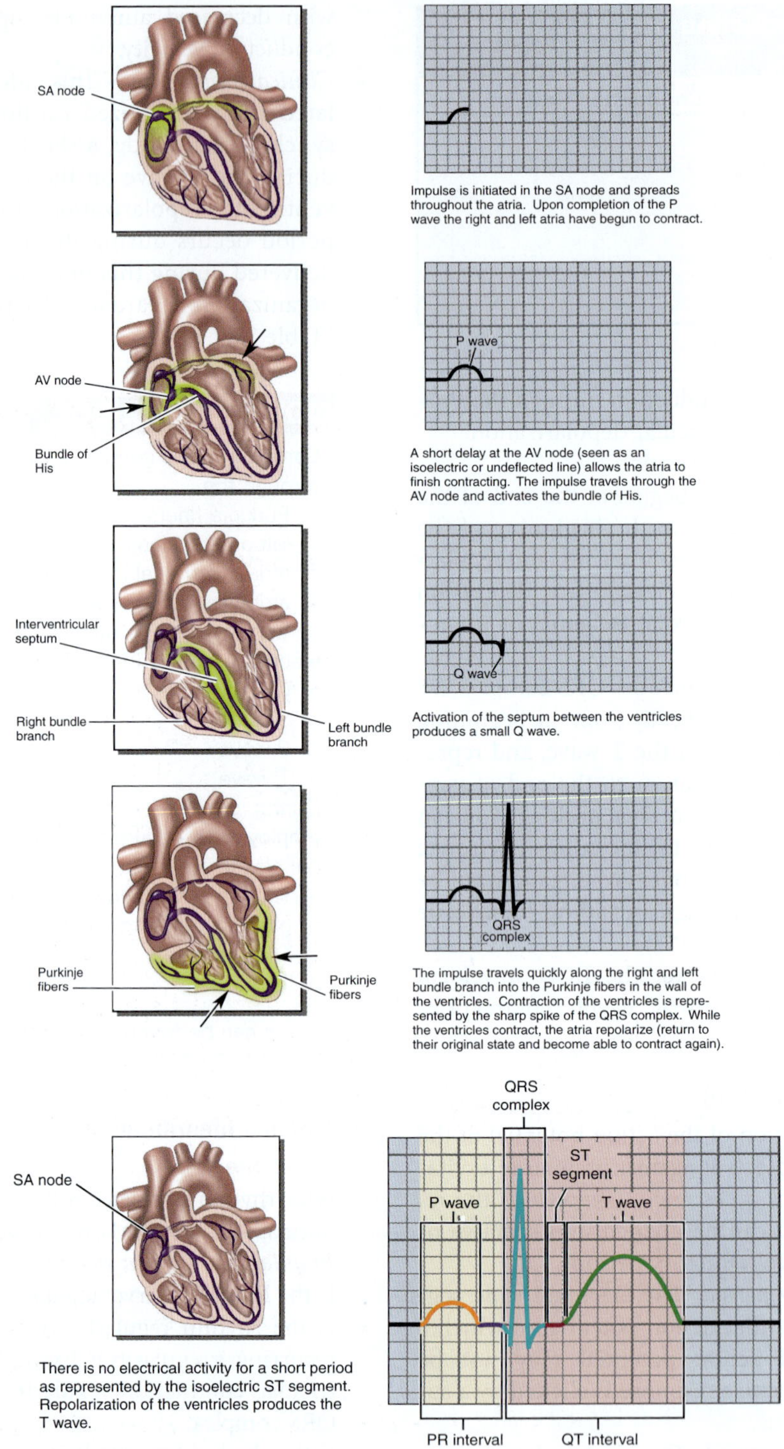

Fig. 3.9 Electrical conduction system of the heart. *AV*, Atrioventricular; *SA*, sinoatrial. (From Hunt SA. *Saunders Fundamentals of Medical Assisting*. Saunders; 2007; Proctor D, Niedzwiecki B, Pepper J, Garrels M, Mills H. *Kinn's The Clinical Medical Assistant: An Applied Learning Approach*. 13th ed. Elsevier: 2017.)

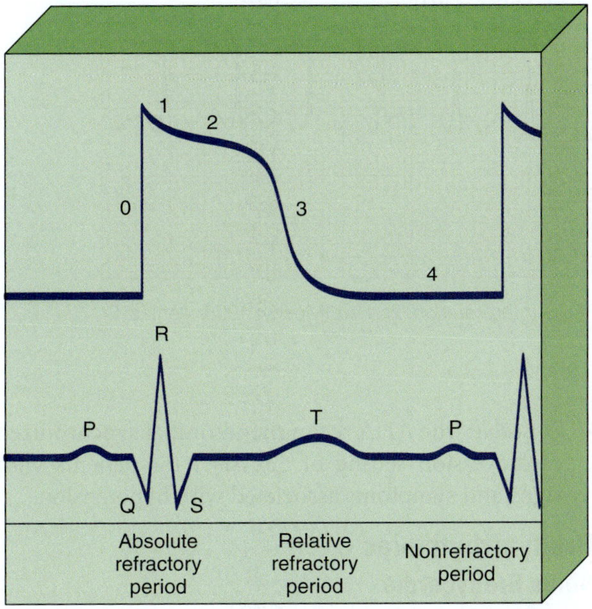

Fig. 3.10 The phases of the cardiac action potential and their relationship to the heart's refractory periods. Phase 0: Depolarization with rapid influx of sodium. Phase 1: Rapid repolarization with rapid efflux of potassium ions and decreased sodium conductance. Phase 2: Plateau with slow influx of sodium and calcium ions. Phase 3: Repolarization with continued efflux of potassium ions. Phase 4: Resting phase with restoration of ionic balance by sodium and potassium pumps. (From Urden LD, Stacy KM, Lough ME. *Priorities in Critical Care Nursing.* 9th ed. Elsevier; 2024.)

TABLE 3.8 Recommendation for Synchronized Cardioversion (Biphasic)

SVT Morphology	Joule Settings
Narrow complex, regular	50–100 J
Narrow complex, irregular	120–200 J
Wide complex, regular	100 J
Wide complex, irregular	Defibrillation

P waves

- Are P waves present?
- Do all the P waves look the same?
- Is there one P wave before each QRS complex?
- Is the PR interval constant or variable?

PR interval

- Is the PR interval between 0.12 and 0.20 seconds?
- Is the PR interval consistent throughout the ECG strip?
- If the PR interval is varied, is there a pattern to the variability?

QRS complex

- Do all the QRS complexes look the same?
- Are the QRS complexes narrow or wide?
- Are the QRS complex intervals regular?
- Is the QRS duration between 0.04 and 0.12 seconds?

Frequent Causes of Dysrhythmias

- ACLS H's
  1. Hypovolemia
  2. Hypoxia
  3. Hyper-/hypokalemia
  4. Hydrogen ion (e.g., hypercarbia and acidosis)
  5. Hypothermia
- ACLS T's
  1. Thrombosis (e.g., pulmonary or coronary)
  2. Tamponade (cardiac)
  3. Tension pneumothorax
  4. Toxicity (e.g., anaphylaxis, local anesthetic toxicity)

Atrial Tachyarrhythmias

Atrial Flutter

***Identification** (Fig. 3.11)*

- Rate: Atrial 240–350 BPM
- Rhythm: Frequently regular
- P wave: None, "sawtooth" pattern
- P:QRS ratio: Most commonly 2:1
- QRS width: Normal
- PR interval: Variable

Treatment

- Atrial flutter: The AHA recommends initial synchronized cardioversion setting of 50–100 joules (J) for patients with signs and symptoms associated with hypotension.

Atrial Fibrillation

***Identification** (Fig. 3.12)*

- Rate: Variable
- Rhythm: Irregularly irregular
- P wave: None discernible, aberrant atrial activity
- P:QRS ratio: None
- QRS width: Normal
- PR interval: None

Treatment

- *Stable:* Rapid rate; β-blocker, calcium channel blocker, digoxin
- *Unstable:* The AHA recommends initial synchronized cardioversion setting of 120–200 J for patients with signs and symptoms associated with hypotension.

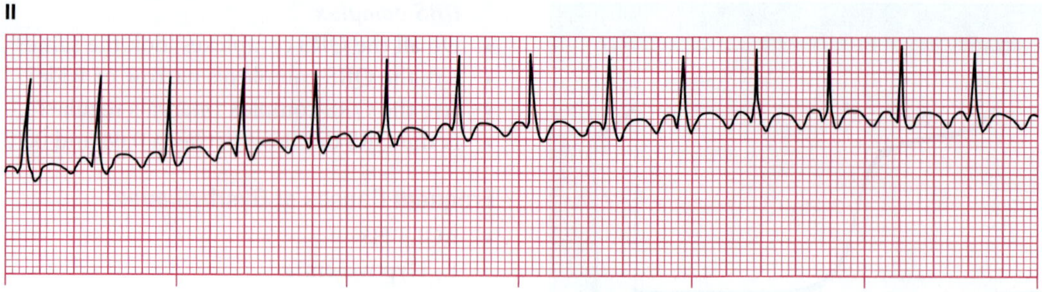

Fig. 3.11 Atrial flutter. (From Grauer K. *A Practical Guide to ECG Interpretation*. 2nd ed. Mosby; 1998; Aehlert B. *ECGs Made Easy*. 6th ed. Elsevier; 2018.)

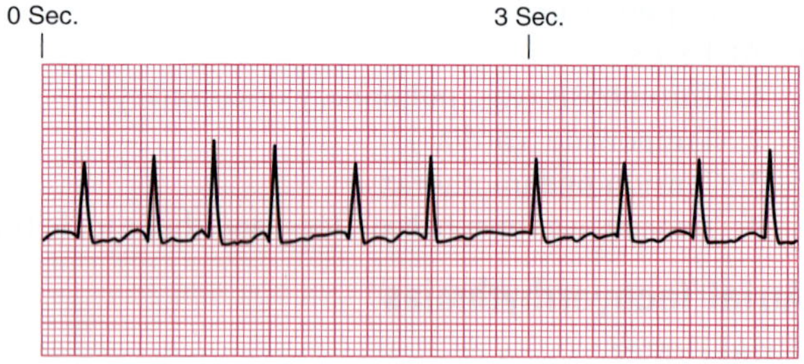

Fig. 3.12 Atrial fibrillation. Notice the irregular ventricular rhythm. (From Urden LD, Stacy KM, Lough ME. *Priorities in Critical Care Nursing*. 9th ed. Elsevier; 2024.)

Supraventricular Tachycardia

Identification (Fig. 3.13)

- Rate: Variable, 140–250 BPM
- Rhythm: Regular
- P wave: Frequently obscured by QRS complex
- P:QRS ratio: None
- QRS width: Typically narrow
- PR interval: None
- If SVT is episodic, it is termed *paroxysmal* SVT.

Treatment

- *Stable:* Vagal maneuvers, adenosine 6 mg rapid IV push; if unsuccessful, adenosine 12 mg rapid IV push, consider calcium channel or β-blocker
- *Unstable:* The AHA recommends initial synchronized cardioversion setting of 50–100 J for patients with signs and symptoms associated with hypotension.

Bradyarrhythmias

Sinus Bradycardia

Identification

- Rate: <60 BPM
- Rhythm: Regular
- P wave: Present
- P:QRS ratio: 1:1
- QRS width: Normal
- PR interval: Normal

First-Degree AV Block

Identification

- Rate: May be greater or less than 60 BPM
- Rhythm: Regular
- P waves: Present, regular, ratio 1:1
- P:QRS ratio: 1:1
- QRS width: Normal
- PR interval: Prolonged, >0.20 seconds

Treatment

- It is rare that first-degree AV block is associated with hemodynamic compromise.

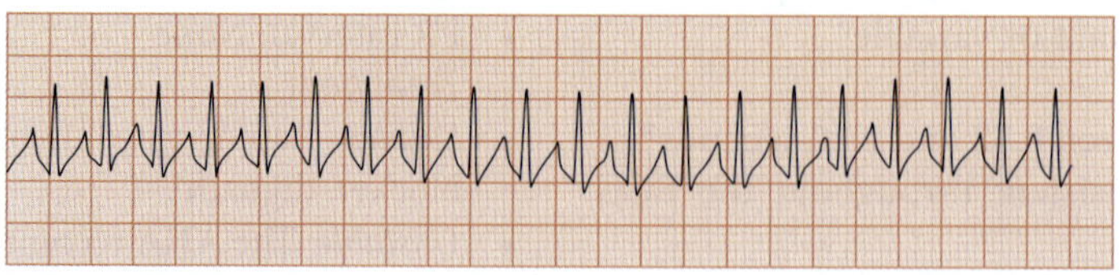

Fig. 3.13 Supraventricular tachycardia. (From the University of Cincinnati Residents: *The Mont Reid Surgical Handbook: Mobile Medicine Series*. 7th ed. Elsevier; 2018.)

Second-Degree Heart Block (Mobitz Type I or Wenkebach)

Identification

- Rate: Frequently <60 BPM
- Rhythm: Regularly irregular
- P waves: Present
- P:QRS ratio: Progressively greater, ratio 1:1 for two, three, or four cycles
- QRS width: Normal
- PR interval: Progressively lengthening until a QRS complex is absent, then repeats

Treatment for second- and third-degree heart block

- Stable: Monitor for signs and symptoms of hypotension.
- Unstable: Atropine 0.5 mg IV, repeat every 3–5 minutes, maximum dose 3 mg
- Consider dopamine or epinephrine infusion, transcutaneous pacing.
- Expert consultation

Second-Degree Heart Block (Mobitz Type II)

- Rate: Frequently <60 BPM
- Rhythm: Regular
- P waves: Present
- P:QRS ratio: Regular, ratio 2:1, 3:1 until QRS complex is absent, then repeats
- QRS width: Normal
- PR interval: Normal or prolonged, constant in relation to QRS complex

Third-Degree Heart Block

- Rate: <60 BPM
- Rhythm: Regular
- P waves: Present, unrelated to QRS complex
- P:QRS ratio: Unrelated
- QRS width: Frequently wide complex
- PR interval: Variable

Specific causes related to anesthesia. Ensure adequate oxygenation and normocarbia.

- Cardiac reflex examples
  - Celiac reflex from a pneumoperitoneum
  - Oculocardiac reflex from pressure on the globe/medial rectus muscle
  - Carotid sinus stimulation during carotid endarterectomy (CEA)

Treatment

- If caused by surgical stimulation and is hemodynamically compromising:
  - Stop stimulus.
  - Consider an anticholinergic (atropine, glycopyrrolate) and/or a sympathomimetic (ephedrine/epinephrine).
- *Unstable:* The AHA recommends transcutaneous pacing or an infusion of a sympathomimetic (epinephrine or dopamine) (Fig. 3.14).

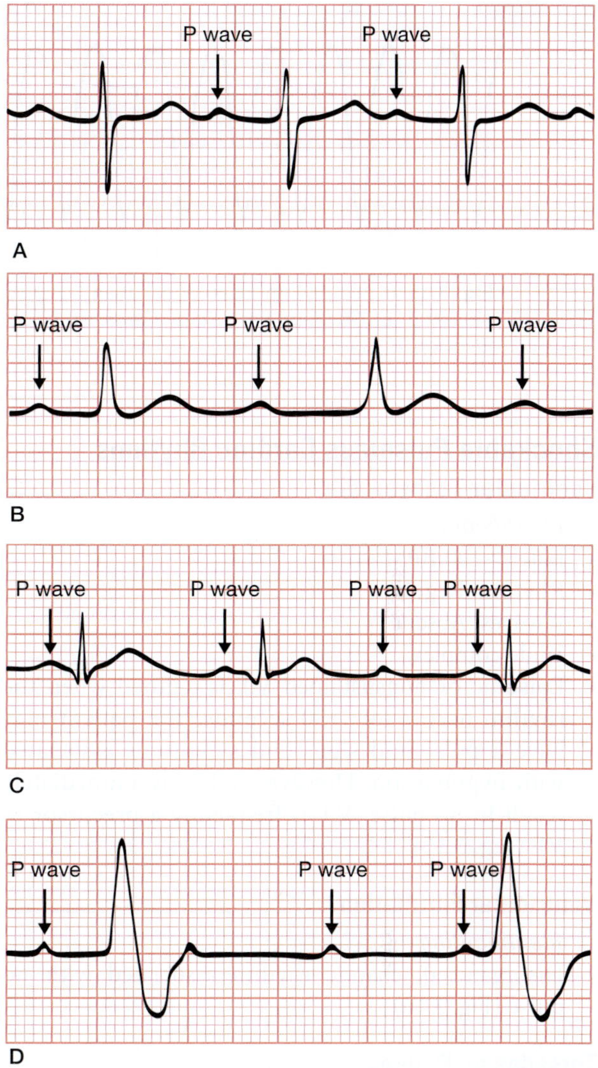

Fig. 3.14 Conduction blocks. (A) First-degree heart block. (B) Second-degree heart block (Mobitz type I [Wenckebach] block). (C) Second-degree heart block (Mobitz type II block). (D) Third-degree (complete) heart block. (From Lim EKS, Loke YK, Thompson AM. *Medicine and Surgery: An Integrated Textbook.* Churchill Livingstone; 2007.)

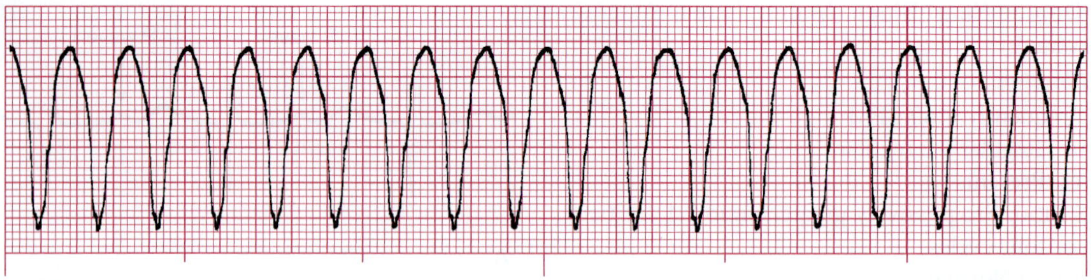

Fig. 3.15 If this rhythm lasts longer than 30 seconds, it is called *sustained ventricular tachycardia*. (From Aehlert B. *ECGs Made Easy Study Cards*. St. Louis, MO: Mosby; 2004; Aehlert B. *ECGs Made Easy*. 6th ed. Elsevier; 2018.)

Shockable Pulseless Cardiac Rhythms

Ventricular Tachycardia

Identification

- Rate: >120 BPM
- Rhythm: Regular
- P waves: Absent
- Wide complex
- Episodic or nonsustained VT is defined when the rhythm occurs for >30 seconds. The patient may have a pulse and signs and symptoms associated with hypotension. However, VT may immediately result in no pulse. VT is frequently a precursor to VF (Fig. 3.15).

Ventricular Fibrillation

Identification

- Disorganized, chaotic rhythm associated with no pulse (Fig. 3.16)

Torsades de Pointes

Identification

- Rate: 200–250 BPM
- Rhythm: Irregular
- Twisting of QRS complexes along an isoelectric line
- QT interval prolongation is associated with torsade de pointes.
- Associated with hypomagnesemia (Fig. 3.17)

Treatment

- Defibrillation: Biphasic 120–200 J, monophasic 360 J
- Cardiopulmonary resuscitation (CPR) for 2 minutes
- Rhythm unchanged: Defibrillation (subsequent defibrillation energy level equal to or greater than previous)

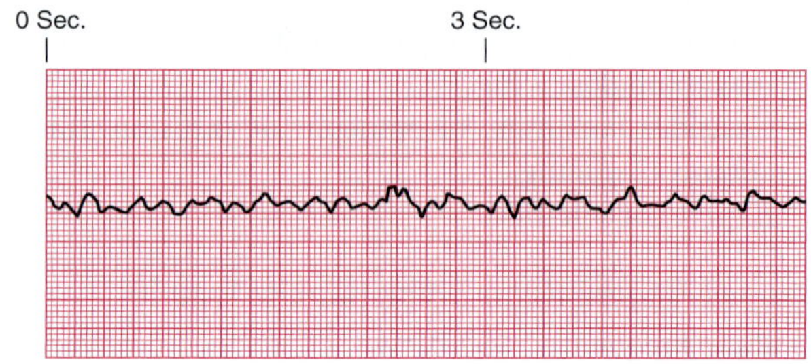

Fig. 3.16 Ventricular fibrillation. (From Urden LD, Stacy KM, Lough ME. *Priorities in Critical Care Nursing*. 9th ed. Elsevier; 2024.)

- CPR for 2 minutes, epinephrine 1 mg IV/IO every 3–5 minutes, securing airway
- Rhythm unchanged: Defibrillation
- CPR for 2 minutes, amiodarone 300 mg IV/IO; if a second dose is needed, 150 mg IV/IO
- Continue with defibrillation, CPR, and epinephrine.

Nonshockable Pulseless Cardiac Rhythms

Identification

- *PEA:* Any organized cardiac rhythm that does not produce a pulse. The most common causes of PEA are hypoxia and hypovolemia.
- *Asystole:* Absence of electrical activity on the ECG
- Treatment
  - Continuous CPR, epinephrine IV/intraosseous (IO) 1 mg every 3–5 minutes, securing airway
  - Assess rhythm change.
  - Consider terminating resuscitative efforts.

See Table 3.9 for a summary of cardiac dysrhythmias, including symptoms, differential diagnosis, and treatment.

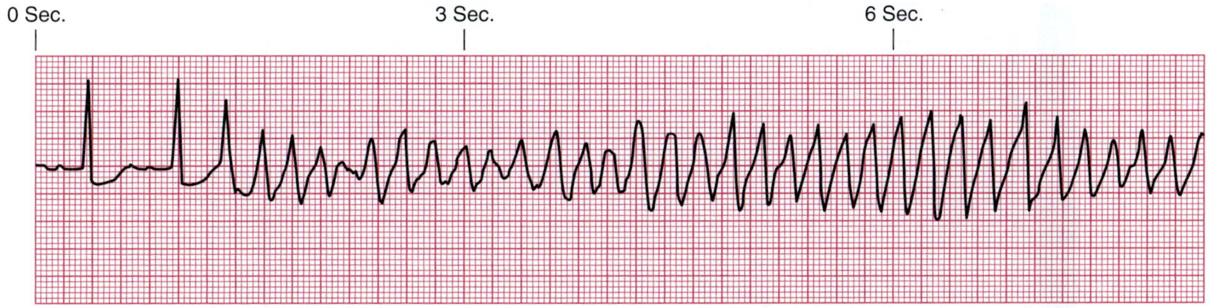

Fig. 3.17 Torsades de pointes. (From Urden LD, Stacy KM, Lough ME. *Priorities in Critical Care Nursing*. 9th ed. Elsevier; 2024.)

KNOWLEDGE CHECK

1. Which cardiac rhythm is associated with hypomagnesemia?
   a. AF
   b. Sinus bradycardia
   c. Second-degree AV block
   d. Torsades de pointes
2. What is the initial treatment for a patient exhibiting signs and symptoms of hypotension and a palpable pulse associated with the following cardiac rhythm?

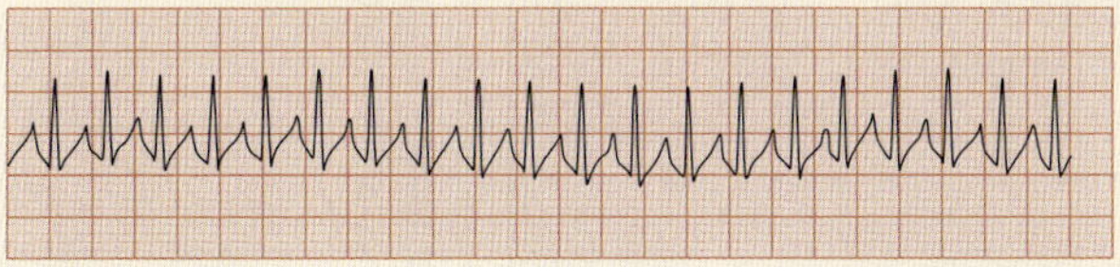

   a. Defibrillation 100 J
   b. Synchronized cardioversion 50 J
   c. Amiodarone 300 mg IV/IO
   d. Epinephrine IV/IO 1 mg
3. After abdominal insufflation to create a pneumoperitoneum, the following changes occur: End tidal carbon dioxide decreases from 38 to 12 mm Hg, BP from 110/58 to 76/38 mm Hg, and pulse oximetry from 97% to undetectable. Which cardiac rhythm is the most likely cause of this scenario?
   a. Bradycardia, heart rate 28 BPM
   b. AF, heart rate 127 BPM
   c. First-degree AV block, heart rate 56 BPM
   d. PEA, heart rate 108 BPM
4. What is the most likely cause of the scenario in question 3?
   a. Acute coronary syndrome
   b. Excessive administration of anesthetic medications
   c. Medication error
   d. Celiac reflex from increased intraabdominal pressure

Answers can be found in Appendix A.

Acute Coronary Syndrome

Atherosclerosis is the most common cause of peripheral vascular occlusive disease. This degenerative process involves the formation of atheromatous plaques that may obstruct the vessel lumen, resulting in a reduction in distal blood flow. The pathophysiologic process is systemic and progressive and primarily affects the arteries as a result of plaque formation, which can lead to stenosis and potentially occlusion of the vascular lumen; thrombosis from hypercoagulability, resulting in acute organ ischemia; embolism from microthrombi or atheromatous debris; and weakening of the arterial wall, resulting in decreased distal blood flow and aneurysm formation (Fig. 3.18). Atherosclerosis is an inflammatory condition that is partially caused by presence of cholesterol plaques within arteries. In response to cholesterol plaques, immune cells such as macrophages and monocytes liberate proinflammatory cytokines, which leads to the progressively increasing size of a plaque. The lipid cap that envelops the plaque can rupture, resulting in intraluminal thrombosis or plaque emboli. Endothelial dysfunction is a potential cause of increased hemodynamic variability during anesthesia.

During anesthesia and surgery, hemodynamic variability commonly occurs throughout the perioperative period. SNS predominance causes cardiac stimulation, resulting in increased inotropy (contractility), chronotropy (heart rate), and dromotropy (speed of cardiac

TABLE 3.9 Cardiac Dysrhythmias

Cardiac Dysrhythmia	Bradycardia	Tachycardia	Atrial Tachyarrhythmias	Ventricular Tachyarrhythmias	Pulseless Electrical Activity (PEA) and Asystole
Signs and symptoms	• Sinus bradycardia HR < 60 BPM • First-, second-, third-degree AV nodal block	• Sinus tachycardia HR >100 BPM	• Atrial fibrillation and flutter • Supraventricular tachycardia	• Ventricular tachycardia and fibrillation • Torsades de pointes	• PEA • Asystole
Differential diagnosis	• Perioperative stress • Structural disease • Conduction disease • H's and T's	• Perioperative stress • Structural disease • Conduction disease • H's and T's	• Perioperative stress • Structural disease • Conduction disease • H's and T's	• Perioperative stress • Structural disease • Conduction disease • H's and T's	• Perioperative stress • Structural disease • Conduction disease • Hs and Ts
Treatment	• ACLS or PALS • Atropine • Transcutaneous pacing • Dopamine • Epinephrine	• Increased depth of anesthesia • Provide analgesia • Maintain euvolemia • Assess for hypermetabolic pathological state	• ACLS or PALS • Atrial fibrillation and flutter • Rate control with diltiazem, β-blockers, or digoxin • Synchronized cardioversion • SVT • Vagal maneuvers (e.g., Valsalva maneuver) • Rate control with adenosine, diltiazem, β-blockers • Synchronized cardioversion	• ACLS or PALS • VT/VF • Defibrillation • Epinephrine • Vasopressin • Amiodarone • Lidocaine • Torsades de pointes • Treatment as above • Consider magnesium sulfate	• ACLS or PALS • Epinephrine • Vasopressin • Atropine

ACLS, Advanced cardiac life support; *AV*, atrioventricular; *BPM*, beats per minute; *H's and T's*, causes of dysrhythmias (H's: hypovolemia, hypoxia, hyper-/hypokalemia, hydrogen ion, hypothermia; T's: thrombosis, tamponade, tension pneumothorax, toxicity); *HR*, heart rate; *PALS*, pediatric advanced life support; *SVT*, supraventricular tachycardia; *VF*, ventricular fibrillation; *VT*, ventricular tachycardia.

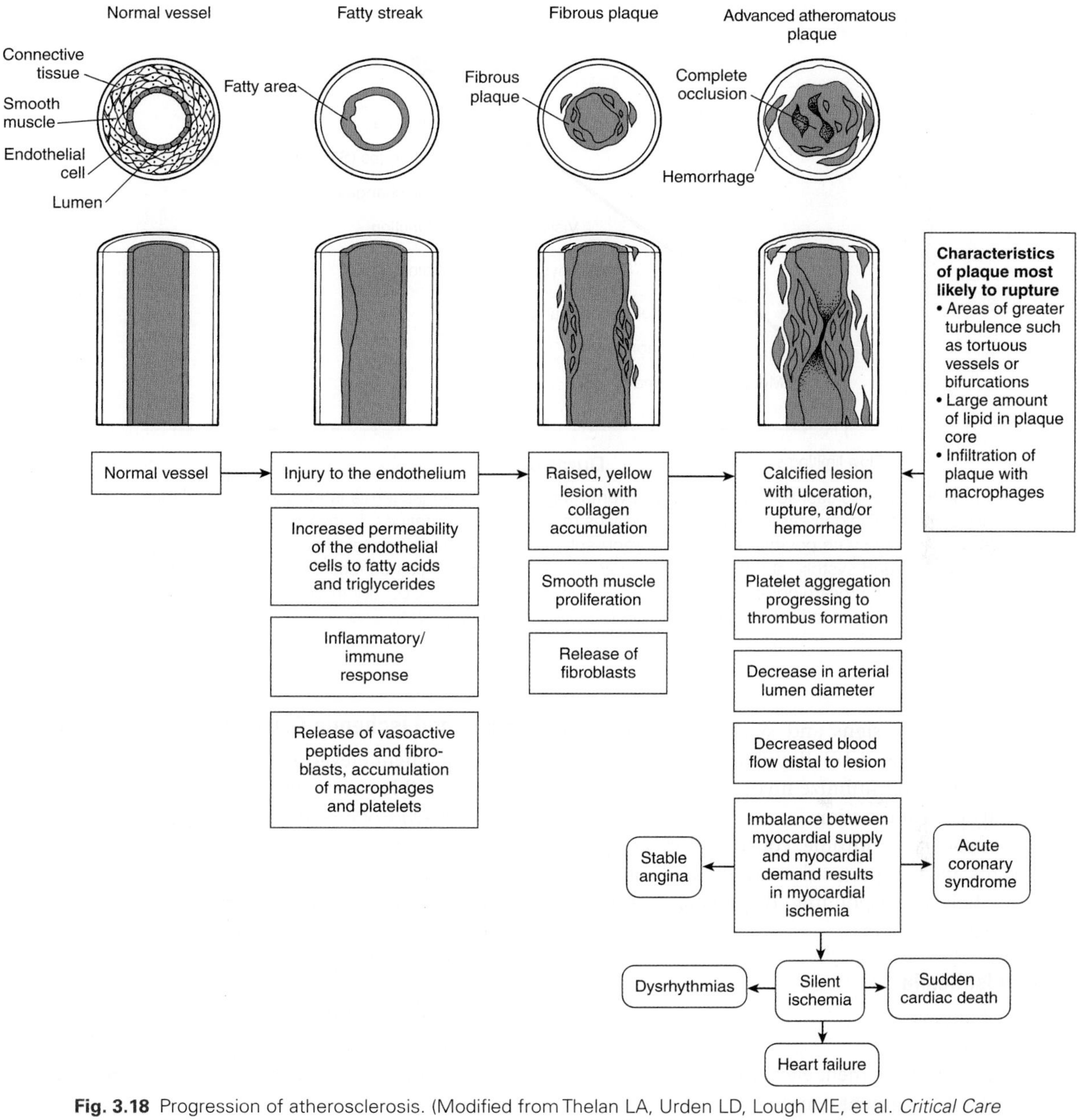

Fig. 3.18 Progression of atherosclerosis. (Modified from Thelan LA, Urden LD, Lough ME, et al. *Critical Care Nursing: Diagnosis and Management*. 3rd ed. Mosby; 1998; Dennison RD. *Pass CCRN [Adult]*. 6th ed. Elsevier; 2024.)

conduction). Also, preload and afterload are increased, further elevating myocardial oxygen demand. SNS inhibition resulting from an increased anesthetic depth can result in decreased myocardial perfusion. When factors increase myocardial oxygen demand greater than oxygen supply, acute coronary syndrome can occur. Myocardial oxygen deprivation causes myocardial excitation-contraction coupling inhibition (decreased cardiac contractility) as a result of a lack of ATP production. This is the reason that increased ventricular volume, decreased ventricular compliance, and ventricular wall hypokinesis resulting in hypotension frequently precede ST-segment

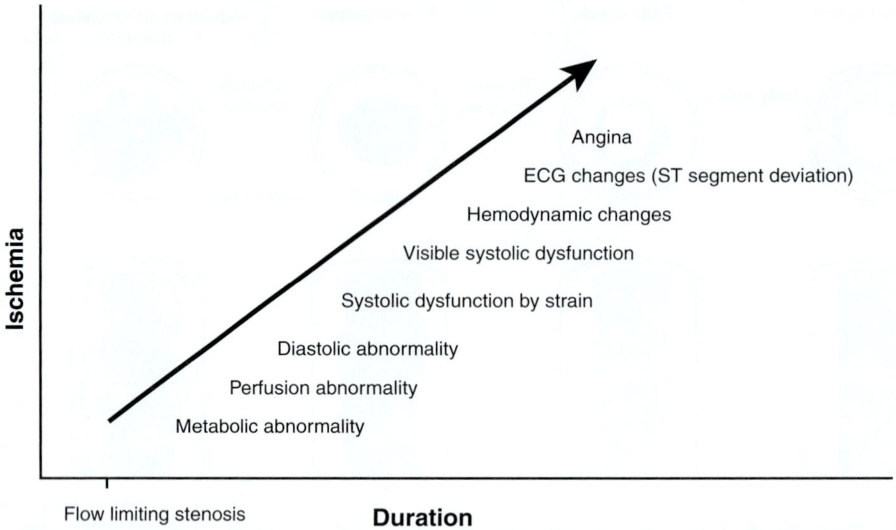

Fig. 3.19 Ischemic cascade: Sequence of events that occur when ischemia is induced in flow-limiting coronary stenosis. The decrease in flow first produces metabolic abnormalities, followed by perfusion defects that can be detected with positron emission tomography or single-photon emission computed tomography. Next are diastolic and systolic abnormalities that can be detected by stress echocardiography, eventually leading to ischemic electrocardiographic changes and angina symptoms. *ECG*, Electrocardiogram. (From Lang RM, Goldstein SA, Kronzon I, et al. *ASE's Comprehensive Echocardiography*. 2nd ed. Elsevier; 2016.)

elevation/depression, signs and symptoms, CHF, and cardiogenic shock (Fig. 3.19). Rapid diagnosis and treatment are essential to minimize myocardial damage and preserve myocardial function.

Acute coronary syndrome constitutes a group of clinical signs and symptoms that are divided into categories by their corresponding diagnostic factors, as outlined next.

Transient Ischemia

- Unstable angina
  - Chest pain
  - *Absence* of ST-segment elevation
  - Possible ST-segment depression
  - Normal cardiac biomarkers (troponins/creatine kinase-MB [CK-MB])
  - Possible findings: T-wave inversion
- Non–ST-segment elevation MI (NSTEMI)
  - Possible chest pain
  - *Absence* of ST-segment elevation
  - Possible ST-segment depression
  - Elevated cardiac biomarkers (troponins/CK-MB)
  - Possible findings: T-wave inversion

Sustained Ischemia Causing Injury/Infarction

- ST-segment elevation MI (STEMI)
  - Possible chest pain
  - *Presence* of new-onset ST-segment elevation ≥1 mm, new-onset left bundle branch block
  - Development of pathologic Q waves
  - Elevated cardiac biomarkers (troponins/CK-MB)
  - Evidence of MI or wall motion abnormalities from imaging

Signs and Symptoms

The only initial sign that may be observed during general anesthesia is hypotension that does not respond to vasopressor therapy.

Respiratory

- Hypercarbia
- Hypoxia
- Rales
- Respiratory arrest
- Shortness of breath
- Tachypnea

Cardiovascular

- Chest pain with or without radiation

- Pain to jaw and/or left arm
- CHF
- Decreased capillary refill
- Decreased peripheral pulses
- Diaphoresis
- ECG
  - Dysrhythmias
  - ST-segment elevation/depression
  - New-onset AV or bundle branch block
  - New-onset T-wave inversion
- Elevated cardiac troponin and CK-MB
- Hemodynamic profile
  - Tachycardia/bradycardia
  - Hypertension/hypotension
  - Increased PCWP
  - Increased CVP
  - Increased SVR
- New-onset cardiac murmur
- TEE/transthoracic echocardiography (TTE): ventricular wall motion abnormalities
- Cardiogenic shock
- Cardiac arrest

Neurologic

- Altered/loss of consciousness
- Dizziness
- Syncope

Treatment of Acute Coronary Syndrome

- Inform the surgeon.
- MONA: Morphine, oxygen (100% during general anesthesia), nitroglycerin, aspirin (PO or nasogastric tube)
- Cardiology consultation
- Invasive monitoring (e.g., arterial line)
- Prepare for higher level of cardiac care.
  - Heparin
  - Consider short-acting β-blockade.
  - Consider clopidogrel and/or glycoprotein IIb/IIIa inhibitor.
  - Fibrinolytic therapy (within 30 minutes of onset)
  - PCI (within 90 minutes of onset)
- Consider external cardiac pacing for bradycardia.
- Perform cardiac resuscitation per AHA ACLS protocol as necessary.

Anesthetic Considerations

- Pharmacologic optimization
  - Continue β-blocker and statins.
  - Hold ACEIs/ARBs and diuretics for 24 hours preoperatively.
- Strategies to minimize perioperative hemodynamic variability
  - Fluid bolus before induction
  - Preoperative multimodal analgesia as appropriate (acetaminophen, meloxicam, gabapentin)
  - Preoperative regional nerve block if applicable
  - Controlled induction, divided doses of induction agent, or lower dose of induction agent and higher doses of narcotics
  - Maintenance: Higher doses of narcotics compared with inhalational agent
  - For spinal/epidural anesthesia, preblock fluid bolus, and minimize height of dermatome blockade necessary for surgical procedure.
  - Treat periods of tachycardia/hypertension/hypotension expeditiously.
  - If reversal of neuromuscular blockade is accomplished with neostigmine/glycopyrrolate, titrate over several minutes to avoid tachycardia.

Treatment of Intraoperative Myocardial Ischemia (Table 3.10)

KNOWLEDGE CHECK

1. Which is a component of NSTEMI? *(Select all that apply.)*
   a. New-onset ST-segment elevation
   b. T-wave inversion
   c. Normal cardiac biomarkers (troponins/CK-MB)
   d. ST-segment depression
2. Fibrinolytic therapy used to treat acute coronary syndrome should be initiated within
   a. 30 minutes.
   b. 45 minutes.
   c. 60 minutes.
   d. 90 minutes.

Answers can be found in Appendix A.

Heart Failure

The term *heart failure* is simply defined as the inability of the heart to adequately fill and/or eject blood in sufficient quantities to meet the metabolic demands of tissues. This pathophysiologic process most often occurs over time, and there is a significant continuum from least to most severe. The cardiac structural or functional

TABLE 3.10 **Treatment of Intraoperative Myocardial Ischemia**

Hemodynamic Event	Therapy	Pharmacologic Action
Hypertension/tachycardia	• Increase anesthetic depth • IV β-blockade • IV nitroglycerin	• ↓ Inotropy/chronotropy • ↓ Preload/wall tension, dilates epicardial vessels
Normotension/tachycardia	• Adequate anesthetic depth? • IV β-blockade	• ↓ Inotropy/chronotropy
Hypertension/normal HR	• Increase anesthetic depth • IV nitroglycerin or nicardipine	• ↓ SVR, myocardial depression • ↓ Preload/wall tension, dilates epicardial vessels
Hypotension/tachycardia	• Volume • Decrease anesthetic depth • Phenylephrine • IV nitroglycerin when normotensive	• ↑ Intravascular volume • ↑ SVR • ↓ Preload/wall tension, dilates epicardial vessels
Hypotension/bradycardia	• Decrease anesthetic depth • IV ephedrine • IV epinephrine • IV atropine • IV nitroglycerin when normotensive	• Hypoxia cardioaccelerator center • ↑ SVR • ↑ Inotropy/chronotropy • ↓ Preload/wall tension, dilates epicardial vessels

IV, Intravenous; *HR*, heart rate; *SVR*, systemic vascular resistance.

limitations affect the endocardium, myocardium, and cardiac valves. Because of the stresses of pumping blood against the pressure exerted by SVR, most cases of heart failure involve left ventricular impairment (Fig. 3.20). The causes of heart failure include the following:

- Decreased myocardial contractility (e.g., ischemic heart disease, cardiomyopathy)
- Valvular abnormalities (e.g., AS)
- Systemic hypertension (e.g., increased SVR)
- Pulmonary hypertension (increased pulmonary vascular resistance)

Heart failure results in hypoperfusion, leading to a neurohumoral imbalance. Activation of the SNS and the renin–angiotensin–aldosterone system induces a host of pathologic responses. Many patients with heart failure will receive multimodal drug therapy aimed at interrupting the response and slowing disease progression. When combined with anesthetics, β-blockers, ACEIs, ARBs, and aldosterone antagonists can have a synergistic effect that leads to intraoperative hypotension. Nevertheless, it is recommended that medications used to control the patient's heart failure be continued in the perioperative period because their benefit is well documented. The preoperative functional cardiac status is presented in Table 3.11.

- *Systolic heart failure* results from decreased systolic wall motion (impaired contractility).
- *Decreased myocardial oxygen supply, causes:* Ischemic heart disease, dilated cardiomyopathy, chronic pressure overload (e.g., AS), chronic volume overload (e.g., AR)
  - Impaired left ventricular EF
    1. ≥55%: normal EF
    2. 45%–54%: mild dysfunction
    3. 30%–44%: moderate dysfunction
    4. <30%: severe dysfunction
- *Diastolic heart failure* results from decreased ventricular relaxation and compliance.

  Increased myocardial oxygen demand, causes: Myocardial edema, fibrosis, ventricular hypertrophy. Associated with preserved EF >40% (Table 3.12).

Anesthetic Considerations

- Preoperative optimization
  - Continue preoperative medication; consider holding ACEI or ARB for 24 hours before surgery and anesthesia.
  - Consider/assess hypovolemia, hyponatremia, and hypokalemia caused by chronic diuretic therapy.

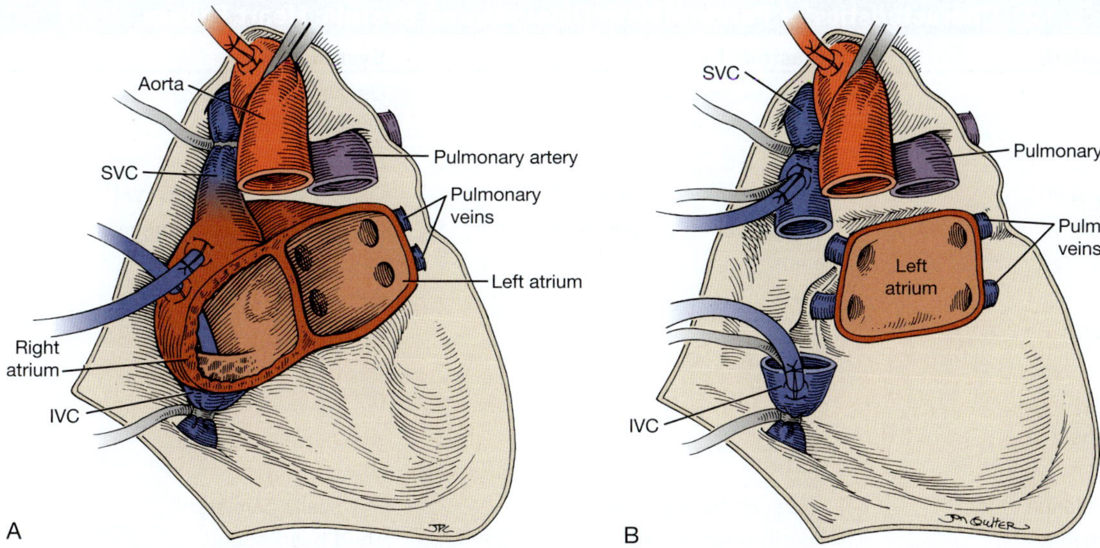

Fig. 3.20 Left ventricular (LV) pressure and volume overload produce compensatory responses based on the nature of the inciting stress. Wall thickening reduces (−) and chamber dilation increases (+) end-systolic wall stress, as predicted by Laplace's law. LV pressure overload hypertrophy has been linked to heart failure with normal ejection fraction, but LV volume overload most often causes heart failure with reduced ejection fraction. *IVC*, Inferior vena cava; *SVC*, superior vena cava. (From Kaplan JA, ed. *Kaplan's Cardiac Anesthesia: For Cardiac and Noncardiac Surgery*. 7th ed. Elsevier; 2017.)

TABLE 3.11 New York Heart Association Functional Classification of Cardiovascular Disability

Classification	Cardiovascular Status
Class I	*Patients with cardiac disease*
	No functional limitations to physical activity, such as walking or climbing stairs. Ordinary physical activity is not associated with undue fatigue, palpitations, dyspnea, or angina.
Class II	*Patients with cardiac disease who are comfortable at rest*
	Slight functional limitations to physical activity, such as walking or climbing stairs rapidly, or during emotional stress. Patients are comfortable at rest. Ordinary physical activity results in fatigue, palpitation, dyspnea, or angina.
Class III	*Patients with cardiac disease resulting in marked limitations to physical activity*
	Patients are comfortable at rest. Less than ordinary physical activity causes fatigue, palpitations, dyspnea, or angina.
Class IV	*Patients with cardiac disease resulting in inability to carry on any physical activity without discomfort*
	Symptoms of cardiac insufficiency or angina syndrome may be present even at rest. If any physical activity is undertaken, discomfort is increased.

Modified from Horak J, Mohler ER, Fleisher LA. Assessment of cardiac risk and the cardiology consultation. In Kaplan JA, Reich DL, Savino JS, eds. *Kaplan's Cardiac Anesthesia: The Echo Era*. 6th ed. Elsevier; 2011:2–15.

- Intraoperative management
  - Consider invasive monitoring: Arterial line and TEE.
  - Cautious/incremental IV fluid management
  - Minimize direct myocardial depression: Dose and time interval dependent (e.g., inhalation agents, propofol). Consider higher doses of narcotics.
- Use caution with neuraxial anesthesia because of potential for severe uncontrolled hypotension associated with hypovolemia and myocardial dysfunction.
- Assess for acute heart failure (hypotension not responsive to vasopressors; new-onset rales; pink,

TABLE 3.12 Characteristics of Patients With Diastolic and Systolic Heart Failure

Characteristic	Diastolic HF	Systolic HF
Age	Often in the elderly	Usually 50–70 years
Sex	Often in females	Often in males
LV EF	Preserved, ≥40%	Depressed, ≤40%
LV cavity size	Normal with concentric LVH	Dilated with eccentric LVH
Chest x-ray	Congestion ± cardiomegaly	Congestion + cardiomegaly
HTN	+++	++
DM	+++	++
Previous MI	+	+++
Obesity	+++	+
COPD	++	0
Sleep apnea	++	++
Dialysis	++	0
Atrial fibrillation	+ Usually paroxysmal	+ Usually persistent
Gallop rhythm	Fourth heart sound	Third heart sound

+, Occasionally associated with; ++, often associated with; +++, usually associated with; 0, no association; *COPD*, chronic obstructive pulmonary disease; *DM*, diabetes mellitus; *EF*, ejection fraction; *HF*, heart failure; *HTN*, hypertension; *LV*, left ventricle; *LVH*, left ventricular hypertrophy; *MI*, myocardial infarction.

Modified from Popescue WM. Heart failure and cardiomyopathies. In Hines RL, Jones SB. *Stoelting's Anesthesia and Co-Existing Disease*. 8th ed. Elsevier; 2022.

frothy sputum; decreased peripheral capillary oxygen saturation [Spo_2]).

- Use caution with events that acutely and significantly increase afterload (e.g., pneumoperitoneum, phenylephrine) (Table 3.13).

KNOWLEDGE CHECK

1. Systolic heart failure is associated with
   a. increased myocardial oxygen demand.
   b. decreased EF.
   c. increased myocardial oxygen supply.
   d. decreased end-diastolic pressure.
2. For each anesthetic consideration, indicate whether the characteristic is associated with *systolic* or *diastolic* heart failure.
   a. Afterload reduction will enhance left ventricular SV.
   b. Left ventricular SV is most dependent on "atrial kick."
   c. The MAC of sevoflurane is 1.5 and is most likely to cause hypotension.
   d. Administering IV fluids before induction is needed to maximize left ventricular preload.

Answers can be found in Appendix A.

Carotid Endarterectomy

Patients who are scheduled to undergo CEA are at high risk for the presence of other vascular lesions/occlusions.

- Patients with a history of peripheral vascular disease have a 60- to 15-fold increase in mortality rate compared with patients undergoing nonvascular surgery (Box 3.3).
- The presence of carotid artery stenosis (CAS; >25%) in patients with peripheral vascular disease over the age of 65 is approximately 40%.
- The prevalence of perioperative cardiac morbidity is 10 times greater in vascular surgery patients than in nonvascular surgery patients.
- Less than 10% of patients who present for vascular surgery have normal coronary arteries.
- Stroke is the fourth leading cause of mortality in the United States.
- For every 1 million people, each year 1600 will have a stroke, and 55% will survive for 6 months.
- There are over 100,000 CEAs performed in the United States per year.
- The severity of carotid artery atherogenesis parallels that in other major vessels.

TABLE 3.13 Anesthetic Considerations for Systolic and Diastolic Dysfunction

	Systolic Dysfunction	Diastolic Dysfunction
Preload	Already ↑, avoid overload, especially coming off pump NTG helps reduce preload and ↑ subendocardial perfusion	Volume will be needed to stretch noncompliant LV Evaluate with TEE as PaEDP ↑ and >LVEDV
Contractility	Reduced, avoid agents that cause further reductions May need inotropic support	Usually good, but caution with agents that depress function
Afterload	Reductions will enhance forward flow as long as coronary perfusion pressure is maintained SNP works well if volume is adequate	Already ↑ Higher MAP needed to perfuse thick myocardium Treat hypotension aggressively with phenylephrine
Heart rate	Usually high normal because of sympathetic activation	Slow normal to maximize diastolic time for coronary perfusion and ↓ MVO_2 Prone to ischemia Maintain SR; dependent on atrial kick (cardiovert early)
CPB	Expect large pump volumes Consider ultrafiltration, diuretic	Pump volume normal

↓, Decreased; ↑, increased; *CPB*, cardiopulmonary bypass; *LV*, left ventricle; *LVEDV*, left ventricular end-diastolic volume; *MAP*, mean arterial pressure; *MVO_2*, myocardial oxygen consumption; *NTG*, nitroglycerin; *PaEDP*, pulmonary artery end-diastolic pressure; *SNP*, sodium nitroprusside; *SR*, sinus rhythm, *TEE*, transesophageal echocardiography.

BOX 3.3 Coexisting Disease and Risk Factors for Patients With Peripheral Vascular Disease

Patient Factors

- Age >60 years: 68%
- History of cigarette smoking: 88%
- Coexisting disease:
  - Hypertension: 40%–68%
  - Previous MI: 40%–60%
  - CAD: 40%–60%
  - Angina: 10%–20%
  - Dysrhythmia: 36%
  - Diabetes mellitus: 8%–44%
  - COPD: 25%–50%
  - CHF: 5%–20%
  - Renal insufficiency: 5%–15%

Surgical Factors

- Expertise of surgeon
- Emergency/semi-emergent state
- Major fluid shifts
- Clamping and unclamping major vessels
- Intraoperative hypertension/hypotension

CAD, Coronary artery disease; *CHF*, congestive heart failure; *COPD*, chronic obstructive pulmonary disease; *MI*, myocardial infarction.

Indications for CEA

- Asymptomatic carotid bruit
- Transient ischemic attack (TIA)
- Reversible ischemic neurologic deficits with >70% stenosis of the vessel wall or an ulcerated plaque, with or without stenosis
- TIAs lasting longer than 1 hour with angiographic evidence of CAS
- Unstable neurologic status, evidence of CAS that persists despite anticoagulation

Preoperative Period

- A thorough history and physical assessment should be completed for each patient receiving anesthesia. Preoperative optimization in patients with vascular disease should focus on the cardiovascular and neurologic systems.
- **Cardiovascular:** Useful data, ECG, echocardiogram, cardiac catheterization (Table 3.14)
  History: Chest pain, palpitations, shortness of breath, syncopal episodes, METs
  Pharmacologic: Patients should continue taking β-blockers, statins
  - Consider holding ACEIs/ARBs for 24 hours preanesthesia and surgery to avoid refractory hypotension.

TABLE 3.14 American College of Cardiology Foundation/American Heart Association Recommendations for Perioperative Cardiac Assessment

	Scenario	Recommendation
Class I	Patients in need of emergency noncardiac surgery	Proceed directly to the operating room.
	Patients with active cardiac conditions, unstable or severe angina (not stable angina), decompensated heart failure, significant dysrhythmia (high-grade AV block, Mobitz type II block, third-degree AV block, symptomatic ventricular arrhythmias, symptomatic bradycardia, and supraventricular arrhythmias [including atrial fibrillation with HR >100 beats/min]), and severe valvular disease	Provide perioperative surveillance, risk stratification, and risk factor management.
	Patients undergoing low-risk procedures	Proceed with planned surgery.
	Patients with poor (<4 METs) or unknown functional capacity and no clinical risk factors	
Class IIa	Patients with functional capacity ≥4 METs without symptoms	Proceed with planned surgery.
	Patients with poor (<4 METs) or unknown functional capacity and three or more clinical risk factors* who are undergoing intermediate-risk surgery	Proceed with planned surgery with heart rate control.
	Patients with poor (<4 METs) or unknown functional capacity and one or two clinical risk factors* who are undergoing vascular surgery or intermediate-risk surgery	
	Patients with poor (<4 METs) or unknown functional capacity and three or more clinical risk factors* who are undergoing vascular surgery	Consider further testing if it will change management.
Class IIb	Patients with poor (<4 METs) or unknown functional capacity and three or more clinical risk factors* who are scheduled for intermediate-risk surgery	Consider noninvasive testing if it will change patient management.
	Patients with poor (<4 METs) or unknown functional capacity and one or two clinical risk factors* who are scheduled for vascular surgery or intermediate-risk surgery	
Class I recommendations suggest that procedures/treatments should be performed; class IIa recommendations suggest that it is reasonable to perform the procedure/treatment; class IIb recommendations imply that the procedure/treatment should be considered; and in class III, the intervention should not be performed, because it may not be helpful and may potentially be harmful to the patient.		

AV, Atrioventricular; *HR,* heart rate; *METs,* metabolic equivalents.
*Clinical risk factors include ischemic heart disease, compensated or prior heart failure, diabetes mellitus, renal insufficiency, and cerebrovascular disease.
From Cronenwett JL, Johnston KW. *Rutherford's Vascular Surgery*. 8th ed. Elsevier; 2014.

- Consider ongoing anticoagulation therapy. If held, restart after surgery after the risk of bleeding has decreased.

Laboratory results: Hemoglobin/hematocrit, electrolyte panel, coagulation panel, glucose, blood urea nitrogen/creatinine

- Blood glucose should be maintained at <200 mg/dL.
- **Neurologic:** Useful data, including carotid Doppler results for CAS in operative carotid artery and contralateral carotid artery, imaging results of existing neurologic infarcts

  History: TIAs, syncopal episodes, CVA

  Physical examination: Pupils equal size and reactive to light, current motor deficits, dizziness when turning head from side to side or during extension

Intraoperative Period

Anesthetic technique

- General versus regional anesthesia
  - Currently, there is a lack of scientific evidence to suggest that the outcomes associated with general anesthesia are definitively improved compared with regional anesthesia.

Monitoring

- Standard monitors/arterial line necessary
- Cerebral blood flow (CBF) monitoring during carotid artery cross-clamping
- Awake patient (regional anesthesia)
- Electroencephalographic monitoring
- Somatosensory evoked potential monitoring
- Transcranial Doppler ultrasonography
- Cerebral oximetry
- Stump pressures

Anesthesia considerations

- *Goals:* Minimize hemodynamic variability; optimize cerebral/cardiac perfusion pressures.

General anesthesia

Advantages

- Use of mild hypothermia
- Decreased cerebral metabolic rate of oxygen consumption by inhalational agent
- Immobility
- Maintenance of a patent airway control
- Patient comfort
- Hemodynamic control
- Monitoring and control of carbon dioxide

Disadvantages

- Hypertensive/hypotensive episodes
- Loss of consciousness with general anesthesia
- General anesthesia with coexisting disease

Considerations

- Avoid cervical hyperextension.
- Intravascular volume repletion
- Controlled induction
- Consider balanced technique.
- Mild hypothermia, active rewarming after reperfusion occurs
- Maintenance of MAP $\geq$20% above preoperative baseline for contralateral carotid stenosis immediately before carotid artery cross-clamping
- Surgical manipulation of the carotid sinus causing baroreceptor stimulation and bradycardia/asystole
- Protamine administration (potential for hypotension, anaphylaxis, thrombus formation)
- Nitrous oxide should be avoided because of enlargement of microbubbles during carotid artery unclamping.
- Tight hemodynamic control during perioperative phase
- Rapid emergence to assess neurologic integrity

Regional anesthesia

Advantages

- Neurological monitoring: Awake patient
- Decreased incidence of hypotension
- Decreased incidence of shunting

Disadvantages

- Increased levels of catecholamines
- Patient cooperation mandatory
- Emergent airway management possible
- Inadvertent phrenic nerve anesthesia
- Hematoma
- Carotid artery cannulation
- Pneumothorax
- Local anesthetic systemic toxicity
- Inadequate anesthesia

Considerations

- Patient acceptance and education
- Deep and superficial cervical plexus block of C2–C4 and wound infiltration
- Conscious sedation as needed
- *Cerebral steal phenomena*: Cerebral arteries are maximally dilated in areas where stenosis exists in order to meet the metabolic demands of brain tissue. When **arterial vasodilation** occurs (e.g., inhalational agents, vasodilators, decreased MAP), cerebral arteries dilate and create a pressure gradient that minimizes or "steals" blood flow from those areas where stenosis is present and blood flow is compromised. Cerebral ischemia and infarction are then possible.
- *Inverse steal phenomenon (Robin Hood syndrome)*: Cerebral **artery vasoconstriction** (e.g., phenylephrine) causes increased pressure in the cerebrovasculature. The increased pressure in areas of stenosis maximizes blood flow in these areas that are at risk for developing cerebral ischemia and infarction.

Postoperative Period

- Postoperative respiratory insufficiency
- Carotid body dysfunction
- Recurrent/superior nerve damage
- Cranial nerve injury: Occurs in 10% of patients after CEA
- Postoperatively, surgeons ask patients to swallow (cranial nerve [CN] IX, glossopharyngeal nerve), say "EEE" (CN X, vagus nerve, specifically superior and recurrent laryngeal nerves), and stick out their tongue (CN XII, hypoglossal nerve) (Table 3.15)
- Cardiovascular instability
  - Hypertension (common), recommended to keep BP $\leq$140/80 mm Hg

TABLE 3.15 Cranial Nerve Function and Assessment

CN	Function	Assessment
VII (facial)	Muscles of facial expression	Smile, frown
IX (glossopharyngeal)	Muscles of pharynx, swallowing	Swallowing reflexes
X (vagus)	Laryngeal muscles	Speech
XII (hypoglossal)	Muscles of the tongue	Stick out tongue, side to side

CN, Cranial nerve.

- Hypotension
- MI
- Pneumothorax/tension pneumothorax
- Hematoma
- Hyperperfusion syndrome
  - *Cause:* As a result of altered cerebral autoregulation (inadequate vasoconstriction during hypertension) caused by increased CBF postoperatively, cerebral edema can occur.
  - *Signs and symptoms:* altered level of consciousness, seizures
- Postoperative stroke
  - Immediate reexploration of wound
  - Cerebral angiogram
  - Anticoagulation

Summary of Anesthetic Management for Carotid Endarterectomy

Indications

- Asymptomatic patients with CAS >60%
- Symptomatic patients with CAS >50%

Preoperative concerns

- Hypertension
- Coronary artery disease
- Diabetes mellitus
- Renal insufficiency
- Coagulation status
- Active neurologic process

Anesthetic technique

- Regional anesthesia *may* be associated with the following:
  - Decreased cardiac morbidity
  - Decreased stroke
  - Fewer shunts
  - Quick recognition of shunt dysfunction
  - Decreased perioperative hypertension
  - Shorter operating room times
  - Decreased postoperative stay
  - Decreased cost

Postoperative concerns

- Hypertension
- Hypotension
- Stroke
- MI
- Wound hematoma
- Cranial nerve injury
- Carotid body damage
- Hyperperfusion syndrome

KNOWLEDGE CHECK

1. Which nerve block is necessary to provide regional anesthesia during CEA?
   a. Supraclavicular
   b. Axillary
   c. Recurrent laryngeal
   d. Cervical plexus
2. Which medication should the anesthetist consider holding for 24 hours to avoid hypoperfusion?
   a. Angiotensin-converting enzyme inhibitor
   b. β-Blocker
   c. Statin
   d. Anticoagulant
3. Which postoperative complication is specifically associated with CEA? *(Select all that apply.)*
   a. Hemorrhage
   b. Hypoglossal nerve injury
   c. Hyperperfusion syndrome
   d. Pneumothorax
   e. Ulnar nerve injury
   f. MI
   g. Cerebral steal phenomena
4. Monitoring for neurologic integrity during CEA is most effectively assessed
   a. by stump pressures.
   b. by near-infrared spectrometry.
   c. in an awake patient.
   d. by electroencephalogram monitoring.

Answers can be found in Appendix A.

Abdominal Aortic Aneurysm

Patients who are scheduled to undergo abdominal aortic aneurysm (AAA) repair are at high risk for the presence of other vascular lesions/occlusions.

- The incidence of AAA is estimated to range between 3% and 10% for patients older than 50 years of age who reside in the Western world.
- AAAs are two to six times more common in males than in females and are two to three times more common in White males than in Black males.
- In males, AAAs most frequently begin to occur at 50 years of age and then peak at 80 years of age.
- As a result of increased wall stress at the bifurcation of the aorta and the iliac arteries, AAAs most frequently develop below the renal arteries (infrarenal), but about 5%–15% of AAAs are juxtarenal or suprarenal. Juxtarenal or suprarenal AAAs are associated with a higher incidence of acute kidney injury postoperatively.

Preoperative Period

- See all preoperative concerns for CEA listed earlier.
- Preoperative renal function is the most indicative factor determining the potential for acute kidney injury postoperatively.
- Type and cross-match for blood and blood products is essential for open AAA repair because of the potential for rapid massive hemorrhage (Box 3.4).

Intraoperative Management

Traditional open AAA repair

Epidural catheter placement before induction:

- *Advantages:* Decreased hypertensive response, decreased inflammatory mediator release, decreased anesthetic requirement, postoperative pain relief
- *Disadvantages:* Hypotension that is minimally responsive to vasopressors especially during massive rapid hemorrhage, minuscule potential for epidural hematoma as a result of anticoagulation
- *Monitoring:* Standard monitors, arterial line mandatory, TEE if available, two large-bore IV catheters, CVP catheter if peripheral venous access is inadequate
- *Anticoagulation:* Heparin 50–100 units/kg

BOX 3.4 Optimization of Body Systems Before Abdominal Aortic Aneurysm Repair

Cardiac Evaluation
- Quantify risk factors and optimize cardiac function.
- Institute appropriate β-blocker.
- Institute statin therapy.
- Control hypertension.
- Institute appropriate anticoagulation therapy.

Pulmonary Evaluation
- Advise smoking cessation.
- Perform radiologic tests and pulmonary function testing as indicated.
- Institute pharmacologic therapy, which may include corticosteroids and bronchodilators.

Renal Evaluation
- Assess electrolytes, creatinine, and glomerular filtration rate.

Adrenal Evaluation
- Provide steroid supplementation for patients at risk for acute adrenal crises.

Deep Vein Thrombosis Prophylaxis
- Administer pharmacologic prophylaxis.
- Provide graduated compression stockings.
- Provide intermittent pneumatic compression.
- Provide venous foot pumps.

Musculoskeletal Evaluation
- Assess range of neck motion before airway management.
- Assess functional limitations for positioning to avoid postoperative paresthesia.

Endocrine Evaluation
- Provide short- and long-term glycemic control (mandatory) because of the increased incidence of diabetes.

Miscellaneous Considerations
- Order laboratory assessments—complete blood count, coagulation panel, electrolyte panel, blood urea nitrogen, creatinine, albumin, blood sugar, liver function tests, type and cross-match 6 units of packed red blood cells

From Thompson A, Fleischmann KE, Smilowitz NR, et al. 2024 AHA/ACC/ACS/ASNC/HRS/SCA/SCCT/SCMR/SVM guideline for perioperative cardiovascular management for noncardiac surgery: A report of the American College of Cardiology/American Heart Association Joint Committee on Clinical Practice Guidelines. *Circulation*. 2024;150(19):e351-e442.

- The most dramatic hemodynamic events include aortic cross-clamping and unclamping (Tables 3.16 and 3.17).
- Renal dose dopamine and/or mannitol administration has not been scientifically proven to improve postoperative renal function.
- Protamine administration at the conclusion of surgery: Not to exceed 50 mg, administration should proceed as slow IV push to avoid hypotension. There is the potential for anaphylaxis.

Postoperative Period

- Consider postoperative ventilation if patient's physical condition is in question (e.g., severe chronic obstructive pulmonary disease [COPD]), large fluid or blood infusion, hemodynamic variability, or inability to meet extubation criteria (Box 3.5).

Endovascular Aortic Repair

- The first successful endovascular stent placement for AAA was performed in 1999.
- Thirty percent of patients with AAA are not candidates for surgery with a traditional open approach.
- It is estimated that 75% of AAAs are repaired via endovascular aneurysm repair (EVAR).
- In high-risk patients having elective AAA repair, the 30-day and 1-year mortality rates are significantly decreased with EVAR compared with open surgical repair.
- Endovascular aneurysm repair is associated with improved 30-day outcomes (reduced all-cause mortality; fewer readmissions; reduced surgical site infection, pneumonia, hemorrhage, acute kidney injury, MI, and sepsis) compared with open surgical repair.

TABLE 3.16 Physiologic Changes Associated With Aortic Cross-Clamping

Hemodynamic Changes	Metabolic Changes	Intraoperative Interventions
Increased arterial blood pressure above the cross-clamp	Decreased total body oxygen consumption	*Reduce afterload* Sodium nitroprusside Inhalation anesthetics Milrinone Shunts and aorta to femoral bypass
Decreased arterial blood pressure below the cross-clamp	Decreased total body carbon dioxide production	*Reduce preload* Nitroglycerin Atrial to femoral bypass
Increased wall motion abnormalities and left ventricular wall tension	Increased mixed venous oxygen saturation	*Renal protection* Fluid administration Mannitol Furosemide Dopamine *N*-acetylcysteine Cold renal perfusion
Decreased ejection fraction and cardiac output	Decreased total body oxygen extraction	*Miscellaneous* Hypothermia Decrease minute ventilation Sodium bicarbonate
Decreased renal blood flow	Increased catecholamine release	
Increased pulmonary occlusion pressure	Respiratory alkalosis	
Increased central venous pressure	Metabolic acidosis	
Increased coronary blood flow		

Modified from Norris EJ. Anesthesia for vascular surgery. In Miller RD, Cohen NH, Eriksson LI, et al, eds. *Miller's Anesthesia*. Vol. 2. 8th ed. Elsevier; 2015:2106–2157; Holt PJE, Thompson MM. Abdominal aortic aneurysms: evaluation and decision making. In Cronenwett JL, Johnston KW, eds. *Rutherford's Vascular Surgery*. Vol. II. 8th ed. Elsevier; 2014:1999–2023.

TABLE 3.17 Hemodynamic Responses to Aortic Unclamping and Therapeutic Interventions

Hemodynamic Changes	Metabolic Changes	Intraoperative Interventions
Decreased arterial blood pressure	Increased lactate	Decrease anesthetic depth
Decreased myocardial contractility	Increased total body oxygen consumption	Decrease vasodilators
Decreased systemic vascular resistance	Decreased mixed venous oxygen saturation	Increase fluids
Decreased central venous pressure	Increased prostaglandins	Increase vasoconstrictor drugs
Decreased preload	Increased activated complement	Reapply cross-clamp for severe hypotension
Decreased cardiac output	Increased myocardial depressant factors	Consider administration of mannitol and sodium bicarbonate
Increased pulmonary artery pressure	Decreased temperature	
	Metabolic acidosis	

Modified from Norris EJ. Anesthesia for vascular surgery. In Miller RD, Cohen NH, Eriksson LI, et al, eds. *Miller's Anesthesia*. Vol. 2. 8th ed. Elsevier; 2015:2106–2157; Holt PJE, Thompson MM. Abdominal aortic aneurysms: evaluation and decision making. In Cronenwett JL, Johnston KW. *Rutherford's Vascular Surgery*. Vol. II. 8th ed. Elsevier; 2014:1999–2023.

BOX 3.5 Postoperative Considerations for Patients Having Abdominal Aortic Aneurysm Repair

- Continue invasive hemodynamic monitoring.
- Treat acute blood pressure extremes, arrhythmias (atrial fibrillation).
- Assess for postoperative myocardial infarction.
- Provide ventilatory management with weaning and extubation.
- Assess for abdominal compartment syndrome.
- Evaluate hemoglobin, hematocrit, coagulation status, and adequacy of volume replacement.
- Assess blood urea nitrogen/creatinine and urine output.
- Institute deep vein thrombosis prophylaxis per protocol.

- Endoleak is the most frequently occurring complication, which may require a second surgical intervention (Box 3.6).
- Major surgical advantages to EVAR include no large incision and no cross-clamping/unclamping of the aorta (Fig. 3.21).

Anesthetic technique

- Local sedation or neuraxial anesthesia is associated with fewer intensive care unit (ICU) admissions, decreased length of hospitalization, and fewer systemic complications compared with general anesthesia, with no difference in 30-day mortality associated

BOX 3.6 Potential Complications Associated With Endovascular Aneurysm Repair

Graft and Deployment Complications

- Failed deployment
- Microembolization
- Migration/occlusion of major branch arteries (e.g., renal, mesenteric)
- Aortic perforation/aneurysm rupture
- Aortic dissection
- Hematoma formation
- Endoleak
- Stenosis/kink/thrombosis
- Graft tear
- Damage to access arteries (femoral → iliac)
- Infection

Radiologic Implications

- Radiation exposure
- Allergy to contrast dye
- Renal insufficiency from contrast dye

Systemic Complications

- Neurologic (CVA, paraplegia)
- Cardiac morbidity/mortality
- Pulmonary insufficiency
- Renal insufficiency
- Postimplantation syndrome

CVA, Cerebrovascular accident.

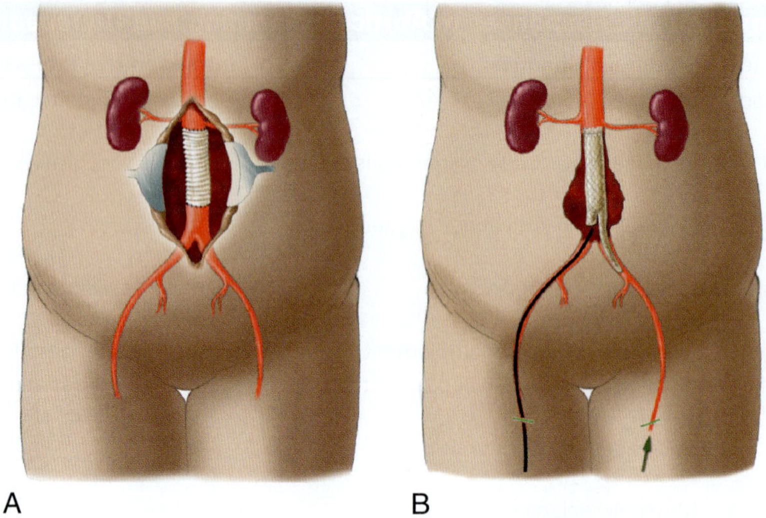

Fig. 3.21 Comparison of (A) open surgical repair and (B) endovascular aneurysm repair (EVAR). (From Elisha S, Heiner JS, Nagelhout JJ. *Nurse Anesthesia*. 7th ed. Elsevier; 2023.)

with either local sedation or general anesthesia provided for EVAR.

- Shorter operative time, shorter length of hospitalization, and fewer postoperative complications are associated with local sedation than with neuraxial or general anesthesia.

KNOWLEDGE CHECK

1. Which hemodynamic effect occurs with cross-clamping of the aorta? *(Select all that apply.)*
   a. Increased arterial pressure above the level of the cross-clamp
   b. Decreased CVP
   c. Increased afterload
   d. Increased EF
2. Which hemodynamic effect occurs with unclamping of the aorta? *(Select all that apply.)*
   a. Decreased PA pressure
   b. Decreased lactate
   c. Decreased myocardial contractility
   d. Decreased ABP
3. Which adverse reaction is associated with protamine administration? *(Select all that apply.)*
   a. Acute hemorrhage
   b. Anaphylaxis
   c. Lactic acidosis
   d. Hypotension

Answers can be found in Appendix A.

RESPIRATORY SYSTEM

The respiratory system is a vital life-sustaining organ system. It consists of both the upper and lower respiratory airways. The upper respiratory airway begins at the nasal and mouth opening and contains the nasal and oral cavities, which lead to the pharynx. The pharynx is a fibromuscular tube that extends from the base of the skull to the cricoid cartilage. It is divided into the nasopharynx, oropharynx, and laryngopharynx (also known as the *hypopharynx*). The upper respiratory airway ends at the cricoid cartilage, where the larynx meets the trachea (Fig. 3.22). The upper respiratory airway's primary functions are to conduct gases toward the lower airway and to protect the lower airway from food, liquid, debris, and other contaminants. The lower respiratory airway begins at the cricoid cartilage and ends at the alveoli. It consists of both conduction and gas exchange areas. The lower airway conduction zones include the trachea, bronchi, and bronchiole generations up to the terminal bronchioles. The gas exchange zones within the lower respiratory airway start with the respiratory bronchioles, where limited gas exchange occurs. These bronchioles then lead to alveolar ducts and alveolar clusters, where the majority of gas exchange and ventilation occurs. For a more detailed review of both upper and lower respiratory airway anatomy and function, see Chapter 1 Airway Management.

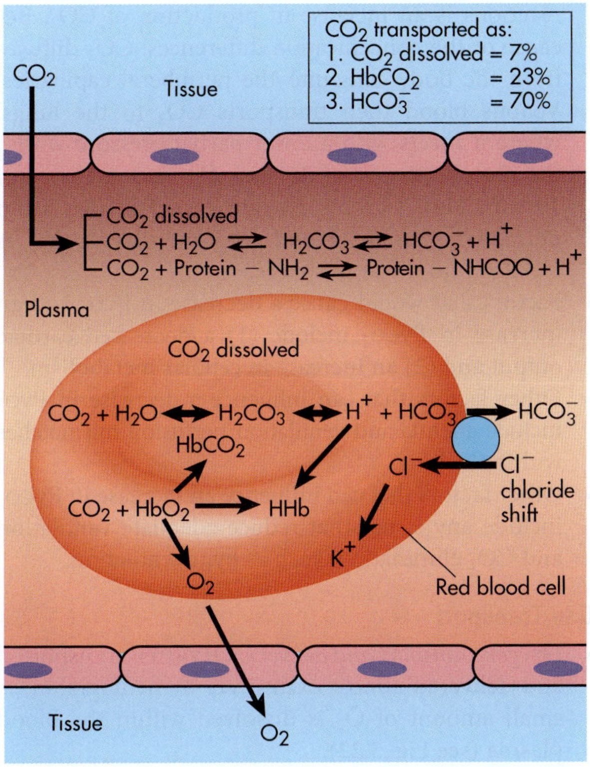

Fig. 3.22 Buffering of hydrogen with hemoglobin and carbon dioxide (CO_2) transport. CO_2 is produced in tissue cells and diffuses to plasma, where it is transported as dissolved CO_2, or it combines with water to form carbonic acid (H_2CO_3), or it combines with protein from which hydrogen has been released. Most of the CO_2 diffuses into the red blood cells and combines with water to form H_2CO_3. The H_2CO_3 dissociates to form hydrogen (H^+) and bicarbonate. Bicarbonate shifts into the plasma, and chloride (Cl^-) shifts into the red blood cell to maintain electroneutrality. Hydrogen combines with hemoglobin that has released its oxygen to form deoxyhemoglobin, which buffers the hydrogen and makes venous blood slightly more acidic than arterial blood. (From McCance KL, Huether SE. *Pathophysiology: The Biologic Basis for Disease in Adults and Children*. 6th ed. Elsevier; 2010.)

Physiology of Breathing

The quality of respiration depends on pulmonary ventilation, gas diffusion, gas transport, and regulation of respiration.

Pulmonary Ventilation

Pulmonary ventilation is the total volume of gas flow into the lungs per minute that is inspired (VI) or expired (VE), expressed in liters per minute. It refers to the process by which oxygen is brought into the lungs from the atmosphere and carbon dioxide is expelled from the body. Pulmonary ventilation differs from alveolar ventilation by including the exchange of dead space gas.

- Alveolar ventilation is the amount of air that reaches the gas exchange areas, such as the respiratory bronchioles, alveolar ducts, and alveoli. Whereas *pulmonary ventilation* refers to the total gas flow (including dead space gas volume), *alveolar ventilation* refers to the effective ventilation of the alveoli where gas exchange takes place with the blood.
- Alveolar ventilation is calculated by subtracting the anatomic dead space from the tidal volume (V_t) and multiplying it by the respiratory rate:
  Alveolar ventilation = (Tidal volume − Anatomic dead space) × Respiratory rate
  Thus, a change in respiratory rate or V_t will either increase or decrease alveolar ventilation. Conversely, impairment of alveolar ventilation will increase the retention of carbon dioxide.
- Slower, deep respirations produce better alveolar ventilation than rapid, shallow breathing. If the respiratory frequency doubles, then both dead space volume and alveolar volume double. However, if V_t increases, then alveolar volume increases, and dead space volume remains the same, allowing for an increase in ventilation of gases within the alveoli. Thus, an increase in V_t is a more effective way to increase alveolar ventilation.

Gas Diffusion

Gas diffusion is the net passive movement of particles (atoms, ions, or molecules) from a region of higher concentration to regions of lower concentration. It continues until the concentration of substances is uniform throughout.

- *Partial pressure:* Each gas has a partial pressure, which is the total pressure of that gas if it alone occupied the entire volume of the original mixture at the same temperature. Gases dissolve, diffuse, and react according to their partial pressures and not according to their concentrations in gas mixtures or liquids. The speed at which gases diffuse across membranes is controlled by several factors, the most important of which is their partial pressure within each compartment. For example, the partial pressure of oxygen within the alveolus is 103 mm Hg, whereas within the pulmonary capillary it is only 40 mm Hg.

Because of the partial pressure difference, oxygen easily diffuses from the alveolus into the capillary.

- Gases within the alveoli are separated from the capillaries by approximately 1–2 mm of tissue: the mucinous covering of the alveolus, the alveolar epithelium (which in some places is incomplete), an interstitial layer, and the endothelium covering the pulmonary capillary.
- Several disease states influence the diffusion of gases within the lungs:
  - *Emphysema:* Total surface area of the alveolar membranes is decreased.
  - *Pneumonia:* Alveolar walls become thickened, thereby prolonging diffusion.
  - *Asthma:* Increase in bronchial secretions acts to impede the exchange of gases.
  - *Methemoglobinemia:* O_2-carrying capacity of the blood is decreased.
- *Oxygen diffusion*: Atmospheric oxygen content at sea level is estimated at 159 mm Hg. This is 21% of the atmospheric pressure (760 mm Hg), which is the total sum of all the partial pressures of gas in the atmosphere. Because of water vapor within the conducting airways, by the time the oxygen reaches the alveoli, it is reduced to a partial alveolar pressure (P_{AO_2}) of 103–105 mm Hg. Oxygen then diffuses into the pulmonary capillaries because of the large difference in partial pressures between alveoli and pulmonary venous blood. As blood returns to the left heart and is circulated to body tissues, the partial pressure of oxygen in arterial blood (Pa_{O_2}) is between 95 and 100 mm Hg. This is due to the physiologic shunt that occurs from both bronchial and thebesian venous drainage into the left heart and aorta. As arterial blood reaches peripheral capillaries and body cells, the difference in oxygen partial pressures between arterial blood (95 mm Hg) and body cells (5–20 mm Hg) causes oxygen to diffuse into cells. What results from this diffusion into body cells is a lower oxygen partial pressure in venous blood (Pv_{O_2} of 40 mm Hg) that is then circulated back to the right heart and into the lungs.
- *Carbon dioxide diffusion:* This begins at the cellular level. The partial pressure of carbon dioxide (Pa_{CO_2}) within the cells is higher than in arterial blood (50 mm Hg versus Pa_{CO_2} of 40 mm Hg) because of the metabolic reactions and energy produced at the cellular level. The byproduct of these cellular metabolic reactions is an increase in production of CO_2. Because of the concentration differences, CO_2 diffuses from the body cells into the peripheral capillaries. Venous blood then transports CO_2 to the lungs, where it meets with a lower partial pressure within the alveoli (Pv_{CO_2} of 45 mm Hg versus P_{ACO_2} of 40 mm Hg). Carbon dioxide easily diffuses from pulmonary venous blood into the alveoli and is exhaled into the atmosphere.
- Factors that would cause a decrease in Pv_{O_2} and an increase in Pv_{CO_2} include (1) a decreased cardiac output and (2) an increase in cellular metabolism.
- Other factors that can influence a decrease in Pv_{O_2} include anemia and ventilation/perfusion mismatches within the lung.
- Other factors that can influence an increase in Pv_{CO_2} include any issues that reduce adequate ventilation and CO_2 elimination, such as hypoventilation.

Gas Transport

- *Oxygen transport and delivery:* Oxygen is transported and delivered almost exclusively by hemoglobin. A small amount of O_2 is dissolved within the blood plasma (see Fig. 3.22).
- Approximately two-thirds of every breath reaches the terminal airways to participate in alveolar ventilation in normal lungs. The majority of O_2 within the alveoli diffuses through the alveolar epithelium, across the interstitial space, and through the capillary endothelium; crosses a small amount of plasma; and enters into the RBCs to combine with hemoglobin. A small amount of O_2 diffuses into the plasma and maintains an arterial O_2 partial pressure. The majority of O_2 is bound to and transported to body cells by hemoglobin. Hemoglobin can hold and carry 1.34 mL of O_2 per gram. Thus by taking the hemoglobin value and multiplying it by the total percentage of O_2 saturation (Sa_{O_2}) and O_2-carrying constant, then adding it to the amount of O_2 dissolved in the blood plasma, a calculation can be made for O_2-carrying capacity:

$$(Pa_{O_2} \times 0.003) + (1.34 \times Hgb \times Sa_{O_2})$$

The following example is a calculation of total O_2-carrying capacity from breathing room air with an Sa_{O_2} of 98%, a Pa_{O_2} of 100 mm Hg, and a normal hemoglobin of 15 g/dL:

$$CaO_2 = (100\ mm\ Hg \times 0.003) + (1.34 \times 15\ g/dL \times 0.98) = 20\ mL\ O_2$$

Thus 20 mL of O_2 is transported in hemoglobin per 100 mL of blood. Assuming a cardiac output of 5 L/min, the total O_2 transported would equal 1000 mL/min. In order to calculate how much oxygen is delivered to the body cells, a venous blood gas is required. Assuming normal venous blood gas values of SvO_2 of 70% and PvO_2 of 40 mm Hg, a calculation can be made using the same formula:

$$CvO_2 = (40\ mm\ Hg \times 0.003) + (1.34 \times 15\ g/dL \times 0.70) = 14.2\ mL\ O_2$$

Subtracting 14.2 from 20 demonstrates that just over 5 mL of O_2 per 100 mL of blood (one-fourth or 250 mL/min total) is picked up and used by the body cells. Factors that can reduce DO_2 to the body cells are (1) decrease in oxygen supply within the lungs (e.g., hypoventilation or pulmonary obstruction), (2) a decrease in cardiac output (e.g., pump failure, shock state), (3) a decrease in O_2-carrying capacity (e.g., hemorrhage or anemia), or (4) an increase in O_2 consumption without adequate O_2 supply (e.g., hypermetabolic states).

- *Carbon dioxide transport and removal:* CO_2 is transported within the blood in three ways: (1) 5%–10% is dissolved in blood plasma, (2) 5%–10% undergoes a rapid nonenzymatic reaction to combine with terminal amine groups of plasma proteins (especially hemoglobin) to become carbamino compounds or carbaminohemoglobin, and (3) 80%–90% is in the form of bicarbonate (see Fig. 3.22). Within the RBCs, CO_2 encounters carbonic anhydrase and combines with water to form carbonic acid. Carbonic acid then dissociates into bicarbonate (HCO_3^-) and hydrogen (H^+) ions. As bicarbonate leaves the RBCs, it is exchanged with chloride ions (Cl^-) to maintain electrical neutrality. This is known as the *chloride shift* or *hamburger shift*. This process is then reversed within the RBCs when bicarbonate reaches the lungs, resulting in CO_2 and H_2O. Carbon dioxide then diffuses out of the RBCs and into the alveoli to be exhaled.

Regulation of Respiration

There are several mechanisms that influence the regulation of respiration, including the cerebral cortex and brainstem, central and peripheral chemoreceptors, and sensory inputs from outside the CNS (Fig. 3.23).

KNOWLEDGE CHECK

1. Which structure marks the transition from the upper to the lower respiratory airway?
   a. Pharynx
   b. Larynx
   c. Cricoid cartilage
   d. Trachea
2. Which change is most effective to increase alveolar ventilation?
   a. An increase in the respiratory rate
   b. A prolonged expiratory phase
   c. Rapid, shallow breathing
   d. An increase in the tidal volume
3. Gas diffusion across the alveolar–capillary membrane is primarily driven by differences in
   a. concentration gradients.
   b. partial pressures.
   c. blood flow.
   d. temperature differences.
4. The majority of carbon dioxide is carried in the blood as
   a. dissolved CO_2.
   b. carbaminohemoglobin.
   c. bicarbonate.
   d. carbonic acid.
5. Which condition causes a decrease in PvO_2 and an increase in $PvCO_2$?
   a. Increased cardiac output
   b. Decreased cardiac output
   c. Hyperventilation
   d. Anemia

Answers can be found in Appendix A.

Brainstem and cerebral cortex control. The brainstem and the cerebral cortex are two groups of neurons within the medulla and two groups of neurons within the pons that are the primary centers for unconscious respiratory control within the brainstem. An individual can also consciously control respiration from neurons located within the cerebral cortex.

- Medullary respiratory control is conducted by the dorsal and ventral respiratory groups.
  - *The dorsal respiratory group* (DRG) is a group of respiratory neurons that is located within the nucleus tractus solitarii. These neurons generate the basic rhythm of respiration by stimulating an inspiratory signal every 5 seconds. These neurons are considered the pacemaker of the respiratory system because they continuously send impulses

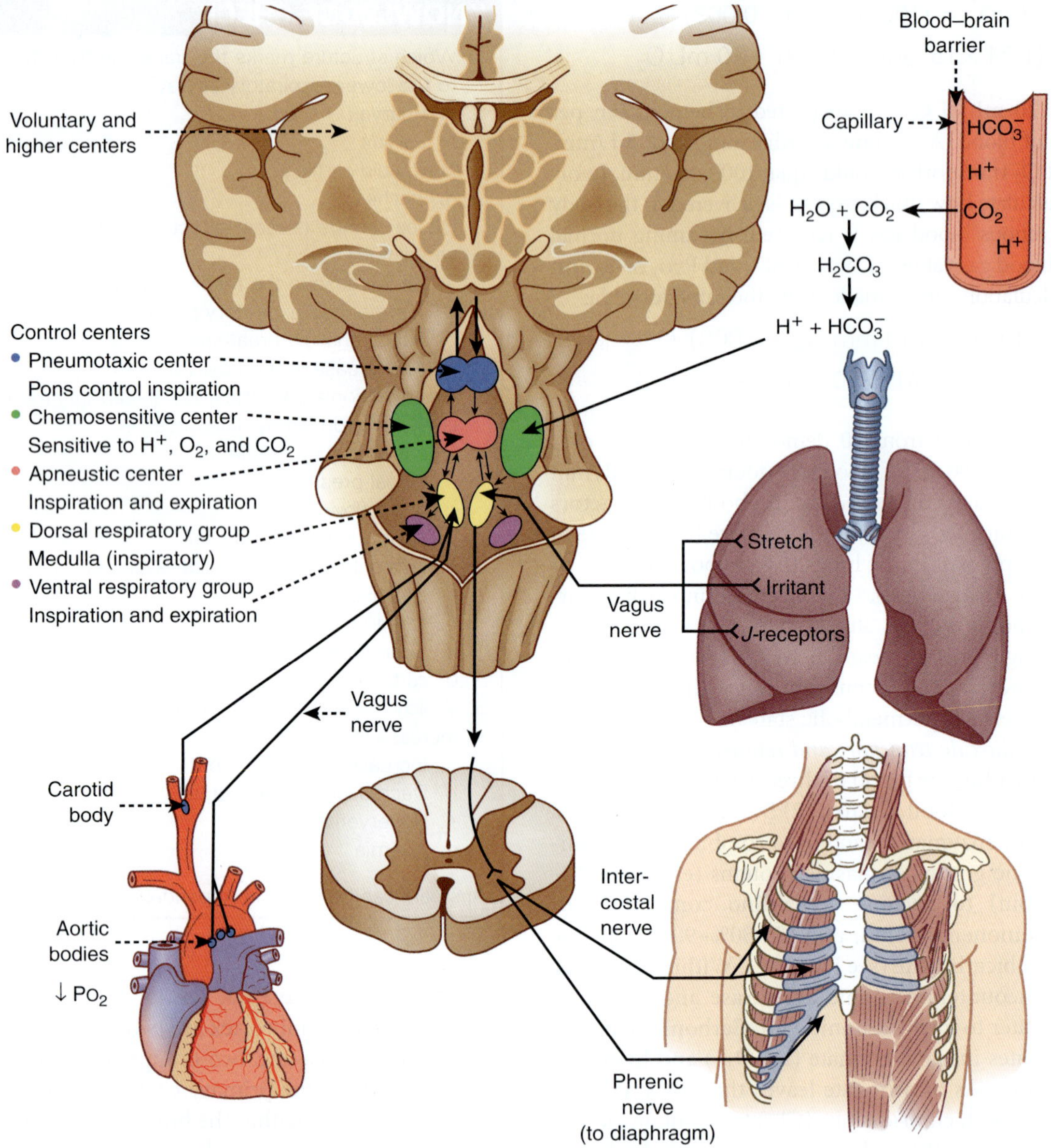

Fig. 3.23 Neurochemical respiratory control system. (From Rogers JL. *McCance and Huether's Pathophysiology: The Biologic Basis for Disease in Adults and Children*. 9th ed. Elsevier; 2023.)

to breathe to the diaphragm (via the phrenic nerves) and external intercostal muscles (via thoracic nerves). Sensory input from the periphery provides information that regulates the inspiratory effort and comes from the vagus nerve (CN X) and glossopharyngeal nerve (CN IX).

- The *ventral respiratory group* is another group of neurons located within the medulla that activate when there is an increased need for pulmonary ventilation (e.g., exercise). These neurons are known as the *overdrive mechanism* that stimulates expiratory muscles for faster and more powerful exhalation, as well as inspiratory accessory muscles for added inspiratory effort.

- Pontine respiratory control is mediated by the pneumotaxic and apneustic centers.
  - The *pneumotaxic center* is located in the upper pons. It acts on the DRG to inhibit inspiration. In other words, it provides an inspiratory "off switch." This center helps regulate the inspiratory rate and prevents overdistention of the lung. It may also play a role in switching from inspiration to expiration.
  - The *apneustic* center acts on the DRG to stimulate an inspiratory effort. This center helps adjust respiratory rate by sending inspiratory stimulant impulses to the DRG. It may also delay or interrupt the "off-switch" signal from the pneumotaxic center to the DRG. Pulmonary stretch receptors directly inhibit this center.
- Conscious control of respiration occurs in the cerebral cortex. This can occur from behavioral or voluntary causes. Activation of the cerebral cortex allows voluntary control of respiration, such as vocalization, hyperventilation, or even apnea. Other brain structures (e.g., hypothalamus) can alter respiration in response to pain and emotions.

Central and peripheral chemoreceptors. Central and peripheral chemoreceptors help regulate respiration based on blood CO_2, H^+, and oxygen levels.

- *Central chemoreceptors* are located in the medulla of the brainstem and are reactive to changes in blood levels of CO_2, O_2, and H^+ ions. The receptors in this chemosensitive area of the medulla sense changes in CO_2 and pH disturbances and activate areas of the respiratory center. These receptors are most responsive to changes in H^+ ion concentrations. However, H^+ ions do not easily cross the blood–brain barrier because it is not very permeable to charged substances. It does become more permeable over time when pH falls or if there is a large increase in blood H^+ ion concentration. Conversely, CO_2 easily passes through the blood–brain and blood–cerebrospinal fluid (CSF) barriers and reacts with H_2O to form carbonic acid. Carbonic acid then dissociates into H^+ and bicarbonate ions within the medulla, resulting in direct stimulation of chemoreceptive neurons by H^+ ions. Thus it is the H^+ ions that provide direct respiratory stimulation, whereas CO_2 is the most potent indirect stimulant for increased respiration. Excitation of the respiratory center by CO_2 is extensive for the first few hours, but then it gradually declines over the next 1–2 days. Finally, the central chemoreceptors have such a powerful response toward normalizing CO_2 that in a disease process such as pneumonia, the $Paco_2$ will correct before the Pao_2 will.
  - Increases in $Paco_2$ cause a rapid ventilatory response (increase in V_t and respiratory rate) within 1–2 minutes. Conditions that can elevate CO_2 include exercise, fever, substance/food ingestion, hypoventilation, or a hypermetabolic state. Additionally, more H^+ ions are released into the chemoreceptive areas of the medulla when there is an increase in blood CO_2 than when there is an increase in blood H^+ ion concentration.
  - Decreases in $Paco_2$ levels decrease the inspiratory effort. For example, while a patient is under general anesthesia and spontaneously breathing, if the breaths are augmented and then overcome with hyperventilation, the patient's intrinsic drive to breathe will decline because of the resulting hypocapnea. Conversely, incentive to begin a respiratory effort after a patient has received assisted or mechanical ventilation is facilitated by allowing the patient to hypoventilate and build up $Paco_2$ levels.
- *Peripheral chemoreceptors* are located within both the carotid and aortic bodies. They primarily respond to changes in Pao_2 and, to a lesser extent, in CO_2 and H^+. These chemoreceptors are known more as an accessory system for controlling ventilation. When the Pao_2 decreases to 60 mm Hg or less, stimulation of the peripheral chemoreceptors occurs, and there is a markedly increased ventilatory response.
  - The afferent response from carotid bodies travels to the medulla respiratory center via the glossopharyngeal nerve, whereas afferent transmission from aortic bodies travels via the vagus nerve. Carotid bodies are thought to have the highest amount of chemoreceptors, more so than the aortic bodies. It has been shown that patients who have had bilateral carotidectomies have a blunted response to hypoxemia.

Other Sensory Inputs. Other sensory inputs outside the CNS help regulate respiration. These include receptors and reflexes that are in the airway, lungs, and joints.

- *Irritant receptors* in the upper airway and tracheobronchial tree send afferent impulses to the brainstem when stimulated. Mechanical or chemical irritation of the nasal mucosa can induce coughing and sneezing reflexes. Sensory impulses here are transmitted via the olfactory (CN I) and trigeminal (CN V) nerves. In the upper airway and tracheobronchial tree, irritant receptors within the mucosa stimulate coughing and bronchoconstriction. The sensory response here is via the vagus (CN X) nerve.

- *Hering-Breuer stretch reflex* is a protective reflex and is known as the *stopping reflex.* Mechanoreceptors are embedded within the smooth muscles of the airway. These are stretch receptors within the lungs and bronchi that, when stimulated (e.g., lungs are overstretched), send signals to inhibit inspiration at the DRG and apneustic centers. This reflex prevents overinflation of the lungs. Both afferent and efferent transmission is via the vagus nerve. In a normal adult, this reflex will occur when inhalation exceeds approximately 1500 mL. This reflex is an important and basic reflex for neonates to help regulate respiration because many of their regulatory systems are still developing.
- *Juxtacapillary* or *"j" receptors* are located within the alveolar septum and are juxtaposed to pulmonary capillaries. They are sensory cells that are stimulated by pulmonary capillary engorgement or increased pulmonary interstitial volume (e.g., pulmonary edema) or specific chemicals in the pulmonary circulation. Afferent signals are sent via the vagus nerve to the medulla to stimulate tachypnea and/or dyspnea.
- *Joint proprioceptors and mechanoreceptors* are located within joints. These receptors are stimulated with the movement of joints, even passive movement. When stimulated, they send excitatory signals to the medulla, which increases pulmonary ventilation. An example would be the movement of joints (knees, hips, elbows, etc.) after several hours of sleep that sends stimuli to begin increasing pulmonary ventilation.

KNOWLEDGE CHECK

1. Which is the most effective intervention to improve alveolar minute ventilation?
   a. Apply PEEP.
   b. Increase tidal volume.
   c. Increase respiratory rate.
   d. Administer a β_2-agonist.
2. Which factor can result in an increase in both venous and arterial carbon dioxide?
   a. Hypovolemia
   b. Hypothermia
   c. Hyperventilation
   d. Hypertension
3. Which is the primary mechanism that facilitates the transport of carbon dioxide in the blood?
   a. Conversion to bicarbonate
   b. Dissolves in blood plasma
   c. Combines with plasma proteins
   d. Combines with hemoglobin
4. Which is the only respiratory area that plays a role in the inhibition of respiration?
   a. DRG
   b. Ventral respiratory group
   c. Pneumotaxic center
   d. Apneustic center
5. Which respiratory center is primarily responsible for generating the basic rhythm of breathing?
   a. VRG
   b. Pneumotaxic center
   c. DRG
   d. Apneustic center
6. What is the primary stimulant that causes peripheral chemoreceptors to significantly increase ventilation?
   a. Decrease in Pao_2 to below 60 mm Hg
   b. Increase in cerebrospinal fluid (CSF) H^+ concentration
   c. Slight increases in $Paco_2$
   d. Lung overinflation
7. What is the main function of the Hering-Breuer stretch reflex?
   a. Stimulate increased respiratory rate during exercise
   b. Prevent overinflation of the lungs
   c. Initiate coughing in response to airway irritants
   d. Switch breathing from voluntary to involuntary control

Answers can be found in Appendix A.

Mechanisms of Pulmonary Function

Muscles of Respiration

Respiratory muscles provide the mechanical breathing support for the lower respiratory system and include the inspiratory and expiratory muscles. During a breathing cycle, the lungs can be expanded in two ways. First, contraction of the diaphragm causes a lengthening of the chest cavity; second, contraction of intercostal muscles leads to an increase in the chest's anteroposterior diameter by elevating the rib cage. Simple relaxation of these muscles and the elastic recoil force of the lung tissue are enough to cause lung deflation.

Inspiratory muscles. These muscles consist of the diaphragm, external intercostals, and accessory muscles (sternocleidomastoid, scalene, pectoralis major, serratus anterior, latissimus dorsi, and serratus posterior superior) (Fig. 3.24).

- The diaphragm accounts for 75% of the breathing effort. It is a dome-shaped muscle that separates the thoracic and abdominal cavities. It consists of a right and left dome that rise all the way to the level of the fourth intercostal space. As it contracts, it flattens, causing a lengthening of the thorax and a negative intrapulmonary pressure. It is the primary muscle of inspiration; thus during quiet breathing, the diaphragm is probably the only muscle of respiration working. During normal exhalation, the diaphragm relaxes (along with the external intercostal muscles if contracted). The thoracic cavity and lungs decrease in size, and air is expelled. In normal breathing, a 1-cm downward movement of the diaphragm causes 350 mL of air to enter the lung. The normal 500-mL V_t will therefore require approximately a 1.5-cm downward movement of the diaphragm. The diaphragm receives its nerve supply from the phrenic nerves, which descend from cervical segments C3–C5.
- *External intercostal muscles* account for the remaining 25% of inspiratory effort. They effect an upward and outward movement of the chest, causing an increase in the anterior-posterior diameter of the chest cavity. The external intercostals are the most superficial layers of the intercostal muscles. There are 11 pairs of external intercostal muscles, extending between the tubercles of the ribs and the costochondral joints. Alone, contraction of the external intercostals would produce very shallow respirations, but it would be enough to sustain life. External intercostals are very sensitive to the neuromuscular blocking effects of anesthetic inhalation agents. Thus, when someone is spontaneously breathing under general anesthesia with inhalation agents, frequently only abdominal breathing is noted and not chest excursion because the diaphragm is the inspiratory muscle providing the respiratory effort.
- *Accessory muscles* are used when additional inspiratory effort is needed. This occurs in situations in which there is labored respiration, such as exercise or pathologic respiratory conditions. They include muscles of the neck and thorax. Within the neck, the sternocleidomastoid and scalene muscles help elevate the thoracic cavity. The two sternocleidomastoid muscles originate from the mastoid process of the temporal bone and the superior nuchal line of the occipital bone. They have attachments at both the clavicle and the sternum. Scalene muscles consist of anterior, medial, and posterior muscles. The pectoralis major, serratus anterior, latissimus dorsi, and serratus posterior superior of the chest and back help elevate and expand the chest during respiratory distress or when additional respiratory effort is needed.

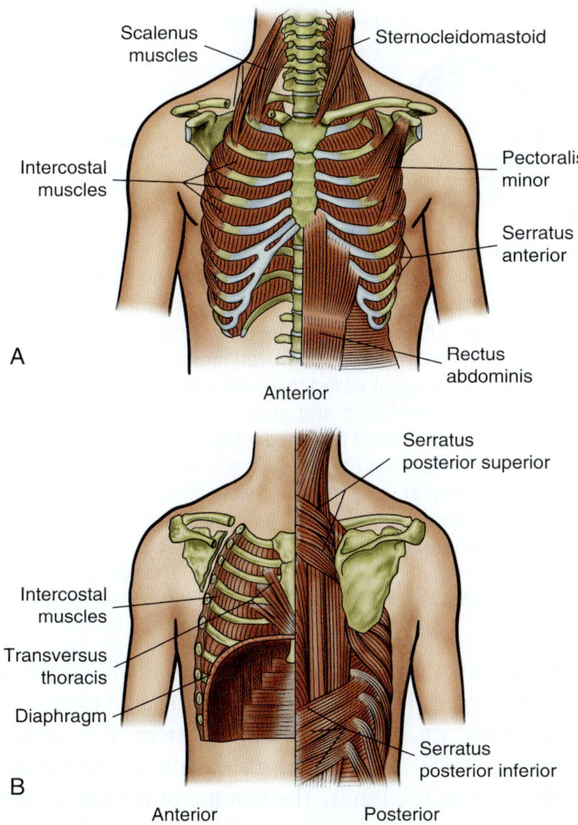

Fig. 3.24 Muscles of respiration. (A) Anterior view. (B) Posterior view. (Modified from Ball JW, Dains JE, Flynn JA, Solomon BS, Stewart RW. *Seidel's Guide to Physical Examination: An Interprofessional Approach*. 9th ed. Elsevier; 2019.)

Expiratory muscles. These muscles consist of the internal intercostal and abdominal muscles (see Fig. 3.24). These muscles are used during rapid labored breathing when passive recoil is not powerful enough to cause rapid exhalation. Their purpose is to contract and forcefully expel air out of the lungs before inspiration.

- *Internal intercostal muscle* contraction decreases the anteroposterior dimension of the chest cavity. The internal intercostal muscles consist of 11 pairs that attach between the costal groove and the superior border of two different ribs within the intercostal spaces.
- *Abdominal muscles* include the transverse abdominis, rectus abdominis, and internal/external oblique muscles (see Fig. 3.24). The abdominal muscles contract and forcefully push abdominal contents against the diaphragm during active expiration. This abdominal force against the diaphragm helps the lungs empty at a faster rate. The abdominal muscle point of origin is the pubic symphysis and pubic crest, and these attach to the xiphoid process and the fifth to seventh costal cartilages. The abdominal muscles initiate as the volume of inspired air increases above 90 L/min, such as during strenuous exercise.

Lung Volumes, Functional Residual Capacity, and Closing Capacity

Lung volumes. *Lung volumes* are the various volumes that exist in the lung (Fig. 3.25 and Table 3.18).

- *Tidal volume (V_t)* is the volume of air that is inspired and expired during normal quiet breathing. Estimated volumes are around 500 mL.
- *Inspiratory reserve volume (IRV)* is the maximum amount of air that can be inspired beyond a normal V_t inspiration and requires patient effort. Estimated volumes are between 3000 and 3300 mL.
- *Expiratory reserve volume (ERV)* is the additional gas volume in excess of normal V_t breathing that can be forcefully exhaled. Estimated volumes are between 1000 and 1200 mL.
- *Residual volume (RV)* is the minimum volume of gas left within the lung at the end of a forced expiratory volume breath. The estimated volumes are approximately 1200 mL. This is the only lung volume that cannot be measured with simple spirometry. However, RV can be estimated using an inert gas dilution technique or by using a nitrogen washout test. The most accurate way of measuring RV is by conducting a body plethysmography exam.
- *Inert gas dilution test:* This method frequently uses helium as the inert gas because it will not dissolve at the alveolar–capillary membrane and will remain at a constant pressure within the lungs. A spirometer is

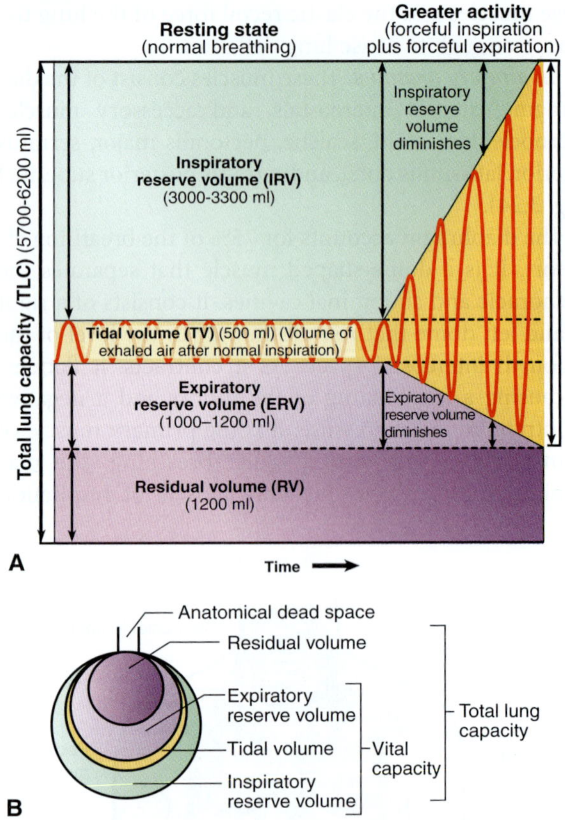

Fig. 3.25 Pulmonary ventilation volumes. The chart in (A) shows a tracing like that produced with a spirometer. The diagram in (B) shows the pulmonary volumes as relative proportions of an inflated balloon. During normal, quiet breathing, approximately 500 mL of air is moved into and out of the respiratory tract, an amount called the *tidal volume*. During forceful breathing (like that during and after heavy exercise), an extra 3300 mL can be inspired (the inspiratory reserve volume), and an extra 1000 mL or so can be expired (the expiratory reserve volume). The largest volume of air that can be moved in and out during ventilation is called the *vital capacity*. Air that remains in the respiratory tract after a forceful expiration is called the *residual volume*. (From Patton KT, Bell F, Thompson T, et al. *The Human Body in Health and Disease*. 8th ed. Elsevier; 2024.)

filled with a predetermined volume of helium mixed with oxygen. The patient is then instructed to breathe normally on a closed-circuit system for several breaths to facilitate equal dispersion of the helium throughout the lungs. The volume of helium is then measured within the spirometer. Based on measured volume within the spirometer, estimations of RVs can then be calculated. This technique is unreliable in patients with obstructive lung disease because the

TABLE 3.18 **Glossary of Static Lung Volumes and Capacities**

Measurement	Symbol	Definition	Capacity (mL)
Volumes			
Residual volume	RV	Volume of air remaining in the lungs after maximum respiration	1200
Expiratory reserve volume	ERV	Maximum volume of air expired from the resting end-expiratory level	1200
Tidal volume	V_t	Volume of air inspired or expired with each breath during quiet breathing	500
Inspiratory reserve volume	IRV	Maximum volume of air inspired from the resting end-inspiratory level	3100
Capacities			
Inspiratory capacity	$IC = IRV + V_t$	Maximum volume of air inspired from the end-expiratory level (the sum of IRV and V_t)	3600
Vital capacity	$VC = IRV + V_t + ERV$	Maximum volume of air expired from the maximum inspiratory level	4800
Functional residual capacity	$FRC = RV + ERV$	Volume of air remaining in the lungs at the end of expiration (the sum of RV and ERV)	2400
Total lung capacity	$TLC = IRV + V_t + ERV + RV$	Volume of air in the lungs after maximum inspiration (the sum of all volumes)	6000

helium is unable to fully equilibrate within the lungs.

- *Nitrogen washout test:* This method begins by allowing the patient to breathe room air, which contains approximately 79% nitrogen, 21% oxygen, and minimal carbon dioxide and methane. After several room air breaths, 100% oxygen is administered. Each breath then subsequently measures the amount of exhaled nitrogen. The patient continues V_t breathing until the exhaled nitrogen level is less than 2% for several breaths. The initial alveolar nitrogen concentration and the amount of nitrogen washed out can then be calculated to determine the RV within the lungs. Similar to the helium dilution test, this exam is unreliable in patients with obstructive lung disease.
- *Body plethysmography:* This test is conducted as a patient breathes through a mouthpiece in a patient-sized sealed chamber. Body plethysmography is based on Boyle's law, which states that for a fixed amount of gas in a closed space, the changes in volume are equal in magnitude but opposite to the changes in pressure. Because the chamber is sealed, the volume and pressure within can be measured. Thus the volumes and pressures within the sealed chamber directly correlate with intrapulmonary volumes and pressures. It is possible to calculate RV, functional residual capacity (FRC), and total lung capacity using a system of calculations and looking at volumes and pressures during the inspiratory cycle.

Functional lung capacities. *Lung capacities* include two or more lung volumes.

- *Inspiratory capacity (IC)* is a combination of the IRV and the V_t. It is the maximum amount of air that can be inspired after a normal V_t expiration. Estimated volumes are between 3500 and 3800 mL.
- *Vital capacity (VC)* is the sum of the IRV, V_t, and ERV. The VC includes the volume of air from a maximal inspiratory effort to a maximal expiratory effort. In essence, the VC combines all of the lung volumes except for the RV. Estimated volumes are between 4500 and 5000 mL.
- *Functional Residual Capacity (FRC)* is a combination of the RV and the ERV. It is the volume of gas that remains in the lungs at the end of a normal expiration (V_t breathing). At FRC, elastic lung recoil forces and chest wall expansive forces are in equal opposition to each other and are connected by the pleural surfaces. These opposing forces, in combination with alveolar air pressure and alveolar surfactant, keep the small airways open and create the FRC. The FRC is an important lung capacity because this is the volume

of air that hemoglobin can draw on during times of apnea. Estimated volumes are 2200–2400 mL.

- Factors that reduce FRC include those that reduce the ERV and the RV, such as obesity, pregnancy, alterations in position (supine, Trendelenburg, lithotomy, etc.), general anesthesia, mechanical ventilation, intrinsic restrictive lung diseases (pulmonary edema, acute respiratory distress syndrome [ARDS], aspiration pneumonia, pulmonary fibrosis, alveolar proteinosis, sarcoidosis, etc.), and extrinsic restrictive diseases (ascites, scoliosis, flail chest, pneumothorax, pleural effusion, spinal cord damage, Guillain-Barré syndrome, etc.)

- *Total lung capacity (TLC)* includes the IRV, Vt, ERV, and RV. This is the total volume contained within the lung after a maximal inspiration. Estimated volumes are between 5700 and 6200 mL.

Closing volume and closing capacity. *Closing volume* is the volume within the lung at which small airways begin to close. It occurs because of a lack of air pressure within the small airways, causing them to collapse during exhalation. *Closing capacity* is the sum of the closing volume plus the RV. It is the total volume within the lungs when the small airways close during exhalation. In healthy individuals, the closing volume is below RV and is not clinically observed. The closing volume normally increases with age as a result of loss of elastic tissue within the lung. It will also increase in certain conditions, such as smoking, COPD, obesity, pregnancy, supine position, asthma and bronchospasm, atelectasis, pneumonia, and pulmonary edema. Closing volumes can be measured using the washout characteristics of tracer gases such as xenon or helium or with body plethysmography.

Thoracic Forces

Thoracic forces include various intrathoracic pressures and lung and chest wall recoil, which work together to keep the lungs open. Elastic forces within lung tissue favor contraction, whereas the recoil forces within the chest wall favor expansion. This creates a balance that provides patency to the lungs. There are also several important pressures that are involved with both intrapulmonary and extrapulmonary opening.

- *Pleural pressure* is the pressure that exists within the pleural space outside the lung between the visceral pleura of the lung and the parietal pleura of the inner chest wall. Pleural pressure is slightly less than atmospheric pressure and is thus a negative pressure. This negative pressure acts like a suction cup to keep the lungs inflated.
  - The negative intrapleural pressure is created by three factors: (1) the surface tension of the fluid within the alveoli causes an inward-pulling pressure of each alveolus and thus the entire lung (surfactant reduces this force); (2) the lungs contain a large amount of tissue that have elastic properties, which causes a strong inward-recoiling force; and (3) the chest wall contains highly elastic lung tissue and provides an opposing outward-recoiling force. The balance of these inward and outward recoil forces is what creates the negative intrapleural pressure. A small amount of pleural fluid creates a surface tension between the inner chest wall and

KNOWLEDGE CHECK

1. Which respiratory muscle is responsible for 75% of the inspiratory effort during normal quiet breathing?
   a. External intercostals
   b. Diaphragm
   c. Sternocleidomastoid
   d. Scalene muscles
2. Which statement about the external intercostal muscles is true?
   a. They assist in forceful expiration.
   b. They are highly resistant to volatile anesthetic agents.
   c. Their contraction increases the anteroposterior diameter of the chest.
   d. They alone can generate full tidal volume breathing under normal conditions.
3. Which muscles are activated during forced expiration when passive lung recoil is insufficient?
   a. Diaphragm and external intercostals
   b. Sternocleidomastoid and scalene muscles
   c. Internal intercostals and abdominal muscles
   d. Latissimus dorsi and serratus anterior
4. Which lung volume cannot be measured with standard spirometry and must be estimated with other techniques, such as helium dilution, nitrogen washout, or body plethysmography?
   a. Tidal volume
   b. IRV
   c. ERV
   d. Residual volume

Answers can be found in Appendix A.

the surface of the lung that prevents separation. In addition, the extensive lymphatic network and drainage that exist within the pleural space augment intrapleural negative pressure.

- In the upright position, intrapleural pressure is more negative at the apex of the lung than at the base. This is because the weight of the lung tissue, blood, lymphatic drainage, and other intrapulmonary and chest contents exerts a positive pressure on the pleural space, making the pressure within the intrapleural space less negative as it travels toward the lung base.
- During inspiration, the chest wall expands, creating a greater intrapleural volume and thus a decreased (more negative) intrapleural pressure. Conversely, during expiration, the intrapleural volume decreases, resulting in an increased (less negative) intrapleural pressure. It is important to note that the pressure within the intrapleural space during the respiratory cycle is always negative.

- *Alveolar pressure* is also known as *intrapulmonary pressure,* which is the pressure within the inside of the alveoli. To understand the pressures that occur within the alveoli during respiration, it is important to note that between each inspiratory and expiratory cycle, there is no air movement, and the intraalveolar pressure is the same as atmospheric pressure (760 mm Hg). This pressure is referred to as *zero.*
  - During inspiration, and with diaphragmatic contraction, intrapulmonary volume increases, causing intrapulmonary pressure to decrease (become negative) and fall below atmospheric pressure. This causes air to flow from an area of high pressure (atmosphere) to an area of low pressure (alveoli). At the end of inspiration, when intrapulmonary pressure again equals atmospheric pressure, the airflow stops.
  - During expiration, the diaphragm and other respiratory muscles relax, and intrapulmonary volume decreases, causing an increase in intrapulmonary (alveolar) pressure. At this point, intrapulmonary pressure is greater (becomes positive) than atmospheric pressure, causing air to flow out of the alveoli and back into the atmosphere. Airflow stops at the end of expiration when, again, intrapulmonary pressure is equal to atmospheric pressure.
- *Transpulmonary pressure* is the difference between alveolar and pleural pressure. Normally, alveolar pressure is greater than pleural pressure, and thus transpulmonary pressure is the alveolar pressure minus the pleural pressure. This pressure difference creates a type of distending pressure or suction pressure that keeps the lungs inflated. If alveolar pressure increases or intrapleural pressure diminishes, the transpulmonary pressure increases, resulting in alveoli that are less able to expand. In other words, the greater the transpulmonary pressure, the greater the distending pressure of the alveoli and the less compliant the alveoli.
  - Alveoli at the apices of the lung may be more inflated (and less compliant) because they have a greater alveolar volume (pressure) and because the intrapleural pressure is more negative at this location. Conversely, as a result of fluid and tissue weight compressing the lungs, the alveoli at the bases are less inflated, with a lower alveolar pressure and a less negative intrapleural pressure. This creates a decreased transpulmonary pressure with alveoli that are more able to expand.
  - Each lung is isolated with its own protective pleural covering. Thus if there is a breach of the chest wall, high atmospheric pressure will be drawn into the low pressure of the pleural space of the side that is breached while the other remains intact. As intrapleural pressure equilibrates to atmospheric pressure, that lung loses the pressure difference (transpulmonary distending pressure) between the alveolar and intrapleural pressures. Transpulmonary pressure goes to zero, and the lung collapses, resulting in a pneumothorax.

Lung Zones

The concept of lung zones considers the effects of gravity and intraalveolar pressure on pulmonary blood flow (Fig. 3.26). It divides the lung into four vertical regions, based on the relationship between the pressures within the alveoli (PA), the arteries (Pa), the veins (Pv), and within the pulmonary interstitium (Pi). The basic idea is that in zone 1: PA > Pa > Pv; in zone 2: Pa > PA > Pv; in zone 3: Pa > Pv > PA; and in zone 4: Pa > Pi > Pv > PA. The hydrostatic pressure of a liquid increases with depth. Thus blood within the lung mimics a single body of liquid, consequently leading to a gradual increase in BP as one travels down the lung's vertical axis. This vertical gradient of BP can result in a variation of nearly 20 mm Hg in pressure between the vasculature in

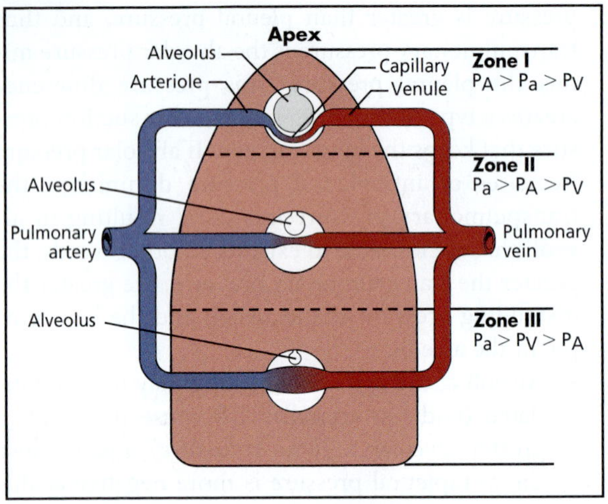

Fig. 3.26 Gravity and alveolar pressure. Effects of gravity and alveolar pressure on pulmonary blood flow in the three lung zones. In zone 1, alveolar pressure (PA) is greater than arterial and venous pressure, and no blood flow occurs. In zone 2, arterial pressure (Pa) exceeds alveolar pressure, but alveolar pressure exceeds venous pressure (PV). Blood flow occurs in this zone, but alveolar pressure compresses the venules (venous ends of the capillaries). In zone 3, both arterial and venous pressures are greater than alveolar pressure, and blood flow fluctuates, depending on the difference between arterial and venous pressures. (From Rogers JL. *McCance and Huether's Pathophysiology: The Biologic Basis for Disease in Adults and Children.* 9th ed. Elsevier; 2023.)

the apex compared with that in the base of the lung. Alveolar pressure is also a major factor governing blood flow. Given these unique considerations, physiologists have divided the lung into three basic zones (with a fourth if the pulmonary interstitium is considered). The lung zones are a representation of the differentiation of blood flow within the upright lung. Pulmonary vascular (and bronchiolar) architecture is the most important factor that determines the distribution of perfusion within the lungs, such that these anatomic and physiologic mechanisms may lead to regional perfusion differences based on the lumen of the pulmonary arterial vessels as they bifurcate down the tracheobronchial tree. There is also evidence that the lung zones may behave in a more concentric fashion, instead of in a vertical fashion, because of the location of the pulmonary arteries and heart within the thorax. Zone 3 would exist nearer the center of the lungs and at the bases, whereas zone 2 would exist concentrically outward nearer the apex and periphery. The vertical model is used to present a clearer understanding of the differences in pressures. Finally, zone 1 and zone 4 do not exist in a healthy lung.

- *Zone 1:* PA > Pa > Pv. Limited blood flow occurs in this zone because the alveolar pressure is greater than both the arterial and venous pressures. Thus alveolar dead space occurs. In healthy individuals, zone 1 does not exist. Decreased BP or a decrease in blood flow (hypovolemia or pulmonary embolism [PE]) and emphysema create zone 1.
- *Zone 2:* Pa > PA > Pv. Blood flow fluctuates because of the relevant pressure gradient between the arterial pressure and the alveolar pressure. Changes in blood flow are based on ventilation pressures. This usually includes the top and middle portions of the lung in a healthy, upright individual at rest. Because pulmonary pressures increase during exercise, zone 2 may begin to rise during periods of heavy breathing with large lung volumes.
- *Zone 3:* Pa > Pv > PA. This zone represents the areas that receive the greatest rates of pulmonary blood flow. The relevant pressure gradient is between the arterial and venous pressures. The best-matched ventilation to perfusion occurs in this zone because of constant perfusion (assuming that there is continuous ventilation).
- *Zone 4:* Pa > Pi > Pv > PA. This zone can be seen at the lung bases at very low lung volumes or in situations that cause pulmonary edema. Interstitial pressure can rise as a result of an increased volume of "leaked" fluid from the pulmonary vasculature (pulmonary edema).

Oxygen Extraction Ratio

The oxygen extraction ratio (O_2ER) measures the ratio of oxygen delivered to that consumed. Do_2 is the total amount of oxygen delivered to the tissues per minute (see earlier Oxygen Transport and Delivery section). Oxygen consumption (Vo_2) is the total amount of oxygen removed from the blood per minute for tissue metabolic needs. Consequently, the oxygen extraction ratio is the amount of oxygen consumed over that delivered ($O_2ER = Vo_2/Do_2$). Under resting conditions and with a normal cardiac output, the amount of oxygen delivered to the body tissues (Do_2) is more than sufficient for cellular needs. Oxygen that is not extracted from the blood is returned via venous circulation to the right heart.

- The *normal requirement* for Vo_2 is 250 mL/min (3–4 mL/kg/min in a normal-sized adult). Normal Do_2 is approximately 1 L/min. The oxygen extraction ratio at rest is 25%, although this can be increased up to 70% during exercise. A mixed venous oxygen saturation (Svo_2) of 70% is normal and indicates adequate Do_2 and extraction.

- *Organs consume different amounts of oxygen.* Each organ has its own Do_2 requirement, and some organs will extract greater amounts of oxygen from the blood, depending on their metabolic needs. For example, cardiac and neurologic cells extract more than 60% of the oxygen from circulating blood, whereas liver cells will extract 40%–50% and renal cells less than 20%.
- *Abnormal oxygen extraction ratios* can be explained by either an inadequate Do_2 or an increase in Vo_2.
  - Inadequate Do_2 can result from decreased oxygen delivery (low Fio_2, high altitude, lung disease), low hemoglobin, decreased contractility with decreased cardiac output, or shock and hypoperfusion from other causes.
  - An increased Vo_2 can be caused by an increased metabolic rate (hyperthermia, hyperthyroid, burns, adrenergic drugs), fever or inflammatory states (sepsis, trauma, surgery), or increased muscular activity (exercise, shivering, seizures).
- *FRC and apnea:* During periods of apnea, oxygen is available and drawn from the FRC. A normal FRC is approximately 2200 mL. A 70-kg adult requires roughly 250 mL of oxygen per minute. Therefore if a person is breathing room air (Fio_2 of 21%), they would have an estimated 462 mL of oxygen available in the FRC (2200 mL × 0.21 = 462 mL). Consequently, this same person would have 1.8 minutes of available oxygen (462 mL available O_2÷50 mL/min Vo_2 = 1.8 minute). If this same person were to breathe 100% oxygen for several minutes to the point of adequate denitrogenation, then the total oxygen availability would rise to over 8 minutes (2200 mL of available O_2÷50 mL/min Vo_2 = 8.8 minutes).

Oxyhemoglobin Dissociation Curve

A graphic depiction of how blood and hemoglobin carry and release oxygen can be seen in Fig. 3.27. The vertical axis portrays hemoglobin's saturation with oxygen, and the horizontal axis shows the related oxygen tension. The curve can move to the left or to the right, depending on several different environmental conditions. Hemoglobin has the ability to alter its structure in relation to the body's metabolic needs. For example, in

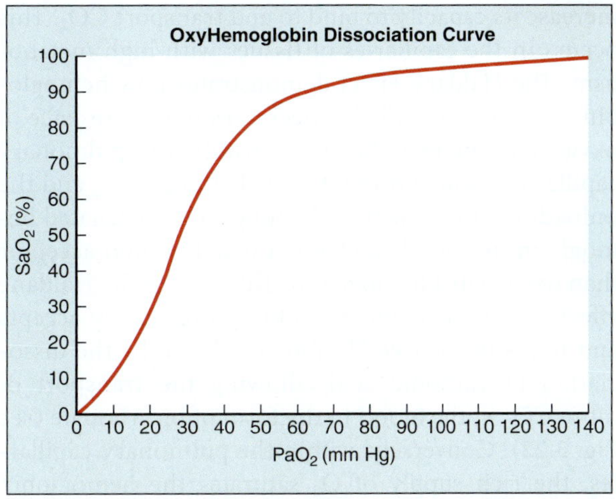

Fig. 3.27 This oxyhemoglobin dissociation curve shows the relationship between the arterial hemoglobin oxygen saturation (Sao_2 in percent) and the arterial partial pressure of oxygen (Pao_2 in mm Hg). Note that the Pao_2 can drop significantly while the patient is breathing supplemental O_2 before there is a noticeable change in Sao_2.(From Hemmings HC Jr, Egan TD. *Pharmacology and Physiology for Anesthesia: Foundations and Clinical Application.* 2nd ed. Elsevier; 2019.)

situations where there is an increase in temperature, 2,3-diphosphoglycerate (DPG; produced in RBCs in response to anemia/hypoxia), and $Paco_2$, or a decrease in pH, hemoglobin will allow oxygen to be more easily released, causing a rightward shift of the curve. Different conditions can cause a decrease in temperature, DPG, and $Paco_2$, or an increase in pH, which promotes a different conformational change in the hemoglobin molecule that makes it bind more tightly to oxygen, leading to a leftward shift in the curve. A rightward shift promotes a decreased affinity for O_2 binding to hemoglobin, so less O_2 is bound and more is unloaded at the tissues.

Haldane and Bohr effects. The oxyhemoglobin dissociation curve represents the association of the percentage saturation of hemoglobin by O_2 with the Pao_2. Similarly, the total CO_2 in blood is related to the $Paco_2$, representing a CO_2 dissociation curve. When hemoglobin saturation is 90%, the approximate corresponding Pao_2 is 60%.

The *Haldane effect* describes how the oxygenation of hemoglobin affects CO_2 transport and elimination. When blood contains primarily deoxygenated hemoglobin, the molecule alters its CO_2 binding sites to increase its capacity to bind to and transport CO_2. This occurs in the capillaries of tissues with high metabolism. The Haldane effect demonstrates how hemoglobin's capacity to hold CO_2 decreases in the presence of oxygenated hemoglobin (e.g., within the pulmonary capillaries), which promotes the loading of O_2 and the unloading of CO_2 within the lungs. Deoxygenated hemoglobin is a weak acid and a better proton acceptor than oxygenated hemoglobin. This sets up the Haldane effect because deoxyhemoglobin more readily accepts and binds to the free H^+ ions produced by the dissociation of carbonic acid, allowing the transport of more CO_2 in the blood in the form of bicarbonate (see Fig. 3.22). Conversely, within the pulmonary capillaries, the rich supply of O_2 saturates the hemoglobin molecule (causing oxyhemoglobin) and stimulates the separation of H^+ from hemoglobin. Bicarbonate then reenters the RBC (in exchange for Cl^-) and combines with H^+ to produce CO_2 and H_2O. At the same time, the CO_2 bound to proteins within the RBC and the CO_2 dissolved in blood plasma all diffuse into the alveoli.

The *Bohr effect* describes the impact that $Paco_2$ and H^+ ions have on hemoglobin's ability to carry and transport O_2. In situations of low pH (acidosis) or high $Paco_2$ (hypercapnia), the excess H^+ ions affect the amino acids of hemoglobin, lowering its affinity for O_2, shifting the oxyhemoglobin dissociation curve to the right, and thus releasing more O_2 to peripheral capillaries and tissues. The Bohr effect is the reason why hemoglobin will deliver and release O_2 more readily to cellular areas that have higher concentrations of CO_2, such as the heart and brain. A suppressed Bohr effect is seen in situations that cause a lower CO_2 (hypocapnia) concentration, such as hyperventilation. Hypocapnia resulting in a higher pH (lower H^+ ions) causes the oxyhemoglobin dissociation curve to shift to the left, which promotes hemoglobin to tightly bind O_2 and prevents effective oxygen delivery. The result is hypoxia and decreased tissue cellular oxygenation.

Gas Laws

- *Boyle's law* is a gas law stating that pressure and volume are inversely proportional. As long as temperature is held constant, when the volume of a container increases, the pressure of a gas within that container decreases. The converse is true: When the volume of a container decreases, the pressure of a gas within the container increases. This law is only true if both the concentration of gas within the container and the temperature are unchanged. Boyle's law can be applied to help understand pulmonary ventilation. Upon inspiration and diaphragmatic contraction, lung volume increases, causing the pressure within the lungs to decrease. Now the air from the atmosphere will travel from a higher pressure to where the pressure is lower (negative) within the alveoli until the pressure equilibrates at end inspiration. At this point, the diaphragm relaxes, and lung recoil decreases lung volume, leading to an increase in pressure. Thus this positive expiratory pressure pushes air from the alveoli back into the atmosphere.
- *Dalton's law* states that the total pressure exerted by a mixture of gases in a fixed volume and at a constant temperature is the sum of each of their individual partial pressures. In other words, each gas's partial pressure can be added to determine the total pressure within a container. For example, an E-cylinder of air that is filled to 1900 psi contains approximately 21% oxygen and 79% nitrogen. Thus oxygen would exert 21% of the 1900 psi (399 psi) within the E-cylinder, and nitrogen would exert 80% of 1900 psi (1501 psi).
- *Henry's law* states that the mass of a gas that will dissolve into a solution is directly proportional to the partial pressure (concentration) of that gas above the solution. The main application of Henry's law in respiratory physiology is to predict how gases will dissolve from the alveoli into the bloodstream. If the pressure (concentration) is increased, then the solubility will increase. The amount of oxygen that dissolves into the bloodstream is directly proportional to the partial pressure of oxygen in the alveoli as long as that concentration is maintained. The same can be said for anesthetic gases. Increasing the concentration (pressure) within the alveoli will increase the diffusion and concentration into the blood. Gas can then diffuse out of solution and back into the air when pressure is released.
- *Fick's law* states that the rate of diffusion of a gas across a permeable membrane is determined by the following:
  - Partial pressure gradient (the driving force) of the gas across the membrane
  - Chemical nature of the membrane
  - Surface area of the membrane
  - Thickness of the membrane

This law relates to how gases behave at the alveolar–capillary membrane. The concept relates how a gas will move from a region of high concentration to a region of low concentration across a concentration gradient based on the previously listed factors. For example, conditions such as a low FiO_2, bronchospasm, atelectasis, or pulmonary edema each affect the surface area of the alveolar–capillary membrane, the thickness of the membrane, or the concentration gradient. Thus a gas such as O_2 will have a reduced ability to diffuse at the membrane, and therefore a decreased amount will enter the pulmonary circulation, leading to a decreased PaO_2 in the arterial blood.

The main difference between Henry's law and Fick's law is that Henry's law is specific for a gas's partial pressure that causes the gas to diffuse and dissolve into a liquid compartment. It describes the gas's solubility at equilibrium. Fick's law describes how substances (e.g., gases, molecules, drugs) move through membranes, dependent on their concentration gradient and the characteristics of the membrane itself. Henry's law is often used to illustrate how oxygen moves from the alveoli into the pulmonary capillary blood, whereas Fick's law describes how drugs such as sevoflurane would enter the pulmonary bloodstream based on their concentration within the alveoli.

Pulmonary Dead Space and Pulmonary Shunt (Hypoxic Pulmonary Vasoconstriction)

Anatomic and alveolar dead space. Physiologic dead space is the sum of the anatomic dead space plus the alveolar dead space and is defined as gases that do not participate in gas exchange with perfused blood. Anatomic dead space consists of the volume of gas that travels through the conducting airways (upper airway, trachea, main bronchi, segmental bronchi, and bronchioles) during an inspiratory breath. Anatomic dead space is approximately 2 mL/kg of ideal body weight and can vary with lung size. Alveolar dead space is the volume of gas contained in nonperfused alveoli; thus O_2 is not delivered to the bloodstream, and CO_2 is not removed. In healthy individuals, approximately two-thirds of the volume of inhaled gas fills the alveoli for ventilation, and the remaining third is located within the conducting airways, representing the anatomic dead space. Furthermore, alveolar dead space is close to zero, and thus physiologic dead space equals anatomic dead space (volume contained within the conducting airways). The $PaCO_2$ is higher than the $ETCO_2$ as a result of CO_2 dilution within the anatomic dead space. Thus, because of CO_2 dilution within the gases of the anatomical dead space, the $ETCO_2$ value is estimated at 5 mm Hg lower than the actual $PaCO_2$ in healthy individuals.

- *Conditions that lead to alveolar dead space:* Clinical examples of alveolar dead space include conditions that disrupt perfusion. These can include PE, hydrostatic pressure failure (e.g., severe hypotension), obliteration of pulmonary capillaries (e.g., COPD), pulmonary vascular vasoconstriction, and high intrathoracic pressure compressing pulmonary vasculature or inhibiting venous return (e.g., PEEP, excessive positive-pressure ventilation).
- *Mechanical dead space:* Any ventilation provided by artificial means. This primarily includes mechanical ventilation with either an endotracheal or a tracheal tube inserted into the airway. An endotracheal tube (ETT) by itself will reduce dead space within the upper airway, and a tracheal tube even more so. This is because the volume within these tubes (because of their limited lengths and diameters) is less than the volume within the upper airway. Normal extrathoracic dead space volume (e.g., tracheal and oropharyngeal volume) is between 70 and 75 mL. The volume of an 8-mm ETT that is 27 cm in length can be calculated using the formula for cylindrical volumes as follows: Volume $= \pi(\text{radius}^2 \times \text{length})$. This calculates to approximately 14 mL, which is a significant decrease in the amount of dead space when using an ETT. The use of a tracheotomy tube would further increase dead space because these tubes are even shorter. Extensions or Y-pieces added to the circuit and attached to the ETT would increase the amount of mechanical dead space.

Pulmonary shunt. A *pulmonary shunt* occurs when the lung is perfused but poorly ventilated. Consequently, blood passes through the pulmonary system and is not oxygenated, causing what is known as a *right-to-left* intrapulmonary shunt. The result is deoxygenated blood being circulated to body tissues.

- Pulmonary shunting relates to alveoli that receive perfusion but, for one reason or another, do not receive adequate ventilation. Blood flowing past areas of nonfunctional or collapsed alveoli is unable to pick up O_2 and release CO_2.

- The larger the shunt, the lower the Pao_2 and the greater the $Paco_2$, which increases the degree of respiratory acidosis.
- Examples of pulmonary shunting include pneumonia, pulmonary edema, tissue trauma causing alveolar swelling, atelectasis, mucus plugging, gastric aspiration, foreign body obstruction, and pulmonary arteriovenous fistula.
- A normal physiologic shunt known as *venous admixture* occurs. Bronchial veins empty into the pulmonary vein, and thebesian veins empty directly into the LA. An estimated 2%–5% of the cardiac output makes up this normal physiologic shunt.

Hypoxic pulmonary vasoconstriction. *Hypoxic pulmonary vasoconstriction (HPV)* is a protective physiologic reflex that occurs in situations that lead to decreased alveolar ventilation and hypoxia. The overall purpose of HPV is to distribute blood flow regionally to increase the overall efficiency of gas exchange between air and blood. Alveolar hypoxia (low oxygen levels) causes contraction of pulmonary vascular smooth muscle within small pulmonary arteries and arterioles, causing them to divert blood to oxygenated lung regions to improve blood oxygenation. This phenomenon is different from peripheral capillaries that vasodilate in response to regional hypoxia. HPV is thought to be the primary mechanism that best matches ventilation to perfusion.

- HPV is the primary mechanism that maintains oxygenation during one-lung ventilation. However, the HPV reflex can persist after about 1 hour of hypoxia, resulting in several hours of pulmonary vasoconstriction even when normal oxygenation returns.
- Several different classes of medications inhibit HPV, including calcium antagonists, ACEIs, inhalation anesthetics agents (>1 MAC), vasodilators, phosphodiesterase inhibitors, prostacyclin, and nitric oxide.

KNOWLEDGE CHECK

1. Which respiratory muscle is responsible for an estimated 25% of the respiratory effort?
   a. Diaphragm
   b. Abdominal rectus
   c. External obliques
   d. External intercostals
2. Which factor reduces the FRC?
   a. Reverse Trendelenburg positioning
   b. Sarcoidosis
   c. Continuous positive airway pressure
   d. Negative-pressure ventilation
3. A decrease in pleural pressure results in a transpulmonary pressure that is
   a. increased.
   b. decreased.
   c. unchanged.
4. In which lung zone can the alveolar pressure exceed the pulmonary capillary arterial pressure?
   a. 1
   b. 2
   c. 3
   d. 4
5. Which Svo_2 value indicates adequate oxygen delivery and extraction?
   a. 50%
   b. 60%
   c. 70%
   d. 80%
6. On the oxyhemoglobin dissociation curve, when the hemoglobin saturation is 90%, what is the corresponding Pao_2?
   a. 20
   b. 40
   c. 60
   d. 80
7. A patient with negative-pressure pulmonary edema has a decreased Pao_2 despite receiving 100% Fio_2. Which gas law is representative of this scenario?
   a. Dalton's
   b. Boyle's
   c. Henry's
   d. Fick's
8. Which gas law describes how the concentration of a gas influences the rate of gas diffusion?
   a. Dalton's
   b. Fick's
   c. Henry's
   d. Laplace's
9. Which best describes the primary purpose of HPV?
   a. Increase blood flow to poorly ventilated regions of the lung
   b. Distribute blood flow away from hypoxic alveoli and toward better-ventilated areas
   c. Cause systemic vasodilation during hypoxia
   d. Enhance oxygen binding to hemoglobin in hypoxic tissues

KNOWLEDGE CHECK—cont'd

10. Which condition causes a rightward shift of the oxyhemoglobin dissociation curve?
    a. Decreased temperature
    b. Decreased 2,3-DPG levels
    c. Increased pH
    d. Increased $Paco_2$
11. Which class of medications inhibits HPV?
    a. Aminoglycoside antibiotics
    b. Inhaled anesthetics
    c. Anticholinergics
    d. α-Adrenergic agonists
12. According to the lung zone model, in which lung zone is alveolar pressure greater than both arterial and venous pressures, leading to alveolar dead space?
    a. Zone 1
    b. Zone 2
    c. Zone 3
    d. Zone 4

Answers can be found in Appendix A.

Pulmonary Pathophysiologic Concepts

Obstructive Versus Restrictive Lung Disease

Conditions that impede gases from being fully exhaled from the lungs and those that result in decreased functional lung volumes and exhaled flow rates are termed *obstructive diseases*. Characteristics include a normal or even larger TLC, a narrowing of bronchioles, and pulmonary inflammation with excessive mucus production that obstructs gas flow and increases the work of breathing. Common examples of obstructive diseases include asthma, COPD, bronchiectasis, and cystic fibrosis. Alternatively, those conditions that hinder the lungs' ability to fully expand and result in an overall decrease in lung volumes are termed *restrictive diseases* (Fig. 3.28). Restrictive disease is characterized by a reduction in both TLC and lung compliance. This can occur as a result of skeletal abnormalities, limited chest/diaphragm movement, pleural disorders, neuromuscular diseases, and/or an increase in alveolar or interstitial fluid. Examples of restrictive diseases are intrinsic restrictive disease (e.g., pulmonary fibrosis, sarcoidosis), extrinsic restrictive disease (e.g., skeletal deformities, pleural disorders, and neuromuscular disorders), pulmonary edema, ARDS, and obesity. Differentiation between obstructive and restrictive diseases can be assessed with pulmonary spirometry. Each condition has varying signs and symptoms and requires specific management strategies.

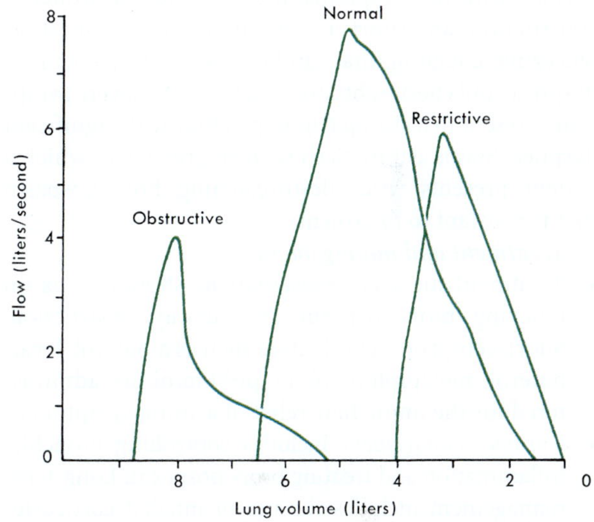

Fig. 3.28 Maximum expiratory flow–volume curve comparing normal with obstructive and restrictive disorders. Displayed as flows at actual lung volumes. (From Wilkins RL, Stoller JK, Kacmarek RM. *Egan's Fundamentals of Respiratory Care.* 9th ed. Mosby; 2009.)

Obstructive pulmonary diseases

Asthma. Asthma is a chronic inflammatory obstructive pulmonary disease affecting the bronchi and small airways. It is characterized by bronchial inflammation and hyperreactivity with airway thickening, excess mucus production, and bronchoconstriction. Specific inflammatory mediators linked to the development of asthma include histamine, prostaglandins, and leukotrienes. The airflow obstruction is reversible, depending on endogenous and exogenous factors.

Etiology. Genetic, environmental, and individual host factors all influence the etiology and severity of asthma. Family member associations with asthma are well documented, and there are several genes and genomic regions within chromosomes that have been identified and linked to both allergies and asthma. Several prenatal risk factors have been linked to early childhood wheezing that may or may not develop into true asthma. Prenatal risk factors include maternal smoking, diet and nutrition, stress, and antibiotic usage.

During childhood, viral infections (e.g., rhinovirus, respiratory syncytial virus) and exposure to smoking or other environmental pollutants can affect the development of asthma, especially in individuals who are predisposed to the disease. Adult-onset asthma is likely due to exercise, occupational hazards, or specific drug treatments (e.g., β-blockers, nonsteroidal antiinflammatory drugs [NSAIDs], or hormone replacement therapy).

Signs and symptoms. Bronchial hyperreactivity, bronchoconstriction, and airway inflammation frequently accompany an exacerbation of asthma. Symptoms are variable depending on times of acute exacerbation and periods with no symptoms. Most periods of bronchoconstriction are short in duration and manifest as wheezing, coughing that can be productive, tachypnea, dyspnea, and chest tightness. Patients with severe symptoms present in a sitting tripod position with significant dyspnea. Status asthmaticus is an emergency in which a patient presents with life-threatening bronchospasm that is resistant to treatment.

Treatment and management

- Treatment for *acute exacerbations* should focus on relieving bronchospasm and airway obstruction. Short-acting bronchodilators such as albuterol, levalbuterol, metaproterenol, or pirbuterol are administered for the immediate relief of asthma symptoms.
- *Chronic management* includes controlling bronchial inflammation and treating bronchospasm. Long-term management includes the use of inhaled corticosteroids (e.g., fluticasone, budesonide, beclomethasone), long-term bronchodilators (e.g., salmeterol, formoterol), a combination of inhaled corticosteroids and long-term bronchodilators, leukotriene modifiers (e.g., montelukast), methylxanthines (e.g., theophylline, aminophylline), anti-IgE monoclonal antibodies, and/or mast cell stabilizers (e.g., cromolyn).
- The treatment of *status asthmaticus* centers on aggressive management of bronchospasm using a β_2-agonist with a metered-dose inhaler or with a continuous nebulizer. Epinephrine in titratable doses (e.g., 10–100 mcg IV) should be considered in patients who do not respond to albuterol or other inhaled bronchodilators. Supplemental oxygen is given to keep the saturation above 90%. IV hydrocortisone or methylprednisolone is administered to help decrease inflammation. Secondary treatments include inhaled ipratropium (Atrovent), IV magnesium sulfate, and oral leukotriene inhibitors. If the condition becomes severe enough, intubation and mechanical ventilation may be required, and general anesthesia with a volatile agent to promote bronchodilation can be administered. Extracorporeal membrane oxygenation (ECMO) can be used as a last resort.

Anesthetic considerations. Evaluation of a patient with a history of asthma should assess the severity of the disease. This includes determining information regarding triggering agents, allergies, previous hospitalizations and intubations, current medications, auscultation for current wheezing, and a review of recent pulmonary function tests (PFTs). A reduced ratio of forced expiratory volume in 1 second (FEV_1) to forced vital capacity (< 65% predicted) is a risk factor for respiratory complications. Preoperative administration of a β_2-agonist is encouraged. When general anesthesia is indicated, efforts to reduce airway reflex stimulation and hyperreactivity include IV administration of lidocaine, opioids, and propofol or ketamine. Sevoflurane is recommended because it is less irritating to the airway. Supraglottic devices should be used whenever possible because they allow for less airway stimulation. Airway humidification will help warm gases, and the patient should receive adequate IV fluid to prevent viscous airway secretions.

- The signs and symptoms of an *intraoperative bronchospasm* include high peak airway pressures, lower V_t, an upslope of the $ETco_2$ waveform, wheezing, increased $Paco_2$, and decreased Pao_2 and O_2 saturation. Causes are listed in Box 3.7. Initial management steps include increasing the Fio_2 and inhalation agent concentration, hand-ventilating to assess bag compliance, propofol IV to deepen the plane of anesthesia, and inhaled β_2-agonists (albuterol, four to eight puffs) through the ETT. If bronchospasm persists, then IV epinephrine (10–100 mcg IV push doses) is indicated. Corticosteroids (methylprednisolone 125 mg), magnesium (1–2 gm), and inhaled ipratropium can also be considered.

Chronic obstructive pulmonary disease. COPD is the result of progressive bronchiolar and alveolar tissue destruction and increased airflow obstruction. Traditionally, COPD represents both emphysema and chronic bronchitis. The characteristics of COPD include the following:

1. Deterioration of functional lung tissue, causing a decrease in lung elasticity (recoil), which diminishes the lungs' ability to remain open

BOX 3.7 Causes of Intraoperative Bronchospasm

Nonpathological
- ETT kinking
- ETT too deep, stimulating the carina
- Endobronchial intubation
- ETT obstruction by secretions
- Overinflation of the ETT cuff
- Inadequate depth of anesthesia

Pathological
- Acute asthma attack
- Pulmonary edema
- Pulmonary embolus
- Pulmonary aspiration
- Pneumothorax
- Anaphylaxis
- Chronic obstructive pulmonary disease

ETT, Endotracheal tube.

2. A reduction in bronchiolar wall rigidity, allowing these airways to collapse more easily during exhalation
3. Narrowed bronchioles that allow for an increase in gas velocity, which results in a lower intraluminal air pressure, prompting airway collapse
4. Increase in mucus production, causing bronchiolar obstruction and provoking bronchospasm
5. As lung functional tissue (parenchyma) is destroyed, there is a creation and enlargement of air sacs.

Unlike asthma, this condition is irreversible.

Etiology. COPD usually develops from environmental factors, or it can occur as an inherited disorder. There are several risk factors for its development, including (1) cigarette smoking, (2) frequent inhalation of dust or chemicals from occupational exposure (e.g., mining, textile manufacture), (3) recurrent childhood infections, and (4) air pollution. An inherited α_1-antitrypsin deficiency can also result in COPD.

Signs and symptoms. Signs and symptoms can vary depending on the progression of COPD that results in obstructive disease. They include dyspnea (on exertion or at rest), chronic cough with sputum production, tachypnea, breathing through pursed lips to prolong expiratory times, and wheezing. As COPD progresses, with chronic hyperinflation from obstructions to exhaled airflow, the chest wall becomes elevated and barrel-shaped. Blood gas abnormalities do not appear until the FEV_1 is less than 50% predicted. Cor pulmonale can occur as a later, more progressive symptom of severe COPD from pulmonary hypertension, potentially causing peripheral edema.

Treatment and management. The most important long-term treatments for COPD are smoking cessation and oxygen administration. Additional medical treatments can include combinations of long-acting β_2-agonists, inhaled corticosteroids, and anticholinergics. Vaccinations against influenza and pneumococcus are suggested in the elderly population. If a patient has signs and symptoms of right heart failure with peripheral edema, then diuretics are recommended. Lung volume reduction surgery is an option in selected patients who have severe COPD with regions of poorly functioning, overdistended lung tissue. Finally, when a patient experiences an acute exacerbation of COPD, the goals of treatment are to provide supplemental oxygen and bronchodilator therapy with noninvasive positive-pressure ventilation (continuous positive airway pressure [CPAP] or bilevel positive airway pressure [BiPAP]). Corticosteroids and antibiotics can help with inflammation and infection. If the episode is severe enough, intubation and mechanical ventilation may be needed.

Anesthetic considerations. Anesthetic considerations focus on preoperative optimization, management of pain, prevention of respiratory decompensation, and promotion of good pulmonary function postoperatively.

- *Preoperative considerations:* Often, patients with COPD have associated comorbidities, and these should be assessed, along with the severity of COPD. Cessation of smoking should always be encouraged for at least 6 weeks before surgery. Education regarding the use of incentive spirometry and voluntary deep breathing in the preoperative area may help motivate the patient to perform these maneuvers in the postoperative period. Dyspnea and wheezing can be managed with bronchodilator therapy, anticholinergics, and corticosteroids. If the patient is already taking these medications, they should continue them until the morning of surgery. Respiratory infections should be managed with antibiotics before surgery. The patient should be given information about the possibility of intubation and mechanical ventilation or CPAP in the postoperative period. If the patient manifests with advanced pulmonary disease, an echocardiogram can help determine the extent of right heart failure. PFTs are used to optimize pulmonary function and are an unreliable tool for assessing risk.
- *Intraoperative considerations:* Regional anesthesia should be considered whenever possible for anesthesia

management and pain control. Nitrous oxide should be avoided to prevent enlargement of air sacs. Inhalation anesthetics can help with bronchodilation; however, their effects may be prolonged if there is a severe expiratory obstruction. Anything that has the potential to cause respiratory depression should be used with caution; this includes opioids, benzodiazepines, and muscle relaxants. Suction equipment for both oropharyngeal and tracheal tube suctioning should be readily available. The goals for mechanical ventilation include the prevention of dynamic hyperinflation and avoidance of barotrauma. Thus mechanical ventilation strategies include limiting peak airway pressures to 30 cm H_2O, V_t of 6–8 mL/kg, Fio_2 titrated to maintain an O_2 saturation above 90%, and adjusting the inspiratory/expiratory ratio to account for adequate exhalation time.

- *Postoperative considerations:* These focus on lung expansion maneuvers, appropriate mechanical ventilation strategies, and pain management. Deep breathing exercises, incentive spirometry, chest physiotherapy, and positive-pressure breathing techniques are all strategies that promote lung expansion and lung volumes and prevent atelectasis. When postoperative mechanical ventilation is indicated, similar intraoperative strategies can be employed. Many patients with COPD benefit from CPAP or a trial of BiPAP immediately after extubation. Both regional nerve blocks (intercostal or paravertebral) and neuraxial analgesia are effective methods for pain management because they do not cause respiratory depression.

Bronchiectasis. Bronchiectasis is a chronic condition characterized by localized bronchial wall scarring and destruction caused by repeated infection and inflammation. As a result, bronchial airways can become dilated, obstructed with mucus, and collapse.

Etiology. There are several potential causes of bronchiectasis. Infection is the most common. However, immune deficiency, cystic fibrosis, aspiration, bronchial tumors, focal bronchial obstructions, inflammatory bowel disease, and several respiratory syndromes can also cause this condition.

Signs and symptoms. The hallmark symptom is a chronic cough with purulent sputum. Hemoptysis, dyspnea, wheezing, and pleuritic chest pain can also occur. Significant bronchiectasis can cause clubbing of the fingers, which differentiates it from COPD. Hemoptysis can occur in severe conditions. Radiographic studies show dilated bronchi that are much larger than their adjacent blood vessels.

Treatment and management. Antibiotics specific to cultured pathogens, chest physiotherapy with mucus clearance, long-acting β_2-agonists, inhaled corticosteroids, and oxygen are primary treatments. Massive hemoptysis may require localized bronchial arterial embolization and lung resection.

Anesthetic considerations. Interventions are similar to those used for other obstructive airway conditions. Surgery should be delayed if there is evidence of an active pulmonary infection. These patients present with significant airway secretions and require repeated oral and tracheal tube suctioning throughout the perioperative period. A double-lumen tube is required for lung isolation in patients undergoing surgery for an empyema or hemoptysis. Nasotracheal intubation or instrumentation through the nasal passages should be avoided because these patients frequently have associated sinus infections.

Cystic fibrosis. Cystic fibrosis is a genetic, autosomal recessive disorder that causes a dysfunction in a protein that helps salt and water move into and out of cells. What results is the formation of viscous secretions and scarring of various glands and tissues. It primarily affects the lungs but can also affect the pancreas, liver, kidneys, and intestines.

Etiology. Cystic fibrosis is a genetic disease caused by a mutation in the cystic fibrosis transmembrane conductance regulator. The regulator fails to produce a protein that allows for the passage of salt and water through an anion channel found within the membrane of epithelial cells. Instead, the dysfunctional regulator blocks this movement, resulting in abnormally thick mucus outside the epithelial cell. Chronic respiratory infections occur because of the obstructive mucus, resulting in bronchiectasis, COPD, and sinusitis.

Signs and symptoms. Chronic cough with productive purulent sputum, dyspnea on exertion, wheezing, frequent lung infections, and pansinusitis (infection of all sinuses) are primary symptoms. High chloride concentrations ($>$70 mEq/L) in sweat and a high percentage of neutrophils from bronchoalveolar lavage are also signs. Most adult patients eventually develop COPD from this disease. Diabetes, cirrhosis, and meconium ileus can all result from cystic fibrosis affecting other organ systems.

Treatment and management. Primary treatments include antibiotics specific to cultured pathogens, long-acting β_2-agonists, and chest physiotherapy or high-frequency chest compression with an inflatable vest to promote mucus clearance. Additionally, recombinant human deoxyribonuclease I can help increase sputum clearance. Management of other organ dysfunctions, enhancing nutrition, providing adequate fluids, and monitoring for intestinal obstruction are also recommended treatments.

Anesthetic considerations. A primary goal is optimal preoperative pulmonary function. This is achieved by providing effective antibiotic therapy and removal of airway secretions. Inhalation anesthetics provide bronchodilation and decrease bronchial hyperreactivity. Secretions can be managed by humidifying anesthetic gases, providing adequate IV fluid, avoiding anticholinergic medications, and frequent tracheal tube suctioning. Postoperative pulmonary complications (e.g., pneumonia, hypoxia, and atelectasis) can be avoided with effective pain control, deep breathing exercises, coughing, full reversal of neuromuscular blockade, adequate postoperative respiratory function, and early ambulation.

KNOWLEDGE CHECK

1. If bronchospasm during anesthesia persists after administration of a β_2-agonist and sevoflurane, which treatment is indicated for progressive desaturation?
   a. Epinephrine IV
   b. Inhaled ipratropium
   c. Inhaled corticosteroids
   d. Magnesium IV
2. Which is the most effective long-term treatment for COPD?
   a. Long-acting β_2-agonists
   b. Corticosteroids
   c. Smoking cessation
   d. Lung volume reduction
3. Which is the most common cause of bronchiectasis?
   a. Immune deficiency
   b. Cystic fibrosis
   c. Aspiration
   d. Infection
4. Management of secretions for a patient with cystic fibrosis includes
   a. administering glycopyrrolate.
   b. humidifying inhaled gases.
   c. promoting head-down position.
   d. limiting administration of IV fluids.
5. Which intraoperative finding is most indicative of bronchospasm in a patient with a history of asthma?
   a. Low peak airway pressures and low tidal volume
   b. High peak airway pressures and an upslope in the $ETCO_2$ waveform
   c. Flat $ETCO_2$ waveform with low $PaCO_2$
   d. Sudden drop in BP without changes in airway pressures

Answers can be found in Appendix A.

Restrictive diseases

Intrinsic restrictive pulmonary diseases. Intrinsic restrictive pulmonary diseases affect the lung parenchyma (functional lung tissue). Lung tissue inflammation and/or scarring or a filling of the air spaces with fluid or exudate are consequences of these diseases that result in restricted lung expansion, lower lung volumes, and reduced pulmonary compliance (see Fig. 3.28). Etiology, signs and symptoms, treatment and management, and anesthetic considerations of chronic intrinsic lung diseases can be found in Table 3.19.

Acute respiratory distress syndrome. ARDS is an acute intrinsic restrictive lung disorder. It is caused by either a direct (pulmonary) or indirect (extrapulmonary) injury to the lungs, triggering an inflammatory injury and acute hypoxemic respiratory failure. Direct lung injury causes damage to the alveolar epithelium, whereas indirect injuries damage the pulmonary capillary endothelium.

Etiology. Direct lung injury can result from pneumonia, aspiration of gastric material, PE, trauma to the lung, smoke inhalation, near drowning, and reperfusion injury after cardiac bypass or ECMO. Indirect causes include sepsis, systemic trauma, burns, blood transfusions, drug overdoses, and acute pancreatitis.

Signs and symptoms. The most significant risk factor associated with the development of ARDS is sepsis. Tachypnea, dyspnea, tachycardia, increased respiratory effort with rapid onset of respiratory failure, and progressive hypoxemia are all signs of ARDS. CXR shows bilateral opacities not explained by other lung pathology. Radiology also demonstrates features that resemble cardiogenic pulmonary edema, except there is respiratory failure without heart failure or volume overload.

TABLE 3.19 **Chronic Intrinsic (Interstitial) Restrictive Pulmonary Diseases**

Restrictive Disease/ Disorder	Pathophysiology and Etiology	Signs and Symptoms	Treatment and Management	Anesthetic Considerations
Pulmonary fibrosis	Scarring and fibrosis of interstitial lung tissue. Initial lung injury can result from exposure to chemicals, radiation, allergens, or environmental factors. As the lung attempts to heal, a dysfunction of inflammation and other factors can lead to interstitial fibrosis and tissue remodeling.	Dyspnea, tachypnea, shallow breathing, nonproductive cough, fatigue, unexplained weight loss, and clubbing of the fingertips and toes. Progressive loss of pulmonary vasculature and development of tissue fibrosis cause pulmonary hypertension and cor pulmonale	Oxygen therapy for saturations <90% or Pa_{O_2} <55 mm Hg. Encourage cessation of smoking if applicable. Treat infections with antibiotics. Provide vaccinations against influenza and pneumococcal pathogens. Encourage clearance of secretions.	Preoperative echocardiogram to assess for right heart function. PFTs are all low. Apneic periods are poorly tolerated because of a low or nonexistent FRC. Avoid high PIP to decrease risk of barotrauma. Keep tidal volumes 4–6 mL/kg and adjust respiratory support according to Pa_{CO_2} levels. Titrate PEEP to keep plateau pressures <30 cm H_2O. DLT may be required for VATS procedure or lung resection.
Pulmonary sarcoidosis	Inflammatory disease that causes noncaseating (nonnecrotizing) granulomas to develop. Granulomas are collections of exhausted inflammatory cells and macrophages surrounded by lymphocytes and collagen. Affects many tissues, particularly intrathoracic lymph nodes and the lungs. Etiology is unknown.	Dyspnea on exertion, nonproductive cough, and auscultated crackles. Fatigue, weakness, weight loss, and a low grade fever may also occur. Can be difficult to diagnosis without lymph node biopsy. Hypercalcemia is only seen in a minority of patients but is a classic manifestation of sarcoidosis. Pulmonary hypertension can occur with cor pulmonale.	NSAIDs for discomfort. Inhaled and oral corticosteroids suppress sarcoidosis and treat hypercalcemia. Immunosuppressants (e.g., azathioprine, cyclophosphamide, methotrexate) may be used if patients are unresponsive or cannot tolerate corticosteroids. The severity of the disease can be assessed with PFTs and exercise pulse oximetry.	Preoperative echocardiogram to assess for right heart function. PFTs are all low. Apneic periods are poorly tolerated because of a low or nonexistent FRC. Avoid high PIP to decrease risk of barotrauma. Keep tidal volumes 4–6 mL/kg and adjust respiratory support according to Pa_{CO_2} levels. Titrate PEEP to keep plateau pressures <30 cm H_2O. Mediastinoscopy for lymph node biopsy confirms diagnosis. Laryngeal sarcoidosis can inhibit ETT passage.

Hypersensitivity pneumonitis (allergic alveolitis)	Hypersensitivity immune response within the alveoli and pulmonary interstitial space in response to inhaled antigens (e.g., fungus, spores, bacteria, protozoa, animal or insect proteins, or other organic compounds). Causes the development of interstitial inflammation and noncaseating interstitial granulomas. Repeated pneumonitis from exposure can develop into pulmonary fibrosis.	Symptom severity depends on the amount of exposure to an antigen, the frequency of exposure, and genetic predisposition. Acute onset of dyspnea, dry cough, chest tightness, fatigue, fever and chills after exposure to an antigen. High white cell count (leukocytosis), an increase in circulating eosinophils (eosinophilia), and arterial hypoxemia. Pulmonary infiltrates on chest x-ray.	Remove offending antigen or completely avoid exposure. Oxygen therapy and corticosteroids (prednisone). Immunosuppressants (azathioprine, mycophenolate). If the disease is severe enough with pulmonary fibrosis then lung transplantation may be indicated.	Preoperative echocardiogram to assess for right heart function. PFT assessment may indicate low values. Apneic periods are poorly tolerated because of a low or nonexistent FRC. Avoid high PIP to decrease risk of barotrauma. Keep tidal volumes 4–6 mL/kg and adjust respiratory support according to $Paco_2$ levels. Titrate PEEP to keep plateau pressures <30 cm H_2O. DLT may be required for VATS procedure.
Pulmonary alveolar proteinosis	Accumulation of protein-rich exudate within the alveoli. A dysfunction in alveolar macrophages may lead to decreased removal of surfactant and other protein-containing materials, causing a buildup of these within the alveoli. Etiology is unknown, but it may occur with chemotherapy, AIDS, or mineral dust inhalation.	Dyspnea with hypoxemia and cough are primary symptoms. Chest discomfort, fatigue, fever, weight loss, and clubbing of the fingertips and toes may be present.	In severe cases, lung lavage may help remove alveolar material and improve macrophage function. Lung transplant has been successfully used in infants and children.	Preoperative echocardiogram. PFTs are all low. Apneic periods are poorly tolerated because of a low or nonexistent FRC. Avoid high PIP to decrease risk of barotrauma. Keep tidal volumes 4–6 mL/kg and adjust respiratory support according to $Paco_2$ levels. Titrate PEEP to keep plateau pressures <30 cm H_2O. DLT is required for pulmonary lavage to isolate affected lung.

DLT, Double-lumen tube; *ETT*, endotracheal tube; *FRC*, functional residual capacity; *NSAIDs*, nonsteroidal antiinflammatory drugs; *PEEP*, positive end-expiratory pressure; *PFT*, pulmonary function test; *PIP*, peak inspiratory pressures; *VATS*, video-assisted thoracic surgery.

Breath sounds are altered to absent in this condition. Pulmonary hypertension leading to right-sided heart failure can occur from severe HPV and the destruction of portions of the pulmonary capillary bed.

Treatment and Management. Primary treatment should focus on correcting the offending insult. Supplemental oxygen, tracheal intubation with mechanical ventilation, PEEP, neuromuscular blockade, IV fluid administration, diuretic therapy, inotropic support, inhaled β_2-agonists, corticosteroids (sometimes used), frequent suctioning (needed), antibiotic therapy (required for identified pathogens), thromboembolism prophylaxis, stress ulcer prophylaxis, and adequate nutritional support are all treatments that are used. Patients are at risk for ventilator-associated lung injury and atelectrauma; therefore recommended tidal volumes for mechanical ventilation should be limited to 4–6 mL/kg of ideal body weight. Respiratory rates are generally increased to keep $Paco_2$ levels within normal and can range from 14 to 24 breaths per minute. PEEP is titrated to keep plateau pressures less than 30 cm H_2O. Common management strategies include prone positioning and inhaled nitric oxide; surfactant replacement therapy and IV prostacyclin are less common. ECMO can be used for those patients with life-threatening hypoxemia and/or hypercarbia who are unresponsive to other treatments.

Anesthetic Considerations. Elective procedures are not performed in patients with ARDS. Anesthesia may be required for patients who have developed ARDS secondary to bowel necrosis or an abscess or for patients who have developed a pneumothorax. Hemodynamic monitoring is frequently required because these patients most often require vasopressor and/or inotropic support. Ventilation strategies are discussed in the treatment and management section below. These patients often have an exaggerated response to anesthetic medications; therefore careful titration is recommended.

Pulmonary edema. Pulmonary edema is another acute intrinsic restrictive lung condition. It is characterized by leakage of fluid from the pulmonary vasculature into the interstitium and alveoli. Pulmonary edema can result from increased capillary permeability or pressure (Table 3.20). An important distinction between the two causes is the presence of protein in the alveolar fluid. Protein is only noted in those types of pulmonary edema that cause an increase in capillary permeability because the respiratory membrane has been disrupted, and protein can leak through along with fluid. Causes that result in an increase in pressure do not generally disrupt the alveolar–capillary membrane.

KNOWLEDGE CHECK

1. Which is the most common trigger for the development of ARDS?
   a. Systemic trauma
   b. Sepsis
   c. Aspiration
   d. Pulmonary embolism
2. Mechanical ventilation strategies for patients with restrictive lung disease should consist of
   a. tidal volume of 8–10 mL/kg.
   b. little or no PEEP.
   c. plateau pressure $<$35 cm H_2O.
   d. respiratory rate of 14–24/min.
3. Which causes pulmonary edema due to increased pulmonary capillary pressures?
   a. High altitude
   b. ARDS
   c. Metabolic alkalosis
   d. Aspiration
4. Which is a distinguishing feature of pulmonary edema caused by increased capillary permeability compared with pulmonary edema caused by increased hydrostatic pressure?
   a. Presence of bilateral opacities on CXR
   b. Protein-rich fluid in the alveoli
   c. Rapid onset of respiratory failure
   d. Absence of breath sounds
5. Which of the following management strategies is most appropriate for a patient with ARDS to minimize ventilator-associated lung injury?
   a. Mechanical ventilation with tidal volumes of 8–10 mL/kg ideal body weight
   b. Prone positioning to improve oxygenation
   c. Use of diuretics to maintain a negative fluid balance
   d. Administration of high tidal volumes to normalize $Paco_2$ quickly

Answers can be found in Appendix A.

TABLE 3.20 Causes of Pulmonary Edema

	Pathophysiology and Etiology	Signs and Symptoms	Treatment and Management	Anesthetic Considerations
Increased Capillary Permeability Pulmonary Edema				
Aspiration	Acidic gastric fluid and/or solids damage pulmonary endothelium and surfactant-producing cells, causing a breakdown in the alveolar–capillary membranes and atelectasis. Aspiration can occur for several reasons.	Tachypnea, dyspnea, bronchospasm, cough, hypoxemia, acute pulmonary hypertension, and sympathetic stimulation. Auscultated crackles. Pulmonary infiltrates may be seen on chest x-ray several hours after the event.	Supplemental oxygen and CPAP for nonintubated patients and PEEP for intubated patients. Bronchodilators help with bronchospasm. Antibiotics should only be used if there is evidence of infection and an identified pathogen. Corticosteroids are reserved for severe aspiration cases that are refractory to other treatments.	Elective surgery should be delayed in anyone with pulmonary edema. End the current procedure as soon as possible and make arrangements for an ICU bed. Identify and treat the underlying cause. Arterial blood pressure and CVP monitoring are useful. Patients may arrive for surgery with vasoactive medication infusions. Ventilator management should focus on strategies to maintain oxygenation while limiting high inspiratory pressures (<30 cm H_2O plateau pressures). Thus smaller tidal volumes (4–6 mL/kg) with higher respiratory rates (14–18/min) and PEEP are indicated. These patients are at risk for barotrauma and pneumothorax. Diuretics should be given to offload fluid from the lungs. Consider ECMO in cases that are severe and refractory to medical management.
Drug or toxin induced	Can occur after the use of some medications, especially opioids and cocaine, or the inhalation of toxic fumes.	Tachypnea, dyspnea, cough, and hypoxemia. Auscultated crackles. Chest x-ray shows bilateral pulmonary infiltrates that are indistinguishable from other causes of pulmonary edema.	Treatment is supportive and may require intubation with mechanical ventilation.	
ARDS	Direct or indirect lung injury causes alveolar damage and capillary permeability. Several causes are discussed in the previous ARDS section.	Tachypnea, dyspnea, tachycardia, hypotension, altered or decreased lung sounds, and hypoxemia. Depending on the cause, the patient may be febrile or even hypothermic.	Requires supplemental oxygen. Intubation, mechanical ventilation, and PEEP frequently needed. Hemodynamic monitoring commonly required. Identify the cause and treat accordingly.	

Continued

TABLE 3.20 **Causes of Pulmonary Edema—cont'd**

	Pathophysiology and Etiology	Signs and Symptoms	Treatment and Management	Anesthetic Considerations
Increased Capillary Pressure Pulmonary Edema				
Ischemic heart disease, CHF, or cardiomyopathy causing left ventricular failure	Decrease in left ventricular contractility results in a reduction of stroke volume and cardiac output. Because of this failure, left ventricular end-diastolic volume and pressure are increased. This causes an elevation in pressures back through the left atrium and pulmonary circulation, resulting in high pulmonary capillary hydrostatic pressure, failed lymphatic draining, and alveolar flooding.	Tachypnea, dyspnea, cough, and hypoxemia. Auscultated crackles. Altered hemodynamics with tachycardia and hypotension. Altered ECG. Elevated cardiac filling pressures (PCWP and CVP). Jugular venous distention. Pulmonary infiltrates and cardiomegaly on chest x-ray.	Requires supplemental oxygen. Assist spontaneous ventilation with CPAP or BiPAP. Intubation and mechanical ventilation as needed. Obtain cardiac markers, ECG and ABG. Assess myocardial function with TEE. Reduce cardiac preload with furosemide (10- to 20-mg bolus), nitroglycerine (0.25–1 mcg/kg/min) unless the patient is hypotensive, and morphine (2-mg increments). Provide inotropic support with dopamine (3–10. mcg/kg/min), dobutamine 5–10 mcg/kg/min), milrinone (50 mcg/kg loading dose, then 0.375–0.75 mcg/kg/min) or epinephrine (0.05–1 mcg/kg/min).	Discontinue cardiac depressive drugs. Elective surgery should be delayed in anyone with pulmonary edema. End the current procedure as soon as possible and make arrangements for an ICU bed. Identify and treat the underlying cause. Arterial blood pressure and CVP monitoring are useful. Patients may arrive for surgery with vasoactive medication infusions. Ventilator management should focus on strategies to maintain oxygenation while limiting high inspiratory pressures (< 30 cm H_2O plateau pressures). Thus smaller tidal volumes (4–6 mL/kg) with higher respiratory rates (14–18/min) and PEEP are indicated. These patients are at risk for barotrauma and pneumothorax. Diuretics should be given to offload fluid from the lungs. Consider ECMO in cases that are severe and refractory to medical management.
Neurogenic	Can occur due to acute brain injury (e.g., trauma, CVA). Massive sympathetic stimulation can cause systemic and pulmonary vasoconstriction, resulting in a shift of peripheral blood into the pulmonary circulation causing pulmonary hypertension and an increase in pulmonary capillary hydrostatic pressure.	Signs and symptoms are similar to other pulmonary edema causes. This type of pulmonary edema is generally diagnosed by an accompanying brain injury.	Treatment and management are supportive with supplemental oxygen, vasodilators, and airway management.	

Negative pressure	Occurs in the spontaneously breathing patient when a forceful inspiration is conducted against a closed glottis. This can be from a laryngospasm, epiglottitis, upper airway tumor, or upper airway redundant tissue. The high negative intrathoracic and intrapleural pressures cause an engorgement of pulmonary vascular volume and subsequent interstitial volume. Lymphatic drainage becomes overwhelmed, and fluid overflows into the alveoli. Hypoxia further aggravates the movement of fluid through the pulmonary circulation by causing systemic vasoconstriction.	Acute upper airway obstruction. Stridorous breath sounds may be present in a partial obstruction. Decreasing saturation. Acute tachycardia and hypertension. After the obstructive event, tachypnea, cough, and hypoxemia are seen.	Prompt identification and intervention to relieve the airway obstruction are essential. Positive-pressure ventilation, propofol, or succinylcholine is used to relieve a laryngospasm. Postobstruction management is supportive with supplemental oxygen, diuretics, and airway management as needed.
High altitude	The exact mechanism is unknown. However, the causes seem to include intense hypoxic pulmonary arterial vasoconstriction and cerebral hypoxia from a lower oxygen content at high altitudes. The result is massive sympathetic discharge and systemic and pulmonary vasoconstriction causing increased pulmonary vascular pressure and congestion.	Tachypnea, dyspnea, low oxygen saturation, tachycardia, headache, nausea/vomiting, and fatigue.	Primary management is to descend from altitude as soon as possible and provide supplemental oxygen. Nifedipine may help decrease arterial pressure. Prophylactic and early use of acetazolamide and dexamethasone help prevent and treat the disorder, respectively.

ABG, Arterial blood gas; *ARDS*, acute respiratory distress syndrome; *BiPAP*, bilevel positive airway pressure; *CHF*, congestive heart failure; *CPAP*, continuous positive airway pressure; *CVA*, cerebrovascular accident; *CVP*, central venous pressure; *ECG*, electrocardiogram; *ECMO*, extracorporeal membrane oxygenation; *ICU*, intensive care unit; *PCWP*, pulmonary capillary wedge pressure; *PEEP*, positive end-expiratory pressure; *TEE*, transesophageal echocardiogram.

Extrinsic restrictive pulmonary disease. Extrinsic restrictive pulmonary diseases are extrapulmonary in nature. Conditions or diseases that affect the chest wall, pleura, or respiratory muscles cause an extrinsic restriction to proper lung expansion and ventilation, leading to reduced lung volumes (see Fig. 3.28). Etiology, signs and symptoms, treatment and management, and anesthetic considerations can be found in Table 3.21.

KNOWLEDGE CHECK

1. The most effective initial intervention for treatment of a tension pneumothorax during anesthesia is
   a. placing the patient on 100% FiO_2.
   b. inserting a chest tube.
   c. performing a needle thoracotomy.
   d. administering epinephrine.
2. One of the most important things to avoid in a patient with extrinsic restrictive pulmonary disease is
   a. nitrous oxide.
   b. prone position.
   c. apnea.
   d. opioids.

Answers can be found in Appendix A.

Obstructive Sleep Apnea

Obstructive sleep apnea (OSA) is a disorder that occurs when pharyngeal muscles relax and allow airway tissues to collapse against the posterior pharyngeal wall during sleep. Repeated collapse of these tissues causes slow and apneic breathing patterns. Hypercapnia and hypoxemia occur, resulting in SNS activation. Obese adults with a large neck circumference are likely to have some degree of OSA. Children with adenotonsillar hypertrophy, altered craniofacial development (e.g., Pierre Robin sequence, Treacher Collins syndrome, or Crouzon syndrome), or neuromuscular anomalies (e.g., cerebral palsy, encephalopathy) are at risk of OSA. Patients should be encouraged to use their CPAP machines before and after surgery if available.

Etiology. Several different predisposing factors can result in OSA. These include obesity, genetics, upper airway narrowing, male sex, use of alcohol or other sedative drugs, and cigarette smoking.

Signs and symptoms. Snoring that progresses to periods of apnea and then arousal is common. Patients often experience daytime sleepiness, a decrease in cognition, and decreased overall performance. Airway-related symptoms include airway obstruction, hypoxemia, regurgitation, pulmonary aspiration, laryngospasm, and bronchospasm. Cardiovascular consequences can occur secondary to OSA and include hypercoagulation, tachycardia, hypertension, increased transmural pressures on the heart and great vessels, increased right and left ventricular afterload, RVH, dysrhythmias, and cardiac dysfunction.

Treatment and management. Detection and identification are important because many individuals with this condition go undiagnosed. Positive airway pressure is the primary treatment. This can be CPAP, BiPAP, or autotitrating pressure. The goal of positive airway pressure is to identify the lowest pressure that eliminates apnea, arousals, snoring, and hypopneas. Oral appliance therapy using mandibular advancement devices is also used. Other treatments include weight loss, exercise, diet control, avoidance of alcohol and other sedative drugs, and head elevation during sleep. Bariatric surgery can be performed in the severely obese patient, which frequently helps with weight loss and results in a decrease in OSA symptoms.

Anesthetic considerations. The STOP-BANG scoring model is used in any patient suspected of having OSA, and it is a good predictor of severe OSA (see Chapter 1, Box 1.3). Opioids should be avoided or limited in the perioperative period, and regional anesthesia or peripheral nerve blocks should be considered as much as possible. Patients who have a CPAP machine are encouraged to bring it for use in the postoperative period.

Anterior Mediastinal Mass

An anterior mediastinal mass occurs when a mass of tissue or cancer forms within the anterior mediastinal compartment of the chest. This compartment is anterior to the pericardium and contains the thymus, lymphatic tissue, distal trachea, and potentially some thyroid tissue.

Etiology. The etiology of an anterior mediastinal mass is benign or malignant tumor formation within the anterior mediastinal compartment (anterior to the heart). These masses include thymomas, germ cell tumors, lymphomas, or even thyroid or parathyroid tissue lesions. These masses have the potential to dangerously compress the trachea, bronchi, heart, and/or great vessels.

Signs and Symptoms. Large mediastinal masses can cause severe airway obstruction and decreased venous return and/or cardiac output. Symptomatic compression of these structures would include edema formation within the upper extremities from vena cava compression. Cardiac compression can result in cough, chest pain, syncope, dysrhythmias, and/or hypotension. Airway manifestations

TABLE 3.21 Extrinsic Restrictive Pulmonary Diseases

Restrictive Disease/Disorder	Pathophysiology and Etiology	Signs and Symptoms	Treatment and Management	Anesthetic Considerations
Costovertebral skeletal deformities	These are skeletal structural deformities that compress the lung and decrease lung volumes. They include scoliosis (lateral spinal curvature and rotation) and kyphosis (anterior spinal flexion). Kyphoscoliosis is a combination of the two and can severely restrict the lungs. Other disorders include ankylosing spondylitis, pectus excavatum (concave chest), and pectus carinatum (outward protrusion of chest).	Visualized skeletal deformity. Reduced PFT lung volumes. Increased work of breathing, especially on exertion. Hypoxemia with secondary erythrocytosis in severe disease. Compression on the pulmonary vessels can lead to pulmonary hypertension and right ventricular dysfunction. Pulmonary infections can reoccur more frequently because of a poor cough effort.	Surgery to correct skeletal deformities is an option in some patients. Oxygen therapy and CPAP are provided to those patients with severe deformities who have nightly apneic episodes.	Patients with these restrictive disorders have a severely reduced FRC and do not tolerate apneic periods. Several airway adjuncts of choice should be immediately available, and the means to ventilate continuously should be supplied. Have a plan for airway failure (e.g., cricothyrotomy). Avoid medications that cause prolonged respiratory depression. Regional anesthesia should be limited to T10 level to avoid any respiratory involvement. Peripheral nerve blocks are encouraged. Mechanical ventilation may require higher inspiratory pressures necessitating vigilant monitoring for a potential pneumothorax. Patients with severe restrictive disease likely will require postoperative mechanical ventilation. Nitrous oxide should be avoided because of the risk of pneumothorax and to be able to increase the amount of inspired O_2. Consider hemodynamic monitoring for long cases, thoracic cases, or ones that have the potential for blood loss.
Flail chest	This is a skeletal structural deformity that compresses the lung and decreases lung volumes. Usually occurs from a traumatic injury. Occurs when three or more ribs fracture in a parallel vertical fashion, causing a paradoxical inward movement during inhalation of the isolated fractured portion and a paradoxical outward motion on exhalation.	Pain, dyspnea, increased respiratory effort, splinting on the side of injury. Atelectasis on the injured side and decreased ability to cough and clear secretions. Reduced PFT lung volumes. Decreased tidal volumes and hypoxemia. Potential lung contusion at the site of injury.	Intubation with positive-pressure ventilation and pain control using opioids and/or regional anesthesia. Stabilization of broken section externally or surgically.	

Continued

TABLE 3.21 **Extrinsic Restrictive Pulmonary Diseases—cont'd**

Restrictive Disease/Disorder	Pathophysiology and Etiology	Signs and Symptoms	Treatment and Management	Anesthetic Considerations
Pleural effusion	Fluid that has accumulated within the pleural space. Effusions can occur from various fluids that collect within the pleural space and include blood (hemothorax), pus (empyema), lipids (chylothorax), or serous liquid (hydrothorax).	Pleural fluid is best identified by chest CT or ultrasound. Bloody pleural effusions are common in patients who have experienced trauma or pulmonary infarction or who have a malignant disease.	Thoracentesis is performed to obtain fluid for diagnosis. Surgery may be required for effusions that cannot be drained with a needle or small catheter. Other surgical options for recurrent effusions include pleuroperitoneal shunt, pleurodesis, decortication, or closure of a diaphragmatic defect.	
Pneumothorax/ tension pneumothorax	Disruption of either the parietal or visceral pleura can cause air to enter the pleural space, causing a pneumothorax. A tear in the parietal pleura is the result of an external penetrating traumatic injury. A visceral pleural tear can happen spontaneously (e.g., spontaneous pneumothorax) or as the result of functional lung tissue pathology (e.g., emphysema, cystic fibrosis, lung abscess). A tension pneumothorax is a medical emergency and occurs when air continues to enter the pleural space but does not exit. Intrathoracic pressure increases with every breath causing compression on the heart, mediastinum, great vessels, and contralateral lung.	Tachypnea, dyspnea, respiratory distress, decreasing O_2 saturation, cyanosis, and/or hypoxemia are respiratory symptoms. Pleuritic chest pain may be present. Decreased or absent breath sounds on the affected lung. Hyperresonance on percussion. Tracheal deviation to the opposite side of injury may be noted in a tension pneumothorax. Hypoxemia, tachycardia, hypotension, and hypercarbia are noted during general anesthesia. Increased inspiratory pressures, decreased tidal volumes, and decreased bag compliance are noted during mechanical ventilation. Bronchospasm may occur.	Prompt recognition and administration of 100% Fio_2. Placement of a large-bore needle thoracotomy at the second intercostal space at the midclavicular line or at the fourth intercostal space at the midaxillary line. Place needle cephalad to rib to avoid neurovascular bundle. Chest tube placement on the affected side. IV fluid bolus, vasopressor, and inotropic agents to treat hypotension.	

Neuromuscular disorders	Occur as a result of a disruption or interruption of nervous transmission from the CNS to respiratory muscles. Nerve transmission disturbance to the respiratory muscles is what causes the restrictive disease. Can result from a spinal cord transection, muscular dystrophies, neuromuscular transmission disorders (e.g., myasthenia gravis, multiple sclerosis), or Guillain-Barré syndrome.	Decrease in inspiratory effort leads to alveolar hypoventilation. Decreases in expiratory airflow and effort results in an ineffective coughing which allows pneumonia to develop. May have decreased PFT values and vital capacity. Breathing may be by diaphragm only.	Abdominal binders to help increase abdominal tone in quadriplegic patients. Anticholinergics for patients with altered sympathetic tone. Mechanical ventilation in patients unable to maintain adequate ventilation (e.g., Guillain-Barré syndrome, multiple sclerosis). Antibiotics for pulmonary infections. Limit or avoid neuromuscular blockade. Decrease the dose of any medication that causes CNS and respiratory depression.
Obesity, ascites, and term pregnancy	External compression on the thoracic cavity causes lung restriction. Excessive abdominal adipose tissue, fluid, or a gravid uterus impairs diaphragmatic function and basal lung opening and compresses lung tissue, promoting closure.	Large abdominal girth. Decrease in PFT values, FRC, and TLC. Snoring and sleep apnea. Hypoxemia. Tachypnea and dyspnea on exertion.	Weight loss by diet, exercise, and/or surgery. Delivery of baby. Abdominal tap or paracentesis to drain excess ascites fluid. Perioperative supplemental oxygen. Maintain spontaneous ventilation when possible.

CNS, Central nervous system; *CPAP*, continuous positive airway pressure; *CT*, computed tomography; *FRC*, functional residual capacity; *IV*, intravenous; *PFT*, pulmonary function test; *TLC*, total lung capacity.

include shortness of breath, dyspnea, hoarseness, cough, stridor, difficulty in advancing or inability to advance ETT, and hypoxemia. Position changes with worsening of symptoms or improvement should be evaluated.

Treatment and management. Many mediastinal masses may require a mediastinoscopy for biopsy and identification. Treatment depends on the pathology and may require surgical resection, radiation, or chemotherapy. Surgical bleeding may be greater than normal as a result of vena cava compression and increased CVP.

Anesthetic considerations. Airway and cardiac compression are primary concerns. Thorough airway assessment with review of imaging and discussion of an airway plan with the perioperative team should occur. Lower extremity IV and arterial lines should be used for symptomatic venous compression. Awake flexible video laryngoscopy (fiberoptic intubation) in the sitting position should be used if there is evidence of airway compression. Avoidance of neuromuscular blockade is recommended to avoid the potential for partial or complete airway obstruction by the mediastinal mass. A patient who experiences a severe airway obstruction should be placed in the lateral or prone position, and a rigid bronchoscope should be used to ventilate. Cardiopulmonary bypass or ECMO may be prepared as a standby option in patients with severe symptoms or large masses.

Upper Respiratory Infection

Upper respiratory infections (URIs) occur because of bacterial or viral infections that affect the tissues of the nasopharyngeal, oropharyngeal, and/or hypopharyngeal airways.

Etiology. The majority of URIs are nasopharyngeal infections. Viral pathogens are the most common cause of an acute URI and can include rhinovirus, influenza virus, coronavirus, and respiratory syncytial virus.

Signs and symptoms. Nonproductive cough, rhinorrhea, and sneezing are the most common URI symptoms. Bacterial infections seem to produce more severe symptoms, such as fever, productive cough, fatigue, malaise, tachypnea, and pulmonary wheezing. Blood cultures identify specific pathogens. URIs can cause laryngospasm, bronchospasm, excessive mucus production, postintubation croup, atelectasis, and airway obstruction.

Treatment and management. Antihistamines, antitussives, antipyretics, and NSAIDs are used to manage viral infection symptoms. Bacterial infections should be treated with antibiotics.

Anesthetic considerations. Elective surgery should be delayed 2–6 weeks, depending on the severity of the URI. Perioperative laryngospasm bronchospasm, as well as postoperative respiratory obstruction from mucus and inflamed airway tissues, can occur as a result of a hyperreactive infected airway. Adequate IV hydration should be provided. Preoperative inhaled bronchodilation with β_2-agonists and racemic epinephrine can help open the upper and lower airways. Airway manipulation should be minimized (laryngeal mask airway preferred over ETT), and attempts at intubation should be limited. Atomized or nebulized lidocaine can decrease laryngeal and tracheal stimulation.

Pulmonary Embolism

PE is a blockage within the right heart and pulmonary arterial vasculature, causing a right ventricular outflow obstruction that impedes blood oxygenation and cardiac output. The result is ventilation/perfusion abnormalities and severe hypoperfusion with the potential for cardiopulmonary collapse.

Etiology. Substances that can cause a PE include a blood clot thrombus, air or gas from surgery, amniotic fluid, or fat particles released from trauma or surgery to a long bone or the pelvis.

Signs and symptoms. A massive PE can cause severe hemodynamic compromise and even cardiac arrest that manifests as PEA or asystole. Other signs and symptoms include tachypnea, dyspnea, hypoxemia, pleuritic chest pain, cough, hemoptysis, fatigue, syncope, wheezing, tachycardia, cyanosis, dysrhythmias, and hypotension.

- Signs and symptoms specifically related to a fat embolism generally do not appear until 24–72 hours after the bone injury. They include hypoxemia; altered mental status; a petechial rash that covers the upper body and neck; thrombocytopenia; and fat globules in the urine, sputum, or retinal vessels.
- Amniotic fluid embolism signs and symptoms manifest during or shortly after labor. These can be severe and include hypoxemia, respiratory failure, disseminated intravascular coagulation (DIC), seizures, coma, and hemodynamic failure from cardiogenic shock.
- Signs and symptoms of a PE under anesthesia may include tachycardia, hypotension, altered or absent $ETco_2$ waveform, hypoxemia, increase in CVP and PA pressures, dysrhythmias, millwheel murmur (air embolism), and/or increased inspiratory pressures. Echocardiography shows hypokinesis of the ventricles.

Treatment and management. Prophylactic therapy includes administration of subcutaneous heparin (5000 units) 1–2 hours before surgery and then every 6–8 hours until the patient is walking. Subcutaneous enoxaparin (30–40 mg) is another option. Warfarin is still another option and should be monitored with serial international normalized ratio levels. Compression stockings and intermittent pneumatic compression boots should be used in most surgical patients. Those most at risk for deep venous thrombosis or PE may benefit from the placement of an inferior vena cava filter, especially if oral anticoagulation is contraindicated.

- If a PE is suspected, administer 100% FiO_2, secure the airway with an ETT and provide mechanical ventilation with PEEP, obtain ABG values, administer an IV crystalloid bolus, place a CVP and arterial line, and support cardiovascular function with inotropic agents (e.g., ephedrine, epinephrine, dopamine, dobutamine, and/or milrinone). If cardiac arrest occurs, begin CPR and follow ACLS protocols.
- Thrombotic therapy is indicated for patients who exhibit hemodynamic compromise or right ventricular dysfunction as a result of a PE. Interventional radiological catheter-directed thrombolytic therapy may be indicated in some surgical patients. Patients with life-threatening PE with hemodynamic collapse may be considered for cardiopulmonary bypass or ECMO, or they may receive a thoracotomy with pulmonary embolectomy if systemic thrombolysis or interventional radiological catheter-directed therapy are not options.

Anesthetic considerations. Management of an intraoperative PE includes many of the management strategies just discussed, with an emphasis on cardiovascular support, pulmonary support with mechanical ventilation and PEEP, and communication with the surgical team. In addition, there are some management plans that are specific to the type of embolism.

- *Venous air embolism (VAE)* and *CO_2 gas embolism:* Communicate with surgeon to flood the field with saline (VAE) or turn off CO_2 gas and exsuf CO_2 gas embolism is suspected based on sig symptoms. Call for assistance. Administer FiO_2, turn off anesthesia gases, avoid N_2O, and ate fluid bolus/vasopressor administration. Turn patient to the left lateral position and place the he below the heart. Provide cardiovascular support an CPR as indicated.
- *Blood clot embolism:* Perform similar management strategies as just discussed for venous air and CO_2 gas embolism. Positioning can remain supine. Obtain consultation with pulmonary or critical care expert. Provide PEEP with mechanical ventilation. Place arterial line and CVP if not already done, and obtain initial ABG results. Begin heparin anticoagulation if not contraindicated (5000 unit bolus followed by 1000 unit/h infusion). Consider thrombolytic therapy.
- *Fat embolism:* Management strategies are similar to those discussed previously, with an emphasis on cardiovascular support and mechanical ventilation with PEEP. Inotropic agents that can be considered include infusions of ephedrine (5–20-mg bolus doses); epinephrine (10–50-mcg bolus doses); and dopamine, dobutamine, milrinone, or epinephrine.
- *Amniotic fluid embolism:* Delivery of the fetus should occur as fast as possible if this type of embolism is suspected. These embolic events often cause severe cardiopulmonary collapse with concurrent DIC. Interventions include obtaining a coagulation panel and requesting type and cross-matched blood, fresh frozen plasma, and platelets based on values. Consider uterotonic agents for uterine atony. Administering atropine 0.2 mg to decrease hypotension caused by increased vagal tone, ondansetron 8 mg to inhibit serotonin and decrease pulmonary vasoconstriction and platelet activation, and ketorolac 15 mg to inhibit thromboxane and the release of inflammatory mediators has been used with success (A-OK protocol).

KNOWLEDGE CHECK

1. Which preoperative question is vital during patient assessment for OSA?
   a. Do you snore loud enough to be heard through a door?
   b. Is your body mass index above 30 kg/m^2?
   c. Do you have diabetes?
   d. Do you have a decreased amount of energy?

2. A primary anesthetic consideration for mediastinoscopy for biopsy of a mediastinal mass is
   a. review of airway imaging with surgeon.
   b. alleviation of preoperative anxiety.
   c. administration of antihypertensive medications.
   d. placement of an IV line in a lower extremity.

Continued

K—cont'd

intervention for both VAE and
(Select all that apply.)

ntrainment into the venous system.
nitrous oxide
20-mL/kg IV fluid bolus.
ntinue sevoflurane administration.
ert a central line in the femoral vein.

ch is the most appropriate initial airway management strategy for a patient with a large anterior mediastinal mass exhibiting signs of airway compression?

a. Rapid sequence induction with muscle relaxant
b. Awake flexible (fiberoptic) intubation in the sitting position
c. Deep sedation followed by mask ventilation
d. Intubation after full paralysis in the supine position

5. A patient undergoing surgery suddenly develops tachycardia, hypotension, hypoxemia, and an abrupt decrease in $ETco_2$. What is the most likely diagnosis?
   a. Acute MI
   b. Upper respiratory infection
   c. OSA
   d. Pulmonary embolism

Answers can be found in Appendix A.

NEUROLOGIC SYSTEM

The *CNS* includes the brain and spinal cord. The *peripheral nervous system* includes the cranial and spinal nerves and their receptors and is divided into the somatic nervous system and the ANS. The *somatic nervous system* contains sensory neurons for the skin, muscles, and joints. The *ANS*, which consists of the sympathetic and parasympathetic nervous systems (PNS), is responsible for involuntary innervation of various organ systems (Fig. 3.29).

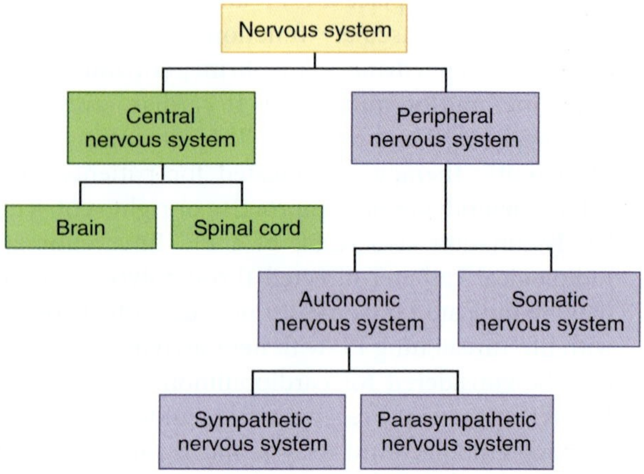

Fig. 3.29 Nervous system: division and function.

Autonomic Nervous System

The SNS and the PNS function in opposition to maintain homeostasis and are responsible for the fight-or-flight response. The SNS and PNS originate within the CNS and require two efferent neurons: a preganglionic neuron originating within the CNS and a postganglionic neuron terminating within the effector organ (smooth muscle, cardiac muscle, or sweat gland). The ANS is controlled by the hypothalamus (Fig. 3.30). Autonomic fibers originating in the brain arise from cell bodies located in the brainstem. Autonomic functions include control of respiration, cardiac regulation (cardiac accelerator and inhibitory centers), and vasomotor activity, which are located within the medulla oblongata.

Sympathetic Nervous System

The SNS response occurs via the thoracolumbar vertebrae, resulting in efferent impulse outflow from the following:

- Preganglionic neurons of the SNS originate in the intermediolateral gray horn of the spinal cord between the first thoracic (T1) and second or third lumbar vertebrae (L2 or L3).
- The postganglionic fibers of the postganglionic neurons may either exit the gray ramus to enter a spinal nerve or extend through a connection between the paravertebral ganglion and one of the three (celiac, superior, or inferior) mesenteric ganglia.
- *Clinical application:* SNS innervation from T1 through T4–T5 innervates the heart and lungs. Stimulation produces an increased heart rate (positive chronotropic effect), an increase in conduction (positive dromotropic effect), and an increase in myocardial contractility (positive inotropic effect). With SCIs that extend above T1, bradycardia caused by SNS denervation of the cardioaccelerator nerve fiber innervation and PNS predominance occurs, resulting in bradycardia.

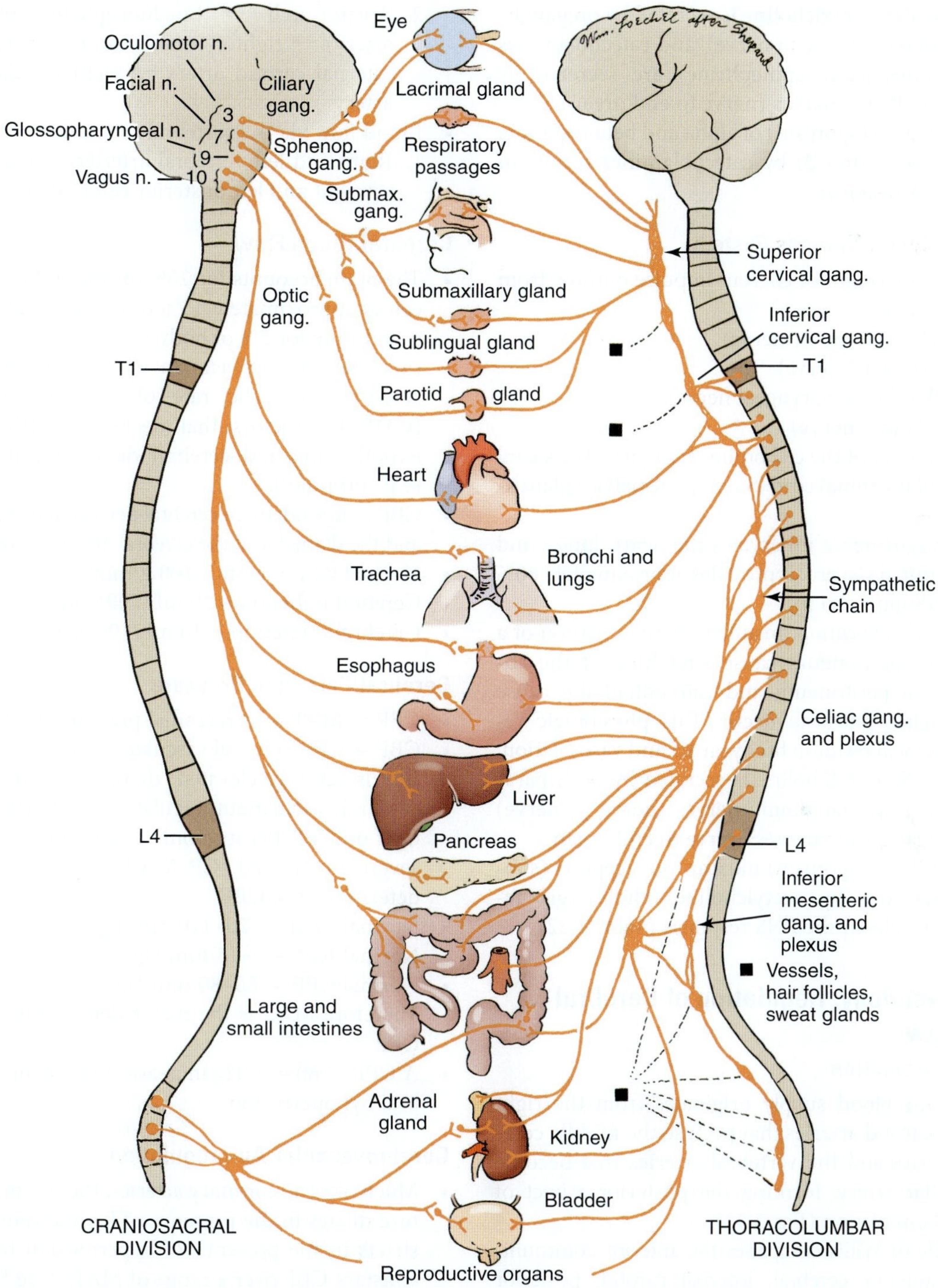

Fig. 3.30 Both divisions of the autonomic nervous system. *gang.*, Ganglion; *n*, nerve. (From Elisha S, Heiner JS, Nagelhout JJ. *Nurse Anesthesia*. 7th ed. Elsevier; 2023.)

- In the SNS, acetylcholine is secreted by preganglionic nerves (nerve to nerve), and catecholamines (norepinephrine, epinephrine) are secreted by postganglionic nerves (nerve to end organ).
- Stimulation (agonism) of alpha and beta receptors (subtypes 1 and 2) by catecholamines results in the SNS response.

Parasympathetic Nervous System

- Craniosacral origin of efferent impulse outflow from the following:
  - *CN III* (oculomotor nerve)
  - *CN VII* (facial nerve)
  - *CN IX* (glossopharyngeal nerve)
  - *CN X* (vagus nerve)
- The remainder of the cell bodies arise from the sacral portion of the spinal cord (S2–S4), the pelvic splanchnic nerves.
  - The vagus nerve innervates the heart, lungs, and abdominal viscera. It provides approximately 80% of PNS innervation.
  - *Clinical application:* Insufflation and creation of a pneumoperitoneum cause stretching of the abdominal peritoneum and can potentially cause the celiac reflex to occur. This physiologic response will result in bradycardia and vasodilation.
- In the PNS, acetylcholine is secreted by both parasympathetic preganglionic nerves (nerve to nerve) and postganglionic nerves (nerve to end organ).
- Stimulation of (agonism) muscarinic receptors (subtypes M1–M5) by acetylcholine (cholinergic response) results in the PNS response (Table 3.22)

Neurophysiology: Regulation of Cerebral Blood Flow

Cerebral Circulation

- The brain's blood supply originates from the right and left carotid arteries that perfuse the middle cerebral arteries and the vertebral arteries that become the basilar artery, forming the posterior aspect of cerebral circulation (Fig. 3.31).
- The circle of Willis comprises the anterior communicating, anterior cerebral, internal carotid, posterior communicating, posterior cerebral, and basilar arteries.
- Blood flow via the internal carotid arteries:
  1. Aortic arch → left common carotid artery → left internal carotid artery → left middle cerebral artery
  2. Aortic arch → brachiocephalic (innominate artery) → right common carotid artery → right internal carotid artery → right middle cerebral artery
- Blood flow via the vertebral arteries:
  1. Right and left vertebral arteries → basilar artery → right and left posterior cerebral arteries

Cerebral Blood Flow

- The brain accounts for 20% of resting V_{O_2}, and it receives approximately 15% of cardiac output despite accounting for 2% of body weight.
- Increases or decreases in CBF are determined by cerebral metabolic rate of oxygen consumption ($CMRO_2$). Factors that decrease $CMRO_2$ include hypothermia and cerebral depressant medications (e.g., propofol).
- CBF is dependent on cerebral perfusion pressure (CPP) and the diameter of the cerebral arteries (Box 3.8).
- Normal CBF ≈ 50 mL/100 g/min
- Cerebral ischemia ≈ 20 mL/100 g/min
- Cerebral infarction ≈ 10 mL/100 g/min

Cerebral Perfusion Pressure

- CPP = MAP – Intracranial pressure (ICP).
- CBF = CPP/cerebral vascular resistance. Therefore if ICP is severely elevated, there is an uncoupling of cerebral vascular autoregulation. CBF will be dependent on CPP. Because only craniotomy can decrease severely increased ICP, MAP becomes the primary determinant of CBF.
- Normal MAP = 70–110 mm Hg.
- Normal ICP = 5–15 mm Hg.
- Normal CPP = 60–80 mm Hg.
- Therefore MAP is the major determining factor for CPP.
- A CPP < 60 mm Hg increases the potential for cerebral hypoperfusion.

Cerebrovascular Autoregulation

- Much like the coronary arteries, the cerebral vasculature dilates in the presence of hypotension and constricts in the presence of hypertension to maintain constant CBF over a range of MAPs (see Fig. 3.1).
- Cerebrovascular autoregulation occurs between MAPs of 60–140 mm Hg.
- Patients with cerebrovascular disease have cerebral autoregulation curves that are shifted to the right.

TABLE 3.22 **Typical Autonomic Influences on Peripheral Effector Organs**

Organ System	Sympathetic Effect	Adrenergic Receptor Type	Parasympathetic Effect	Cholinergic Receptor Type
Eye				
Radial muscle, iris	Contraction (mydriasis)	α_1		
Sphincter muscle, iris			Contraction (miosis)	M_3, M_2
Ciliary muscle	Relaxation for far vision	β_2	Contraction for near vision (accommodation)	M_3, M_2
Heart				
Sinoatrial node	Increase in heart rate	β_1	Decrease in heart rate	M_2
Atria	Increase in contractility and conduction velocity	β_1	Decrease in contractility	M_2
Atrioventricular node	Increase in automaticity and conduction velocity	β_1	Decrease in conduction velocity; atrioventricular block	M_2
His-Purkinje system	Increase in automaticity and conduction velocity	β_1	Little effect	M_2
Ventricle	Increase in contractility, conduction velocity, automaticity	β_1	Slight decrease in contractility	M_2
Arteries and Veins				
Coronary	Constriction; dilation	α; β_2	None	—
Skin and mucosa	Constriction	α_1; β_2	None	—
Skeletal muscle	Constriction; dilation	α_1; β_2	None	—
Cerebral	Constriction (slight)	α_1	None	—
Pulmonary	Constriction; dilation	α_1; β_2	None	—
Abdominal viscera	Constriction; dilation	α_1; β_2	None	—
Salivary glands	Constriction and reduced secretions	α_1; α_2	Dilation and increased secretions	M_3
Renal	Constriction; dilation	α_1, α_2; β_1, β_2	None	—
Veins	Constriction; dilation	α_1, α_2; β_2	None	—
Lung				
Tracheal and bronchial smooth muscle	Relaxation	β_2	Contraction	M_2, M_3

Continued

TABLE 3.22 Typical Autonomic Influences on Peripheral Effector Organs—cont'd

Organ System	Sympathetic Effect	Adrenergic Receptor Type	Parasympathetic Effect	Cholinergic Receptor Type
GI Tract				
Motility and tone	Decrease	α_1, α_2; β_1, β_2	Increase	M_2, M_3
Sphincters	Contraction	α_1	Relaxation	M_3, M_2
Secretion	Inhibition	α_2	Stimulation	M_3, M_2
Gallbladder and ducts	Relaxation	β_2	Contraction	M
Kidney				
Renin secretion	Increase	β_1	None	—
Urinary Bladder				
Detrusor	Relaxation	β_2, β_3	Contraction	M_3, M_2
Trigone and sphincter	Contraction	α_1	Relaxation	M_3, M_2
Uterus	Contraction (pregnant)	α_1	None	—
	Relaxation (pregnant and nonpregnant)	β_2		
Liver	Glycogenolysis and gluconeogenesis; increased blood sugar	α_1; β_2		
Pancreas				
Islets cells	Decreased insulin secretion	α_2	None	—
	Increased insulin secretion	β_2	None	—
Adipocytes	Lipolysis	α_1; β_1, β_2, β_3	None	—

GI, Gastrointestinal; *M*, muscarinic receptor.

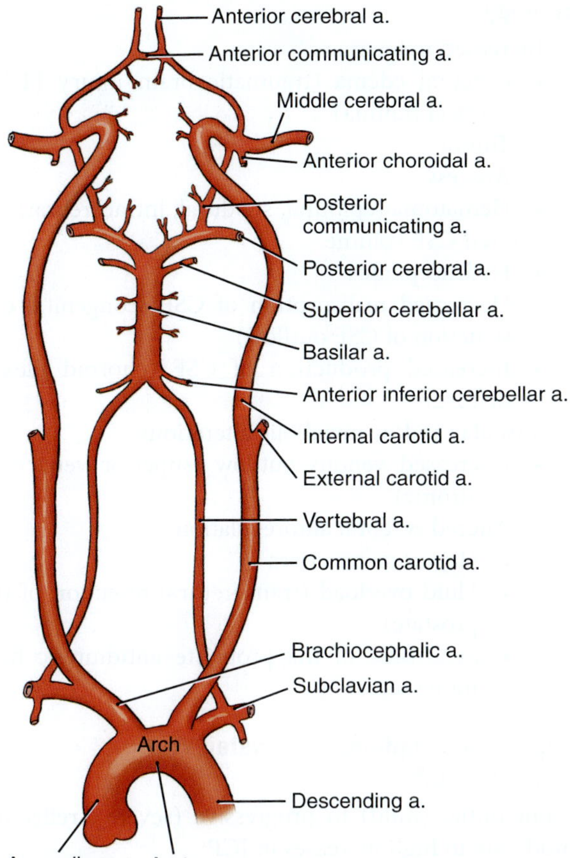

Fig. 3.31 Cerebral vasculature. *a*, Artery. (From Elisha S, Heiner JS, Nagelhout JJ. *Nurse Anesthesia*. 7th ed. Elsevier; 2023.)

BOX 3.8 Factors That Affect Cerebral Blood Flow

Increase	Decrease
• Hypoxia • Hypercarbia • Increased intracranial pressure (early) • Metabolic (acidosis, hyperkalemia, free adenosine, phospholipid metabolites)	• Hyperoxia • Normocarbia/hypocarbia • Cerebral depressant anesthetic medications

Therefore they will need a higher MAP to maintain an adequate CPP.

- *Cerebral steal phenomena:* When decreased cerebral artery blood flow to a tissue segment exists (e.g., plaque), those arteries are maximally dilated to meet the metabolic demands of the tissues that they perfuse. *Cerebral steal* refers to blood flow that is decreased or "stolen" from areas at risk for developing ischemia as a result of vasodilation and decreased perfusion pressure to the vasculature that supplies the compromised tissue region. An example is administration of anesthetic medications that cause vasodilation of arteries in the circle of Willis, decreasing perfusion to compromised collateral arteries that are maximally dilated, thereby causing ischemia.
- *Inverse steal phenomenon (Robin Hood syndrome)*: Vasoconstriction in proximal tissue beds increases the perfusion pressure in distal tissue beds. Therefore in areas where angiopathology and compromised blood flow resulting from intrinsic vasodilation exist, increased blood flow occurs.

KNOWLEDGE CHECK

1. Which factor increases CBF? *(Select all that apply.)*
   a. Hypoxia
   b. Hypocarbia
   c. Acidosis
   d. Propofol
2. Which factor is the main determinant of CPP?
   a. Intracranial pressure
   b. SVR
   c. CVP
   d. MAP
3. Which factor decreases the cerebral metabolic rate of oxygen consumption? *(Select all that apply.)*
   a. Septicemia
   b. Hypothermia
   c. Most anesthetic medications
   d. Decreased CPP
4. Cerebral autoregulation occurs with MAPs of
   a. 70–110 mm Hg.
   b. 60–100 mm Hg.
   c. 60–150 mm Hg.
   d. 50 mL/100 g/min.

Answers can be found in Appendix A.

Intracranial Hypertension

- Intracranial hypertension (IH) occurs with a sustained increase in ICP above 20–25 mm Hg. It develops from expanding tissue or a fluid mass that causes cerebral edema. Often, multiple factors are responsible for the development of IH.
- When ICP exceeds 30 mm Hg, CBF progressively decreases. Ischemia produces brain edema, which in turn increases ICP, further precipitating ischemia.

- When ICP exceeds 40–50 mm Hg, decreased cerebral perfusion causes progressive neurologic damage and/or cerebral herniation.
- *Monro-Kellie hypothesis:* The brain is enclosed within the cranium, a rigid structure that is not expandable. Thus, any increase in intracranial volume produces an accompanying increase in ICP. The intracranial space is occupied by three constituent compartments: the brain (80%), blood volume 10%, and CSF volume (10%). If ICP is to remain constant during increased cerebral mass, compensatory changes occur: (1) Cerebral blood volume (CBV) decreases as a result of compression of veins that shunt blood to venous sinuses and into central circulation, and (2) there is increased reabsorption and decreased production of CSF.
- As intracranial volume initially increases, ICP does not increase dramatically, primarily because there is space within the cranium to accommodate the increased mass. However, when intracranial mass has expanded to the point that there is limited space within the cranium, small increases in intracranial volume rapidly and dramatically increase ICP (Fig. 3.32). It is at this point that patients have significant signs and symptoms associated with increased ICP. The result of extreme and sustained increases in ICP is cerebral herniation.

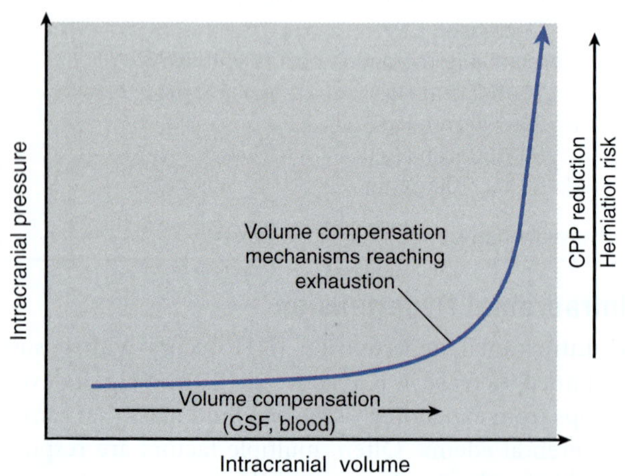

Fig. 3.32 The intracranial pressure–volume relationship. *CPP,* Cerebral perfusion pressure; *CSF,* cerebrospinal fluid. (From Miller RD, et al, editors. *Miller's Anesthesia.* 8th ed. Elsevier; 2015:2160.)

Etiology

- Increased tissue mass
  - Cerebral edema (traumatic brain injury [TBI], surgical trauma)
  - Tumor
  - Abscess
  - Hematoma (epidural, subdural, intracerebral)
- Altered CSF volume
  - Hydrocephalus
  - Decreased reabsorption of CSF (congenital obstruction of CSF outflow)
  - Increased production of CSF (choroid plexus disease)
- Vascular and/or metabolic alterations
  - Decreased venous outflow (superior vena cava syndrome)
  - Altered cerebral autoregulation
    - Hypertensive crises
    - Fluid overload (transurethral resection of the prostate)
    - Syndrome of inappropriate antidiuretic hormone secretion

Signs and Symptoms Associated With Increased ICP

From initial (mild) to progressive (severe), reflecting moderate to high increases in ICP:

- Headache
- Nausea and vomiting
- Papilledema
- Pupillary dilation
- Focal neurologic deficits
- Altered ventilatory function
- Altered hemodynamic function
- Decreased consciousness
- Seizures
- Coma
- *Cushing's response or reflex* is associated with a triad of symptoms. It is a late sign of exceedingly high ICP. The restriction of cerebral flow results in massive SNS stimulation. Signs include hypertension, irregular respirations, and bradycardia. Cushing's triad precedes cerebral herniation.

Treatment

- Treatment of definitive causative disease process: Remove tumor/abscess; stop intracranial hemorrhage (interventional radiology).

- Additional treatments are aimed at the following:
  - Decreasing CBV and CSF volume
  - Decreasing $CMRO_2$
- Treatment for IH:
  - *CBF*: Ensure SBP > 100 mm Hg, MAP ≥ 60 mm Hg, CPP > 60 mm Hg, CVP 5–10 mm Hg to maximize perfusion.
  - Patient's head of bed 15 degrees to maintain venous drainage
  - *Temperature:* $CMRO_2$ decreases 7% for each 1°C decrease.
  - *Ventilation:* Mild to moderate IH: controlled hypocapnia ($Paco_2$ 35–40 mm Hg). Severe IH: controlled hypocarbia ($Paco_2$ ≤ 30 mm Hg). CBF decreases by 4% for every 1-mm Hg decrease in $Paco_2$. The effect of hyperventilation is temporary because bicarbonate excretion through renal compensation allows for normalization of pH within 2 days. Poor outcomes are associated with IH and prolonged periods of hypocarbia.
  - Minimize PEEP to ≤5 mm Hg to maximize cerebral venous drainage.
  - Medication-induced coma to decrease $CMRO_2$
  - Hyperosmolar therapy (mannitol, hypertonic saline) to decrease brain parenchyma volume and vasogenic edema.
  - Diuretic therapy (furosemide) to decrease blood volume
  - CSF drainage via intraventricular catheter for ICP > 20 mm Hg
  - Decompressive craniectomy

Anesthetic Considerations

- Avoid movement of cervical spine during intubation: manual inline axial stabilization.
- Specialized monitoring: arterial line, CVP, possibly ICP
- Inhalational anesthetic agents:
  - All decrease $CMRO_2$.
  - All increase ICP in a dose-dependent manner as a result of cerebral vascular dilation, resulting in increased CBF.
  - It is recommended to administer ≤1 MAC.
  - The use of nitrous oxide is contraindicated because of the potential for expansion of air, causing or exacerbating a pneumocephalus.
- With the exception of ketamine, other IV anesthetic medications decrease $CMRO_2$. As a result, vasoconstriction causes decreased CBF, CPP, and ICP in a dose-dependent manner (Table 3.23).

KNOWLEDGE CHECK

1. Which change in cerebral physiology is associated with inhalation agents? *(Select all that apply.)*
   a. Decreased $CMRO_2$
   b. Decreased CBF CPP
   c. Increased ICP
   d. Cerebrovascular constriction
2. Which sympathetic response is consistent with the following signs for a patient with IH: BP 186/110 mm Hg, heart rate 42, spontaneous/irregular respirations, and widening pulse pressure?
   a. Beck's triad
   b. Celiac reflex
   c. Oculocardiac reflex
   d. Cushing's response
3. Which is an intervention that may improve neurologic outcomes after severe IH? *(Select all that apply.)*
   a. Episodic hyperventilation
   b. Sevoflurane >1 MAC
   c. Hyperthermia
   d. Head of bed at 10-degree elevation
   e. CPP >60 mm Hg
4. Which are the anatomic components of the Monro-Kellie hypothesis?
   a. Brain tissue, intraparenchymal fluid, CBV
   b. Brain tissue, cerebrospinal fluid, amygdala
   c. Brain tissue, CBV, cerebrospinal fluid
   d. Brain tissue, cerebral ventricles, infratentorial structures

Answers can be found in Appendix A.

Seizures

A seizure is a sudden onset of excessive cerebral neuronal activity resulting in an altered level of conscious and/or tonic-clonic muscular activity.

Etiology

Epilepsy

Eclampsia

Metabolic

- Hypoglycemia
- Hypoxia
- Hyperosmolar nonketotic hyperglycemia
- Hyperthermia (e.g., febrile seizures)
- Dehydration
- Uremia

TABLE 3.23 Effects of Anesthetics on Cerebral Hemodynamics

Drug	Cerebral Blood Flow	$CMRO_2$	Intracranial Pressure	Cerebral Perfusion Pressure
Inhalation				
Nitrous oxide	↑	↑↓	0/↓	↓
Sevoflurane	↑	↓	↑	↓
Isoflurane	↑	↓	↑	↓
Desflurane	↑	↓	↑	↓
IV				
Barbiturates	↓↓	↓↓	↓↓	0/↓
Etomidate	↓↓	↓↓	↓	0
Propofol	↓	↓	↓	↓
Ketamine	↑	↑	↑↑	↓
Benzodiazepines	↓	↓	↓	0/↓
Dexmedetomidine	↓	0/↓	0	0/↓
Morphine	0/↓	0/↓	↓	↑↓
Fentanyl	0/↓	0/↓	↓	0/↓
Alfentanil	0/↓	0/↓	↓	↓
Sufentanil	0/↓	0/↓	↓	↓
Remifentanil	0/↓	0/↓	↓	↓

CMRO2, Cerebral metabolic rate of oxygen; *IV,* intravenous.
From Zaglaniczny KL, Aker J, eds. *Clinical Guide to Pediatric Anesthesia.* Saunders; 1999; Sakabe T, Matsumoto M. Effects of anesthetic agents and other drugs on cerebral blood flow, metabolism, and intracranial pressure. In Cottrell JE, Young WL, eds. *Cottrell and Young's Neuroanesthesia.* 5th ed. Elsevier; 2010:78–94.

- Porphyria
- Electrolyte disorder
  - Hypocalcemia
  - Hyponatremia (e.g., transurethral resection of prostate syndrome)
  - Hypomagnesemia

Intracranial

- Hemorrhagic/ischemic stroke
- Increased ICP
- Uncontrolled hypertension
- Neurotrauma
- Mass lesion
- Meningitis
- Abscess

Medications/Drug Misuse

- Omission of antiseizure medication
- Withdrawal from medication (e.g., antipsychotics, antidepressants)
- Acute alcohol withdrawal
- Sympathomimetic drug withdrawal (e.g., methamphetamines)
- Medication toxicity
  - Local anesthetics
  - Meperidine (metabolite: normeperidine toxicity)
  - Atracurium/cisatracurium (metabolite: laudanosine toxicity)

Signs and Symptoms

- *Status epilepticus:* A convulsive or nonconvulsive seizure that lasts for ≥5 minutes or two or more seizures within a 5-minute period. There is a continued loss of consciousness after the seizure has stopped.
- *Focal (partial) seizures:* Begin in a single hemisphere, and approximately 60% progress to a generalized seizure. Frequently preceded by an "aura": sensory, autonomic, visual, and olfactory sensations.
- *Generalized seizures:* Rapid onset and involve loss of consciousness. Various types and their characteristics are presented in Table 3.24.
- *Postictal phase:* After the seizure has stopped and the patient regains consciousness, the patient exhibits a period of mental confusion hallmarked by difficulty speaking, slurred speech, headache, and generalized

TABLE 3.24 Types of Seizures

Type	Features	Duration
Generalized: Loss of consciousness		
Absence (petit mal)	Momentary loss of consciousness	Seconds
	Blank stare, cessation of activity	
	Eye blinking, lip smacking may occur	
	May lose muscle tone	
Tonic-clonic (grand mal)	May be preceded by an aura and a cry from forced expiration	3–5 minutes
	Loss of consciousness	
	Symmetrical tonic-clonic extremity movements	
	May experience apnea with cyanosis until tonic phase ends	
	May bite tongue, may be incontinent	
	Postictal fatigue, muscle soreness, confusion, lethargy, and/or headache	
Myoclonic	Short, abrupt muscle contractions of arms, legs, and torso	Seconds
	Contractions may be symmetric or asymmetric	
Clonic	Muscle contraction and relaxation but slower than with myoclonic seizure	Several minutes
Tonic	Abrupt increase in muscle tone of torso and face	Seconds
	Flexion of arms; extension of legs	
Atonic	Abrupt loss of muscle tone	Seconds
	May cause falling and injuries related to fall	
Partial: Focal at onset but may evolve into a generalized seizure		
Simple partial	Consciousness not impaired	Seconds to minutes
	Abnormal unilateral movement of arm, leg, or both	
	Patient may sense abnormal smell, sound, or sensation, such as numbness, tingling, or burning	
	Tachycardia or bradycardia, tachypnea, skin flushing, epigastric discomfort	
Complex partial	Loss of consciousness, but eyes may be open	Minutes
	Lip smacking, chewing, picking at clothing	
	Mumbling, speaking in repetitive phrases	
	Posturing or jerking movements	
	Postictal confusion, amnesia common	

confusion. The postictal phase can range from minutes to hours in duration.

Treatment

If seizures are tonic-clonic, protect patient from injury, treat acute seizure activity, and provide airway management as needed. Treat a potential definite cause (e.g., hypoglycemia-dextrose IV 10–25 g [20–50 mL 50% solution]) (Table 3.25).

Initial medication: benzodiazepine

- Lorazepam (Ativan)
- Midazolam (Versed)

Medications to prevent additional seizure activity

- Phenytoin (Dilantin)
- Fosphenytoin (Cerebyx)
- Phenobarbital
- Levetiracetam (Keppra)
- Lacosamide (Vimpat)

TABLE 3.25 **Anticonvulsant Drugs**

Drug	IV Dosage	Time to Stop Seizure/Duration of Anticonvulsant Effect	Adverse Effects
Lorazepam (Ativan)	0.1 mg/kg IV (not to exceed 8 mg/kg IV) at a rate no faster than 2 mg/min	6–10 minutes/12–24 hours	• Respiratory depression • Tachycardia • Hypotension • Dysrhythmias
Midazolam (Versed)	0.2 mg/kg IV	1–3 minutes/30 minutes	• Respiratory depression • Tachycardia • Hypotension • Dysrhythmias
Phenytoin sodium (Dilantin)	10–20 mg/kg IV at a rate no faster than 50 mg/min; must be mixed in saline	30 minutes/24 hours	• Hypotension • Dysrhythmias; blocks • Hepatitis • Nephritis • Blood dyscrasias
Fosphenytoin (Cerebyx)	15–20 mg/kg IV phenytoin equivalent (PE) at a rate no faster than 150 mg/min; may be administered intramuscularly	15 minutes/24 hours	• Hypotension (less risk than phenytoin) • Dysrhythmias (less risk than phenytoin) • Nephritis • Blood dyscrasias
Phenobarbital (phenobarbital sodium; Luminal)	20 mg/kg IV at a rate no faster than 50 mg/min (not actively seizing) or 100 mg/min (actively seizing)	20–30 minutes/48 hours	• Respiratory depression • Hypotension • Angioedema • Thrombophlebitis
Levetiracetam (Keppra)	500–1500 mg over 15 minutes; must be diluted	15–30 minutes/6–30 hours	• Somnolence • Dizziness, vertigo • Vomiting, diarrhea • Irritability
Lacosamide (Vimpat)	200–400 mg over 30–60 minutes	1–4 hours/13 hours	• Dizziness • Ataxia • Diplopia • Cardiac rhythm and conduction abnormalities

IV, Intravenous.

Medications for refractory status epilepticus

- Valproic acid
- Propofol (Diprivan)
- Inhalational anesthetics

Anesthetic Considerations

- In patients with a known seizure disorder, ensure therapeutic blood levels of antiseizure medications.
- Continue antiseizure medications until the time of surgery and then postoperatively.
- Avoid medications that decrease seizure threshold:
  - Etomidate
  - Ketamine
- Avoid medications with metabolites that induce seizure activity:
  - Atracurium/cisatracurium—laudanosine
  - Meperidine (Demerol)—normeperidine

- Antiseizure medications (phenytoin) cause enzyme induction, resulting in increased hepatic degradation of opioids and neuromuscular blocking drugs.

KNOWLEDGE CHECK

1. Which medication has the potential to cause seizures? *(Select all that apply.)*
   a. Lidocaine
   b. Rocuronium
   c. Remifentanil
   d. Meperidine
2. Which medication is considered a first-line treatment for an active tonic-clonic seizure?
   a. Etomidate
   b. Ketamine
   c. Midazolam
   d. Fosphenytoin
3. Which medication can increase ICP caused by increased CBF?
   a. Zofran
   b. Decadron
   c. Ketamine
   d. Propofol

Answers can be found in Appendix A.

Cerebrovascular Accident

- For every 1 million people, 1600 will have a stroke each year, and 55% will survive for 6 months.
- Annually, there are 500,000 hospitalizations and 150,000 deaths caused by CVA in the United States.
- Patients with cardiovascular and/or neurovascular disease are at increased risk of perioperative CVA. A perioperative CVA is associated with an eight times greater risk of death within 30 days postprocedure.

Etiology

Hemorrhagic cerebrovascular accident. Impaired CBF due to vasculature rupture (accounts for approximately 8%–12% of all CVAs)

- Subarachnoid hemorrhage into the subarachnoid space
- Intracerebral
  - Intraparenchymal (hemorrhage within brain tissue)
  - Intraventricular (hemorrhage within cerebral ventricles)

Ischemic cerebrovascular accident. Impaired CBF due to intravascular thrombosis or embolism (accounts for approximately 80%–90% of CVAs)

- Thrombosis
- Embolism
- Systemic hypotension

Transient ischemic attack

- Typical duration is several minutes.
- Etiology: temporary disruption of CBF caused by microemboli
- Referred to as *ministrokes*, the incidence of CVA after TIA is 50%. Approximately one-third of patients will have a CVA within 1 year.

Risk Factors Associated With Cerebrovascular Accident

- Advanced age
- Angiopathology (e.g., smoking, diabetes, hypertension, hypercoagulability, hyperlipidemia, coronary artery disease, family history)
- Dysrhythmias (e.g., AF)
- Valvular heart disease
- Arteriovenous malformation
- Traumatic head injury

Signs and Symptoms

- *"FAST"*: facial droop, arm weakness, speech difficulties, time (time to definitive treatment is critical)
- Headache
- Dizziness
- Syncope
- Aphasia
- Diplopia
- Blurred vision
- Hemiplegia
- Irregular respirations
- Seizures
- Loss of consciousness

Treatment

Hemorrhagic cerebrovascular accident (assuming loss of consciousness)

- Airway management/ventilation to protect from aspiration and maintain Spo_2 >95%
- Expert consultation
- Sedation

TABLE 3.26 Guidelines for Blood Pressure Management in Common Neurologic Conditions

Diagnosis	Recommendation
Acute ischemic stroke	Keep <180/110 mm Hg if thrombolysis; treat only BP >220/120 mm Hg if no thrombolysis
Intracerebral hemorrhage	Keep SBP <180 mm Hg and MAP <30 mm Hg (ideal SBP <160 and MAP <110 mm Hg)
Subarachnoid hemorrhage	Keep SBP <160 mm Hg before aneurysm treated; do not lower BP after aneurysm treated
Traumatic brain injury	Keep MAP to maintain CPP >60 mm Hg

BP, Blood pressure; *CPP*, cerebral perfusion pressure; *MAP*, mean arterial pressure; *SBP*, systolic blood pressure.
Modified from Rabinstein AA, Fugate JE. Principles of neurointensive care. In Daroff RB, Jankovic J, Mazziotta JC, Pomeroy SL, editors. *Bradley's Neurology in Clinical Practice*. 7th ed. Elsevier; 2016:742–757.

- BP management (Table 3.26)
  - Hypertension increases the potential for rebleeding (most common).
    - Calcium channel blocker: Nicardipine
    - α-/β-blockade: Labetalol
    - Direct vasodilator: Nitrates/hydralazine
  - Hypotension further decreases CBF and oxygenation.
    - Phenylephrine
- Maintain blood glucose < 200 mg/dL.
- Treat/prevent cerebral artery vasospasm.
  - Nimodipine
- Surgical intervention
  - Aneurysm
- Clipping, ligation, endovascular: Coil/intravascular balloon
  - Arteriovenous malformation
- Excision, glue or bead embolization

Ischemic CVA (assuming loss of consciousness)

- See previously described treatment for hemorrhagic stroke.
- If a hemorrhagic etiology is excluded on the basis of brain computed tomography, tissue plasminogen activator is administered within 1 hour in-hospital time and 3 hours from initial symptoms (Box 3.9).

BOX 3.9 Absolute Contraindications to Tissue Plasminogen Activator Administration

- Subarachnoid hemorrhage
- Acute head injury or CVA within previous 3 months
- Active bleeding
- Prior intracranial hemorrhage
- Arterial puncture within previous 3 months
- Hypertension: SBP >185 mm Hg or DBP >110 mm Hg
- Platelet count <100,000/mm^3
- Heparin administration within 48 hours with elevated aPTT
- Hypoglycemia: blood glucose <50 mg/dL
- Use of anticoagulants with evidence of increased coagulation test values
- Multilobar cerebral infarction

aPTT, Activated partial thromboplastin time; *CVA*, cerebrovascular accident; *DBP*, diastolic blood pressure; *SBP*, systolic blood pressure.

Anesthetic Considerations

Ventilation

- Titrate FiO_2 to maintain SpO_2 ≥90%.
- Avoid hypocarbia unless ICP from hemorrhagic CVA is greatly increased.
  - Hypocarbia decreases CBF, which decreases CBV and decreases ICP. However, by decreasing CBF, cerebral ischemia can occur.
  - Profound hypercarbia increases CBF and ICP.

Pharmacology. With increased ICP:

- Inhaled agents should be maintained at ≤1 MAC because they increase CBF and ICP.
- Ketamine should be avoided.
- Fasciculations caused by succinylcholine cause transient increases in ICP. If succinylcholine is to be used, consider a defasciculating dose of a nondepolarizing muscle relaxant.
- If evacuation of a cerebral hematoma via craniotomy is required, avoid nitrous oxide because of the potential for pneumocephalus and/or venous air embolus. Additionally, nitrous oxide may increase CBF and $CMRO_2$.
- Consider administration of an antiseizure medication for increased ICP and craniotomy.

Fluids

- Restrictive fluid administration is warranted unless severe hypotension from hypovolemia (e.g., massive hemorrhage) is present.
- Isotonic crystalloid such as normal saline is appropriate.
- Mannitol, an osmotic diuretic, redistributes fluid from tissues into the intravascular space. It may also decrease organ injury as a free radical scavenger. The diuretic effect associated with mannitol causes diuresis and potentially hypotension.

Blood glucose

- Blood glucose should be monitored and treated with insulin for levels >200 g/dL.

Temperature

- Avoid hyperthermia because it increases $CMRO_2$.

KNOWLEDGE CHECK

1. Which is a sign or symptom associated with acute CVA? *(Select all that apply.)*
   a. Facial droop
   b. Trousseau's sign
   c. Diplopia
   d. Hypertension
   e. Aphasia
2. Which is the *ideal* BP after intracerebral hemorrhage?
   a. <180/100 mm Hg
   b. <100/60 mm Hg
   c. <140/90 mm Hg
   d. <160/90 mm Hg
3. Which effect does hypocarbia have on CBF?
   a. Decreases
   b. Increases
   c. Remains unchanged
4. Which is true regarding increased ICP after hemorrhagic CVA?
   a. Isoflurane should be administered at <1.3 MAC.
   b. Ketamine can be safely administered in small doses.
   c. Vecuronium 0.01 mg/kg should be administered if succinylcholine is used.
   d. Deliberate hypotension should be employed.

Answers can be found in Appendix A.

Traumatic Brain Injury

- TBI is a contributory factor in up to 50% of deaths resulting from trauma.
- It is estimated that 10%–40% of patients with TBI have other associated injuries (e.g., cervical spine, thoracic/intraabdominal, skeletal fractures).
- Systemic factors such as hypoxemia, hypercapnia, and hypotension contribute to mortality.
- Sustained increases in ICP of approximately 60 mm Hg result in irreversible brain edema.

Etiology

Primary causes of TBI:

- Falls 35%
- Struck by/against object 17%
- Motor vehicle–related 17%
- Unknown 12%
- Assault 10%
- Other 9%

Signs and Symptoms

- The Glasgow Coma Scale (GCS) assesses the degree of consciousness of a patient.
- GCS is scored in three domains:
  1. **Verbal response**
     - None = 1
     - Sounds = 2
     - Inappropriate words = 3
     - Confused speech = 4
     - Appropriate = 5
  2. **Eye opening**
     - None = 1
     - Opens to pain = 2
     - Opens to voice = 3
     - Spontaneous = 4
  3. **Motor response to painful stimuli**
     - None = 1
     - Extends extremities = 2
     - Flexes extremities = 3
     - Withdraws extremities = 4
     - Localizes with extremities = 5
     - Obeys commands = 6
- Severe injury, GCS <8
- Moderate injury, GCS 9–12
- Minor injury, GCS ≥13
- Cushing's triad (hypertension, bradycardia, irregular respirations)
- Airway management to prevent hypoxia and aspiration common with GCS <8

Treatment

- Emergency therapy for TBI should begin before hospital admission because a large proportion of deaths occur in the prehospital phase.

- Prevention of secondary brain injury resulting from the following:
  - Increased ICP from worsening cerebral edema and/or hemorrhage
  - Hypoxia
  - Hyper-/hypocapnia
  - Hypotension
  - Anemia
  - Hyperthermia
  - Hyper-/hypoglycemia
  - Acidosis
  - Cerebral artery vasospasm
  - SIRS
- Diabetes insipidus

Airway management

- As many as 70% of patients with TBI have concurrent hypoxemia.
- Airway obstruction, inadequate ventilation, and vomiting/aspiration resulting in hypoxia commonly occur with moderate to severe TBI. Airway management is warranted.
- Cervical spine injury occurs in approximately 10% of patients with TBI.
- Airway management must occur with the patient's head in a neutral position using inline manual axial stabilization.
- A rapid sequence induction with cricoid pressure is required.
- Video laryngoscopy or fiberoptic-assisted intubation as standby equipment or as initial intubation attempt is appropriate.
- Nasal intubation should be avoided in the presence of suspected basilar skull fracture, bleeding diathesis, suspected upper airway foreign body, or facial fractures.

Anesthetic Considerations

- See previous section on treatment for hemorrhagic CVA (Box 3.10).

BOX 3.10 Management of Increased Intracranial Pressure

- Secure the airway; ventilate with 100% O_2.
- Determine whether problem is hemorrhagic or occlusive (see text).
- *Hemorrhagic:* Immediate heparin reversal (1 mg protamine for each 50–100 units of heparin given) and low normal mean arterial pressure
- *Occlusive:* Deliberate hypertension, titrated to neurologic examination, angiography, or physiologic imaging studies or to clinical context
- Head up 15 degrees in neutral position, if possible
- $Paco_2$, manipulation consistent with clinical setting, otherwise normocapnia
- Mannitol 0.5 g/kg, rapid IV infusion
- Titrate IV agent to electroencephalogram burst suppression
- Passive cooling to 33°C–34°C
- Consider ventriculostomy for treatment or monitoring of increased ICP.
- Consider anticonvulsants (e.g., phenytoin or propofol).

ICP, Intracranial pressure; *IV,* intravenous; *$Paco_2$,* partial pressure of arterial carbon dioxide.

Autonomic Hyperreflexia

Etiology

- Associated with patients who have an existing SCI; 85% of episodes occur when the SCI is above T6.
- Autonomic hyperreflexia (AH) has occurred in patients with SCIs as low as T10.
- May occur weeks to years after an SCI that resulted in neurogenic shock.
- *Mechanism for AH:* Noxious cutaneous or visceral (most commonly bladder distention and/or fecal impaction) stimulation below the level of the SCI creates nerve impulses that are transmitted to the spinal cord. This results in an exaggerated SNS response, causing hypertension. The hypertension initiates the baroreceptor response, potentially causing bradycardia. If the spinal cord were intact, parasympathetic nervous system activation (baroreceptor response) would result in vasodilation and decreased BP. However, because of the SCI, this vasodilatory response does not occur, and potentially life-threatening hypertension persists.

Signs and Symptoms

- Extreme hypertension resulting in bradycardia
- Dysrhythmias
- Headache
- Blurred vision
- Cerebral hemorrhage
- Pupillary constriction

KNOWLEDGE CHECK

1. Which three categories are components of the GCS?
   a. Verbal response, eye opening, motor response
   b. Eye opening, hemodynamic stability, pupillary reactivity
   c. Oxygen saturation, respiratory rate, MAP
   d. Respiratory rate, Cushing's triad, verbal response
2. A GCS score of 7 is suggestive of
   a. mild injury.
   b. moderate injury.
   c. severe injury.
3. Which airway management technique is warranted for a patient involved in a motor vehicle crash with a GCS score of 3?
   a. Video laryngoscopy
   b. Inline manual axial stabilization
   c. Fiberoptic intubation
   d. Nasal intubation
4. Which medication is *contraindicated* for a patient with increased ICP?
   a. Fentanyl
   b. Dexmedetomidine
   c. Ketamine
   d. Midazolam

Answers can be found in Appendix A.

- Nasal stuffiness
- Pulmonary edema
- Above the level of the SCI: flushing from vasodilation (PNS response)
- Below the level of the SCI: pale and cool skin from vasoconstriction (SNS response)

Treatment

- Remove the stimulus: bladder catheterization or fecal disimpaction.
- For severe, persistent hypertension:
  - Vasodilators: Clonidine, hydralazine, nitroglycerin, nitroprusside
  - Ganglionic blockers: Phentolamine, trimethaphan

Anesthetic Considerations

- *Goal:* Prevent/inhibit SNS stimulation
- Deep plane: General anesthesia
- Neuraxial anesthesia
  - Spinal
  - Epidural: May be less effective than spinal anesthesia because of sacral nerve sparing
- Regional anesthesia
- May occur during the postoperative period

KNOWLEDGE CHECK

1. AH is most likely to occur with an SCI above
   a. T5.
   b. T6.
   c. T7.
   d. S2.
2. Which sign is associated with AH?
   a. Flushing from vasodilation below the level of the SCI
   b. Peaked T waves on ECG
   c. Bradycardia
   d. Circumoral numbness
3. Which stimulus most often causes AH to occur?
   a. Increased intravascular volume
   b. Bladder distention
   c. Extreme hypertension
   d. Baroreceptor activation
4. Which anesthetic technique can allow AH to occur as a result of sacral nerve sparing?
   a. Epidural anesthesia
   b. Deep general anesthesia
   c. Spinal anesthesia
   d. Regional anesthesia

Answers can be found in Appendix A.

Postoperative Visual Loss

Etiology

- Postoperative visual loss (POVL) is an uncommon but devastating complication associated with nonophthalmologic surgery.
- It may occur in one or both eyes
- The result can range from decreased visual acuity to complete blindness (Box 3.11).
- Five distinct causes of POVL:
  1. Ischemic optic neuropathy (ION)
     - Anterior ION
     - Posterior ION
  2. Central retinal artery occlusion (CRAO)
  3. Central retinal vein occlusion
  4. Cortical blindness
  5. Glycine toxicity
- Patient positioning may be a contributing factor for ION and CRAO.
- Greater association in prone spinal operations, steep Trendelenburg position, cardiopulmonary bypass surgery, and head and neck procedures

BOX 3.11 Perioperative Blindness

- Providers should consider informing patients who are having spinal surgery in the prone position with prolonged duration and/or substantial blood loss that they have a small but unpredictable risk of perioperative visual loss (POVL).
- POVL can be caused by direct pressure on the globe, resulting in central retinal artery occlusion (CRAO).
- Ischemic optic neuropathy (ION) is the most common cause of POVL associated with prone spinal surgery procedures.
- Factors that significantly and independently increase the risk of ION associated with spine surgery in the prone position include male sex, obesity, use of Wilson frame, longer surgical duration, larger blood loss, and a lower percentage of colloid in the nonblood fluid administration.
- Risk reduction strategies include the following:
  - Avoid the horseshoe headrest, which has a small margin of error, or any headrest that does not allow adequate assessment of the eyes during the procedure.
    - Avoid direct pressure on the eyes.
  - Perform and document periodic eye checks throughout the perioperative period.
  - Minimize venous pressure and congestion in the head.
  - Minimize bleeding.
    - Avoid coagulopathy
    - Modify surgical technique
  - Decrease the duration of the prone position.
    - Stage prolonged procedures if possible.
  - Avoid significant hemodynamic changes as much as possible.
    - Closely monitor blood pressure.
    - Monitor hemoglobin and hematocrit periodically throughout surgery.
    - Use colloid along with crystalloid for nonblood fluid resuscitation.
    - Resume normotension after turning patient supine unless medically contraindicated.
    - Keep the head in a neutral position at or above the heart level.
    - Avoid using the Wilson frame if possible.
    - Assess patient vision when the patient becomes alert.
    - An urgent ophthalmologic consultation should be obtained if there is concern for postoperative visual loss.
- Prognosis is poor for POVL due to ION and CRAO and usually results in permanent visual loss.
  - Consider magnetic resonance imaging to rule out intracranial causes of visual loss.
  - Antiplatelet agents, steroids, or medications to decrease intraocular pressure have not been shown to be effective for treatment of perioperative ION.
  - Hyperbaric oxygen therapy treatment has been proposed for CRAO, with the highest chance of significant improvement in visual acuity resulting when treatment is started within 6 hours of the onset of symptoms.

Modified from American Society of Anesthesiologists Task Force on Perioperative Visual Loss. Practice advisory for perioperative visual loss associated with spine surgery: an updated report by the American Society of Anesthesiologists Task Force on Perioperative Visual Loss. *Anesthesiology*. 2012;116:274–278; Kla KM, Lee LA. Perioperative visual loss. *Best Pract Res Clin Anaesthesiol*. 2016;30:69–77.

- POVL may occur in any patient. There is a higher incidence in males, anemia, blood loss greater than 1 L, surgery lasting over 5 hours, diabetes, hypertension, vascular disease, open-angle glaucoma, sickle cell disease, smoking, obesity, intraoperative hypotension, steep Trendelenburg, and prone positioning.
- According to the American Society of Anesthesiologists Postoperative Visual Loss Registry, ION and CRAO accounted for 81% of all cases, with ION accounting for 89% of POVL after prone spinal procedures.

Anesthetic Considerations

- Because the causes resulting in ION are not fully understood, there are no scientific guidelines for instances that increase the risk (e.g., degree of hypotension, hemoglobin level).
- Interventions are used to decrease intraocular pressure and increase/maintain optic nerve perfusion. Avoid periods of the following:
  - Extreme hypotension (decreased optic nerve perfusion)
  - Hemorrhage associated with significant anemia (decreased optic nerve perfusion)
  - Fluid overload (optic nerve edema and decreased optic nerve perfusion)
  - Increased venous pressure (e.g., steep Trendelenburg position, prone position with excessive pressure on the abdomen; decreased optic nerve perfusion)

- Direct ocular pressure (increased intraocular pressure and decreased optic nerve perfusion)
- *Prone positioning:* Head should be in a neutral position while avoiding flexion to decrease edema formation. Pressure on the eye(s) should be assessed, and documentation of the assessment should occur every 15 minutes.

KNOWLEDGE CHECK

1. Which pathological states are associated with POVL? *(Select all that apply.)*
   a. Diabetes
   b. Hypertension
   c. Peripheral vascular disease
   d. Open-angle glaucoma
   e. Sickle cell disease
   f. Obesity
2. Which factor increases the possibility of POVL? *(Select all that apply.)*
   a. Hypervolemia
   b. Hemoglobin 13.8 g/dL
   c. Head flexion during prone positioning
   d. MAP 58 mm Hg
   e. Direct ocular pressure
   f. Surgical procedure 1.5 hours in duration

Answers can be found in Appendix A.

Peripheral Nerve Injuries

Etiology

- *Transection:* Partial or complete destruction (e.g., inadvertent surgical resection of a peripheral nerve)
- *Compression:* Pressure on nerve from bony prominence pressing against an internal (e.g., cervical plexus is compressed by stenotic interlaminar space from arthritis) or external surface (e.g., ulnar nerve compression with arms supinated)
- *Traction:* Stretching of a nerve against immobile surface (e.g., femoral nerve stretching under the inguinal ligament when the thighs are flexed on the abdomen, as in the exaggerated lithotomy position)
- The mechanism associated with peripheral nerve injury
  - *Ischemia* associated with compression, traction, and/or edema formation
  - *Structural disruption* of one or more of the following: Axon (nerve fiber), endoneurium (connective tissue covering axons), perineurium (connective tissue covering nerve fascicles), epineurium (connective tissue covering external surface of the nerve)
  - *Transection:* Complete or partial destruction of axons (Box 3.12)

Signs and Symptoms

- *Algesia:* Increased sensitivity to pain
- *Algogenic:* Pain producing
- *Allodynia:* A normally nonharmful stimulus is perceived as painful.
- *Analgesia:* Absence of pain in the presence of a normally painful stimulus
- *Dysesthesia:* Unpleasant, painful, abnormal sensation, whether evoked or spontaneous

BOX 3.12 Factors Associated With Position-Related Injuries

Positioning Devices
- Table straps
- Leg holders and stirrups
- Axillary roll
- Bolsters
- Fracture table post
- Shoulder braces
- Positioning frames
- Headrests

Length of Procedure
- Longer than 4 hours

Body Habitus
- Obesity
- Malnutrition
- Bulky musculature

Preexisting Pathophysiology
- Anemia
- Diabetes mellitus
- Peripheral vascular disease
- Liver disease
- Peripheral neuropathies
- Alcoholism
- Limited joint mobility
- Smoking

Anesthetic Technique
- General anesthesia
- Hypotension
- Neuromuscular blockade

- *Hyperalgesia:* Heightened response to a normally painful stimulus
- *Neuralgia:* Pain in the distribution of a peripheral nerve(s)
- *Neuropathy:* Abnormal disturbance in the function of a nerve(s)
- *Paresthesia:* Abnormal sensation, whether spontaneous or evoked

Anesthetic Considerations

Common nerve injuries, including etiology and prevention, are listed in Table 3.27.

TABLE 3.27 Common Nerve Injuries: Etiology and Prevention

Nerve/Nerve Group Injured	Potential Cause	Positioning Recommendation
Brachial plexus	*Supine, Trendelenburg, lithotomy*	
	Arm abducted more than 90 degrees on armboard	Do not abduct arm more than 90 degrees.
	Arm falls off table edge and is abducted and externally rotated.	Ensure arms are adequately secured.
	Arm abduction and lateral flexion of the head to the opposite side	Support head to maintain neutral alignment.
	Trendelenburg	
	Shoulder braces placed too medial or lateral	Place well-padded shoulder brace over the acromioclavicular joint.
		Avoid use if possible.
	Lateral	
	Thorax pressure exertion on dependent shoulder and axilla	Place roll caudad to the axilla supporting the upper part of the thorax.
	Prone	
	Arms abducted more than 90 degrees	Abduct arms minimally.
Ulnar nerve	Arm pronated on arm board	Supinate forearm on padded arm board.
	Arms folded across abdomen or chest with elbows flexed more than 90 degrees	Do not flex elbows more than 90 degrees.
	Arms secured at side with inadequate padding at the elbow	Place sufficient padding around elbow.
	Arms inadequately secured at side, elbows extend over table edge	Draw sheet should extend above the elbow and be tucked between the patient and the mattress.
Radial nerve or circumflex nerve	Arm pressed against vertical positioning or retractor post or pole securing ether screen	Place adequate padding between or ensure arm is not pressing against vertical posts or pole.
Suprascapular nerve	Patient in lateral position rolls semiprone onto dependent arm with shoulder circumduction	Stabilize patient in lateral position.
Sciatic nerve	Malnourished/emaciated patient supine or sitting on inadequately padded table	Generous soft padding under buttock
	Legs straight in sitting position	Flex table at knees
	Lithotomy	
	Legs externally rotated with knees extended	Minimal external rotation of legs; knees should be flexed

TABLE 3.27 Common Nerve Injuries: Etiology and Prevention—cont'd

Nerve/Nerve Group Injured	Potential Cause	Positioning Recommendation
Common peroneal nerve	*Lithotomy*	
	Fibular neck rests against vertical bar of lithotomy stirrup	Adequate padding between leg and stirrup
	Knees extended, legs externally rotated	Knees flexed with minimal external rotation
	Lateral	
	Undue pressure on downside leg	Padding under the fibular head
Posterior tibial nerve	*Lithotomy*	
	"Knee crutch" stirrups supporting posterior aspect of knees	Generous padding under knees
		Avoid use of this stirrup for prolonged procedures.
Saphenous nerve	*Lithotomy*	
	Foot suspended outside vertical bar, leg rests on bar	Sufficient padding between legs and vertical bar
	Excessive pressure on medial aspect of leg from "knee crutch" stirrups	Sufficient padding between stirrup and leg
Obturator nerve	*Lithotomy*	
	Excessive flexion of the thigh at hip	Minimal hip flexion
Pudendal nerve	Traction of legs against perineal post or orthopedic fracture table	Generous padding between perineum and post

Modified from American Society of Anesthesiologists Task Force on Prevention of Perioperative Peripheral Neuropathies. Practice advisory for the prevention of perioperative peripheral neuropathies: an updated report by the American Society of Anesthesiologists Task Force on Prevention of Perioperative Peripheral Neuropathies. *Anesthesiology.* 2011;114:741–754; Phillips N. *Berry and Kohn's Operating Room Technique.* 13th ed. Elsevier; 2017; Heizenroth PA. Positioning the patient for surgery. In: Rothrock JC, ed. *Alexander's Care of the Patient in Surgery.* 15th ed. Elsevier; 2015:155–185.

KNOWLEDGE CHECK

1. Which term is associated with a heightened response to a normally painful stimulus?
   a. Allodynia
   b. Dysesthesia
   c. Hyperalgesia
   d. Paresthesia
2. Which is a method to decrease common peroneal nerve injury? *(Select all that apply.)*
   a. Do not abduct arms >90 degrees.
   b. Minimal external rotation of the knees.
   c. Minimize hip flexion.
   d. Place padding under ankles.
3. Traction that contributes to a peripheral nerve injury is caused by
   a. stretching of a nerve against immobile surface.
   b. pressure on nerve from bony prominence pressing against an internal or external surface.
   c. partial or complete destruction.

Answers can be found in Appendix A.

Myasthenia Gravis Versus Lambert-Eaton Myasthenic Syndrome

Myasthenia Gravis

- Occurs in approximately 1 in every 40,000 adults
- Females between the ages of 20 and 30 years are most often affected (60%–70%).
- Onset for males/females equally between 60 and 70 years of age
- Patients younger than 16 years of age account for 10% of cases.
- Prevalence of myasthenia gravis (MG) worldwide is increasing.

Lambert-Eaton Myasthenic Syndrome (LEMS)

- Occurs in approximately 3 in every 1 million adults
- Most often occurring in males between 50 and 70 years of age
- Approximately 60% of patients who develop LEMS have an associated malignancy.
- The most common malignancy associated with LEMS is small cell or "oat cell" cancer of the lung.

Etiology

Myasthenia gravis

- *Cause:* Autoimmune disease
- Normal neuromuscular function: Acetylcholine is released and binds (stimulates) to postsynaptic acetylcholine receptors.
- Antiacetylcholine receptor antibodies destroy acetylcholine receptors.
- The result is decreased neuromuscular transmission due to *postsynaptic acetylcholine receptor destruction*, resulting in weakness.
- Exacerbations are caused by stress, infection, aminoglycoside antibiotics, procainamide, lithium, calcium channel blockers, and hypokalemia (diuretics).

Lambert-Eaton myasthenic syndrome

- *Cause:* Autoimmune disease
- Normal neuromuscular function: Calcium binds to presynaptic voltage-gated calcium channel end plates, resulting in acetylcholine release from presynaptic vesicles.
- Antibodies bind to *presynaptic voltage-gated calcium channel end plates*, which decreases the release of acetylcholine at the neuromuscular junction, resulting in weakness (Fig. 3.33).

Signs and Symptoms

Myasthenia gravis

- Hallmarked by generalized muscle weakness and rapid exhaustion of skeletal muscles with repetitive use, followed by partial recovery with rest
- Most common early-onset symptoms are ptosis and diplopia.
- Difficulties with chewing and swallowing
- Facial drooping
- Improvement in muscle strength with anticholinesterase drugs
- Respiratory muscle weakness is rare but occurs with severe MG.
- Myocarditis causing dysrhythmias

Lambert-Eaton myasthenic syndrome

- Hallmarked by proximal limb muscle and shoulder girdle weakness (legs affected more severely than arms)
- Ptosis
- Depressed deep tendon reflexes
- Dysphagia
- Respiratory muscle weakness is rare.
- ANS dysfunction (orthostatic hypotension, dry mouth, constipation, urinary retention)
- Exercise improves strength: Lambert's sign.
- No improvement in muscle strength with anticholinesterase drugs
- May also be associated with sarcoidosis, thyroiditis, or lupus

Treatment

Myasthenia gravis

- Anticholinesterase drug, most commonly pyridostigmine
- Thymectomy: Early thymectomy considered the treatment of choice
- Immunosuppression (IV immunoglobulins/steroids)
- Plasmapheresis

Lambert-Eaton myasthenic syndrome

- Removal, chemotherapy, and/or radiation of the malignancy
- Immunosuppression (IV immunoglobulins/steroids)
- 3,4-Diaminopyridine (stimulates the presynaptic release of acetylcholine by blocking potassium channels) (Table 3.28)
- Anticholinesterase drug, most commonly pyridostigmine

Anesthetic Considerations

Myasthenia gravis

- Assess the patient for disease control and medical treatment several days before surgery and again immediately before surgery.
- Avoid routine premedication with sedatives or opioids.
- If anticholinesterase medication is continued on the morning of surgery, consider cholinergic side effects (e.g., bradycardia, bronchospasm, excessive oral secretions).
- Consider pharyngeal muscle weakness, difficulty eliminating oral secretions, and the risk of pulmonary aspiration in the anesthesia plan of care.
- Opt for local or regional anesthesia if appropriate; in myasthenic parturients, neuraxial anesthesia is preferred for both cesarean and vaginal delivery.

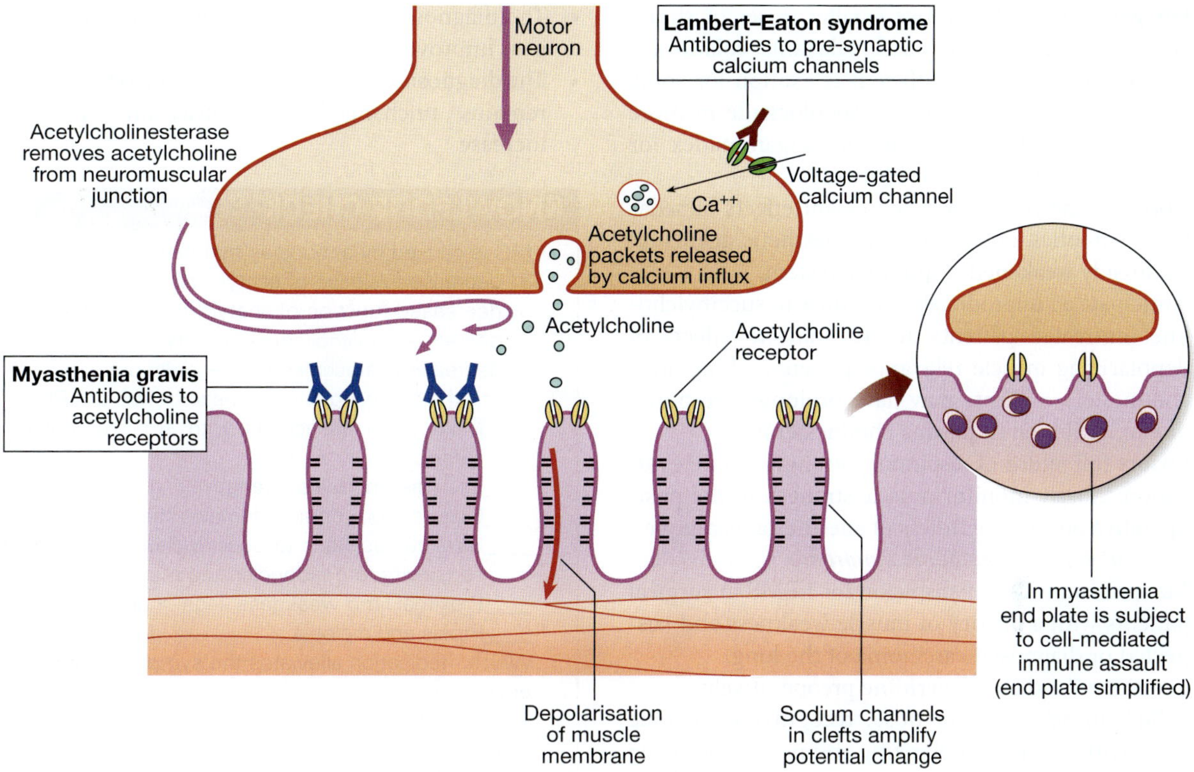

Fig. 3.33 Myasthenia gravis and Lambert-Eaton myasthenic syndrome (LEMS). In myasthenia, there are antibodies to the acetylcholine receptors on the postsynaptic membrane that block conduction across the neuromuscular junction (NMJ). Myasthenic symptoms can be transiently improved by inhibition of acetylcholinesterase (e.g., with Tensilon [edrophonium bromide]), which normally removes the acetylcholine. A cell-mediated immune response produces simplification of the postsynaptic membrane, further impairing the safety factor of neuromuscular conduction. In LEMS, antibodies to the presynaptic voltage calcium channels impair release of acetylcholine from the motor nerve ending; calcium is required for the acetylcholine-containing vesicle to fuse with the presynaptic membrane for release into the NMJ. (From Walker BR, Colledge NR, Ralston SH, Penman ID, editors. *Davidson's Principles and Practice of Medicine*. 22nd ed. Churchill Livingstone; 2014.)

TABLE 3.28 **Summary Comparison of Myasthenia Gravis and Lambert-Eaton Myasthenic Syndrome**

	Myasthenia Gravis	Lambert-Eaton Myasthenic Syndrome
Sex	Female > Male	Male > Female
Presenting symptoms	Extraocular, bulbar, and facial weakness	Proximal limb weakness (legs > arms)
Other symptoms	Fatigue on activity Reflexes normal	Increased strength on activity precedes, reflexes reduced or absent
Response to neuromuscular blocking drugs	Possible resistance to depolarizing neuromuscular blockers Sensitive to nondepolarizing neuromuscular blockers	Sensitive to both depolarizing and nondepolarizing neuromuscular blockers
Pathologic state	Thymoma present in 20%–25% of patients	Small cell AKA oat cell bronchogenic carcinoma

- For general anesthesia, use smaller doses of short-acting nondepolarizing muscle relaxants; volatile anesthetics may provide sufficient relaxation for some patients; monitor neuromuscular blockade in more than one muscle group; consider sugammadex for reversal of neuromuscular blockade.
- Consider the respiratory depressant effects of sedatives, narcotics, and inhalation anesthetic agents on an already weakened respiratory system.
- Anticipate an unpredictable response to succinylcholine; untreated patients are resistant to effects of depolarizing muscle relaxants; patients taking anticholinesterase agents may have prolonged response due to inhibition of plasma cholinesterase.
- Ensure full return of respiratory strength before extubation; closely monitor muscle strength in the postoperative period, regardless of anesthesia technique.

Lambert-Eaton myasthenic syndrome

- Maintain an index of suspicion for LEMS in surgical patients with a history of muscle weakness and suspected or diagnosed carcinoma of the lung.
- Continue 3,4-diaminopyridine preoperatively.
- Adjust muscle relaxant dose, recognizing extreme sensitivity to both depolarizing and nondepolarizing muscle relaxants; assess neuromuscular blockade closely.
- Monitor closely for postoperative respiratory failure, regardless of anesthesia technique.

Differentiating Myasthenic Crises and Cholinergic Crises

Myasthenic crisis (exacerbation of MG)

- Caused by decreased neuromuscular transmission at the postsynaptic junction.
- Causative factors: See previous MG description; omission of anticholinesterase drugs, progression of MG
- Major symptom is muscle weakness.
- Pupillary dilation

Cholinergic crisis

- Caused by an excess of anticholinesterase drug
- Occurrence is rare.
- Major symptom is muscle weakness.
- Other signs and symptoms: Bradycardia, abdominal cramping, pupillary constriction
- Treatment: Anticholinergic medication
- Tensilon test: To differentiate between myasthenic crisis and cholinergic crisis, 1–10 mg of edrophonium IV is administered.
- The diagnosis of *myasthenic* crisis is made if weakness improves.
- The diagnosis of *cholinergic* crisis is made if weakness remains unchanged and muscarinic symptoms increase.

KNOWLEDGE CHECK

1. MG is caused by antibodies that cause
   a. decreased release of acetylcholine.
   b. decreased function of acetylcholine receptors.
   c. decreased anticholinergic activity.
   d. decreased catecholamine degradation.
2. Match the following characteristic to MG or LEMS.
   ____Most often associated with small or oat cell carcinoma
   ____Exercise improves strength
   ____Occurs more often in females than males
   ____May be resistant to succinylcholine, increased sensitivity to nondepolarizing muscle relaxants
   ____Proximal limb weakness (legs > arms)
   ____Ptosis and diplopia
3. Which medication alleviates the symptoms of cholinergic crises?
   a. Pyridostigmine
   b. Ephedrine
   c. Edrophonium
   d. Atropine

Answers can be found in Appendix A.

ENDOCRINE SYSTEM

The endocrine system, which includes the hypothalamus, pituitary gland, and target glands, creates and secretes hormones that have significant physiologic effects throughout the body. Endocrine hormones allow for maintenance of homeostasis and respond to constant changes to the internal and external environments (e.g., insulin levels to maintain blood glucose, thyroid hormone levels to regulate metabolic rate) but also play a vital role during periods of physiologic stress (e.g., adrenocortical hormones increase water reabsorption [aldosterone] and increase vascular tone [cortisol] to increase BP). The metabolic functions associated with the endocrine system include the following:

- Metabolism
- Growth and development
- Acid–base balance
- Reproduction

- Fluid and electrolyte status
- Reproduction

Hormones

Hormones are complex chemical substances secreted directly into the bloodstream that stimulate various physiologic processes in target glands or organs. They are classified as proteins, tyrosine amino acid derivatives, and steroids. Table 3.29 summarizes endocrine glands, the hormones that are synthesized, and their physiologic effect.

- Proteins (growth hormone, follicle-stimulating hormone)
- Amino acids (catecholamines-epinephrine, norepinephrine, dopamine, thyroid hormones)
- Steroids (aldosterone, cortisol, androgens)

TABLE 3.29 Common Endocrine Glands, Hormones, Their Functions, and Structures

Gland/Tissue	Hormones	Major Functions	Chemical Structure
Hypothalamus	Thyrotropin-releasing hormone	Stimulates secretion of thyroid-stimulating hormone and prolactin	Peptide
	Corticotropin-releasing hormone	Causes release of adrenocorticotropic hormone	Peptide
	Growth hormone–releasing hormone	Causes release of growth hormone	Peptide
	Growth hormone–inhibitory hormone (somatostatin)	Inhibits release of growth hormone	Peptide
	Gonadotropin-releasing hormone	Causes release of luteinizing hormone and follicle-stimulating hormone	Peptide
	Dopamine or prolactin-inhibiting factor	Inhibits release of prolactin	Amine
Anterior pituitary	Growth hormone	Stimulates protein synthesis and overall growth of most cells and tissues	Peptide
	Thyroid-stimulating hormone	Stimulates synthesis and secretion of thyroid hormones (thyroxine and triiodothyronine)	Peptide
	Adrenocorticotropic hormone	Stimulates synthesis and secretion of adrenocortical hormones	Peptide
	Prolactin	Promotes development of the female breasts and secretion of milk	Peptide
	Follicle-stimulating hormone	Causes growth of follicles in the ovaries and sperm maturation in Sertoli cells of testes	Peptide
	Luteinizing hormone	Stimulates testosterone synthesis in Leydig cells of testes; stimulates ovulation, formation of corpus luteum, and estrogen and progesterone synthesis in ovaries	Peptide
Posterior pituitary	Antidiuretic hormone (also called vasopressin)	Increases water reabsorption by the kidneys and causes vasoconstriction	Peptide
	Oxytocin	Stimulates milk ejection from breasts and uterine contractions	Peptide
Thyroid	Thyroxine (T_4) and triiodothyronine (T_3)	Increases the rates of chemical reactions in most cells, thus increasing body metabolic rate	Amine
	Calcitonin	Promotes deposition of calcium in the bones and decreases extracellular fluid calcium ion concentration	Peptide

Continued

TABLE 3.29 **Common Endocrine Glands, Hormones, Their Functions, and Structures—cont'd**

Gland/Tissue	Hormones	Major Functions	Chemical Structure
Adrenal cortex	Cortisol	Has multiple metabolic functions for controlling metabolism of proteins, carbohydrates, and fats; also has antiinflammatory effects	Steroid
	Aldosterone	Increases renal sodium reabsorption, potassium secretion, and hydrogen ion secretion	Steroid
Adrenal medulla	Norepinephrine, epinephrine	Same effects as sympathetic stimulation	Amine
Pancreas	Insulin (β cells)	Promotes glucose entry in many cells, and in this way controls carbohydrate metabolism	Peptide
	Glucagon (α cells)	Increases synthesis and release of glucose from the liver into the body fluids	Peptide
Parathyroid	Parathyroid hormone	Controls serum calcium ion concentration by increasing calcium absorption by the gut and kidneys and releasing calcium from bones	Peptide
Testes	Testosterone	Promotes development of male reproductive system and male secondary sexual characteristics	Steroid
Ovaries	Estrogens	Promotes growth and development of female reproductive system, female breasts, and female secondary sexual characteristics	Steroid
	Progesterone	Stimulates secretion of "uterine milk" by the uterine endometrial glands and promotes development of secretory apparatus of breasts	Steroid
Placenta	Human chorionic gonadotropin	Promotes growth of corpus luteum and secretion of estrogens and progesterone by corpus luteum	Peptide
	Human somatomammotropin	Probably helps promote development of some fetal tissues, as well as the mother's breasts	Peptide
	Estrogens	See actions of estrogens from ovaries	Steroid
	Progesterone	See actions of progesterone from ovaries	Steroid
Kidney	Renin	Catalyzes conversion of angiotensinogen to angiotensin I (acts as an enzyme)	Peptide
	1,25-dihydroxycholecalciferol	Increases intestinal absorption of calcium and bone mineralization	Steroid
	Erythropoietin	Increases erythrocyte production	Peptide
Heart	Atrial natriuretic peptide	Increases sodium excretion by kidneys, reduces blood pressure	Peptide
Stomach	Gastrin	Stimulates hydrogen chloride secretion by parietal cells	Peptide
Small intestine	Secretin	Stimulates pancreatic acinar cells to release bicarbonate and water	Peptide
	Cholecystokinin	Stimulates gallbladder contraction and release of pancreatic enzymes	Peptide
Adipocytes	Leptin	Inhibits appetite, stimulates thermogenesis	Peptide

From Hall JE, Hall ME. *Guyton and Hall Textbook of Medical Physiology*. 14th ed. Elsevier; 2021:915–927.

Hormone Receptors

Binding to specific target cell receptors initiates the hormonal response. The hormone receptor is highly specific and has a significant affinity for a particular type of hormone, which is dependent on its chemical structure and lipid solubility. After binding occurs, the hormone receptor complex induces changes in the intracellular functioning of the target organ, which produce a specific physiologic response.

Regulation of Hormone Synthesis

The synthesis and secretion of hormones are regulated by neural control (e.g., SNS releasing catecholamines), biorhythms (circadian rhythm and release of cortisol), or feedback mechanisms (e.g., negative feedback loop). Assuming no pathology, the endocrine system effectively modulates many of the body's homeostatic mechanisms automatically without conscious control. The pathway used to regulate and synthesize most endocrine hormones includes hypothalamic stimulation of the pituitary gland, resulting in specific stimulating factors that enter the blood and target glands to create the specific hormones (e.g., hypothalamus, which releases corticotropin-releasing hormone → anterior pituitary, which releases adrenocorticotropic hormone → adrenal glands, which produce and release aldosterone, cortisol, and androgens).

Hypothalamus

The hypothalamus has many functions in addition to being vital for endocrine system functioning (e.g., temperature regulation, hunger). Nearly all secretion of pituitary hormones is controlled by the hypothalamus, which is located below the thalamus, forming the basal portion of the diencephalon. It is a component part of the limbic system. The hypothalamus receives information from numerous sources within the nervous system. The lower border of the hypothalamus is called the *median eminence*; it connects to the pituitary stalk and contains an intricate network of arteries and veins. Hypothalamic releasing factors/hormones enter the area that forms the superior aspect of the hypothalamic hypophyseal portal system and are transported to the anterior pituitary gland (Fig. 3.34).

The hypothalamus produces releasing hormones or factors that are transported via the hypothalamic-hypophysial portal vessels to the anterior pituitary. However, two areas in the hypothalamus, supraoptic and periventricular nuclei, produce antidiuretic hormone (vasopressin) and oxytocin, which are synthesized in the hypothalamus and then transported via neurons into the posterior pituitary gland.

Anterior Pituitary Gland

The pituitary gland or hypophysis is known as the "master endocrine gland" because of the multiple vital

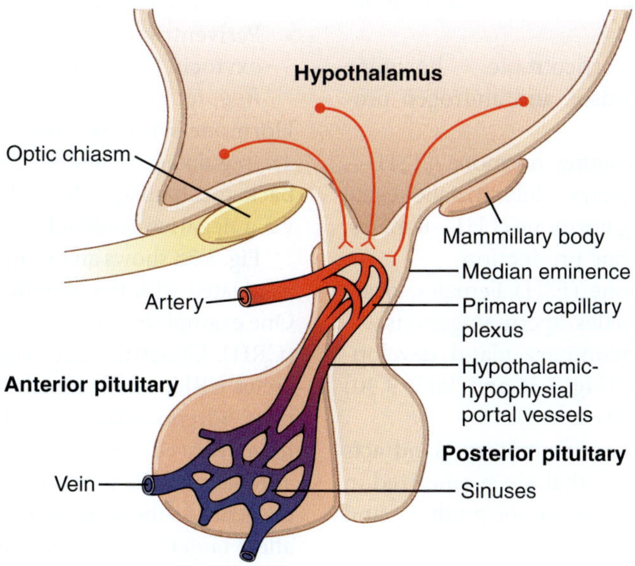

Fig. 3.34 Hypothalamic-hypophysial portal system. (From Hall JE, Hall ME. *Guyton and Hall Textbook of Medical Physiology*. 15th ed. Elsevier; 2026.)

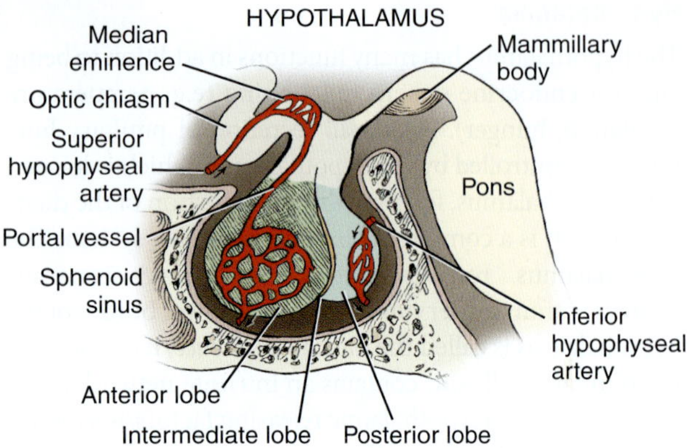

Fig. 3.35 The pituitary gland is located at the base of the brain. It is connected to the overlying hypothalamus by the pituitary or hypophyseal stalk. (From Elisha S, Heiner JS, Nagelhout JJ. *Nurse Anesthesia*. 7th ed. Elsevier; 2023.)

physiologic effects that it controls: homeostatic, reproductive, metabolic, developmental, and ANS. It is approximately the size of a pea and is centrally located at the base of the brain, encased within the bony structure of the sella turcica. The pituitary gland is attached to the hypothalamus via the hypophysial stalk. It is divided into the anterior (adenohypophysis) and posterior (neurohypophysis) (Fig. 3.35).

The anterior pituitary gland constitutes 80% of the pituitary gland by weight and secretes six major peptide hormones.

- Somatotrophs: Growth hormone (GH)—skeletal development and growth
- Corticotropes: Adrenocorticotropic hormone (ACTH)—aldosterone, cortisol, and androgen production
- Thyrotropes: Thyroid-stimulating hormone (TSH)—thyroid hormone regulating intracellular metabolic rate
- Gonadotrophs: Luteinizing hormone (LH)—females, ovulation; males, testosterone production
- Follicle-stimulating hormone (FSH) Females, ovarian follicle development; males, spermatogenesis
- Lactotrophs: Prolactin—mammary gland development and milk production (Fig. 3.36 and Table 3.30)

Posterior pituitary hormones

As previously stated, the posterior pituitary gland acts as a reservoir for two hormones that are synthesized in the hypothalamus, stored in the posterior pituitary, and released into the blood.

- Supraoptic nuclei in the hypothalamus produce antidiuretic hormone (vasopressin). There are three types of vasopressin receptors that have been identified:
  1. V_1 receptors—stimulation results in vasoconstriction.
  2. V_2 receptors—stimulation increases filtrate reabsorption from the kidney tubules.
  3. V_3 receptors—stimulation increases corticotropin-releasing hormone secretion.
- Periventricular nuclei in the hypothalamus produce oxytocin (Fig. 3.37).

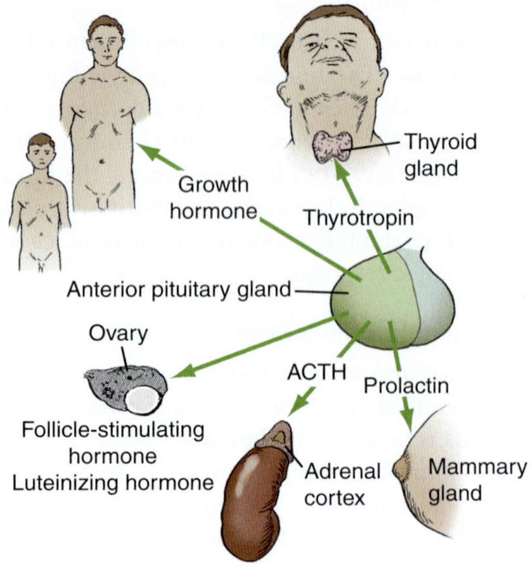

Fig. 3.36 Major target sites for anterior pituitary hormones. *ACTH,* Adrenocorticotropic hormone. (From Elisha S, Heiner JS, Nagelhout JJ. *Nurse Anesthesia*. 7th ed. Elsevier; 2023.)

Regulation of hormone secretion

Hormone synthesis and secretion by endocrine glands are regulated by neural control, biorhythms, and feedback mechanisms. Most hormone levels are regulated via a negative-feedback mechanism or loop.

Fig. 3.38 shows an example of a negative-feedback loop associated with the hypothalamic–pituitary–adrenal axis. One example is corticotropin-releasing hormone or factor (CRH). Under normal conditions, the hypothalamus secretes CRH, which signals anterior pituitary cells to produce adrenocorticotropic hormone (ACTH). ACTH is then released into the blood and stimulates cells in the adrenal medulla to produce aldosterone, cortisol, and androgens. As these hormones are released into the blood to affect target cells throughout the body, they also have an inhibitory effect on both the hypothalamus and anterior pituitary to decrease the rate of synthesis and secretion of

TABLE 3.30 Hypothalamic Hormones and Corresponding Anterior Pituitary Hormones

Hypothalamic Releasing/ Inhibiting Hormones	Anterior Pituitary Target Cell Type	Anterior Pituitary Hormone Produced	Hormone Target Site	Primary Peripheral Hormone Involved in Negative Feedback
Thyrotropin-releasing hormone (TRH)	Thyrotrope	Thyroid-stimulating hormone (TSH; thyrotropin)	Thyroid gland	Triiodothyronine (T_3)
Corticotropin-releasing hormone (CRH)	Corticotrope	Adrenocorticotropic hormone (ACTH; corticotropin)	Zona fasciculata and zona reticularis of adrenal cortex	Cortisol
Gonadotropin-releasing hormone (GnRH)	Gonadotrope	Follicle-stimulating hormone Luteinizing hormone	Gonads (testes, ovaries)	Estrogen, progesterone, testosterone
Prolactin-inhibitory hormone (PIH; dopamine)	Lactotrope	Inhibits prolactin synthesis and secretion		None
Growth hormone–releasing hormone (GHRH)	Somatotrope	Growth hormone	All tissues	Growth hormone, insulin growth factor-1
Growth hormone–inhibitory hormone (somatostatin)	Somatotrope	Inhibits growth hormone secretion		Growth hormone, insulin growth factor-1

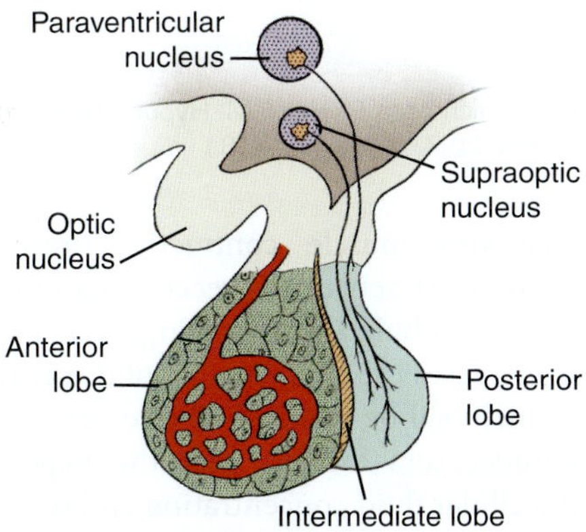

Fig. 3.37 Nerve fibers arising from the supraoptic nucleus and the paraventricular nucleus transport antidiuretic hormone and oxytocin to the posterior pituitary. (From Elisha S, Heiner JS, Nagelhout JJ. *Nurse Anesthesia*. 7th ed. Elsevier; 2023.)

CRH and ACTH. As the levels of these hormones decrease, the stimulatory process to create more hormones ensues. Lastly, physiologic compensation can override this negative-feedback loop. An example is if a patient were to become severely hypotensive from blood loss, the amount of aldosterone and cortisol production would be increased to decrease urine output and increase cardiovascular performance (increased: heart rate, contractility, cardiac conduction, and vascular resistance), respectively.

Endocrine system dysfunction. The endocrine system maintains a steady state of hormones in multiple target organs to ensure that homeostasis is achieved while adapting to constant physical and psychological variability. Endocrine dysfunction is classified as either hypersecretion or hyposecretion of a hormone that either pathologically amplifies or diminishes the normal response. Disorders of the endocrine system are classified as follows.

Example: Hyperthyroidism is caused by a release of excessive thyroid hormone from the thyroid gland.

- Primary endocrinopathy—dysfunction of the target gland
- Secondary endocrinopathy—dysfunction of the anterior or posterior pituitary gland. Example: Pathologically increased TSH synthesis and release cause increased thyroid hormone production by the thyroid gland.
- Tertiary endocrinopathy—dysfunction of the hypothalamus.

Example: Pathologically increased thyrotropin-releasing hormone synthesis stimulates the anterior pituitary to produce excessive amounts of TSH, which increases thyroid hormone synthesis in the thyroid gland.

The onset of physical signs and symptoms of endocrine system dysfunction can occur acutely (e.g., acute

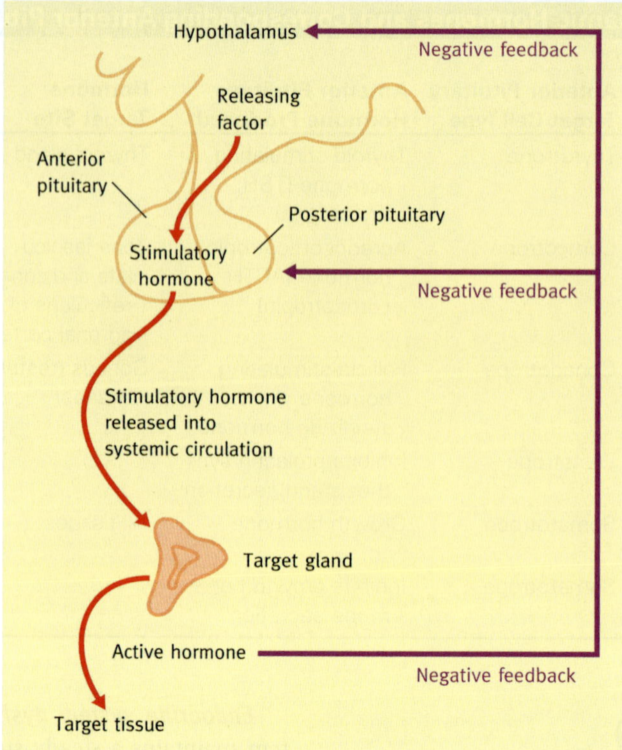

Fig. 3.38 Negative-feedback control of hypothalamic–pituitary axis. (From Nicholson G, Hall GM. Hypothalamic-pituitary-adrenal function: anaesthetic implications. *Anaesth Int Care Med.* 2014;15[10]:473–476.)

adrenal insufficiency) or more often chronically (e.g., excessive growth hormone secretion—acromegaly). Lastly, dysfunction of a particular target gland and/or an abnormality of the target cells' response to a hormone can also cause endocrine pathology.

Posterior pituitary gland dysfunction. The hypothalamus produces antidiuretic hormone (ADH), which is also known as *vasopressin* and *arginine vasopressin.* The synthesis occurs within a collection of specialized cells known as the *supraoptic nuclei.* This hormone is transported via neurons to the posterior pituitary gland. Major physiologic functions of ADH include the following:

- Fluid and electrolyte balance
- Renal tubular permeability
- Maintenance of BP
- Synergistic effect with other hormones (CRH, aldosterone)

The three types of vasopressin receptors and their function were summarized earlier (Posterior Pituitary Hormones section). ADH acts on V_1 receptors, causing vascular smooth muscle contraction, resulting in increased BP. ADH acts on V_2 receptors and primarily affects the distal tubule and collecting ducts in the kidneys. This increases the permeability of these structures to water, which will be reabsorbed into central circulation. Osmoreceptors located near the hypothalamus sense extracellular fluid concentration and release ADH as serum osmolarity increases (hypovolemia). A list of factors that increase the synthesis and release of ADH is presented in Box 3.13.

Diabetes insipidus. Diabetes insipidus (DI) results from either an inadequate amount of ADH synthesis/secretion (neurogenic or central DI) or impaired renal tubular receptor sensitivity to the effects of ADH (nephrogenic DI). The result is decreased water reabsorption by the kidneys, large urine output, and hypovolemia. Common causes of DI include the following:

- Idiopathic (approximately 50% of adult cases)

Neurogenic

- Pituitary gland surgery
- Meningitis/encephalitis

BOX 3.13 Factors That Stimulate the Release of Antidiuretic Hormone

- Increased plasma sodium ion concentration
- Increased serum osmolarity
- Decreased blood volume
- Decreased blood pressure
- Smoking (nicotine)
- Stress
- Nausea
- Vasovagal reaction
- Various medications (chlorpropamide, clofibrate, thiazide diuretics, carbamazepine, nicotine, cyclophosphamide, vincristine, morphine, high-dose oxytocin)
- Angiotensin II
- Positive-pressure ventilation

- Closed head trauma
- Brain lesions

Nephrogenic
- Hypercalcemia
- Hypokalemia
- Pyelonephritis
- Sarcoidosis
- Medications (e.g., lithium, rifampin)

Medications that inhibit ADH secretion
- Phenytoin (Dilantin)
- Chlorpromazine (Thorazine)
- Reserpine (Serpasil)

Medications that inhibit the effect of ADH on renal tubules
- Lithium
- α-Adrenergic agonists (norepinephrine)
- Amphotericin B
- Alcohol

Diagnostic criteria
- Low urine osmolarity (<200 mOsm/L)
- High serum osmolality (>290 mOsm/L)
- Low urine specific gravity (1.010)
- Hypernatremia—serum sodium >145 mEq/L
- Urine volume (8–12 L/day)

Anesthetic Considerations

- Desmopressin (1-deamino-8-D-arginine vasopressin [DDAVP]) infusion (synthetic analog of vasopressin)
- Fluid replacement
- Treat the underlying cause.
- Potential for seizures
- Preoperative assessment of electrolytes, renal function, and plasma osmolarity
- Patients are sensitive to the cardiovascular effects of anesthetic agents as a result of hypovolemia.

Syndrome of Inappropriate Antidiuretic Hormone Secretion

Syndrome of inappropriate antidiuretic secretion (SIADH) results from hypersecretion of ADH. As ADH levels are pathologically high, the kidney tubules reabsorb large amounts of water, causing hypervolemia, dilutional hyponatremia, and plasma hypotonicity. Common causes of SIADH include the following:

Neurogenic
- Pituitary tumor
- Meningitis
- Head trauma
- Neoplasms

Ectopic SIADH production
- Cancer
  1. Lung
  2. Prostate
  3. Pancreatic
  4. Leukemia
  5. Thymoma

Nephrogenic
- General anesthetics
- Thiazide diuretics
- Tricyclic antidepressants
- Beta-adrenergic agonists (e.g., isoproterenol)

Signs and symptoms are associated with dilutional hyponatremia and include the following:

Minor neurologic symptoms—confusion, lethargy, headache, nausea, vomiting

Major neurologic symptoms—seizures, cerebral edema, coma

- Treat the underlying cause.
- Potential for seizures

A comparison of the features associated with DI and SIADH is shown in Table 3.31. The severity of symptoms can be correlated to the degree of hyponatremia and the rapidity of onset.

Anesthesia Case Management

Correct hypervolemia and dilutional hyponatremia.
- Fluid restriction

TABLE 3.31 Syndrome of Inappropriate Antidiuretic Hormone (SIADH) and Diabetes Insipidus (DI)

	SIADH	DI
Serum osmolarity	<270 mOsm/L	>290 mOsm/L
Serum sodium	<135 mEq/L	>145 mEq/L
Urine volume	Low	High
Urine osmolarity	Hypertonic urine relative to plasma	Hypotonic urine relative to plasma
Treatment	Correction of underlying cause, fluid restriction; if patient symptomatic or serum Na^+ <115–120 mEq/L, hypertonic saline may be considered	Correction of underlying cause, fluid replacement Central DI—DDAVP Nephrogenic DI—NSAIDs, thiazide diuretics

DDAVP, 1-deamino-8-D-arginine vasopressin; *NSAID*, nonsteroidal antiinflammatory.

- Diuretic-Lasix and or mannitol
- Hypertonic saline infusion
- Assess urine output, serum sodium, and plasma and urine osmolarity.

KNOWLEDGE CHECK

1. Which factors are associated with DI? *(Select two.)*
   a. Hyponatremia
   b. Low urine osmolarity
   c. Hypokalemia
   d. Proteinuria
2. Which are interventions used to treat SIADH? *(Select two.)*
   a. DDAVP infusion
   b. Lasix
   c. IV fluid bolus
   d. Hypertonic saline infusion

Answers can be found in Appendix A.

Diabetes Mellitus

Diabetes mellitus (DM) is a group of metabolic diseases resulting in hyperglycemia caused by a lack of insulin secretion, insulin resistance, or both. Type 1 diabetes (5%–10% of cases) occurs as a result of destruction of pancreatic B cells, leading to a deficiency of insulin production. Type 2 diabetes (90%–95% of cases) is characterized by insulin resistance of peripheral tissues, with an associated deficiency of insulin and excessive hepatic glucose production. Approximately 80% of patients with type 2 diabetes are obese. The criteria for diagnosis of diabetes are shown in Box 3.14.

BOX 3.14 Criteria for Diagnosing Diabetes: Four Options

1. A_{1c} ≥6.5%
   or
2. Fasting plasma glucose (FPG) ≥126 mg/dL
   Fasting defined as no caloric intake for at least 8 hr
   or
3. 2-hr plasma glucose ≥200 mg/dL during an oral glucose tolerance test
   75 g anhydrous glucose dissolved in water
   or
4. Random plasma glucose ≥200 mg/dL in a patient with classic symptoms of hyperglycemia or hyperglycemic crisis

From American Diabetes Association. Standards of medical care in diabetes—2019. *Diabetes Care*. 2019;42(S1).

Hyperglycemic Crises

Diabetic ketoacidosis. Diabetic ketoacidosis (DKA) occurs as a result of a lack of insulin in both type 1 and type 2 diabetics. It is associated with a triad of signs: (1) hyperglycemia, (2) ketonemia, and (3) acidemia. These most often develop acutely within 24 hours. Precipitating factors include events that cause physiologic stress, such as infections, MI, trauma, or noncompliance with insulin regimen.

Signs and symptoms associated with DKA:

- Blood glucose >250 mg/dL
- Metabolic acidosis—arterial pH <7.3
- HCO_3 <15 mEq/L
- $Paco_2$ <35 mm/Hg

- Anion gap >10 mEq/L
- Serum osmolarity >300 mOsm/L
- Urine glucose and ketones
- Altered level of consciousness/seizures/coma
- Hypotension/compensatory tachycardia
- Fruity ketone odor on breath
- Rapid/deep breaths (Kussmaul respiration pattern)

Anesthesia Case Management

- Identify and treat cause.
- Monitor for dehydration, hypovolemia, and hypoperfusion.
- Assess electrolytes and blood glucose every half hour.
- Normal saline IV infusion 1–2 L
- Regular insulin 10 units IV
- Regular insulin IV infusion—5–10 units/hour (Goal = decrease glucose by 50–100 mg/dL per hour)
- Monitor for complications of DKA—MI, hypovolemic shock, cerebral edema, seizures, stroke, pulmonary embolism, acute renal failure, and septic shock.

Hyperglycemic hyperosmolar state. Hyperglycemic hyperosmolar state (HHS), also known as *hyperosmolar nonketotic coma*, is a life-threatening condition caused by insulin depletion, volume depletion, and acid–base abnormalities. It most commonly occurs in patients with type 2 diabetes and is characterized by blood glucose levels of >600 mg/dL. The amount of insulin secreted is frequently sufficient to avoid ketoacidosis. The signs and symptoms and treatment for HHS are the same as for DKA, described earlier. A comparison of the components of DKA and HHS is presented in Table 3.32.

KNOWLEDGE CHECK

1. Which pathologic state is associated with a blood glucose level of >600 mg/dL?
   a. DKA
   b. Primary hyperaldosteronism
   c. HHS
   d. Hyperparathyroidism

Answers can be found in Appendix A.

Adrenal Gland Dysfunction

The adrenal glands are pyramidal-shaped organs that are anatomically located atop each kidney. There are two distinct layers that comprise the adrenal gland: (1) adrenal cortex (80%, outer layer), which creates and secretes steroid hormones, and (2) adrenal medulla (20%, inner layer), which creates and secretes norepinephrine (80%) and epinephrine (20%). A discussion of pheochromocytoma that involves the adrenal medulla is presented later in this chapter.

The adrenal cortex is composed of three distinct layers:

- Zona glomerulosa: Creates and secretes mineralocorticoids, primarily aldosterone. Primary effect is to

TABLE 3.32 Comparison of Diabetic Ketoacidosis (DKA) and Hyperglycemic Hyperosmolar State (HHS)

	DKA	HHS
Plasma glucose	250–600 mg/dL	600–1200 mg/dL
pH	6.8–7.3	>7.3
Serum bicarbonate	<15 mEq/L	Normal or slightly decreased
Serum osmolarity	300–320 mOsm/L	350–380 mOsm/L
Ketonemia	++++	+/−
Mental obtundation	Variable	Present
Hypovolemia	Present	Present
Serum potassium*	Normal or slight +	Normal
Arterial P_{CO_2}	20–30 mm Hg	Normal

+, Increase; ++++, large increase.

*Plasma levels may be normal or high, but total body stores are usually depleted.

Adapted from Powers AC, Niswender KD, Rickels MR. Diabetes mellitus: management and therapies. In: Jameson J, Fauci AS, Kasper DL et al, eds. *Harrison's Principles of Internal Medicine*. 20th ed. McGraw-Hill; 2018.

increase the reabsorption of sodium from the kidney tubules. As sodium is reabsorbed, water is also reabsorbed back into the peritubular capillary system and central circulation. To maintain electrical neutrality within the body, potassium and hydrogen ions are excreted.

- Zona fasciculata: Creates and secretes glucocorticoids, primarily cortisol. Cortisol has an effect on nearly every cell in the body because it regulates carbohydrate, protein, and fat metabolism. It has potent antiinflammatory and immunosuppressive effects. Cortisol is a stress hormone and has an effect on the maintenance of normal vascular tone and cardiac contractility.
- Zona reticularis: Creates and secretes dehydroepiandrosterone sulfate (precursor to testosterone and estrogen) (Fig. 3.39)

Primary Aldosteronism (Conn Syndrome)

Primary aldosteronism is caused by hypersecretion of aldosterone caused by adrenal adenoma, adrenocortical hyperplasia, or carcinoma. Treatment involves resection of the hypersecreting adenoma or surveillance and medical management. Manifestations include the following:

- Hypertension caused by hypervolemia
- Hypernatremia
- Hypokalemia
- Metabolic alkalosis

Anesthesia Case Management

- Assessment of cardiac status—potential for CHF
- Electrolyte abnormalities
  - Hypokalemia—muscle weakness, potentiation of neuromuscular blockers
- Potential for hypertension

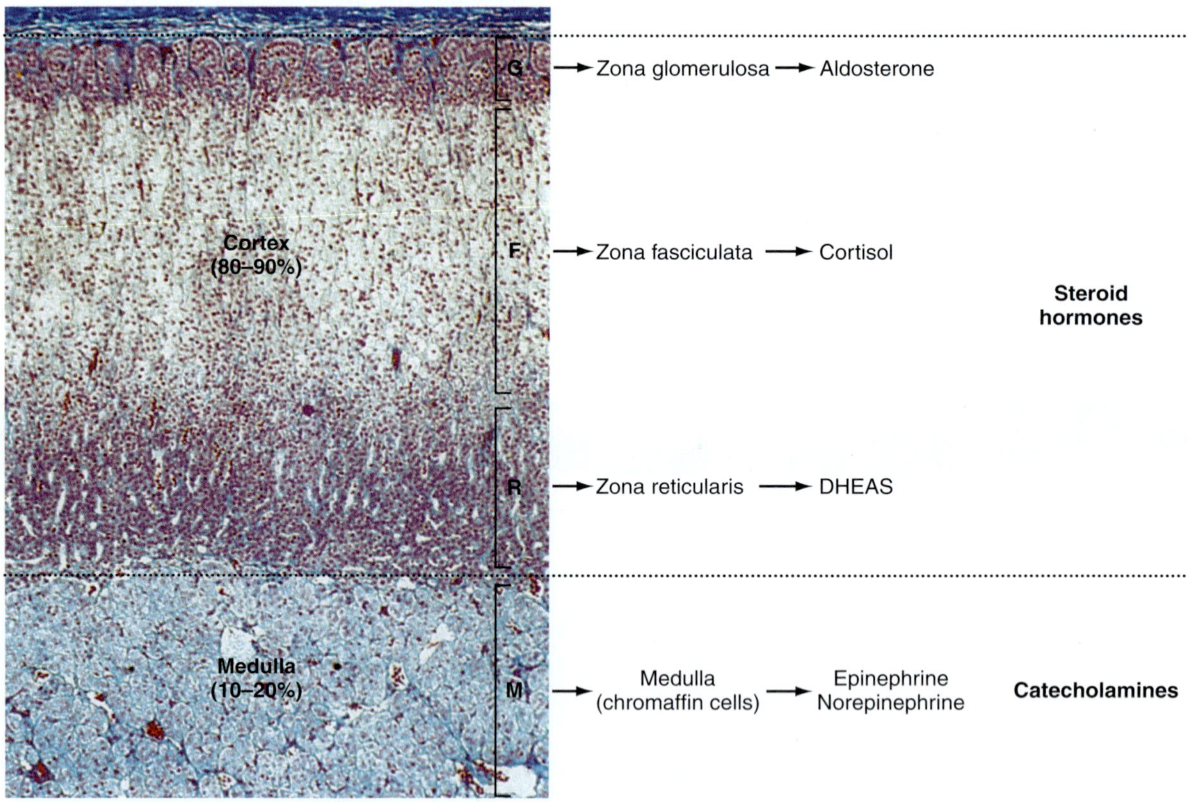

Fig. 3.39 Histology of the adrenal gland. Higher magnification clearly illustrating the zonation of the cortex. The corresponding endocrine function and the different zones of the cortex and the medulla are noted. *DHEAS,* Dehydroepiandrosterone sulfate. (From Koeppen BM, Stanton BA. *Berne and Levy Physiology (Updated).* 7th ed. Elsevier; 2017:768. Modified From Young B, Woodford P, O'Dowd G. *Wheater's Functional Histology.* 6th ed. Elsevier; 2014:328.)

Glucocorticoid Excess—Cortisol (Cushing Syndrome)

Hypercortisolism is caused by either an overproduction of cortisol secretion from the adrenal glands or exogenously administered steroids for medical treatment. Cortisol is a potent stress hormone that has powerful physiologic effects. Acute supraphysiologic concentrations cause the following:

- Maintenance of SVR
- Increasing cardiac contractility
- Promoting gluconeogenesis and glycogenolysis
- Increased mental acuity

The physiologic effects of hypercortisolism are presented in Box 3.15.

Causes of hypercortisolism include neurogenic (pituitary tumor), which accounts for approximately 70% of cases; exogenous steroid use to treat inflammatory conditions (e.g., asthma, arthritis); and adrenal gland tumors.

Anesthesia Case Management

- Normalization of BP
- Monitoring blood glucose levels, treating hyperglycemia as needed
- Assessing electrolyte status—the most common electrolyte abnormalities include the following:
    - Hypervolemia, hypernatremia, hypokalemia, metabolic alkalosis

BOX 3.15 Clinical Features of Glucocorticoid Excess (Cushing Syndrome)

- Hyperglycemia
- Systemic hypertension
- Weight gain; central obesity; fat pad on back of neck (buffalo hump); moon facies
- Increased susceptibility to infection
- Poor wound healing
- Hypokalemia
- Alkalosis
- Hirsutism; acne; loss of libido; menstrual disturbances
- Osteopenia; osteoporosis
- Skeletal muscle weakness (especially proximal muscle weakness)
- Cataracts
- Skin striae; spontaneous ecchymoses; facial plethora
- Depression; cognitive dysfunction; emotional lability

Adrenocortical Insufficiency

Primary Adrenocortical Insufficiency (Addison Disease)

The pathologic process in primary adrenocortical insufficiency is caused by destruction of the adrenal glands as a result of infection, tuberculosis, human immunodeficiency syndrome, and most commonly autoimmune disease, which accounts for 50% of cases. The clinical features are the result of a lack of adrenocortical hormones.

- Hypoglycemia—loss of cortisol
- Hypovolemia/hyponatremia/hyperkalemia—loss of aldosterone
- Hypotension—volume depletion (↓ aldosterone), decreased SVR (↓ cortisol)

A complete description of the clinical features associated with primary adrenocortical disease is presented in Table 3.33.

Secondary adrenocortical disease is caused by a deficiency of ACTH. The primary etiologies are (1) HPA axis suppression caused by long-term supraphysiologic steroid administration and (2) decreased ACTH from hypothalamic (decreased CRH) or anterior pituitary disease (decreased ACTH).

Medical management for adrenocortical dysfunction involves determining the specific cause and treating if possible. Treatment focuses on the degree of the lack of aldosterone and cortisol and providing steroids that have mineralocorticoid and glucocorticoid effects. Patients taking supraphysiologic doses of steroids for more than 3 weeks within 1 year are at risk for acute adrenocortical insufficiency (AAI).

Anesthetic Case Management

- Correct electrolyte and metabolic abnormalities.
- Potential for severe hypotension during intraoperative anesthesia management
- Steroid preparation for patients at risk of AAI:
    - Decadron 4 mg or hydrocortisone 100 mg IV
- If AAI occurs, the drug of choice is hydrocortisone 100 mg IV.
- Etomidate should be avoided in all patients at risk for AAI. One dose of etomidate can cause inhibition of cortisol production for up to 24 hours after administration. Etomidate inhibits 11 *B* hydroxylase, an enzyme necessary to synthesize cortisol (Table 3.34).

TABLE 3.33 Clinical Features of Primary Adrenal Insufficiency

Feature	Frequency (%)
Symptoms	
Weakness, tiredness, fatigue	100
Anorexia	100
Gastrointestinal symptoms	92
Nausea	86
Vomiting	75
Constipation	33
Abdominal pain	31
Diarrhea	16
Salt craving	16
Postural dizziness	12
Muscle and joint pains	13
Signs	
Weight loss	100
Hyperpigmentation	94
Hypotension (<110 mm Hg systolic)	88–94
Vitiligo	10–20
Auricular calcification	5
Laboratory Findings	
Electrolyte disturbances	92
Hyponatremia	88
Hyperkalemia	64
Hypercalcemia	6
Azotemia	55
Anemia	40
Eosinophilia	17

From Newell-Price JDC, Auchus RJ. The adrenal cortex. In: Melmed S, Auchus RJ, Goldfine AB et al, eds. *Williams Textbook of Endocrinology*. 14th ed. Elsevier; 2020: 480–541.

Acute adrenal crisis (addisonian crisis). AAI is a rare but life-threatening condition that is caused by severe hypovolemia from a lack of aldosterone and inhibition of myocardial excitation contractile coupling and decreased SVR from a lack of cortisol. The result is severe hypotension that does not respond to vasopressor therapy. Because of the lack of aldosterone, the electrolyte and metabolic disturbance associated with AAI is hypovolemic, hyponatremic, hyperkalemic, hypoglycemic metabolic acidosis. Cortisol is necessary for normal adrenergic receptor functioning. Thus higher doses of vasopressors may be needed to adequately treat severe hypotension. Vasopressin 1–4 units IV bolus may also be effective (Box 3.16).

KNOWLEDGE CHECK

1. Which abnormalities are associated with acute adrenal crises? *(Select two.)*
   a. Hypernatremia
   b. Hyperkalemia
   c. Metabolic alkalosis
   d. Hypovolemia
2. Which medication should be avoided in patients who are at risk of developing acute adrenal insufficiency?
   a. Fentanyl
   b. Zofran
   c. Lasix
   d. Etomidate
3. Which are anesthetic considerations associated with Cushing syndrome? *(Select two.)*
   a. Hypertension
   b. Decreased SVR
   c. Increased urine output
   d. Hyperglycemia

Answers can be found in Appendix A.

Adrenal Medulla (Inner Layer)

Pheochromocytoma

A pheochromocytoma is a catecholamine-secreting tumor that originates within the adrenal gland in approximately 90% of cases. The tumors are composed of chromaffin cells that can produce, store, and secrete catecholamines. As a result, norepinephrine is secreted at levels above normal. As with many other endocrinopathies, norepinephrine values can be mildly, moderately, or extremely elevated. The more active the pheochromocytoma, the more epinephrine that is secreted and the more dramatic the signs and symptoms associated with SNS predominance.

Less common are extraadrenal pheochromocytomas, which can develop within chromaffin tissue that exists in many areas of the body. Extraadrenal pheochromocytomas are most often located in the abdominal cavity. A pheochromocytoma can also be associated with multiple endocrine neoplasia syndrome (MEN), which is hereditary. The components associated with MEN are shown in Table 3.35. A pheochromocytoma can exist in

TABLE 3.34 Steroid Preparations

Steroid	Glucocorticoid Potency (Antiinflammatory)*	Mineralocorticoid Potency (Salt Retention)	Approximate Equivalent Glucocorticoid Dose
Glucocorticoids			
Short Acting			
Cortisol (hydrocortisone)	1.0	1.0	20 mg
Cortisone	0.8	0.8	25 mg
Intermediate acting			
Prednisone	4.0	0.25	5 mg
Prednisolone	4.0	0.25	5 mg
Methylprednisolone	5.0	0	4 mg
Triamcinolone	5.0	0	4 mg
Long Acting			
Dexamethasone	30	0	0.75 mg
Mineralocorticoids			
Fludrocortisone	12	125	

Fludrocortisone is not used for antiinflammatory effect.
*Glucocorticoid and mineralocorticoid potencies are relative to cortisol, with cortisol being 1.0. When given at replacement doses, triamcinolone and dexamethasone have no clinically important mineralocorticoid activity.
From Wall RT. Endocrine disease. In: Hines RL, Marschall KE, eds. *Anesthesia and Co-Existing Disease*. 7th ed. Elsevier; 2018:449–475.

BOX 3.16 Treatment for Acute Adrenal Crises

- Endotracheal intubation and controlled ventilation for respiratory arrest
- Intravascular volume expansion with isotonic crystalloid (e.g., Ringer's lactate or normal saline)
- Hydrocortisone 100 mg IV bolus, followed by hydrocortisone 50–100 mg every 6 hr for 24 hr (total 300 mg/d)
- Administer D50W bolus if hypoglycemia is present.
- Administer vasopressors or positive inotropes to treat hypotension.
- Invasive monitoring (e.g., arterial line or central venous line) as necessary
- Monitor laboratory values (e.g., electrolytes, cortisol, ACTH, and glucose).
- Perform cardiac resuscitation per American Heart Association ACLS/PALS protocol as necessary.

ACLS/PALS, Advanced cardiac life support/pediatric advanced life support; *ACTH,* adrenocorticotropic hormone; *D50W,* 50% dextrose in water; *IV,* intravenous.

one adrenal gland, in bilateral adrenal glands, or in extraadrenal sites. The incidence of this disease is 0.6 per 100,000 people, and most cases are identified incidentally by either x-ray or imaging studies or during a surgical procedure. This disease state affects males and females equally and most frequently manifests between 30 and 50 years of age.

The clinical manifestations mirror uncontrolled norepinephrine release, resulting in SNS hyperactivity. Examples include the following:

- Triad of signs/symptoms
  1. Headaches resulting from uncontrolled episodes of hypertension
  2. Profuse sweating caused by sympathetic cholinergic stimulation of the sweat glands
  3. Palpitations and tachycardia from β_1 adrenergic receptor stimulation and sensitization of the myocardium from excess catecholamines
- Hyperglycemia from increased gluconeogenesis/glycogenolysis and inhibition of insulin secretion

TABLE 3.35 **Manifestations of Multiple Endocrine Neoplasia***

Syndrome	Manifestations
MEN type 1 (Werner syndrome)	Hyperparathyroidism, pituitary adenomas, pancreatic islet cell tumors
MEN type 2A (Sipple syndrome)	Medullary thyroid cancer, primary hyperparathyroidism, pheochromocytoma, pigmented skin lesions (lichen amyloidosis)
MEN type 2B (Gorlin syndrome or mucosal neuroma syndrome)	Medullary thyroid cancer, pheochromocytoma, mucocutaneous neuromas (typically involving the tongue, lips, and eyelids), skeletal deformities (e.g., kyphoscoliosis, lordosis), intestinal ganglioneuromas

*Multiple endocrine neoplasia (MEN) is a group of rare diseases caused by genetic defects that lead to hyperplasia and hyperfunction of various components of the endocrine system.

BOX 3.17 **Clinical Manifestations of Pheochromocytoma Listed by Frequency of Occurrence**

1. Headaches
2. Profuse sweating
3. Palpitations and tachycardia
4. Hypertension, sustained or paroxysmal
5. Anxiety
6. Pallor
7. Nausea
8. Abdominal pain
9. Weakness
10. Weight loss
11. Paradoxic response to antihypertensive drugs
12. Polyuria and polydipsia
13. Constipation
14. Orthostatic hypotension
15. Dilated cardiomyopathy
16. Erythrocytosis
17. Elevated blood sugar

- Orthostatic hypotension and polycythemia occur as a result of intravascular volume depletion resulting from α_1 adrenergic receptor stimulation, causing increased SVR.
- Cerebral hemorrhage, MI, cardiomyopathy, CHF, and renal insufficiency caused by prolonged undiagnosed hypertension (Box 3.17)

A pheochromocytoma is not directly innervated by the ANS and therefore is not controlled by neural stimulation. Consequently, stimulation of the tumor resulting in catecholamine release is not completely understood, and the precipitating factors are not clearly defined and vary per individual. However, events that are associated with causing tumor activation include hypotension, hypothermia, defecation, physiologic stress, medications, intubation, and surgery.

Factors that increase the potential for morbidity and mortality include the following:

- The activity of the pheochromocytoma—a highly active tumor is associated with increased concentrations of catecholamines and a more dramatic physiologic response.
- Inadequate preoperative α-receptor and then β-receptor blockade
- Advanced end-organ damage
- Whether the pheochromocytoma is malignant or benign—the 5-year survival rate for a patient with a benign tumor is approximately 90%. However, if the pheochromocytoma is malignant, the survival rate dramatically decreases to 10% because of metastasis resulting from the high amount of blood flow that courses through the adrenal glands.

Anesthesia Case Management

- Controlling hemodynamic variability (intraoperative hypertension, postoperative hypotension)
- Assess blood glucose.
- Maintain fluid status.
- Monitor for acute hemorrhage.

Preoperative Period

The goal of preoperative therapy for a patient with a pheochromocytoma includes control of excessive catecholamine release. Preoperative pharmacologic preparation as prescribed by an endocrinologist is essential.

Pharmacologic Therapy

Preoperative pharmacologic management of these patients includes α-receptor blockade, β-receptor blockade, and volume expansion. *α-Receptor blockade is always instituted before β-receptor blockade* and is usually accomplished by the administration of phenoxybenzamine, a noncompetitive α_1 receptor and α_2 receptor antagonist. The patient will take phenoxybenzamine or another α-adrenergic receptor blocker as prescribed for 10–14 days preoperatively. Once adequate α-receptor blockade is established, β-receptor blockade can begin. Initiation of β-receptor blockade before α-receptor blockade can cause a hypertensive crisis and can lead to the development of CHF. The tachycardia that is caused by excessive β-receptor activity or vasodilation caused by phenoxybenzamine is managed with β-receptor blockade, most often propranolol. For a complete list of medications used to pretreat patients with a pheochromocytoma, see Table 3.36.

Another medication that can be administered preoperatively is metyrosine. This medication has an inhibitory effect on the creation of catecholamines, which occurs in adrenergic nerves. This drug decreases the effect of tyrosine hydroxylase, an enzyme that is necessary during the biosynthesis of catecholamines.

The following criteria must be met before surgical intervention and anesthesia administration:

- BP must remain less than 160/90 mm Hg within the 48 hours before surgery.
- Orthostatic hypotension must occur; however, the BP must be greater than 80/45 mm Hg.
- The ECG must not have ST-/T-wave abnormalities for at least 1 week and have no more than one premature ventricular contraction every 5 minutes.
- Adequate hydration is achieved by a decrease in the hematocrit by 5% from baseline values.

Intraoperative Period

Administration of any medications that can cause an increased BP or heart rate or cause the release of histamine should be avoided. Alternative drugs that stimulate the release or inhibit the breakdown of catecholamines should be used. A complete list of anesthetic medications

TABLE 3.36 Drugs Used for Preoperative Management of Pheochromocytoma

Drug	Action	Preoperative Blood Pressure Control	Comments
Phenoxybenzamine	Nonselective α-blocker	Initial oral (PO) dose 10–30 mg/day, daily dosage increased by 30 mg as needed	Long half-life; may accumulate; S/E postural hypotension, nasal congestion, diarrhea, retrograde ejaculation, miosis
Doxazosin	Selective α_1-antagonist	1 mg/day PO up to 8 mg/day PO	First-dose phenomenon; may cause syncope; dizziness; drowsiness
Propranolol	Nonselective β-blocker	40 mg/day PO up to 480 mg/day in divided doses to control tachycardia	Should not be administered without first creating α-blockade
Atenolol	Selective β_1-blocker	PO 50–100 mg/day	Long acting; eliminated unchanged by kidney; should not be administered without first creating α-blockade
Labetalol	α- and β-blocker	PO 200 mg, divided doses Up to 800 mg/day	A much weaker α-blocker than β-blocker; may cause pressor response with pheochromocytoma
Nicardipine sustained release	Calcium channel blocker	30 mg PO twice a day; up to 120 mg/day	Arterial vasodilator; edema; flushing; headache
α-methyltyrosine	Inhibitor of biosynthesis of catecholamines	Initial PO 1 g/day; up to 4 g/day in divided doses	For patients not amenable to surgery; may be nephrotoxic

PO, Per os; *S/E*, symptoms and effects.

Modified from Schwartz JJ et al. Endocrine function. In: Barash PG, Cullen BF, Stoelting RK, et al., eds. *Clinical Anesthesia*. 8th ed. Wolters Kluwer; 2017:1341.

BOX 3.18 Anesthetic Medications That Should Be Avoided in Patients With a Pheochromocytoma

- Desflurane: Sympathomimetic effects
- Pancuronium: Sympathomimetic effects
- Atracurium: Histamine release
- Succinylcholine: Fasciculation causing catecholamine release
- Morphine: Histamine release
- Droperidol: Antidopaminergic effects—neuroleptic malignant syndrome
- Metoclopramide: Antidopaminergic effects—neuroleptic malignant syndrome
- Phenothiazines: Antidopaminergic effects—neuroleptic malignant syndrome
- Ephedrine: Sympathomimetic effects
- Ketamine: Sympathomimetic effects
- Atropine: Produces tachycardia
- Naloxone hydrochloride: Sympathetic nervous system predominance

that should be avoided for these patients is included in Box 3.18.

- Most often accomplished laparoscopically
- Potential for hemorrhage—type and screen obtained
- Standard monitors, one IV hep lock and one functioning IV preferred
- Vasodilator/vasopressor infusions may be necessary.
- Nitrous oxide should be avoided because of the potential for bowel distention and concerns regarding the development of a pneumothorax.
- The administration of succinylcholine for muscle paralysis is controversial because the resulting fasciculation causes abdominal rigidity and can increase the release of catecholamines from the pheochromocytoma.
- The anesthetist should expect BP lability throughout the entire perioperative course.

Hypertension most commonly occurs during intubation, incision, manipulation of tumor, and ligation of the venous drainage of the affected adrenal gland. Hypertension is most effectively managed by the following:

- Increasing the concentration of inhalation anesthetic agent
- Administering narcotics—dexmedetomidine, propofol
- Infusing sodium nitroprusside, nitroglycerine, and/or clevidipine as an IV drip

Hypotension is most common after removal of tumor. Hypotension is most effectively treated by the following:

- Decreasing the anesthetic depth
- Administering crystalloids, colloids, or packed RBCs
- Administering a direct-acting vasopressor, such as phenylephrine

The patient's blood glucose level should be assessed preoperatively and incrementally throughout the surgical procedure. Hyperglycemia commonly occurs before the tumor removal as a result of the inhibition of endogenous insulin release and glycogenolysis by the liver. Conversely, hypoglycemia can develop rapidly during the postoperative period.

Postoperative Period

The following are possible postoperative complications associated with adrenalectomy for pheochromocytoma excision:

- Hypertension from residual pheochromocytoma, pain, hypoglycemia, hypervolemia, and hypoxia
- Hypotension can result from residual α-adrenergic receptor blockade, hypovolemia, myocardial ischemia or infarction, bleeding, or sepsis.
- Pneumothorax
- Hemorrhage
- Sepsis
- Hypoglycemia
- Hypoadrenocorticism

Thyroid Gland Dysfunction

The thyroid gland consists of two lobes connected by an isthmus. It is bound to the anterior and lateral aspects of the trachea, with the superior border of the isthmus located just below the cricoid cartilage. Two pairs of parathyroid glands are located on the posterior aspect of each lobe—one pair that is superior and one pair that is inferior on each lobe—which regulate calcium levels. The posterior aspects of the thyroid gland run alongside the carotid sheath and the esophagus.

The recurrent laryngeal nerve (RLN) is a branch of the vagus nerve that innervates the intrinsic muscles of the larynx, which serve a variety of functions, including adducting and abducting the vocal cords. The RLN can be damaged during resection of the thyroid gland, causing hoarseness, stridor, and/or respiratory distress.

Arterial blood is supplied by the superior and inferior thyroid arteries. A venous plexus is formed by the

KNOWLEDGE CHECK

1. The classic triad of symptoms associated with pheochromocytoma includes
   a. elevated systolic pressure, swelling, and anxiety.
   b. headache, diaphoresis, and tachycardia.
   c. elevated diastolic pressure, diaphoresis, and tachycardia.
   d. mood swings, increased pulse pressure, and arrhythmias.
2. The majority of extraadrenal pheochromocytomas are located in which region of the body?
   a. Thorax
   b. Cranium
   c. Mediastinum
   d. Abdomen
3. Which is true regarding pheochromocytoma excretion of endogenous catecholamines?
   a. Norepinephrine > epinephrine
   b. Norepinephrine < epinephrine
   c. Dopamine > norepinephrine
   d. Epinephrine < dopamine
4. Which of the preoperative vital signs are reflective of adequate for surgery and anesthetic management for a patient scheduled for adrenalectomy for pheochromocytoma?
   a. Heart rate 101, BP 138/66, hematocrit 27
   b. Heart rate 83, BP 149/82, hematocrit 36
   c. Heart rate 96, BP 155/66, hematocrit 48
   d. Heart rate 62, BP 138/112, hematocrit 51
5. Which medication should be initially administered preoperatively to a patient with a pheochromocytoma?
   a. Hydrocortisone
   b. Phenoxybenzamine
   c. Metyrosine
   d. Propranolol

Answers can be found in Appendix A.

superior, middle, and inferior thyroid veins. The thyroid gland lies adjacent to the common carotid artery and the anterior jugular vein, which are potential sources of rapid and massive blood loss.

The hypothalamus secretes thyrotropin-releasing hormone (TRH) and stimulates the anterior pituitary gland to create TSH. The biosynthesis of thyroid hormone created by the thyroid gland is solely controlled by TSH. The thyroid functions to produce and secrete the thyroid hormones T_3 (triiodothyronine) and T_4 (tetraiodothyronine [thyroxine]) in a ratio of 1:10, respectively. When the concentration of thyroid hormone is sufficient, T_3 and T_4 have an inhibitory effect on the hypothalamus and anterior pituitary gland, creating a negative-feedback loop. This process is illustrated in Fig. 3.40.

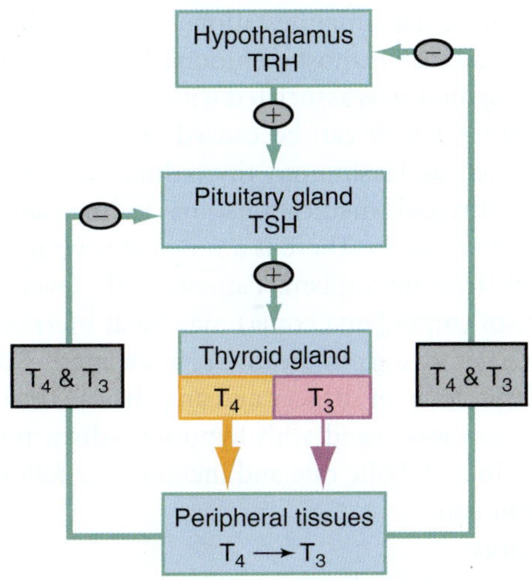

Fig. 3.40 Physiologic control of thyroid hormone secretion. *TRH*, Thyrotropin-releasing hormone; *TSH*, thyroid-stimulating hormone. (From Hall RM, Hockberger RS, Gausche-Hill M. *Rosen's Emergency Medicine: Concepts and Clinical Practice.* 9th ed. Elsevier; 2018.)

Thyroid hormones regulate the metabolic rate of numerous physiologic processes, including tissue growth, oxygen consumption, and the rate at which tissues utilize energy for catabolic processes. The symptomatology associated with thyroid dysfunction is directly related to the increase or decrease in metabolic rate that occurs with hyperthyroid or hypothyroid disease states, respectively. The signs and symptoms associated with these disease states are presented in Box 3.19.

Pathophysiology. *Hyperthyroidism* is a pathologic state in which the thyroid gland secretes an excessive amount of T_3 and T_4, resulting in hypermetabolism. Most cases are a result of Graves disease, toxic multinodular goiter, or toxic adenoma. Common signs and symptoms that are associated with hyperthyroidism include the following:

- Weight loss
- Exophthalmos
- Heat intolerance
- Tachycardia

BOX 3.19 Comparison of Signs and Symptoms of Hyperthyroidism and Hypothyroidism

Hyperthyroidism	Hypothyroidism
• Heat intolerance	• Cold intolerance
• Weight loss	• Weight gain
• Anorexia	• Depression
• Frequent bowel movements	• Constipation
	• Fatigue
• Muscle weakness/ fatigue	• Mood swings
	• Pericardial effusion
• Tremors	• Coronary artery disease
• Tachydysrhythmia (atrial fibrillation)	• Hypoglycemia
	• Peripheral vascular disease

- Muscle weakness
- Hyperglycemia
- Increased deep tendon reflexes
- Fatigue
- Cardiovascular manifestations—tachycardia, dysrhythmias (AF is most common), hypertension

Hypothyroidism is associated with low levels of T_3 and T_4 hormone, which can be caused by an autoimmune disease such as Hashimoto thyroiditis, radioactive iodine, antithyroid medications, or iodine deficiency, among other causes. There is a range of severity associated with hypothyroidism. Patients with severe hypothyroidism (myxedema coma) may be at increased risk for perioperative complications associated with the physiologic stress of surgery and anesthesia. The clinical presentation associated with hypothyroidism reflects a decrease in metabolic rate and includes the following:

- Weight gain
- Lethargy
- Coronary artery disease
- Hypoglycemia
- Peripheral vascular disease
- Cold intolerance
- Constipation
- Depression
- Decreased cardiac output

Anesthesia Case Management

Goals of perioperative management:

- Control hemodynamic variability (intraoperative hypertension).
- Potential for difficult airway
- Monitoring for postoperative respiratory insufficiency
  1. RLN injury
  2. Hematoma that impinges on the trachea
- Increased risk for postoperative nausea and vomiting

Preoperative Period

All elective cases should be postponed until antithyroid medications can allow the patient to achieve a euthyroid state. The patient should be evaluated for signs and symptoms such as tachycardia, fever, dysrhythmias, or agitation. Airway assessment and management may be complicated in patients having a thyroidectomy. The anesthetist must be aware that a potentially difficult intubation may occur in a patient with an enlarged thyroid gland. A nodule or goiter may displace the larynx and distort the normal airway anatomy, thus obscuring the view during laryngoscopy. Additionally, one should note the character of the patient's voice because hoarseness may indicate compression of the trachea or RLN.

Pharmacologic Therapy

- Thioamides

  Propylthiouracil (PTU) and methimazole (Tapazole) are thioamide medications that decrease the formation of thyroid hormone by inhibiting thyroid peroxidase, which catalyzes the conversion of iodide to iodine in the thyroid follicle cell. Additionally, these medications inhibit the organification process and decrease T_3 and T_4 levels.
- Iodides

  Sodium iodide or potassium iodide inhibits the organification process, the production and release of thyroid hormone, and the size and vascularity of the thyroid gland if hyperplasia exists. Because 60% of T_3 and T_4 is composed of iodine, it would seem counterintuitive to administer iodide. However, the Wolff-Chaikoff effect is an autoregulatory process that inhibits thyroid activity for several days to weeks if excessive quantities of iodide are present.
- β-Adrenergic blockade

  β-Blocking medications that do not possess intrinsic sympathomimetic activity inhibit the peripheral conversion of T_4 to T_3 and decrease the cardiac manifestations of enhanced SNS activity.
- Corticosteroids

Steroids have an inhibitory effect on TSH. These medications can be used in conjunction with others to achieve a euthyroid state.

Intraoperative Period

Maintenance of anesthesia should focus on attenuating SNS stimulation. This can be achieved by obtaining adequate depth of anesthesia to prevent an exaggerated response to surgical stimulation while avoiding drugs that excite the SNS. Some anesthetists avoid the use of desflurane because of the potential for SNS activation.

Although hyperthyroidism increases metabolic requirements, clinical evidence does not support an increase in MAC requirements for these patients. MAC requirements may be increased in the presence of hyperthermia; on average, a 4%–5% increase in MAC is seen with every degree that the temperature increases above 37°C. For this reason, continuous monitoring of temperature is essential.

The nerve integrity monitor (NIM) endotracheal tube uses electromyographic (EMG) information to determine the real-time integrity of the right and left RLNs. The electrodes that are present on the proximal end of the tube are inserted into a monitor that interprets the signals, allowing the surgeon to determine whether RLN function remains intact throughout surgery. Neuromuscular blockade and laryngeal tracheal lidocaine instillation will have an inhibitory effect on EMG, and their use is contraindicated if this endotracheal tube is used. If the patient must remain intubated for a prolonged period, the NIM endotracheal tube should be replaced with a standard endotracheal tube because of the potential for kinking and rupturing.

Thyroid storm. Early detection and prevention of thyroid storm is essential, and resuscitative measures should be instituted as soon as possible to prevent circulatory collapse. Thyroid storm is a hypermetabolic state due to an abrupt increase in circulating thyroid hormone. In most cases, diagnosis of thyroid storm is based on clinical findings alone because onset is abrupt, and treatment precludes diagnosis with laboratory tests or other screening measures.

Thyroid Storm—Signs and Symptoms

- Hyperthermia
- Tachycardia
- Tachydysrhythmias
- Hypertension
- Psychosis or altered mental state
- Rhabdomyolysis

Although thyrotoxic crisis can occur intraoperatively, the onset more frequently occurs 6–18 hours postoperatively. Precipitating factors include infection, surgery, DKA, CHF, pregnancy, and extreme physiologic stress. Without early recognition and treatment, thyroid storm can be fatal.

The treatment of thyroid storm involves pharmacologic treatment to decrease circulating thyroid hormone, as well as providing supportive interventions.

- Fluid resuscitation with chilled IV fluids in the presence of hyperthermia
- Serial electrolyte and ABG analysis
- Propylthiouracil or methimazole can be administered to further inhibit the synthesis of thyroid hormone.
- Sodium iodide is given to block the release of hormone from the thyroid gland.
- Acetaminophen is the antipyretic of choice. Aspirin is contraindicated because it can displace thyroid hormone from proteins, thereby increasing the physiologic effect.
- β-Adrenergic antagonists should be administered to control the cardiovascular effects associated with SNS predominance. Propranolol or a continuous infusion of esmolol can be administered.
- Steroid administration, such as dexamethasone or hydrocortisone
- Ruling out the possibility of other hypermetabolic states (e.g., MH, pheochromocytoma)

Postoperative Period

- *RLN damage* can be either unilateral or bilateral. Unilateral damage will manifest as hoarseness, whereas bilateral nerve palsy may result in aphonia, stridor, or respiratory distress. The incidence of permanent vocal cord paralysis is rare (0.5%–2.4%, with incidence of temporary paralysis being 2.6%–5.9%) and can be avoided by surgically identifying the location of the RLN intraoperatively before resection of the thyroid gland. Vocal cord function can be assessed via either direct laryngoscopy after deep extubation or by having the patient phonate "e" postoperatively. RLN dysfunction, whether unilateral or bilateral, may require reintubation and reexploration of the surgical site.

- *Hematoma formation* can cause further compression or collapse of the airway secondary to tracheomalacia (a weakening of the walls of the trachea). This typically occurs within 6–24 hours postoperatively. Inadequate surgical hemostasis, coagulopathy, acute hypertension, and straining from postoperative nausea and vomiting can increase the potential for postoperative bleeding. The definitive treatment involves immediate reexploration and evacuation of the hematoma.
- *Pneumothorax* is a rare complication associated with a thyroidectomy. Because the apices of the lungs extend above the level of the clavicles, very close to the surgical site, there is the potential for air to enter the thoracic cavity.
- *Acute hypocalcemia* resulting from inadvertent removal of the parathyroid glands
  Hypocalcemia is most likely to occur during the postoperative period. It is most likely to occur 24–48 hours after surgery is complete. Parathyroid dysfunction is typically transient, returning to normal in about 4 weeks postoperatively, and is treated with calcium and vitamin D supplementation.
- *Thyroid storm*, as discussed earlier

KNOWLEDGE CHECK

1. Which medication should be administered to treat thyroid storm? *(Select two.)*
   a. Methimazole
   b. Aspirin
   c. Dantrolene
   d. Sodium iodide
2. Which sign is *not* commonly observed during thyroid storm?
   a. Hypertension
   b. Hyperthermia
   c. Tachycardia
   d. Hypocarbia
3. Which best describes the sequence of physiologic stages that leads to the biosynthesis of thyroid hormone?
   a. TSH stimulates the thyroid gland to produce T_3 and T_4.
   b. TRH stimulates the thyroid gland to produce thyroid hormone.
   c. T_3 and T_4 directly stimulate the thyroid gland to produce thyroid hormone.
   d. T_3 and T_4 directly stimulate the hypothalamus to produce TSH.
4. If damaged, which nerve will cause hoarseness, stridor, and/or respiratory distress?
   a. Superior laryngeal
   b. Recurrent laryngeal
   c. Hypoglossal
   d. Facial
5. Because of its proximity to the thyroid gland, accidental removal of the parathyroid gland may result in
   a. hypokalemia.
   b. hypomagnesemia.
   c. hypermagnesemia.
   d. hypocalcemia.

Answers can be found in Appendix A.

Parathyroid Gland Dysfunction

The parathyroid glands are oval-shaped structures located at the four corners of the posterior aspect of the thyroid gland. They regulate calcium levels and produce parathyroid hormone (PTH), which has the effect of increasing blood calcium levels by doing the following:

- Increasing osteoclast activity in bone, causing the release of calcium
- Increasing reabsorption of calcium from the intestines
- Increasing reabsorption of calcium and the excretion of phosphate from the kidney

Approximately 99% of calcium exists within the bony skeleton. Ionized (free) calcium exerts vital physiologic effects, including skeletal, cardiac, and smooth muscle contractility; blood coagulation; and hormone and neurotransmitter release.

Hyperparathyroidism

Hyperparathyroidism results in an excess of PTH secretion, causing increased serum calcium levels. Frequent causes are associated with primary hyperparathyroidism, parathyroid gland adenoma, parathyroid gland hyperplasia, or parathyroid gland cancer. Secondary hyperparathyroidism is associated with chronic renal disease, vitamin D deficiency, and gastrointestinal malabsorption syndromes. With the development of sensitive laboratory assays for measuring PTH and imaging techniques, most patients are diagnosed and treated before the development of severe hypercalcemia.

TABLE 3.37 **Clinical Features of Hyperparathyroidism and Hypoparathyroidism**

System	Hyperparathyroidism	Hypoparathyroidism
Cardiovascular	Hypertension, cardiac conduction disturbances, shortened QT interval	Prolonged QT interval, hypotension, decreased cardiac contractility
Musculoskeletal	Bone pain, pathologic fractures, muscle weakness, muscle atrophy	Neuromuscular excitability; spasms; cramps
Neurologic	Somnolence, cognitive impairment, depression, hypotonia	Tetany, paresthesia, numbness in fingers and toes, seizures
Gastrointestinal	Anorexia, nausea, vomiting, constipation, abdominal pain, pancreatitis, peptic ulcer	Abdominal cramps
Renal	Tubular absorption defects, diminished renal function, kidney stones, polyuria	None significant

The signs and symptoms associated with hyperparathyroidism and hypoparathyroidism are shown in Table 3.37.

Anesthesia Case Management

- Parathyroidectomy is most often performed under general anesthesia; regional anesthesia and sedation can also be used.
- Intraoperative PTH and calcium levels are monitored.
- Consider normal saline as the IV fluid if patients are even mildly hypercalcemic.
- Sensitive to neuromuscular blockade—incremental dosing, neuromuscular blocker monitoring, and reversal with sugammadex are indicated.
- Potential for postoperative hypocalcemia—serial calcium level monitoring prudent
- Potential for RLN injury—postoperative hematoma that impinges on the airway and pneumothorax

Hypoparathyroidism

Hypoparathyroidism results in a deficiency of PTH secretion, causing decreased serum calcium levels. It results from either decreased secretion of PTH or peripheral tissue resistance to the effects of PTH (autoimmune hypoparathyroidism). Surgical procedures (e.g., inadvertent removal of parathyroid glands during thyroidectomy, radical neck dissection) are the most common causes of hypoparathyroidism. Medical treatment for hypoparathyroidism includes vitamin D, calcium, and magnesium supplementation.

Anesthesia Case Management

- Patients with moderate to severe hypocalcemia (ionized calcium levels <4.5 mg/dL) should receive calcium chloride 1 gram IV infusion preoperatively, and ionized calcium levels should be assessed after infusion.
- Hypocalcemia is associated with neuromuscular hyperactivity and is associated with the following:
  1. Chvostek sign—facial muscle hyperexcitability from pressure on the facial nerve
  2. Trousseau sign—carpopedal spasms
  3. Hyperactive deep tendon reflexes
- Patients are at risk for laryngospasm, muscle cramps, paresthesia, and labored respirations.
- If a nondepolarizing neuromuscular blocking medication is administered, careful assessment of neuromuscular functioning is necessary. Reversal with sugammadex is prudent.

KNOWLEDGE CHECK

1. Which mechanism is associated with increased secretion of PTH?
   a. Renal reabsorption of phosphate
   b. Decreased calcium absorption from the intestines
   c. Release of TSH
   d. Calcium release from the breakdown of bone

2. Which form of calcium is used to support normal physiologic functioning?
   a. Calcium phosphate
   b. Calcium gluconate
   c. Ionized calcium
   d. Total calcium

Continued

KNOWLEDGE CHECK—cont'd

3. Which are medical treatments for hypoparathyroidism? *(Select two.)*
   a. Potassium
   b. Vitamin D
   c. Sodium
   d. Magnesium
4. A patient with hyperparathyroidism may be sensitive to the effects of
   a. fentanyl.
   b. propofol.
   c. rocuronium.
   d. dexmedetomidine.
5. Which signs are associated with hypoparathyroidism? *(Select two.)*
   a. Chvostek
   b. Cushing
   c. Trousseau
   d. Beck

Answers can be found in Appendix A.

HEPATIC SYSTEM

Hepatic Anatomy

The liver is the largest abdominal organ and is located in the right upper quadrant (also known as the *right hypochondrium*). It is positioned inferiorly to the diaphragm and right rib cage (from rib 7 to 11 on the midaxillary line) and superiorly to the stomach, right kidney, and intestines. The left lobe of the liver extends into the left side of the abdomen (also known as the *left hypochondrium*).

The liver is a reddish-brown organ that weighs between 3 and 3.5 pounds.

- It is divided into four anatomical lobes:
  - Right lobe, which is the largest lobe and occupies most of the right upper quadrant of the abdomen
  - Left lobe, which is a smaller lobe and extends into the left upper quadrant
  - Caudate lobe, which is located on the posterior side of the liver near the inferior vena cava (IVC) and ligamentum venosum
  - Quadrate lobe, which is located on the inferior surface of the right lobe near the gallbladder fossa and the porta hepatis
- The liver is further divided into eight subdivisions with separate vascular and biliary drainage (Fig. 3.41):
  - I—caudate lobe
  - II—left lateral superior
  - III—left lateral inferior
  - IV—left medial
  - V—right anteroinferior
  - VI—right posteroinferior
  - VII—right posterosuperior
  - VIII—right anterosuperior
- The *falciform ligament* separates the right and left lobes on the anterior side of the liver, whereas the *ligamentum venosum* and *ligamentum teres* (remnants of fetal circulation) divide the posterior portions of the liver.
- The *porta hepatis* is a deep transverse fissure located on the inferior surface of the liver. It is known as the *hilum of the liver* and allows an entryway for passage of the portal vein, hepatic artery, common bile duct, nerves, and lymphatics into the liver.
- The liver contains roughly 50,000–1,000,000 fundamental working components known as *liver lobules*. These are funnel-shaped structures that are several millimeters long and roughly 2 mm wide.
- Each liver lobule consists of several hepatic plates made up of *hepatocytes* arranged two cells thick that sandwich a bile canaliculus and radiate outward from a central vein toward portal tracts within the interlobular septum.
- Hepatocyte cellular plates are separated by *venous sinusoids* (e.g., small venous blood vessels) that lead to a central vein for drainage. Blood flow from the portal tracks follows these sinusoid pathways within the liver lobule, allowing the hepatocytes access to all components within the blood serum.
- Each sequence of plates within a liver lobule is lined externally by *Kupffer cells* and *endothelial cells* that exist with a space between them and the cellular plates known as the *space of Disse*. These cells are the ones that are in contact with the venous sinusoids.
  - Endothelial cells line the sinusoids and have large pores (~1 μm in diameter), which allow plasma substances to pass through.

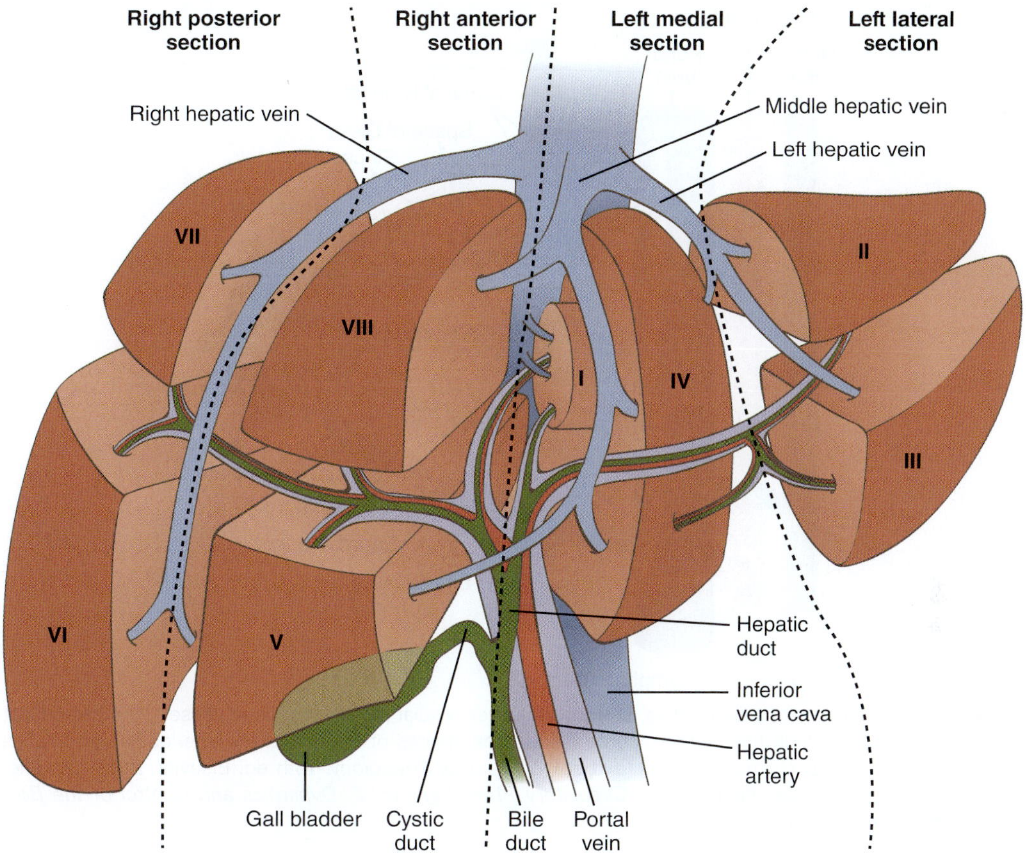

Fig. 3.41 Anatomic and functional subdivisions of the liver. The eight functional anatomic segments of the liver are demonstrated in this drawing. Each segment has its own blood supply and biliary drainage. (From Hines RL, Jones SB. *Stoelting's Anesthesia and Co-Existing Disease*. 8th ed. Elsevier; 2022.)

    - Kupffer cells are resident macrophages that remove bacteria and debris from the bloodstream.
    - Spaces of Disse are spaces that exist between the hepatic cells and endothelial cells and (1) facilitate exchange of plasma substances and (2) drain excess fluid into lymphatic vessels.
- Hepatic blood flow, bile processing, and lymphatic flow support each liver lobule via a portal venule, hepatic arteriole, bile ductule, and lymphatic vessel within the interlobular septum (Fig. 3.42).

Hepatic Blood Flow

- The liver is a highly metabolic organ with a high blood flow. It receives approximately 25% of the cardiac output and accounts for 20% of total body oxygen consumption.
- The liver receives a dual blood supply from the hepatic artery and the portal vein.
    - The *common hepatic artery* provides 25% of hepatic blood flow, transporting oxygenated blood from the celiac trunk, which is a major branch of the abdominal aorta.
        - The hepatic artery provides 50% of the liver's oxygen supply.
    - The *portal vein* provides 75% of hepatic blood flow and carries deoxygenated (but nutrient-rich) blood from the stomach, intestines, spleen, and pancreas to the liver for nutrient processing (Fig. 3.43).
- After entering through the porta hepatis, both the hepatic artery and portal vein branch into each of the liver subdivisions and eventually mix the oxygenated and deoxygenated blood at the hepatic sinusoids,

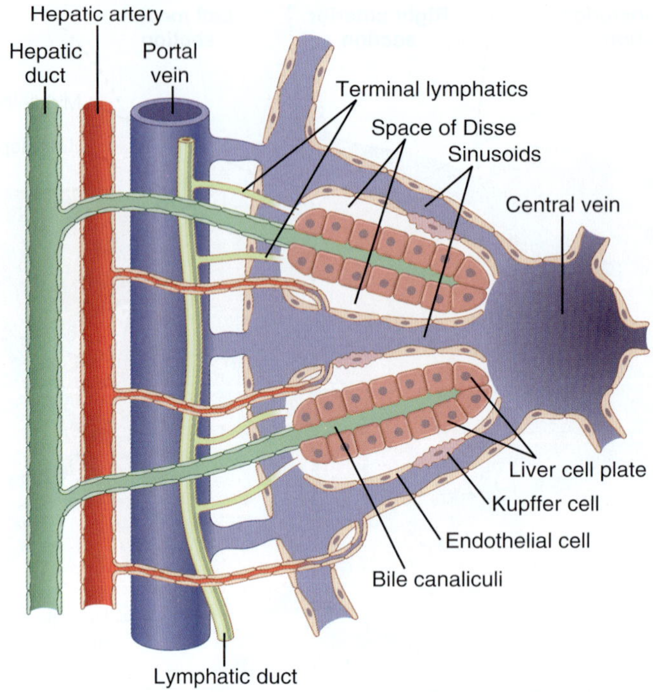

Fig. 3.42 Basic structure of a liver lobule, showing the liver cellular plates, the blood vessels, the bile-collecting system, and the lymph flow system composed of the spaces of Disse and the interlobular lymphatics. (From Hall JE, Hall ME. *Guyton and Hall Textbook of Medical Physiology.* 15th ed. Elsevier; 2026. Modified from Guyton AC, Taylor AE, Granger HJ. *Circulatory Physiology. Vol 2: Dynamics and Control of the Body Fluids.* WB Saunders, 1975.)

where hepatocytes extract nutrients and detoxify substances.

- Blood drains from the hepatic sinusoids into the central vein of each liver lobule, which then converges into hepatic veins and ultimately empties into the IVC.
- A summary of liver blood flow is as follows:
  - Hepatic portal vein (containing deoxygenated blood from the stomach, intestines, pancreas, and spleen) and hepatic artery (carrying oxygenated blood from the LV) enter the liver through the porta hepatis.
  - Blood flow is divided into each of the eight liver subdivisions.
  - Interlobular hepatic arterioles and portal veins direct blood into hepatic sinusoids.
  - Hepatic sinusoids are specialized capillaries located within liver lobules.
    - Within these sinusoids is where blood from the portal vein and hepatic artery mix.
    - The mixture then flows through the sinusoids and drains into the central vein of each liver lobule.
  - The central veins channel blood into the hepatic veins.
  - Hepatic veins empty blood into the IVC.
- Arterial autoregulation of hepatic blood flow ensures a relatively constant blood supply to the liver despite changes in systemic circulation.
  - It requires coordination between hepatic arterial and portal venous blood flow systems.
  - The mean pressure of the hepatic artery is similar to that of the aorta.
  - The *hepatic arterial buffer response (HABR)* causes hepatic artery dilation to increase hepatic blood flow to compensate for decreased portal venous flow.
    - This mechanism is mediated in part by adenosine, which accumulates and causes arterial vasodilation.
  - Conversely, when portal blood flow increases, hepatic arterial flow reflexively decreases.
  - Other factors that assist with the autoregulation of liver blood flow include the myogenic response of

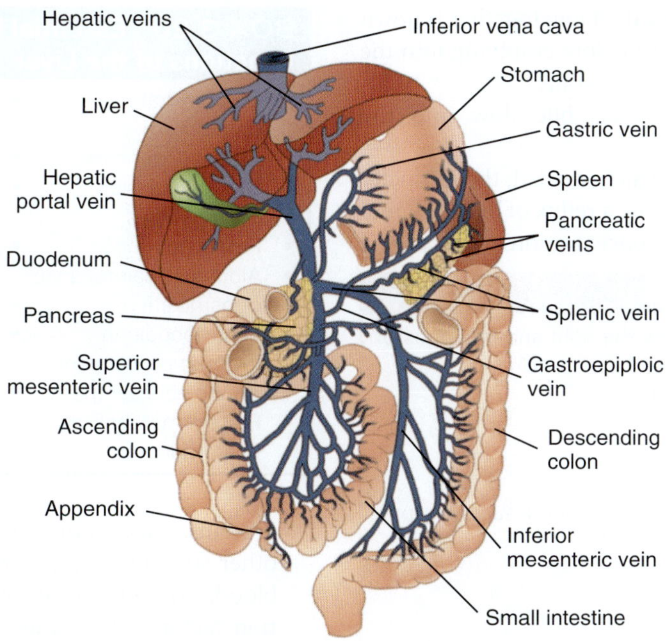

Fig. 3.43 Hepatic portal circulation. In this unusual circulatory route, a vein is located between two capillary beds. The hepatic portal vein collects blood from capillaries in visceral structures located in the abdomen and empties into the liver for distribution to the hepatic capillaries. Hepatic veins return blood to the inferior vena cava. *I,* Inferior; *L,* left; *R,* right; *S,* superior. (From Patton KT, Bell F, Thompson T, et al. *Anatomy & Physiology.* 11th ed. Elsevier; 2022.)

liver arterioles that will constrict or dilate in response to changes in systemic pressure and portal venous pressure.

- Local metabolism and autonomic input fine-tune vascular tone within the hepatic system.

- The liver portal venous pressure is between 6 and 10 mm Hg, which allows for the storage of a significant amount of blood volume, especially in patients with cardiac failure.
  - In a normal and healthy liver, there is a very low pressure through the venous sinusoids.
  - A normal liver blood volume that includes the hepatic veins and sinuses is 450 mL. However, the liver has the ability to expand and allow an additional 500–1000 mL within the venous system in cases of increased right heart pressures.

Hepatic Biliary System

- Liver hepatocytes produce bile, which is moved through the hepatic ducts into the common bile duct and is secreted into the small intestine through the sphincter of Oddi to aid in digestion, absorption, and excretion of substances.
- The biliary system consists of the following (see Fig. 3.41):
  - *Bile canaliculi*, which are very small ducts located between hepatocyte cellular plates and collect bile produced by hepatocytes within liver lobules
  - Bile canaliculi drain into a network of small ducts known as *intrahepatic bile ducts* that merge from each of the liver subdivisions to form the *right and left hepatic ducts.*
  - The right and left hepatic ducts come together to form the *common hepatic duct.*
  - The *cystic duct* connects the gallbladder to the common hepatic duct and transports stored bile into the common bile duct.
  - The *common bile duct* is formed by the union of the common hepatic duct and cystic duct; it transports bile to the duodenum of the small intestine.
  - The *sphincter of Oddi* is a muscular valve that is located at the junction where the common bile

duct and the pancreatic duct join together (known as the *ampulla of Vater*) before emptying into the duodenum of the small intestine.

- This sphincter controls bile flow into the duodenum.
- If bile is not immediately needed, the sphincter of Oddi closes, causing a reflux of bile back into the gallbladder for concentration and storage.

KNOWLEDGE CHECK

1. Which structure separates the right and left lobes of the liver on the anterior surface?
   a. Ligamentum venosum
   b. Falciform ligament
   c. Common bile duct
   d. Hepatic portal vein
2. What percentage of the liver's blood supply is provided by the portal vein?
   a. 25%
   b. 50%
   c. 75%
   d. 100%
3. Which cells in the liver are responsible for phagocytizing bacteria and debris from the bloodstream?
   a. Endothelial cells
   b. Hepatocytes
   c. Kupffer cells
   d. Sinusoidal cells
4. What is the function of the hepatic arterial buffer response?
   a. Increases bile production and flow into intestines during periods of fasting
   b. Maintains consistent hepatic blood flow despite portal vein fluctuations
   c. Stimulates the release of digestive enzymes
   d. Contracts the sphincter of Oddi to concentrate and store bile
5. Which structure controls the flow of bile into the small intestine?
   a. Duodenum
   b. Ligamentum teres
   c. Sphincter of Oddi
   d. Ampulla of Vater

Answers can be found in Appendix A.

Hepatic Physiology

- The liver is a highly metabolic organ that is involved in many biochemical reactions as well as the synthesis of numerous substances (Box 3.20).
- The primary physiologic functions of the hepatic system include (1) metabolism of carbohydrates, proteins, fats, cholesterol, hormones, drugs, and other substances; (2) filtration and detoxification of blood; (3) synthesis of various proteins and coagulation factors; (4) storage of vitamins and iron; and (5) formation of bile.
  - The liver contains hepatocytes that comprise approximately 75%–80% of the liver cellular volume. These hepatocytes are the backbone of the various physiologic functions, including metabolism, detoxification, protein synthesis, and bile production.
- The hepatic system facilitates multiple metabolic processes, including the metabolism of carbohydrates, proteins, fats, hormones, and other foreign chemicals.

BOX 3.20 Essential Physiologic Functions of the Liver

- Carbohydrate metabolism
- Gluconeogenesis
- Glycogenolysis
- Glycogenesis
- Protein synthesis
- Albumin (maintenance of osmolarity)
- Thrombopoietin (platelet production)
- Amino acid synthesis
- Protein metabolism
- Bile production
- Lipid metabolism
- Lipogenesis
- Cholesterol synthesis
- Coagulation factor synthesis
- Production of factors I, II, V, VII, IX, X, and XI
- Insulin clearance
- Drug metabolism/transformation
- Bilirubin metabolism

Carbohydrate Metabolism

- One of the primary functions of the liver is to metabolize carbohydrates into glucose for use by various organs (e.g., brain, kidneys, heart).
- A healthy liver maintains euglycemia (especially during fasting) by storing glycogen and regulating blood glucose levels by means of the following:
  - *Glycogenolysis*, which is the process of breaking down glycogen into glucose.
    - When glucose levels are low, glucagon (and epinephrine) initiates glycogenolysis.
    - This process is facilitated by the enzymes glycogen phosphorylase (key enzyme in glycogenolysis), phosphoglucomutase, and glucose-6-phosphatase.
  - *Gluconeogenesis* is the process of synthesizing glucose from noncarbohydrate sources such as lactate,

glycerol, and glucogenic amino acids when dietary intake is low. This function is especially helpful during fasting, prolonged exercise, or starvation.
- Gluconeogenesis is stimulated by glucagon and cortisol and inhibited by insulin.
- It utilizes precursors such as lactate (from anaerobic glycolysis), glycerol (from fat breakdown), and glucogenic amino acids (from skeletal muscle protein breakdown),
- Several different enzymes are involved in gluconeogenesis.
- The end result is the production and release of glucose into the bloodstream to maintain blood glucose levels, especially for the brain and RBCs.

- Carbohydrate metabolism and the production of glucose are altered in situations of poor liver function or disease, leading to elevated blood glucose levels after meals. This is a result of impaired gluconeogenesis and reduced glycogen stores.

Protein Metabolism

- Several important processes occur in the liver regarding the metabolism of protein. These include amino acid uptake, deamination and catabolism, detoxification of ammonia into urea, and the synthesis of important proteins.
- The liver removes amino acids from the portal blood after digestion.
  - It then uses a process called *deamination* to remove the amino group ($-NH_2$), forming ammonia (NH_3) and a carbon skeleton. Deamination is necessary so that amino acids can be used as energy or converted into carbohydrates or fats.
    - These carbon skeletons are then used for energy production (e.g., conversion into ATP via the citric acid cycle) from gluconeogenesis or lipogenesis.
    - Transamination is a form of deamination that uses transaminase enzymes such as alanine transaminase (ALT) and aspartate transaminase (AST) (Table 3.38) to synthesize ingested amino acids into nonessential amino acids. This process helps with amino acid metabolism and removal of nitrogen from amino acids.
  - Excess amino acids are catabolized, and their energy is converted into glucose, ketone bodies, or fat.
- Ammonia produced from the deamination of proteins and gut bacteria is detoxified and converted into urea via the urea cycle, which occurs in liver hepatocytes.
  - Urea is then excreted by the kidneys.
  - This process prevents the toxic buildup of ammonia in the blood.
- The liver synthesizes several plasma proteins (up to 90% of body's plasma proteins)
  - It produces albumin, complement proteins, and clotting factors.
  - Liver hepatocytes also synthesize acute-phase proteins in response to inflammatory signals that play a role in the body's defense against injury and infection.
  - Protein synthesis helps regulate plasma oncotic pressure and transport molecules within the blood plasma.
  - A loss of plasma proteins during liver disease can result in the following:
    - Lower plasma oncotic pressure
    - Edema and ascites (e.g., cirrhosis)
    - Drug-binding problems resulting in exaggerated and prolonged drug effects
    - Adjustments in drug dosing (e.g., nondepolarizing neuromuscular blockers)
    - Plasma cholinesterase deficiency resulting in prolonged effects of succinylcholine and/or ester local anesthetics

Fat Metabolism

- Liver metabolism of fat is an important function related to the body's energy balance from fatty acid oxidation, lipogenesis, ketone body synthesis (ketogenesis), and cholesterol metabolism.
- Fatty acid uptake and oxidation lead to the production of energy.
  - The liver removes free fatty acids from the blood (e.g., from dietary sources or adipose tissue lipolysis), which are then moved into hepatocytes.
  - Within hepatic cells, acyl-coenzyme A (CoA) synthetases convert free fatty acids into *fatty acyl-CoA* using ATP and Mg^{2+}.
  - β-Oxidation of fatty acyl-CoA within the hepatocyte mitochondria is necessary for the breakdown of fatty acids for energy.
    - Fatty acyl-CoA cannot directly enter the mitochondria for β-oxidation. Instead, it is converted to *acylcarnitine* through the *carnitine*

TABLE 3.38 Liver Laboratory Analysis and Clinical Significance

Test (Normal Range*)	Clinical Significance
Aminotransferases ALT (10–55 units/L) AST (10–40 units/L)	Abnormalities cause leakage from damaged hepatic tissue. ALT is more specific than AST for hepatic injuries. AST/ALT >2 suggests alcoholic liver disease or cirrhosis of any etiology. AST nonspecific: can originate from skeletal muscle, red blood cell, kidney, pancreas, brain, and myocardium
AP (45–115 units/L)	Abnormalities cause overproduction and leakage into serum. Moderate elevations: Many types of liver disease Marked elevations: Extrahepatic and intrahepatic cholestasis, diffuse infiltrating disease (e.g., tumor, MAC), rarely alcoholic hepatitis Extrahepatic origin may be from bone growth or disease (e.g., tumor, fracture, Paget disease), placenta, intestine, and tumors.
GGTP (0–30 units/L)	Abnormalities cause overproduction and leakage into serum. Moderate elevations: Many types of liver disease. Marked elevations: Extrahepatic and intrahepatic cholestasis, diffuse infiltrating disease (e.g., tumor, MAC), ethanol and drugs GGTP/AP >2.5 suggests alcoholic liver disease.
5′ nucleotidase (0–11 units/L)	Abnormalities cause overproduction and leakage into serum. Found in many tissues, but serum elevation is relatively specific for liver disease. Moderate elevations: Many types of liver disease Marked elevations: Extrahepatic and intrahepatic cholestasis, diffuse infiltrating disease (e.g., tumor, MAC), rarely alcoholic hepatitis
Bilirubin (0–1 mg/dL)	Abnormality is related to decreased hepatic clearance. Moderate elevations: Many types of liver disease Marked elevations: Extrahepatic and intrahepatic bile duct obstruction; viral, alcoholic, or drug-induced hepatitis; inherited hyperbilirubinemia
Prothrombin time (PT): (10.9–12.5 seconds) international normalized ratio (INR): (0.9–1.2)	Abnormality is due to a decrease in synthetic capacity from acute or chronic liver failure (prolonged PT unresponsive to vitamin K); biliary obstruction (prolonged PT usually responsive to vitamin K administration) Abnormality may also be the result of vitamin K deficiency (secondary to malabsorption, malnutrition, antibiotics, consumptive coagulopathy).
Albumin (3.5–5.0 g/dL)	Abnormality due to decreased synthesis; increased catabolism from chronic liver failure Abnormalities caused by extrahepatic origins include nephritic syndrome, protein-losing enteropathy, vascular leak, malnutrition, malignancy, infections, and inflammatory states.

*The normal values shown in this table are for adult males and will vary with the methodology used in testing.
ALT, Alanine aminotransferase; *AP*, alkaline phosphatase; *AST*, aspartate aminotransferase; *GGTP*, gamma-glutamyl transpeptidase; *MAC*, *Mycobacterium avium* complex.

shuttle, which facilitates the transport of fatty acyl-CoA across the mitochondrial membrane.
    - Once inside the mitochondria, acylcarnitine is reconverted to fatty acyl-CoA. β-Oxidation of fatty acyl-CoA results in acetyl-CoA for energy.
- Liver lipogenesis converts excess carbohydrates into fatty acids. These are then stored as triglycerides or transported as very-low-density lipoproteins (VLDLs).
- Insulin stimulates lipogenesis, and glucagon inhibits lipogenesis (especially during fasting).
- When energy is abundant, the liver converts excess glucose and acetyl-CoA into fatty acids and triglycerides.
- Triglycerides are stored in the liver (but only in small amounts) or packaged into VLDLs for export into adipose tissue.

- Ketogenesis (ketosis) produces ketone bodies from acetyl-CoA, primarily during periods of prolonged fasting, starvation, low carbohydrate intake, or uncontrolled diabetes.
    - Ketone bodies are water soluble, are easily transported in the blood, and provide an alternative energy source for the brain, heart, and skeletal muscle.
    - Ketosis is a normal adaptive response to fasting or low-carbohydrate diets.
    - In DKA, excessive ketone production leads to metabolic acidosis.

Cholesterol Extraction, Synthesis, Transport, and Elimination

- Cholesterol extraction and uptake, synthesis, storage, transport, and excretion occur primarily in the liver.
- The liver extracts dietary cholesterol from intestinal blood flow.
    - Cholesterol in the liver is primarily used to synthesize bile salts (for digestion). It is also used to build cell membranes, create steroid hormones, facilitate vitamin D conversion, and transport lipoproteins for cell use.
    - Cholesterol is used for the synthesis of vitamin D_3 in the skin. The liver then converts vitamin D_3 (from skin absorption) into the active form 25-hydroxyvitamin D, which then travels to the kidneys for the final conversion to the most active form, 1,25-dihydroxyvitamin D.
- The liver will synthesize cholesterol, especially when dietary intake is low.
    - It begins with acetyl-CoA and uses the enzyme hydroxymethylglutaryl–coenzyme A (HMG-CoA) reductase to convert it to HMG-CoA, which eventually results in mevalonate. Mevalonate then undergoes several steps to form cholesterol.
    - Statin medications target HMG-CoA reductase to lower cholesterol levels.
- The liver plays a key role in cholesterol transport:
    - VLDL carries triglycerides and some cholesterol to peripheral tissues (especially adipose tissue).
    - Low-density lipoprotein (LDL) is formed from VLDL remnants and is a method of cholesterol delivery to tissues.
    - High-density lipoprotein (HDL) originates from excess cholesterol in peripheral tissues, which is returned to the liver (reverse cholesterol transport).
- Cholesterol excretion and elimination from the body occur through the bile. Some cholesterol is secreted directly into bile, but most is converted to bile salts/acids (cholic and chenodeoxycholic acid) and then excreted into the intestine.
- Excess cholesterol is stored in the liver.

KNOWLEDGE CHECK

1. Which is *not* a primary physiologic function of the liver?
    a. Protein synthesis
    b. Filtration and detoxification of blood
    c. Production of insulin
    d. Formation of bile
2. Which metabolic process describes the liver's ability to create glucose from noncarbohydrate sources?
    a. Glycogenolysis
    b. Lipogenesis
    c. Gluconeogenesis
    d. Ketogenesis
3. What enzyme is the rate-limiting step in cholesterol synthesis within the liver?
    a. Glucose-6-phosphatase
    b. HMG-CoA reductase
    c. Glycogen phosphorylase
    d. Acyl-CoA synthetase
4. Which plasma protein, synthesized by the liver, plays a major role in maintaining plasma oncotic pressure?
    a. Fibrinogen
    b. Albumin
    c. Complement proteins
    d. Acute-phase proteins
5. A failure of the liver's ability to convert toxic ammonia into urea can result in what complication?
    a. Hypoglycemia
    b. Hyperbilirubinemia
    c. Hepatic encephalopathy
    d. Hyperlipidemia

Answers can be found in Appendix A.

Hormone, Drug, and Other Substance Metabolism

- The liver metabolizes and inactivates certain endogenous hormones and exogenous compounds such as drugs, alcohol, and toxins.
    - Examples of hormones metabolized by the liver include thyroxine, estrogen, cortisol, and aldosterone.
    - Examples of drugs metabolized include alcohol, sulfonamides, penicillins, opioids, benzodiazepines, volatile anesthetics, propofol, and other anesthetic drugs.

- Liver damage can result in hormone imbalances and altered drug metabolism.
- Metabolism primarily occurs through two enzymatic reaction phases.
  - Phase I reactions are oxidative and hydrolytic to facilitate the inactivation of substances for easier elimination, whereas phase II reactions promote easier excretion of substances via the bile or urine.
    - The main enzyme system involved in phase I reactions is the cytochrome P450 enzyme system (CYP450).
    - Phase I reactions (known as *modification reactions*) can inactivate a substance, bioactivate a substance into a more active form, or produce reactive intermediates that can be further metabolized in phase II reactions.
    - Phase II reactions (known as *conjugation reactions*) help detoxify substances in the liver and involve the conjugation of a substance (attaching a hydrophilic group to a drug or metabolite) by enzymes that convert it into a more excretable form. These reactions generally result in inactive, nontoxic, and hydrophilic metabolites.
    - The major types of conjugation reactions include glucuronidation (most common), sulfation, glutathione conjugation, acetylation, and methylation.

Filtration and Detoxification of Blood

- The liver acts as a central filter and detoxification center for the blood that drains from the intestines, stomach, pancreas, and spleen via the portal vein.
  - The hepatic system ensures that nutrients, toxins, drugs, and microbial byproducts absorbed from the gut are processed before entering systemic circulation.
  - Blood from intestinal capillaries picks up bacteria (e.g., colon bacilli), then travels into the portal venous blood.
- Blood flow from the portal vein and hepatic artery mixes in the hepatic sinusoids, allowing interaction with hepatocytes and immune cells.
- Within the hepatic sinusoids, blood flows through fenestrated capillaries lined by endothelial cells and Kupffer cells.
  - Kupffer cells are resident macrophages that phagocytose pathogens, debris, aged RBCs, and bacteria from the gut.
  - The hepatic macrophage system is very fast and efficient at cleansing the blood: Bacteria contacting Kupffer cells can be captured by these cells in $<$0.01 second and pulled inward to be digested. More than 99% of bacteria from portal blood are eliminated before reaching systemic circulation.
  - Stellate cells are also present and involved in immune signaling.
- Hepatocytes line the sinusoids and perform biochemical detoxification in three main steps:
  1. Uptake: Transporters on hepatocyte membranes import substances from the blood (e.g., bile acids, bilirubin, drugs, toxins).
  2. Biotransformation: They perform phase I reactions that modify compounds (e.g., oxidation by cytochrome P450 enzymes) and phase II reactions that conjugate compounds with polar groups (e.g., glucuronidation, sulfation) to increase solubility.
  3. Excretion: Processed substances are excreted into bile (e.g., bilirubin, drug conjugates) and transported into the intestines for elimination in feces, or they are absorbed in the blood for transport to the kidneys for secretion into the renal tubule and elimination in the urine.
- The liver also processes nutrients from the gut and does the following:
  - Converts glucose to glycogen for storage
  - Converts amino acids to urea and other proteins
  - Converts lipids into lipoproteins or ketone bodies
  - Stores vitamins and minerals
- The hepatic system clears the blood of hormones and ammonia.
  - The liver metabolizes hormones (e.g., insulin, glucagon, estrogen).
  - The ammonia produced by protein catabolism and gut bacteria is converted to urea (via the urea cycle) and excreted by the kidneys.
- The hepatic system processes hemoglobin breakdown from the spleen.
  - Heme from hemoglobin breakdown is converted to unconjugated bilirubin by reticuloendothelial cells in the spleen.
    - Unconjugated bilirubin is water insoluble and neurotoxic at high serum blood levels.
  - Unconjugated bilirubin from the spleen binds to albumin in blood and is transported to the liver.
  - Hepatocytes absorb albumin-bound unconjugated bilirubin from the blood and convert it to conjugated

bilirubin with the enzyme UDP-glucuronosyltransferase (UGT) and glucuronic acid.
- The conjugated form of bilirubin is water soluble and nontoxic, and it is secreted into bile canaliculi in liver lobules and then delivered to the small intestine via the biliary system, where it is metabolized by gut bacterial enzymes and excreted in the feces.
- If the liver fails to process bilirubin (e.g., in liver disease, bile duct obstruction, or hemolysis), bilirubin can accumulate and cause jaundice.

Synthesis of Various Proteins and Coagulation Factors

- The liver plays a central role in the synthesis of plasma proteins and blood coagulation factors.
- Primary plasma proteins that are synthesized within the liver include albumin, transferrin, ceruloplasmin, haptoglobin, alpha-1 antitrypsin, alpha-2 macroglobulin, complement proteins, lipoproteins, and C-reactive proteins (Table 3.39).
- Most blood coagulation factors are synthesized in the liver, including factor I (fibrinogen), factor II (prothrombin), factor V, factor VII, factor IX (Christmas), factor X, factor XI and XII, and factor XIII (fibrin-stabilizing) (Table 3.40).
  - Vitamin K–dependent factors include factors II, VII, IX, and X, as well as protein S and protein C (anticoagulants), which are all vital for the clotting cascade.
  - Warfarin inhibits the vitamin K production of functional vitamin K–dependent factors.
  - Blood coagulation factors not synthesized in the liver are factor VIII (von Willebrand factor), tissue thromboplastin (factor III), and calcium (factor IV).
- Liver dysfunction (e.g., cirrhosis, hepatitis) can lead to the following:
  - Hypoalbuminemia, which can result in edema and/or ascites
  - Reduction in clotting factor synthesis (particularly vitamin K–dependent ones), which can result in coagulopathies with prolonged prothrombin time (PT)/international normalized ratio (INR) values and an increase in bleeding tendencies
- The liver does not primarily regulate calcium; however, it influences calcium homeostasis by activating vitamin D.
  - Vitamin D, either D_2 (ergocalciferol) or D_3 (cholecalciferol), is synthesized by the skin when exposed to ultraviolet (UV) light or obtained from the diet and absorbed from the small intestine.
  - The liver performs the initial hydroxylation of vitamin D (D_2 and D_3) and converts it into 25-hydroxyvitamin D, which is the primary circulating form of vitamin D.
  - 25-hydroxyvitamin D then travels to the kidney, where it undergoes a second hydroxylation and is converted to 1,25-dihydroxyvitamin D (calcitriol), which is the active form of vitamin D.
  - Calcitriol increases intestinal calcium absorption, bone metabolism, and other physiologic activities.

TABLE 3.39 Primary Plasma Proteins Synthesized in the Liver

Plasma Protein	Function/Notes
Albumin	Maintains oncotic pressure, transports hormones, drugs, and fatty acids
Transferrin	Iron transport
Ceruloplasmin	Copper transport
Haptoglobin	Binds free hemoglobin
Alpha-1 antitrypsin	Serine protease inhibitor; protects lung tissue
Alpha-2 macroglobulin	Broad-spectrum protease inhibitor
Complement proteins (C1–C9)	Innate immunity, inflammation, activates complement cascade to target and destroy pathogens
Lipoproteins (LDL, HDL, VLDL)	Lipid transport
C-reactive protein (CRP)	Acute-phase reactant (rises in response to inflammation); rapidly activates the complement system and other immune processes

HDL, High-density lipoprotein; *LDL*, low-density lipoprotein; *VLDL*, very low-density lipoprotein.

TABLE 3.40 Coagulation Factors Synthesized in the Liver

Clotting Factors	Name	Vitamin K Dependent?	Function/Notes
Factor I	Fibrinogen	No	Precursor of fibrin
Factor II	Prothrombin	Yes	Converted to thrombin
Factor V	Proaccelerin	No	Cofactor in prothrombinase complex
Factor VII	Proconvertin	Yes	Activates extrinsic pathway
Factor IX	Christmas factor	Yes	Activates factor X (intrinsic pathway)
Factor X	Stuart-Prower factor	Yes	Common pathway; activates thrombin
Factor XI	Plasma thromboplastin antecedent	No	Intrinsic pathway
Factor XII	Hageman factor	No	Initiates contact activation pathway
Factor XIII	Fibrin-stabilizing factor	No	Cross-links fibrin; also synthesized by platelets
Protein S	Anticoagulant	Yes	Cofactor for the formation of protein C
Protein C	Anticoagulant	Yes	Inhibits coagulation by preventing excessive thrombin generation and clot formation

Hepatic Storage of Vitamins, Iron, and Copper

- The liver plays a major role in the storage, regulation, and release of essential fat-soluble and water-soluble vitamins.
  - Fat-soluble vitamins stored in the liver include the following:
    - Vitamin A (retinol)—used for vision, immune function, and epithelial maintenance. The liver can store enough vitamin A to meet body needs for months to years.
    - Vitamin D—used for calcium and phosphate metabolism, as well as bone health. Vitamin D absorbed from the skin and gut goes through hydroxylation in the liver to become 25-hydroxyvitamin D (calcidiol), and it is stored in this form for several months.
    - Vitamin E (tocopherol)—used as an antioxidant to protect cell membranes and is stored in smaller amounts than vitamin A.
    - Vitamin K—used for the synthesis of clotting factors (II, VII, IX, X, and protein C and S). Vitamin K has a shorter half-life and lower storage capacity than other fat-soluble vitamins.
  - Water-soluble vitamins stored in the liver include the following:
    - Vitamin B_{12} (cobalamin)—used for DNA synthesis, neurologic health and function, RBC production, and cell metabolism. Can be stored for 1–5 years, making B_{12} one of the few water-soluble vitamins with significant storage.
    - Folate (vitamin B_9)—used for DNA synthesis and repair, RBC formation, and white blood cell production and function. The liver stores about half the body's folate for several weeks to months.
    - The liver is primarily involved in the storage and regulation of iron.
  - Iron is stored in the following forms:
    - Ferritin—the safe and bioavailable form that acts as the first-line buffer against iron deficiency
    - Hemosiderin—insoluble and less readily available form that accumulates when iron levels are chronically high
  - Iron is regulated by key liver proteins:
    - Hepcidin is the primary regulator of iron and controls its absorption in the gut and release from macrophages and hepatocytes in the liver.
    - Liver disease causes reduced hepcidin production, leading to iron overload.
    - When hepcidin levels are high because of inflammation, anemia can occur as a result of reduced iron availability despite normal or increased stores.
    - Transferrin is a glycoprotein synthesized by the liver that binds iron in plasma, safely transports it in the bloodstream, and delivers it to hepatocytes.
- The liver plays a central role in the storage, regulation, and excretion of copper.
  - Copper is absorbed in the small intestine, travels to the liver bound to albumin and amino acids, and is then stored in hepatocytes.

- Excess copper is excreted into bile and eliminated in feces.
- Copper is released by the hepatocytes in low states, and more is excreted in the bile in high states.
- Malabsorption syndromes, excess zinc intake (competes with copper), or parenteral nutrition without copper supplementation can lead to copper deficiencies, resulting in anemia, neutropenia, and neurologic issues.

Formation and Function of Bile

- Bile is a fluid produced in the liver and stored in the gallbladder that helps with intestinal absorption, digestion, and excretion of substances.
- Bile has five main functions: (1) fat digestion, (2) absorption of fat-soluble vitamins (vitamins A, D, E, and K), (3) aiding in the excretion of bilirubin and excess cholesterol, (4) neutralizing stomach acid by providing an alkaline solution, and (5) providing bactericidal activity from bile salts.
- Hepatocytes secrete primary bile into bile canaliculi, which then transport it to bile ducts, which then empty into intrahepatic ducts.
  - Bile is modified by biliary epithelial cells known as *cholangiocytes*. Their function is to add water and alkalinity to the bile fluid.
- Bile flows into the gallbladder via the cystic duct between meals for storage and concentration. It is released in response to meals.
  - Cholecystokinin (CCK) is a hormone produced in the small intestine and released in response to fats and proteins. Vagal stimulation (via acetylcholine) will also stimulate its release.
  - One primary function of CCK is to cause gallbladder contraction and the release of bile into the small intestine. It also causes pancreatic enzyme secretion and promotes satiety.
- Bile duct obstructions can be caused by gallstones (the most common), cysts, strictures of the duct, or tumors, which can potentially cause the following:
  - Fat malabsorption (steatorrhea)—results in pale, foul-smelling, oily stools
  - Fat-soluble vitamin deficiencies—vitamin D (hypocalcemia, osteomalacia), vitamin K (coagulopathy)
  - Cholesterol imbalances—may lead to hypercholesterolemia
  - Bilirubin accumulation when bile is completely blocked—can cause jaundice
  - Potential for bacterial overgrowth in the gut

Liver Regeneration

- One characteristic of the liver is its ability to regenerate after significant tissue loss (e.g., partial hepatectomy or after acute injury).
- Remaining lobes can enlarge and, over time, restore the liver to its original size.
- Key factors involved in liver regeneration include hepatocyte growth factor (produced by mesenchymal cells), an increase in liver blood flow, other growth factors, and cytokines.
- Liver regeneration is severely compromised in liver disease (e.g., inflammation, viral infections, fibrosis), which instead causes a deterioration in liver function.

KNOWLEDGE CHECK

1. Which enzyme system is primarily responsible for phase I reactions in the liver?
   a. UGT
   b. Cytochrome P450
   c. Acetylcholinesterase
   d. Aminotransferase
2. Which blood coagulation factors is *not* synthesized in the liver?
   a. Factor II (prothrombin)
   b. Factor VIII (von Willebrand factor)
   c. Factor IX (Christmas factor)
   d. Factor X
3. Which vitamins is stored in the liver in significant amounts and can supply the body's needs for several years?
   a. Vitamin K
   b. Vitamin E
   c. Vitamin B_{12}
   d. Vitamin D
4. Which hormones is primarily metabolized by the liver?
   a. Insulin
   b. PTH
   c. Prolactin
   d. Calcitonin

Continued

KNOWLEDGE CHECK—cont'd

5. Which best describes the role of Kupffer cells in hepatic filtration?
   a. They store glycogen and fat-soluble vitamins.
   b. They synthesize bile acids for fat digestion.
   c. They rapidly phagocytose bacteria and debris from portal blood.
   d. They conjugate bilirubin to increase water solubility.
6. What is the correct sequence of hepatocyte actions during blood detoxification?
   a. Excretion → Uptake → Biotransformation
   b. Biotransformation → Uptake → Excretion
   c. Uptake → Biotransformation → Excretion
   d. Uptake → Excretion → Biotransformation
7. A patient with advanced liver cirrhosis develops significant edema. Which answer best explains this finding?
   a. Decreased transferrin synthesis
   b. Decreased ceruloplasmin synthesis
   c. Decreased albumin synthesis
   d. Decreased C-reactive protein synthesis

Answers can be found in Appendix A.

Hepatic Pathophysiologic Concepts

Liver dysfunction may occur from several different pathophysiologic causes, such as infections, toxins and drugs, metabolic and genetic disorders, and autoimmune diseases. The effects these have on liver function vary depending on the level of damage to the liver, but they could result in hepatitis, portal hypertension, ascites, esophageal varices, jaundice, cirrhosis, and/or liver failure.

- *Hepatitis* is an inflammation of the liver that can be caused by various factors, including infections, alcohol, other toxins, autoimmunity, or ischemia. It can be acute or chronic and has implications for drug metabolism, coagulation, and other body systems.
  - *Acute hepatitis* is a transient liver insult with potential for full recovery but poses short-term risks during active inflammation (Table 3.41).
    - It may have a variable presentation and, in mild forms, can result in high transaminases levels and an elevated INR.
    - The risk of drug-induced liver injury from anesthesia medications is higher.
    - In severe cases, it can result in acute liver failure, encephalopathy, and systemic coagulopathies, which could necessitate urgent liver support and transplant evaluation.
  - *Chronic hepatitis* often manifests with a silent progression and long-term consequences, especially if cirrhosis develops.
    - It is associated with a higher risk of bleeding, infections, hemodynamic instability, and drug sensitivity.
    - The various types of chronic hepatitis include the following:
      - Chronic persistent is mild, limited to portal areas, and rarely results in cirrhosis.
      - Chronic lobular causes recurrent flares and also rarely results in cirrhosis.
      - Chronic active is progressive and severe, causing hepatocyte destruction, cirrhosis, and liver failure. Severe cases can lead to portal hypertension, ascites, hepatorenal syndrome (HRS), encephalopathy, and/or variceal bleeding.
    - Preoperative assessments include evaluating liver function test (LFT) levels, albumin, INR, platelets, and signs of portal hypertension (varices, ascites).
    - Use caution with any agents that require hepatic clearance.
    - Adjustments in drug dosages are common (e.g., opioids, benzodiazepines, neuromuscular blocking agents).
  - *Viral hepatitis* is the most common hepatitis, with five main types: A, B, C, D, and E.
    - Hepatitis A and E are transmitted via the fecal-oral route.
      - Hepatitis A (HAV) transmission can occur with fecal-oral contamination, such as with contaminated food or water.
        - HAV is usually acute and self-limited and rarely leads to fulminant hepatic failure.
      - Hepatitis E (HEV) transmission is similar to that of HAV.

TABLE 3.41 **Comparison Between Acute and Chronic Hepatitis**

	Acute Hepatitis	Chronic Hepatitis
Definition	Liver inflammation lasting <6 months	Liver inflammation persisting for ≥6 months
Common causes	• Viral (HAV, HBV, HEV, HCV early stage) • Drug-induced (e.g., acetaminophen) • Ischemic injury ("shock liver") • Toxins	• Viral (HBV, HCV) • Autoimmune hepatitis • NASH • Metabolic/genetic disorders
Onset	Sudden onset of symptoms	Subtle and insidious, often asymptomatic initially
Symptoms	Fatigue, jaundice, nausea, RUQ pain, fever	Often asymptomatic until advanced (fatigue, pruritus, signs of cirrhosis)
Liver enzymes	ALT and AST often very elevated (>10× normal)	Mild to moderate elevations; can be normal in late-stage disease
Histology	Hepatocyte necrosis with inflammation	Inflammation with fibrosis, possibly progressing to cirrhosis
Coagulation and synthetic function	May be acutely impaired (↑INR, ↓albumin), especially in severe cases	Often progressively impaired (chronic ↓ albumin, ↑INR, ↓platelets)
Progression	Usually resolves or rarely progresses to acute liver failure	Progressively leads to cirrhosis, portal hypertension, ascites, hepatorenal syndrome
Anesthetic considerations	• Delay elective procedures until resolved • Monitor liver function and coagulation • Avoid hepatotoxic drugs	• Adjust drug doses (reduced hepatic metabolism) • Monitor for coagulopathy, ascites, encephalopathy • Avoid hepatotoxic drugs • Higher perioperative risk

ALT, alanine transaminase; *AST*, aspartate transaminase; *HAV*, hepatitis A virus; *HBV*, hepatitis B virus; *HCV*, hepatitis C virus; *HEV*, hepatitis E virus; *INR*, international normalized ratio; *NASH*, nonalcoholic steatohepatitis, insidious; *RUQ*, right upper quadrant.

    - HEV is also typically self-limited, but it can become severe in pregnancy (especially during the third trimester).
- Hepatitis B, C, and D are transmitted via contact with blood or body fluids.
  - Hepatitis B (HBV) can be found in an infected individual's blood, semen, or vaginal fluid and can be transmitted if it comes in contact with a susceptible individual's bloodstream.
    - HBV can progress to cirrhosis and hepatocellular carcinoma.
  - Hepatitis C (HCV) is primarily bloodborne and can be transmitted with blood-to-blood contact, IV drug use, or a contaminated blood transfusion.
  - HCV can progress to cirrhosis and hepatocellular carcinoma, and chronic cases may only reveal subclinical liver dysfunction.
  - Hepatitis D (HDV) requires an HBV coinfection and is associated with a more severe prognosis.
- *Alcoholic hepatitis* can result from excessive alcohol consumption. Too much alcohol overwhelms the liver's metabolic ability to process it, leading to cell damage, inflammation, and an immune response.
  - Resident macrophages of the liver (Kupffer cells) are activated during the metabolism of alcohol and release inflammatory cytokines.
  - This inflammation and immune response can cause swelling and further damage to liver cells.
  - The metabolism of alcohol produces *acetaldehyde*. This is a liver-toxic substance that binds to liver proteins, further triggering an immune response because this binding is recognized as foreign by the immune system.
  - Over time, elevated transaminase levels (AST, ALT), fever, hepatomegaly, portal hypertension, ascites, esophageal varices, jaundice, and cirrhosis can develop.
  - Can be acute or chronic; flare-ups may occur if cirrhosis is present.

- Implications for anesthesia:
  - There will be an increased sensitivity to any medication metabolized by the liver (e.g., opioids, sedatives, neuromuscular blocking agents).
  - Avoid hepatotoxic medications.
  - Coagulopathy and thrombocytopenia can occur.
  - Evaluate for esophageal varices, ascites, and encephalopathy.
- *Nonalcoholic steatohepatitis* (NASH) is a more severe form of *nonalcoholic fatty liver disease* (NAFLD), which is caused by fat accumulation (steatosis) in the liver due to reasons other than alcohol consumption.
  - NAFLD (now also known as *metabolic dysfunction–associated steatotic liver disease* [MASLD]) results from a combination of factors that can include obesity, type 2 diabetes, high cholesterol, high triglycerides, insulin resistance, certain medications, or metabolic syndrome.
  - NAFLD often has no symptoms, but some individuals may experience fatigue, weakness, or discomfort in the upper right abdomen.
  - When it progresses to liver inflammation and damage, then NASH may occur, which can lead to further complications, such as liver scarring and fibrosis, cirrhosis, liver failure, or even liver cancer.
  - Implications for anesthesia:
    - Assess LFTs in obese patients.
    - Potential for reduced hepatic drug metabolism
    - Consider difficulty with airway, OSA, and potential for insulin resistance.
- *Drug-induced hepatitis,* also known as *drug-induced liver injury* (DILI), is primarily caused by harmful or toxic medications, vitamins, herbal remedies, or supplements. This can occur either through direct toxicity or through idiosyncratic (immune response) reactions.
  - Certain drugs taken in high doses can directly damage the liver from metabolites produced through hepatocyte reactions that can be toxic to liver cells.
    - Propofol infusion syndrome can occur in critically ill or pediatric patients who receive prolonged infusions (>4 mg/kg/hr for >48 hr). The mechanism for this syndrome is related to mitochondrial dysfunction that leads to impaired fatty acid oxidation, rhabdomyolysis, lactic acidosis, and hepatic steatosis. Signs and symptoms include hyperlipidemia, acute refractory bradyarrhythmias, metabolic acidosis, and elevated transaminases and bilirubin levels.
    - Acetaminophen toxicity is rare in the perioperative period as long as cumulative dosing is less than 4 g/day. However, it can occur in malnourished or liver-compromised patients or in acetaminophen overdoses. The mechanism causing toxicity includes the conversion of enzymes that reduce glutathione levels (these are important for detoxification reactions and protect against oxidative stressors), which results in centrilobular liver necrosis. Signs and symptoms include right upper quadrant pain, significant ALT/AST elevations, and coagulopathy.
  - Idiosyncratic reactions are more unpredictable and can occur even with normal doses of a drug (e.g., antibiotics, antiepileptics). The exact mechanism is not fully understood, but these reactions are thought to involve activation of the immune system.
  - Older volatile halogenated inhalational anesthetics (e.g., halothane and enflurane, which are not used anymore) have been associated with drug-induced liver injury.
    - "Halothane hepatitis" occurred in approximately 1 in 10,000 adults after a first exposure and up to 1 in 1000 after multiple exposures.
    - Halothane is metabolized by cytochrome P450 (especially CYP2E1) enzymes that are converted into trifluoroacetyl (TFA) intermediates. These substances bind to hepatic proteins and cause an immune-mediated hepatic necrosis.
  - Implications for anesthesia:
    - Evaluate medication history for potential hepatic-toxic substances.
    - Monitor for signs of acute liver failure (encephalopathy, INR elevation) when potential hepatic-toxic substances are administered.
    - Select anesthetic agents with minimal hepatic metabolism in situations where a hepatic insult has occurred.

- *Autoimmune hepatitis* may be caused by a combination of factors that include genetic predisposition, environmental factors, and/or potential triggers that initiate the immune system (specifically T cells) to mistakenly attack hepatocytes within the liver. The exact cause of autoimmune hepatitis is unknown, but these triggers might include viruses, medications, or other environmental factors.
  - Clinical management includes the administration of immunosuppressant medications (e.g., steroids, azathioprine).
  - Implications for anesthesia:
    - Assess immune status.
    - Monitor LFTs and coagulation.
    - Avoid medications that cause immunosuppressive or hepatotoxic effects.
- *Ischemic hepatitis* ("shock liver") is a condition where liver cells are damaged and die as a result of reduced hepatic blood flow. This can lead to liver failure and is often associated with other serious medical conditions, such as shock.
  - Factors that can cause ischemic hepatitis include shock (hypovolemic, septic, or cardiogenic), severe heart failure, respiratory failure, or other conditions that result in low BP or reduced hepatic perfusion, resulting in hypoxia.
  - General signs and symptoms include nausea, vomiting, fatigue, mental confusion, and/or low urine output. Liver tenderness or enlargement may occur, and marked increases in transaminase level (>1000 IU/L) can occur. Liver failure can develop in severe cases.
  - Primary management includes identification and treatment of the underlying condition and restoring hepatic perfusion. Ischemic hepatitis is often reversible with hemodynamic correction. Fluid management, blood product administration, vasopressor therapy, maintaining electrolyte levels, and/or mechanical ventilation may be necessary.
    - If liver failure develops, consultation for a liver transplant may be necessary.
  - Implications for anesthesia:
    - Avoid further hypotension or hepatotoxic drugs.
    - Consider arterial line and central line to monitor BP and provide blood therapy and vasopressor support.
    - Monitor for coagulopathy.

KNOWLEDGE CHECK

1. Which of the following forms of hepatitis is most likely to result in liver failure during pregnancy, particularly in the third trimester?
   a. Hepatitis A
   b. Hepatitis B
   c. Hepatitis C
   d. Hepatitis E
2. A patient with a history of heavy alcohol use presents with jaundice, hepatomegaly, and esophageal varices. Which pathophysiologic mechanism is primarily responsible for the liver damage in alcoholic hepatitis?
   a. Immune-mediated hepatocyte destruction
   b. Direct viral invasion of liver cells
   c. Acetaldehyde-induced injury
   d. Fat accumulation in liver cells without inflammation
3. Which of the following conditions is most associated with the development of NASH?
   a. Chronic alcohol use
   b. Obesity and insulin resistance
   c. Hepatitis B infection
   d. Autoimmune disease
4. Which of the following anesthetic concerns is most appropriate for a patient with ischemic hepatitis ("shock liver")?
   a. Avoiding hypoventilation during anesthesia
   b. Strict avoidance of all IV fluids
   c. Careful maintenance of BP to optimize hepatic perfusion
   d. Maximizing drug doses to overcome liver dysfunction

Answers can be found in Appendix A.

- *Cirrhosis* is a late-stage scarring (fibrosis) of the liver caused by chronic damage. When liver damage is severe enough, fibrosis replaces healthy liver cells, causing a decreased ability of the liver to function properly. Cirrhosis can result from various conditions, including chronic infections (e.g., hepatitis B or C), excessive alcohol consumption, and other liver diseases.
  - Common signs and symptoms of cirrhosis include fatigue, weakness, loss of appetite and unexplained weight loss, nausea and vomiting, abdominal pain or tenderness, itchy skin, leg swelling, and/or dark-colored urine or light-colored stools.
  - Advanced signs of cirrhosis can include portal hypertension, coagulopathy, hypoalbuminemia,

TABLE 3.42 Progressive Complications of Cirrhosis With Corresponding Medical Management

Cirrhosis Complications	Management
Portal hypertension	Nonselective beta-blockers, TIPS, variceal band ligation
Ascites	Sodium restriction, spironolactone and/or furosemide, paracentesis, albumin infusion
Coagulopathy	FFP, platelets if bleeding or invasive procedures, cryoprecipitate for low fibrinogen levels, vitamin K
Jaundice and pruritus	Cholestyramine, antihistamines
Malnutrition	Nutritional support
Hepatic encephalopathy	Correct triggers (e.g., cirrhosis), correct electrolyte imbalances, lactulose, rifaximin
Esophageal varices	Octreotide and/or vasopressin, endoscopic banding, prophylactic antibiotics
Hepatorenal syndrome	Midodrine, octreotide, albumin, terlipressin (if available), dialysis, liver transplant
Liver failure (ESLD)	Avoid hepatotoxic drugs; nutritional support, manage electrolyte imbalances, liver transplant

ESLD, end-stage liver disease; *FFP*, fresh frozen plasma; *TIPS*, transjugular intrahepatic portosystemic shunt

splenomegaly, jaundice, ascites, encephalopathy, esophageal varices, HRS, and/or end-stage liver disease (Table 3.42).
  - Cirrhosis that develops at the cellular level is a result of hepatocyte necrosis caused by a specific hepatic injury that leads to the formation of fibrous tissue (scar tissue) and nodules. At the point of liver cirrhosis, the liver cannot repair itself and instead produces fibrous tissue and nodules, which then replace liver cells, distorting normal liver architecture and function. What results is an impairment of portal blood flow and a reduction of the liver's metabolic and synthetic function.
- *Portal hypertension* occurs when the liver is damaged (e.g., cirrhosis) and hepatic blood flow is obstructed, leading to a buildup of pressure within the portal venous system (e.g., blood flow to the liver from the stomach, intestines, pancreas, and spleen). This increased pressure can lead to various complications, including esophageal varices, ascites, splenomegaly, hepatic encephalopathy, and/or HRS.
  - Cirrhosis-driven remodeling of the liver cells, resulting in fibrosis and nodules, causes an increased resistance to portal blood flow within the liver lobules. This increase in resistance causes a retrograde pressure back into the portal venous circulation, affecting collateral circulation and leading to complications like varices, ascites, and splenomegaly.
  - Medical management:
    - Medications that reduce portal venous pressure, such as nonselective β-blockers (e.g., propranolol, nadolol)
    - Endoscopic variceal ligation (banding) for bleeding varices
    - Diuretics and sodium restriction (if ascites present)
    - Transjugular intrahepatic portosystemic shunt (TIPS) involves the insertion of a stent between the portal veins and adjacent blood vessels with lower pressures. TIPS is used in refractory cases to relieve the backflow pressure within the hepatic vascular system in order to stop bleeding and the backup of fluid.
- *Hypoalbuminemia* is a low blood serum albumin and is a common complication of liver cirrhosis.
  - Progressive liver damage and fibrosis from cirrhosis result in impaired hepatocytes with a reduced capacity to synthesize and produce albumin.
  - Hypoalbuminemia lowers plasma oncotic pressure and contributes to ascites and edema.
  - Additionally, increased capillary permeability caused by cirrhosis can lead to the leakage of albumin into the peritoneal cavity, interstitial spaces, or other body tissues, further contributing to ascites and generalized edema.
  - Cirrhosis is also associated with malabsorption and reduced appetite, which causes nutritional deficiencies that impair albumin production.
  - Signs and symptoms:
    - Low albumin levels
    - Edema
    - Fatigue, muscle weakness, and weight loss
    - Nausea, vomiting, and/or diarrhea
    - Jaundice

- Medical management:
  - Albumin infusions (especially after large-volume paracentesis)
  - Nutritional support (adequate protein intake)
  - Management of ascites (via diuretics, paracentesis)
- *Ascites* is the buildup of fluid within the abdominal cavity and is a complication of cirrhosis.
  - The most frequent cause of ascites is portal hypertension and hypoalbuminemia (also a complication of cirrhosis).
  - Portal hypertension leads to an increase in pressure within the portal veins, and hypoalbuminemia leads to a decreased vascular oncotic pressure. Both can result in fluid leakage into the peritoneal cavity.
    - Other causes include cancer, heart failure, and kidney failure.
  - Ascites fluid often contains protein, further exacerbating osmotic imbalances and fluid retention.
  - In some individuals, the renin–angiotensin–aldosterone system (RAAS) is activated, leading to an increase in sodium and water retention and worsening ascites.
  - Signs and symptoms associated with ascites:
    - Abdominal distention and bloating
    - Weight gain
    - Dyspnea (due to pressure on diaphragm)
    - Dullness on percussion
  - Medical management:
    - Treat the underlying cause of ascites (e.g., liver disease or cancer).
    - Sodium restriction to reduce fluid retention
    - Diuretics to help eliminate excess fluid (e.g., spironolactone, furosemide)
    - Paracentesis to drain excess fluid from the abdomen
    - Albumin infusion after removal of a large fluid volume after paracentesis
    - Consideration of a TIPS procedure for refractory ascites
- *Coagulopathy* can occur as a result of cirrhosis and liver failure. Liver fibrosis leading to hepatocyte scarring and dysfunction impairs the synthesis of fibrinogen (factor I), factor V, vitamin K–dependent clotting factors (II, VII, IX, X), and anticoagulants (protein S and protein C). Splenomegaly can cause a sequestration of platelets, leading to thrombocytopenia, which further affects coagulopathy.
  - Signs and symptoms of an existing coagulopathy:
    - Easy bruising
    - Prolonged bleeding
    - Gastrointestinal (GI) bleeding (e.g., esophageal varices)
    - Prolonged PT/INR and activated partial thromboplastin time (aPTT)
    - Low platelets (thrombocytopenia)
    - Low fibrinogen levels
  - Medical management:
    - Monitoring of PT/INR, aPTT, fibrinogen, platelets
    - Administration of vitamin K
    - Fresh frozen plasma (FFP) infusion for active bleeding or before surgical procedures
    - Platelet transfusions for thrombocytopenia
    - Consider cryoprecipitate for low fibrinogen levels.
    - Avoidance of anticoagulants unless absolutely indicated
- *Jaundice* occurs from an accumulation of bilirubin (byproduct of RBC breakdown) in the blood due to hepatocellular dysfunction and an inability to excrete bilirubin in bile. A buildup of both conjugated and unconjugated bilirubin in the blood causes the skin and the sclera of the eyes to turn yellow.
  - Cirrhosis affects the metabolism and excretion of bilirubin in several ways:
    - First, impaired hepatocyte and enzyme function is unable to conjugate bilirubin, leading to accumulation of toxic unconjugated bilirubin.
    - Second, bile canaliculi within liver lobules become compressed or damaged as a result of fibrosis and nodular regeneration, causing reduced bile flow (intrahepatic cholestasis) and a backup of conjugated bilirubin into the blood.
    - Third, obstruction of bile ducts occurs in advanced cirrhosis from fibrosis, further reducing bilirubin excretion and leading to hyperbilirubinemia.
  - Signs and symptoms:
    - Yellowing of skin and sclera
    - Dark urine
    - Pale stools
    - Pruritus

- Medical management:
  - Correction of the underlying cause (e.g., cessation of alcohol consumption, cessation of hepatotoxic drugs, antiviral medications for viral hepatitis)
  - Cholestyramine and antihistamines for pruritus
  - Monitor progression of liver disease and other symptoms related to cirrhosis.
- *Hepatic encephalopathy* is a neuropsychiatric syndrome that occurs as a result of severe liver dysfunction. It results from decreased clearance of ammonia by the liver and causes mental status changes that can range from subtle cognitive changes to coma or death if left untreated.
  - Ammonia and other neurotoxins accumulate as a result of reduced hepatic clearance and portosystemic shunting.
  - Portosystemic shunting (which often happens spontaneously in cirrhosis) allows toxins to exit the gut and bypass the liver to directly enter systemic circulation.
  - When blood serum ammonia levels are high enough, they can alter neurotransmission within the brain, causing hepatic encephalopathy.
  - Signs and symptoms:
    - Confusion and disorientation
    - Asterixis (flapping tremor of the hands)
    - Personality and mood changes
    - Mild confusion or forgetfulness
    - Slurred speech
    - Drowsiness or lethargy
    - Somnolence progressing to stupor or coma in severe cases
  - Medical management:
    - Identify and treat precipitating causes (e.g., cirrhosis).
    - Lactulose (reduces ammonia absorption in the gut)
    - Rifaximin (nonabsorbable antibiotic that reduces ammonia-producing bacteria)
    - Avoidance of sedatives
    - Correction of electrolyte imbalances
- *Esophageal varices* are abnormally dilated and enlarged veins in the lower part of the esophagus.
  - Cirrhosis causes fibrosis and scarring within the liver lobules, causing reduced hepatic blood flow and resulting in a backflow of blood into the portal venous system. This increase in pressure causes esophageal veins to dilate, swell, and form into varices.
  - Esophageal varices are fragile and prone to rupture, which can lead to life-threatening upper GI hemorrhage.
  - Signs and symptoms:
    - Hematemesis (vomiting blood)
    - Melena (black, tarry stools)
    - Anemia
    - Signs of hypovolemic shock if bleeding is severe (e.g., dizziness, hypotension, tachycardia)
  - Medical management:
    - Prophylactic β-blockers (nonselective)
    - Endoscopic variceal ligation or sclerotherapy
    - Octreotide or vasopressin (both cause splanchnic vasoconstriction, which decreases blood flow in the liver and reduces the pressure within the portal vein).
    - TIPS for recurrent bleeding
    - Antibiotic prophylaxis (e.g., ceftriaxone) in acute bleed
- HRS is characterized by a sudden reduction in kidney function due to prerenal vascular vasoconstriction and reduced renal perfusion. This occurs despite the normal kidney structure and function. It can develop in individuals with advanced liver disease, specifically those with portal hypertension and ascites.
  - The exact mechanism of HRS is not fully understood; however, the primary theories indicate that portal hypertension and ascites have a strong influence.
  - Portal hypertension triggers splanchnic vasodilation (blood vessels supplying the intestines) and results in blood pooling within the splanchnic vessels.
  - This causes a decrease in overall arterial blood volume, despite normal or even increased total blood volume.
  - Activation of the following vasoconstrictor systems occurs in response to low arterial blood volume and perceived hypovolemia:
    - RAAS
    - SNS
    - ADH
  - These systems cause systemic vasoconstriction, particularly in the renal vasculature, in an effort to maintain BP.
  - Persistent vasoconstriction leads to overall reduced renal blood flow and decreased glomerular

filtration, ultimately leading to acute kidney injury (AKI).

- Large-volume ascites and infections (e.g., spontaneous bacterial peritonitis) can also contribute to reduced vascular flow to the kidneys and the development of HRS.
- Signs and symptoms:
  - Oliguria
  - Increased serum creatinine
  - Progressive ascites
  - No improvement with fluid resuscitation
- Medical management:
  - Administer midodrine and octreotide to increase the MAP.
  - Administer albumin to increase blood plasma oncotic pressure.
  - Terlipressin causes vasoconstriction in the splanchnic circulation and reduces blood pooling in the splanchnic area.
  - Avoid nephrotoxic medications (NSAIDs, aminoglycosides).
  - Hepatic transplantation is the only definitive treatment.
  - Dialysis can be used as a bridge to transplant.

- *End-stage liver disease* (ESLD), also known as *liver failure*, is the final stage of chronic liver disease (e.g., cirrhosis) and is the point where the liver is severely and irreversibly damaged.
  - Signs and symptoms:
    - Fatigue, weight loss, muscle wasting
    - Jaundice
    - Ascites
    - Peripheral edema
    - Hepatic encephalopathy
    - Esophageal varices
    - Pruritus
    - Spontaneous bacterial peritonitis
    - Asterixis (flapping tremor)
    - Gynecomastia, spider angiomas (due to estrogen buildup)
    - HRS (oliguria, rising creatinine)
  - Medical management is primarily supportive while waiting for a liver transplant.
    - General supportive care consists of avoiding hepatotoxic drugs (e.g., NSAIDs, acetaminophen in excess), nutrition support, and managing electrolyte imbalances (e.g., hyponatremia, hypokalemia).
    - Definitive treatment is liver transplantation

KNOWLEDGE CHECK

1. Which is a major cause of cirrhosis?
   a. Acute appendicitis
   b. Excessive alcohol consumption
   c. Chronic hyperglycemia
   d. AKI
2. Portal hypertension in cirrhosis primarily results from
   a. increased vascular volume.
   b. excess albumin production.
   c. decreased bilirubin production.
   d. obstruction of hepatic blood flow resulting from fibrosis and nodules.
3. Which medication is used to decrease portal venous pressure and prevent bleeding from esophageal varices?
   a. Lactulose
   b. Furosemide
   c. Propranolol
   d. Ceftriaxone
4. Which intervention is appropriate after a large-volume paracentesis in a patient with significant ascites?
   a. Administering lactulose
   b. Providing albumin infusion
   c. Starting rifaximin
   d. Administering vitamin K
5. What is the definitive treatment for HRS in a patient with cirrhosis?
   a. Dialysis
   b. Midodrine and octreotide
   c. Liver transplantation
   d. Albumin infusions

Answers can be found in Appendix A.

Anesthesia Management for Hepatic Disease

- Patients with liver disease and cirrhosis can present with significant anesthetic challenges due to multiorgan involvement and impaired liver function.
- *Preoperative anesthesia evaluation* should (1) evaluate laboratory values related to the liver, (2) assess the severity of liver disease by assessing the complications related to conditions such as cirrhosis, and (3) optimize comorbid conditions (Table 3.43).
  - Evaluation of blood serum laboratory values before anesthesia care should include the following:
    - Hemoglobin and hematocrit
    - Platelets
    - Electrolyte values (including magnesium and calcium)
    - PT/INR and aPTT
    - Creatinine and creatinine clearance

TABLE 3.43 Anesthesia Management for Patients With Advanced Liver Disease

	Anesthesia Considerations
Preoperative assessment	• Assess degree of liver damage (evaluation of serum transaminase, bilirubin, coagulation, and albumin levels). • Screen for encephalopathy, ascites, esophageal varices, renal function. • Correct coagulopathy, electrolytes, infection. • Obtain baseline liver and kidney function tests. • Evaluate for cardiopulmonary issues (consider echocardiogram, CXR). • Consider nutritional status, muscle wasting, and potential for alcohol dependency.

Intraoperative management	• Maintain MAP and CO to preserve hepatic perfusion.
	• Consider arterial line for blood pressure monitoring, ABG analysis, frequent lab checks, and point-of-care testing.
	   • Central line if appropriate for vasopressor and fluid and/or blood administration
	• Impaired hepatic metabolism and hypoalbuminemia may lead to prolonged drug clearance (e.g., opioids, NMBA).
	   • Use drugs with short half-lives **or** nonhepatic metabolism (e.g., cisatracurium).
	   • Titrate drug doses carefully.
	• Consider reduced pseudocholinesterase activity (succinylcholine may be prolonged).
	• Isoflurane or sevoflurane preferred volatile agents
	   • Avoid halothane because of higher risk for causing liver damage.
	   • No significant clinical toxicity from sevoflurane (fluoride ions)
	• Avoid medications that potentially cause hepatotoxicity or inhibit CYP450:
	   • Acetaminophen, halothane, sulfonamides, tetracycline, penicillin, amiodarone
	• Coagulation abnormalities should be corrected.
	   • Avoid regional anesthesia unless coagulation is corrected.
	   • Consider point-of-care monitoring using TEG/ROTEM.
	   • Monitor blood coagulation values.
	   • Risk of bleeding (especially with varices or large vessels).
	   • Have blood products available in room (PRBCs, FFP, platelets, cryoprecipitate).
	   • Risk of DIC or hyperfibrinolysis
	• Monitor fluid administration.
	   • Potential for third spacing and hypoalbuminemia (risk of ascites and pulmonary edema)
	   • Use albumin or colloids cautiously.
	   • Avoid fluid overload.
	• Maintain cardiovascular status.
	   • Cirrhotic patients have low SVR **and** hyperdynamic circulation.
	   • Prone to hypotension during anesthesia
	   • Use vasopressors (norepinephrine) if needed.
	   • Maintain MAP >65 mm Hg.
	   • Avoid excessive fluid overload (can worsen ascites and pulmonary status).
	• Monitor for respiratory compromise from ascites or edema.
	   • Consider preoperative paracentesis if severe.
	   • Use low tidal volumes, higher PEEP.
	   • Risk of aspiration (delayed gastric emptying, varices)
	   • Perform RSI if indicated.
	• Monitor renal perfusion.
	   • Maintain MAP >65 mm Hg.
	   • Avoid nephrotoxic medications (acetaminophen, halothane, sulfonamides, tetracycline, penicillins).
	   • Monitor for electrolyte disturbances (e.g., hyponatremia, hypokalemia).
	• Consider encephalopathy risk.
	   • Evaluate for elevated ammonia levels.
	   • Avoid benzodiazepines and sedatives unless absolutely needed.
	   • Risk of postoperative mental status decline

TABLE 3.43 Anesthesia Management for Patients With Advanced Liver Disease—cont'd

Postoperative management	• High risk of infection (consider antibiotic therapy) • Provide pain management (avoid regional anesthesia if coagulopathy is present). • Monitor liver and kidney function closely. • Reassess hematological, coagulation, and electrolyte values. • Maintain MAP >65 mm Hg. • Consider ICU admission for close monitoring in moderate to severe cases.

ABG, arterial blood gas; *CO*, cardiac output; *CXR*, chest radiograph; *DIC*, disseminated intravascular coagulation; *FFP*, fresh frozen plasma; *ICU*, intensive care unit; *MAP*, mean arterial pressure; *NMBA*, neuromuscular blocking agents; *PEEP*, positive end-expiratory pressure; *PRBCs*, packed red blood cells; *ROTEM*, rotational thermoelectrometry; *RSI*, rapid sequence induction; *SVR*, systemic vascular resistance; *TEG*, thromboelastography.

- Transaminase levels (ALT/AST)
- Bilirubin levels
- Albumin levels

- Complications of cirrhosis and ESLD may include the following:
  - Ascites
  - Hepatic encephalopathy
  - Coagulopathy
  - Hypoalbuminemia and malnutrition
  - Esophageal varices
  - HRS
  - Cardiomyopathies and/or CHF
  - Alcoholism and potential for withdrawal syndrome
- Optimize comorbid conditions (see Table 3.42).
- Consider cardiopulmonary issues (e.g., hepatopulmonary syndrome), nutritional status and muscle wasting, and potential for withdrawal (e.g., alcohol dependency).

- *Intraoperative anesthesia care* should concentrate on preserving hepatic blood flow; avoiding hepatotoxic medications; and carefully titrating drugs that rely on hepatic clearance, protein binding, or metabolism by blood enzymes produced by the liver (see Table 3.43).
  - Primary goal is to maintain hepatic perfusion.
    - General and regional anesthesia, volatile anesthetics, and depressant anesthetic medications can lead to decreases in MAP and a reduction in hepatic blood flow.
    - Isoflurane and sevoflurane are the preferred volatile agents in patients with liver disease.
  - ABPs and central lines may help with BP monitoring, ABG evaluation, blood sampling, fluid and blood administration, and vasopressor administration/monitoring.
  - Coagulation abnormalities should be corrected.
    - Goal-directed fluid therapy is useful.
    - Cardiovascular, respiratory, renal, and neurologic status should be monitored.
    - Current studies show no significant clinical toxicity from sevoflurane conversion into hexafluoroisopropanol (HFIP) and fluoride ions in the liver.
    - Avoid medications with the potential for CYP450 inhibition or hepatotoxicity, such as acetaminophen, halothane, sulfonamides, tetracycline, penicillin, and amiodarone.
- *Postoperative anesthesia considerations* for patients with advanced liver disease include a high risk of infection, renal failure, and cardiopulmonary decompensation.
  - Provide pain management (avoid regional anesthesia if coagulopathy is present).
  - Monitor liver and kidney function closely.
  - Reassess hematological, coagulation, and electrolyte values.
  - Maintain MAP >65 mm Hg.
  - Consider ICU admission for close monitoring in moderate to severe cases.

Biliary Tract Diseases

- The anatomic and physiologic function of the biliary tract starts within liver lobules and involves a network of ducts that initially collect bile from liver cells and ultimately transport it to the common bile duct. Bile aids in the digestion of fats and fat-soluble vitamins within the intestines.
  - The biliary tract begins with small tubes called *canaliculi* within the hepatocytes, which drain bile produced by hepatocytes into larger ducts within each liver lobule, then into larger ducts between hepatic lobules.

KNOWLEDGE CHECK

1. Which laboratory value assessment is important when evaluating a patient's coagulation status before anesthesia in a patient with liver disease?
   a. AST/ALT
   b. PT/INR
   c. Bilirubin
   d. Albumin
2. A patient with cirrhosis undergoing surgery has significant ascites and coagulopathy. Which intraoperative strategy is most appropriate?
   a. Liberal fluid resuscitation
   b. Aggressive use of spinal anesthesia
   c. Correction of coagulation abnormalities
   d. Administration of acetaminophen for analgesia
3. In patients with liver disease, why should the perioperative use of acetaminophen be avoided?
   a. Tendency to cause hypocalcemia
   b. Impairs clotting function
   c. Potential for hepatotoxicity
   d. Increases ammonia levels, leading to encephalopathy
4. What is the primary intraoperative anesthesia goal when managing a patient with hepatic disease?
   a. Suppress hepatic enzyme activity.
   b. Maintain hepatic perfusion.
   c. Lower portal venous pressure.
   d. Increase hepatic metabolism.
5. Which drug characteristics are most important when selecting anesthetic medications for a patient with cirrhosis?
   a. Drugs highly bound to albumin
   b. Drugs with long half-lives
   c. Drugs with nonhepatic metabolism or short half-lives
   d. Drugs requiring renal excretion

Answers can be found in Appendix A.

- These intrahepatic ducts eventually merge to form the right and left hepatic ducts, then combine to form the common hepatic duct.
- The gallbladder sits inferior to the liver within the right upper quadrant of the abdomen. Its primary function is to store and concentrate the bile produced by the liver (about 30–60 mL).
- Stored bile from the gallbladder is transported through the cystic duct, which connects to the common hepatic duct to form the common bile duct.
- The resulting common bile duct then continues downward toward the small intestine.
- The pancreatic duct meets the common bile duct near the small intestine to form the ampulla of Vater, which is a small reservoir that allows bile and pancreatic juices to mix and then be released into the duodenum to aid in digestion.
- The sphincter of Oddi acts as a valve that is situated at the end of the ampulla of Vater before the duodenum; it controls the flow of bile and pancreatic juices into the duodenum.
- Sphincter of Oddi functions include (1) acting as a barrier to intestinal bacteria, (2) regulating bile/pancreatic juice flow, (3) preventing reflux, and (4) aiding in gallbladder filling of bile for concentration when no bile is needed within the intestines.
  - Relaxation of the sphincter of Oddi is initiated by cholecystokinin (hormone released by the small intestine) and then mediated by vasoactive intestinal polypeptide (VIP). Relaxation can also occur from nitric oxide.
  - Contraction of the sphincter of Oddi is mediated through the parasympathetic nervous system and also by somatostatin and octreotide.
- Primary diseases of the biliary tract include conditions affecting the gallbladder, bile ducts, and related structures.
- Diseases of the gallbladder include cholelithiasis, cholecystitis, and gallbladder cancer.
  - *Cholelithiasis* is a general term for the formation of stones that can be anywhere in the biliary tract. However, they are most commonly found in the gallbladder. Cholelithiasis can lead to cholecystitis and other pain along the biliary tract. Endoscopic retrograde cholangiopancreatography (ERCP) is a surgical procedure that can help remove the stones.
  - *Cholecystitis* is an inflammation of the gallbladder that is most commonly caused by gallstones obstructing the flow out of the gallbladder or cystic duct. When severe obstruction occurs causing pain, the gallbladder can be removed (e.g., cholecystectomy).
  - *Gall bladder cancer* is often associated with prolonged inflammation of the gallbladder by gallstones, gallbladder polyps, or infection. It is

managed with a combination of radiation and chemotherapy and potentially cholecystectomy.

- Diseases of the bile duct include choledocholithiasis, cholangitis, and biliary tract malignancies such as cholangiocarcinoma.
  - *Choledocholithiasis* is the presence of stones (cholelithiasis) in the common bile duct, which can lead to obstruction and/or infection. It is usually diagnosed and can be managed with ERCP.
  - *Cholangitis* is an inflammation of the bile duct that can occur from an autoimmune cause (e.g., primary biliary cholangitis) or an infective cause (e.g., bacterial cholangitis).
  - *Biliary tract malignancies* (e.g., cholangiocarcinoma) are cancers affecting the epithelial lining of the bile ducts.

Anesthesia Management for Biliary Tract Diseases

- Anesthetic considerations for biliary tract surgery generally focus on gallbladder removal (e.g., cholecystectomy) and/or bile duct exploration (Table 3.44).
  - Preoperative considerations include evaluation of the patient's comorbidities and progression of the biliary tract disease (e.g., whether it is affecting the liver and producing jaundice, ascites, or a coagulopathy).
    - Evaluate liver transaminase levels, hematologic values, electrolytes, coagulation status, and imaging.
    - Correct any problems such as coagulation deficiencies, electrolyte imbalances, or fluid deficits.
  - Laparoscopic cholecystectomy and ERCP are the most common types of biliary surgery/procedure,

TABLE 3.44 Anesthesia Considerations for Gallbladder and Biliary Tract Surgery

	Anesthesia Considerations
Preoperative	• Evaluate history of biliary disease and comorbidities, potential for jaundice, pruritus, fever, past ERCP/surgery. • Review medication list. • Evaluate LFTs (AST/ALT, bilirubin), INR/PT, CBC, electrolytes, renal panel. • Review US/CT. • Treat cholangitis (e.g., antibiotics), correct coagulopathy (vitamin K, FFP), optimize fluids/electrolytes.
Intraoperative	• Standard monitors • Arterial line (if indicated) • Foley catheter (if indicated) • Rarely a central line • General anesthesia with ETT • Consider epidural for open procedures. • Consider fascial plane block (TAP, ESP) for cholecystectomy. • Propofol or etomidate (if unstable) • Neuromuscular blockade (e.g., rocuronium, cisatracurium if renal or hepatic disease) with nerve stimulator monitoring • Volatile agents are okay. • Avoid nitrous oxide. • Opioid titration (caution in liver disease) can cause spasm of sphincter of Oddi. • Multimodal analgesia (e.g., ketamine, NSAIDs, acetaminophen, magnesium) • Nausea prophylaxis (e.g., ondansetron, decadron) • Laparoscopic pneumoperitoneum affects ventilation pressures and venous return. • Max abdominal insufflation pressure 15 mm Hg
Postoperative	• Analgesia with IV opioids (adjust for hepatic clearance), acetaminophen (dose-adjusted for liver disease), NSAIDs if no renal compromise • Monitor LFTs, coagulation, respiratory status, signs of bile leak or infection.

ALT, Alanine transaminase; *AST*, aspartate transaminase; *CBC*, complete blood count; *CT*, computed tomography; *ESP*, erector spinae plane; *ERCP*, endoscopic retrograde cholangiopancreatography; *ETT*, endotracheal tube; *FFP*, fresh frozen plasma; *INR*, international normalized ratio; *IV*, intravenous; *LFT*, liver function tests; *NSAIDs*, nonsteroidal antiinflammatory drugs; *PT*, prothrombin time; *TAP*, transvers abdominis plane; *US*, ultrasound.

with a goal of relieving symptoms and preventing further complications. Both require general anesthesia and endotracheal intubation.

- Intraoperative care should consider the following:
  - Appropriate induction agent based on the patient's overall health status (e.g., propofol or etomidate)
  - Neuromuscular blockade monitored with a nerve stimulator
  - Analgesia with a combination of multimodal medications (e.g., opioids, NSAIDs, acetaminophen, ketamine, fascial plane nerve block, epidural in open procedures)
  - Nausea prophylaxis
  - Ventilation strategy that accounts for an increased abdominal pressure that compresses the lungs (e.g., pressure control mode with PEEP)
  - ERCP procedures are conducted in the operating room in the GI lab, and the patient is placed in a lateral position after induction of anesthesia and intubation to allow for upper endoscopy.
  - Provide adequate padding for lateral decubitus position.
- CO_2 insufflation is used to create a pneumoperitoneum in order to perform a laparoscopic cholecystectomy (most common method).
  - Mechanical ventilation can lead to decreases in FRC, increases in peak pressure, and decreases in venous return.
  - Risks include hypercarbia, hypotension, diaphragmatic pressure on lungs, and potential for CO_2 gas embolism.
  - Recommended intraabdominal pressure is 15 mm Hg.
  - Avoid nitrous oxide to prevent bowel distension.
  - Laparoscopic cholecystectomy position is reverse Trendelenburg, with a slight left tilt.
- Postoperative management:
  - Appropriate pain management (e.g., opioids, NSAIDs, fascial plane block)
  - Shoulder tip pain may occur from pneumoperitoneum.
  - Primarily caused by irritation of the phrenic nerve due to CO_2 gas trapped under the diaphragm, leading to referred pain in the shoulder area.
- Opioids can cause spasm of the sphincter of Oddi, leading to an increase in biliary pressure, biliary colic pain, a delay in bile flow into the intestine, and/or a false-positive result on intraoperative cholangiogram.
  - Most often occurs with morphine
  - Consider the use of synthetic opioids (e.g., fentanyl, hydromorphone).
  - Management can include the administration of glucagon, nitroglycerine (contraindicated with low BP), deepening the anesthesia, naloxone, and/or nalbuphine.

KNOWLEDGE CHECK

1. What is the primary function of the gallbladder within the biliary tract system?
   a. Production of bile
   b. Storage and concentration of bile
   c. Absorption of fat-soluble vitamins
   d. Regulation of bile flow into the pancreas
2. Which hormone primarily initiates the relaxation of the sphincter of Oddi to facilitate bile flow into the duodenum?
   a. Somatostatin
   b. Cholecystokinin (CCK)
   c. Acetylcholine
   d. Insulin
3. Which condition refers specifically to the presence of stones in the common bile duct?
   a. Cholelithiasis
   b. Cholangitis
   c. Choledocholithiasis
   d. Cholangiocarcinoma
4. During a laparoscopic cholecystectomy, CO_2 insufflation can lead to which of the following respiratory effects?
   a. Increased FRC
   b. Decreased peak airway pressures
   c. Hypercarbia and decreased venous return
   d. Improvement in oxygenation due to abdominal compression
5. Why should nitrous oxide be avoided during laparoscopic cholecystectomy?
   a. It can cause spasm of the sphincter of Oddi.
   b. It increases the risk of bile duct injury.
   c. It contributes to bowel distention.
   d. It decreases hepatic perfusion.

6. If a patient experiences a sphincter of Oddi spasm after opioid administration, which of the following is an appropriate management strategy?
   a. Increase the opioid dose.
   b. Administer glucagon or nitroglycerin.
   c. Administer acetaminophen.
   d. Use nitrous oxide for relaxation.

7. Which is the correct patient positioning for a laparoscopic cholecystectomy?
   a. Supine with slight jackknife
   b. Reverse Trendelenburg with left tilt
   c. Lateral decubitus with slight reverse Trendelenburg
   d. Trendelenburg with right tilt

Answers can be found in Appendix A.

RENAL SYSTEM

The primary functions of the kidneys are the filtration of blood and concentration of urine in combination with salt and water balance. The kidneys filter a human adult's entire blood volume about 300 times per day (an approximate filtration volume of 1500–1700 L) in an effort to remove toxins, waste products, and excess salt and water.

In addition to the filtration of blood and formation of urine, the kidneys also (1) regulate water and electrolyte balance; (2) excrete metabolic waste, drugs, and hormone metabolites; (3) provide a level of gluconeogenesis; (4) regulate ABP; (5) regulate acid–base balance; (6) regulate erythrocyte production; and (7) regulate 1,25-dihydroxyvitamin D_3 (calcitriol) production.

The human kidneys are a pair of bean-shaped organs that are located outside the peritoneal space and within the retroperitoneal space in the posterior portion of the abdomen on either side of the spine, between the T12 and L3 vertebrae. Each kidney weighs roughly 150 g and measures approximately 10–12 cm in length, has a width of 5–7 cm, and is 3 cm in thickness, or about the size of a clenched fist. The right kidney is typically positioned slightly lower than the left because of the presence of the liver. Each kidney has a convex lateral border and a concave medial border, which contains the renal hilum. The renal hilum serves as both the entry and exit point for the renal artery, renal vein, lymphatics, nerves, and ureter (Figs. 3.44 and 3.45).

The kidney is encapsulated by a fibrous tissue on the outside known as the *capsule of the kidney*, which

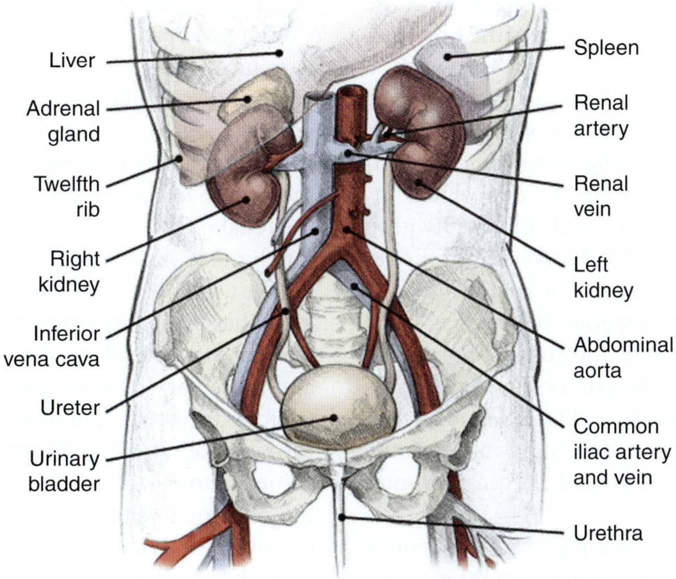

Fig. 3.44 Kidney position. (From Elisha S, Heiner JS, Nagelhout JJ. *Nurse Anesthesia*. 7th ed. Elsevier; 2023.)

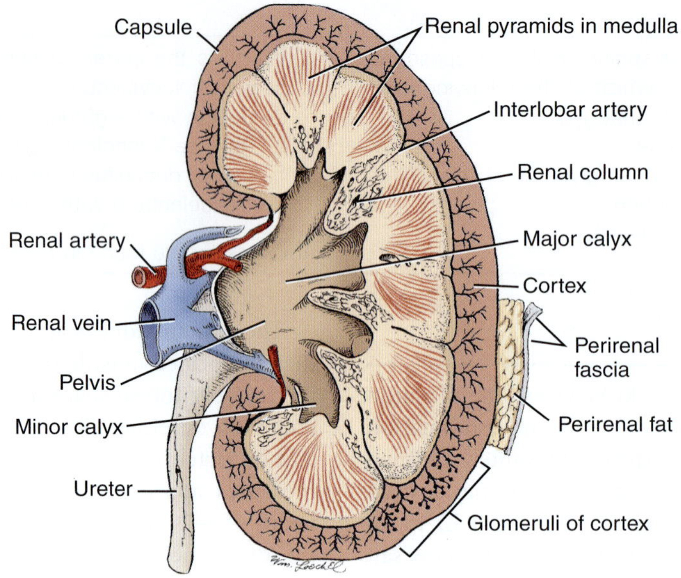

Fig. 3.45 Longitudinal section of the kidney. (From Elisha S, Heiner JS, Nagelhout JJ. *Nurse Anesthesia.* 7th ed. Elsevier; 2023.)

protects the kidneys against other structures within the abdomen while the body is in motion. The internal structure of the kidney is composed of three main regions: the renal cortex, the renal medulla, and the renal pelvis.

The *renal cortex* is the outermost region of the kidney that contains the renal corpuscles, convoluted tubules, distal tubule, and initial "cortical" collecting ducts of the renal nephron. The renal corpuscle houses the tiny clusters of blood vessels known as the *glomeruli* within a glomerular capsule, known as *Bowman's capsule*. The renal corpuscles are the filtration units of the kidney and the starting point of the renal nephron. Immediately after the renal corpuscles are the convoluted tubules of the renal nephron that are also located within the outer layer of the renal cortex. Extensions of the renal cortex (known as *renal columns* or *columns of Bertini*) project downward and separate the various renal pyramids of the renal medulla. The cortical portion of the tubule collecting ducts, blood vessels, and fibrous material make up these columns and function to anchor the cortex in place. The distal convoluted tubule is the other renal tubular structure located within the outer layer of the renal cortex.

The *renal medulla* is the inner region of the kidney and is organized into 8–12 cone-shaped groups of tissue known as *renal pyramids*. The renal medulla's main function is to concentrate urine. Each renal pyramid has a broad base that sits at the borders of the renal cortex and renal medulla and then projects into a pointed renal papilla that extends to the minor calyces of the renal pelvis. The renal medulla contains loops of Henle and "medullary" collecting ducts of the renal nephron, which give it the pyramid-like structure (Fig. 3.46).

The *renal pelvis* is a funnel-shaped structure that collects urine. The outer regions of the renal pelvis are divided into cup-like structures called *minor calyces* that adjoin the renal papillae, allowing urine to drain from the collecting ducts of the nephron. The minor calyces then merge into major calyces, facilitating urine drainage into the renal pelvis, which then funnels urine into the ureter for elimination through the bladder and urethra.

The ureters are muscular tubes approximately 25–30 cm long that transport urine from the renal pelvis to the bladder via peristalsis. The urinary bladder is a hollow and muscular organ located in the pelvis. Its function is to store urine collected from both ureters in preparation for removal. The urge to urinate occurs with a bladder urine volume of 150–250 mL, but it can store up to 500 mL of urine in females and 700 mL in males. The act of urinating or voiding is the process of expelling urine from the bladder, known as *micturition*. The micturition reflex involves both sympathetic and parasympathetic

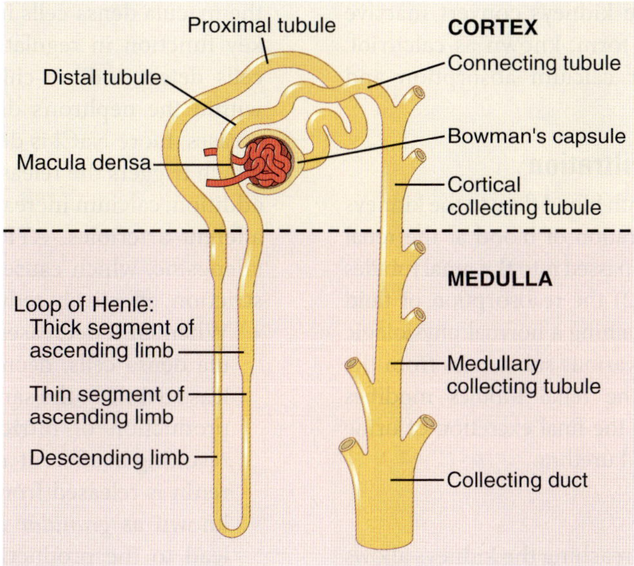

Fig. 3.46 Basic tubular segments of the nephron. The relative lengths of the different tubular segments are not drawn to scale. (From Hall JE, Hall ME. *Guyton and Hall Textbook of Medical Physiology*. 15th ed. Elsevier; 2026.)

controls. The SNS keeps the smooth muscle within the bladder wall (known as the *detrusor muscle*) relaxed and the internal sphincter contracted to allow urine to fill within the bladder. As urine accumulates, the bladder stretches, which is sensed by stretch receptors within the bladder wall and communicated to the brain. Signals from the brain are sent through the sacral spinal cord to initiate bladder contraction via parasympathetic innervation and detrusor (smooth muscle) contraction. The internal sphincter, located at the junction of the bladder and the urethra, also relaxes, opening the passage for urine to flow into the urethra. The urethra is the tube that delivers urine from the bladder to the external environment. The male urethra is approximately 18–20 cm in length and passes through the prostate and penis. The female urethra is shorter, at about 3–4 cm in length, and opens anterior to the vaginal orifice. When the micturition reflex is initiated and the internal "bladder" sphincter opens, urine cannot be eliminated until the external sphincter that surrounds the urethra opens. The external "urethral" sphincter is innervated by the pudendal nerve (S2–S4) and composed of skeletal muscle, which is under conscious control. This is the sphincter we can consciously control to allow for urination when appropriate. Once urination is complete, the bladder relaxes, and sympathetic control reengages to keep the internal "bladder" sphincter closed while the external "urethral" sphincter contracts, restoring continence.

Renal Physiology

The kidneys are vital organs within the human body responsible for blood filtration, the removal of waste via urine, and the regulation of fluid balance. Their primary physiological functions include the following:

- *Filtration of blood*: The kidneys filter approximately 180 L of blood per day in order to remove waste products such as urea, creatinine, and toxins through the formation of urine.
- *Regulation of fluid and electrolyte balance*: The kidneys help maintain water levels and regulate essential electrolytes such as sodium, potassium, and calcium.
- *Regulation of acid–base balance*: The excretion of hydrogen ions and reabsorption of bicarbonate by the kidneys help to maintain proper blood pH.
- *ABP regulation*: The kidneys regulate BP through the RAAS, which controls blood volume and vessel constriction.
- *Erythropoiesis*: The kidneys produce the hormone erythropoietin, which stimulates bone marrow to produce RBCs in response to low oxygen levels.

- *Vitamin D activation*: The kidneys convert inactive vitamin D into its active form, known as calcitriol. Calcitriol is essential for calcium absorption and bone health.

Renal Blood Flow and Filtration

The creation of urine begins with blood flow to the kidneys and then involves (1) the filtration of blood at the renal corpuscle. Fluid filtrate is then passed into the renal tubules and collecting ducts, where (2) the reabsorption of fluid and electrolytes occurs, maintaining a normal physiologic balance. The secretion (3) of various substances from the peritubular capillaries into the renal tubules modifies the urine filtrate, allowing for the final excretion of urine (4) via the ureters, bladder, and urethra.

Renal Blood Flow

- The amount of blood flow reaching the kidneys allows for the filtration of blood by the kidneys. The amount of blood delivered to both kidneys is normally about 20%–25% of the cardiac output, or roughly 1100–1200 mL/min. This results in the entire adult blood volume being filtered by the kidneys about 300 times per day. The kidneys have intrinsic mechanisms that allow for a regular and constant blood flow over a wide range of systemic arterial pressures, known as *autoregulation*. *Renal autoregulation* is the kidney's ability to maintain a relatively constant blood flow and glomerular filtration rate (GFR), despite fluctuations in systemic BP. Renal autoregulation primarily operates within a MAP range of 80–180 mm Hg and involves two key mechanisms known as the *myogenic* and *tubuloglomerular feedback mechanisms*. These two mechanisms work together to protect the kidneys from damage due to fluctuating BPs while at the same time ensuring the steady filtration of blood. In extreme conditions, such as severe hypotension or hypertension, autoregulation may fail, leading to potential kidney injury.
- The *myogenic mechanism* is based on the intrinsic ability of the renal afferent arteriole's smooth muscle to respond to changes in BP. When BP increases and arterial vascular walls stretch, the afferent arterioles vasoconstrict to reduce blood flow to the glomerulus, preventing excessive filtration. When BP decreases, the afferent arterioles dilate to maintain adequate glomerular blood flow and filtration pressure.
- The *tubuloglomerular feedback mechanism* involves the juxtaglomerular apparatus (JGA), particularly the macula densa cells in the renal nephron, and is a key function in regulating the GFR. Macula densa cells detect sodium-chloride (NaCl) concentration within the nephron's distal tubule. When GFR increases, more NaCl is delivered to the macula densa, which triggers the release of ATP from these cells. In addition, calcium increases in smooth muscle cells of afferent arterioles. ATP is then broken down into adenosine, which causes afferent arteriole vasoconstriction, effectively reducing GFR back to normal.
    - When GFR decreases, less NaCl reaches the macula densa cells, decreasing ATP and calcium release, while at the same time causing an increased production of nitric oxide and prostaglandins, resulting in afferent arteriole dilation. In addition, renin is released from juxtaglomerular cells (also known as *granular cells*). Increased renin levels lead to the production of angiotensin II in the lungs and kidneys, which increases ABP, renal blood flow, and GFR. An additional mechanism happens when angiotensin II binds to receptors in the adrenal glands' zona glomerulosa, stimulating aldosterone release and resulting in the reabsorption of sodium and water within the distal tubule and collecting ducts of the nephrons, effectively increasing blood volume.
    - Angiotensin II and nitric oxide influence renal autoregulation to a small degree.
    - Massive sympathetic stimulation, from pathologic states such as systemic shock, can override renal autoregulation, causing significant decreases in renal autoregulation.
- Blood flow to the kidney is also regulated by local renal vascular resistance, which is primarily located in the interlobular arteries and afferent and efferent arterioles. The resistance within these vessels is controlled by the SNS, several hormones, and internal renal control mechanisms. Increased resistance will result in decreased renal blood flow, and a decrease in resistance will result in increased renal blood flow. Glomerular filtration pressure depends not only on the renal artery perfusion pressure but also on the balance between afferent and efferent arteriolar tone.
    - *Afferent arterioles* branch from the interlobular arteries and are the immediate preglomerular arterioles. They regulate blood flow to the glomerular capillaries and help to maintain a steady state blood flow in order to maintain a consistent GFR.

- Systemic and local factors that influence renal afferent arteriole vasoconstriction include sympathetic stimuli (e.g., norepinephrine), increased arteriole capillary BP and the myogenic response, angiotensin II, adenosine released from macula densa cells, and endothelin.
- Systemic and local factors that influence renal afferent arteriole vasodilation include decreased systemic BP and the myogenic response, prostaglandins, nitric oxide, atrial natriuretic peptide (opposite effect on efferent arterioles), and low NaCl delivery to the macula densa.

- *Efferent arterioles* drain the glomeruli and are larger than afferent arterioles. These vessels have an important role in "fine-tuning" glomerular perfusion by their ability to vasoconstrict. The vasoconstrictor response by these vessels is also important in maintaining glomerular perfusion in the presence of decreased afferent arteriolar pressure and/or reduced renal blood flow. Efferent arterioles branch into the vasa recta within the renal medulla and into peritubular capillaries within the renal cortex.
  - Systemic and local factors that influence renal efferent arteriole vasoconstriction include sympathetic stimuli (e.g., norepinephrine), angiotensin II (larger effect on efferent than afferent arterioles), atrial natriuretic peptide, and endothelin.
  - Systemic and local factors that influence renal efferent arteriole vasodilation include increased NaCl at the macula densa (tubuloglomerular feedback), nitric oxide, and exogenous administration of angiotensin-converting enzyme (ACE) inhibitors.
- The functional units within each kidney are the nephrons. By the time each kidney becomes fully formed in utero, it contains approximately 800,000–1,000,000 nephrons. Once developed, no new nephrons can be created, and after the age of 40 years, functional nephrons decrease in number by approximately 10% every 10 years. Each nephron is capable of creating urine, with sections located in both the renal cortex and renal medulla. Even though each nephron contains the same components, there are differences in nephron structure depending on how deep the nephron is located within the kidney. The majority of nephrons are known as *cortical nephrons* (Fig. 3.47), which house their glomeruli in the outer cortex and have short loops of Henle that pass downward within the renal cortex and only a short distance into the renal medulla. Approximately 20%–30% of nephrons have glomeruli that are positioned deep in the renal cortex adjacent to the renal medulla. These are known as *juxtamedullary nephrons*, and they contain longer loops of Henle that pass deep into the renal medulla. The components of each nephron include (see Fig. 3.46):
  1. A renal corpuscle, which is a cluster of glomerular capillaries that are encapsulated within Bowman's capsule
  2. The proximal convoluted tubule
  3. A thin and thick portion on the loop of Henle
  4. The distal convoluted tubule
  5. Collecting ducts

Glomerular Filtration

- Glomerular filtration is the first step in urine formation. Filtration occurs at the renal corpuscle by the glomerular capillaries within Bowman's capsule. Because of the high amount of renal perfusion, an estimated 180 L/day is filtered through the glomerular capillaries and into Bowman's capsule. The structure of the thicker glomerular capillary membrane acts as a filtration barrier with three major layers that prevent proteins and other large molecules from entering the plasma filtrate. Freely filtered substances include water, electrolytes, glucose, urea, creatinine, and amino acids. Partially filtered substances include myoglobin and albumin. Nonfiltered substances include substances such as larger proteins, red and white blood cells, and platelets (Table 3.45). Negatively charged large molecules are less filtered than positively charged molecules of similar size because of the negatively charged glycoproteins contained within each layer. The three layers that make up the glomerular capillary membrane include an endothelial layer, a basement membrane, and podocyte cells.
  - The first inner layer of the glomerular capillary membrane consists of a glomerular capillary *fenestrated endothelial layer* that has pores that are only large enough to allow small molecules to pass through.

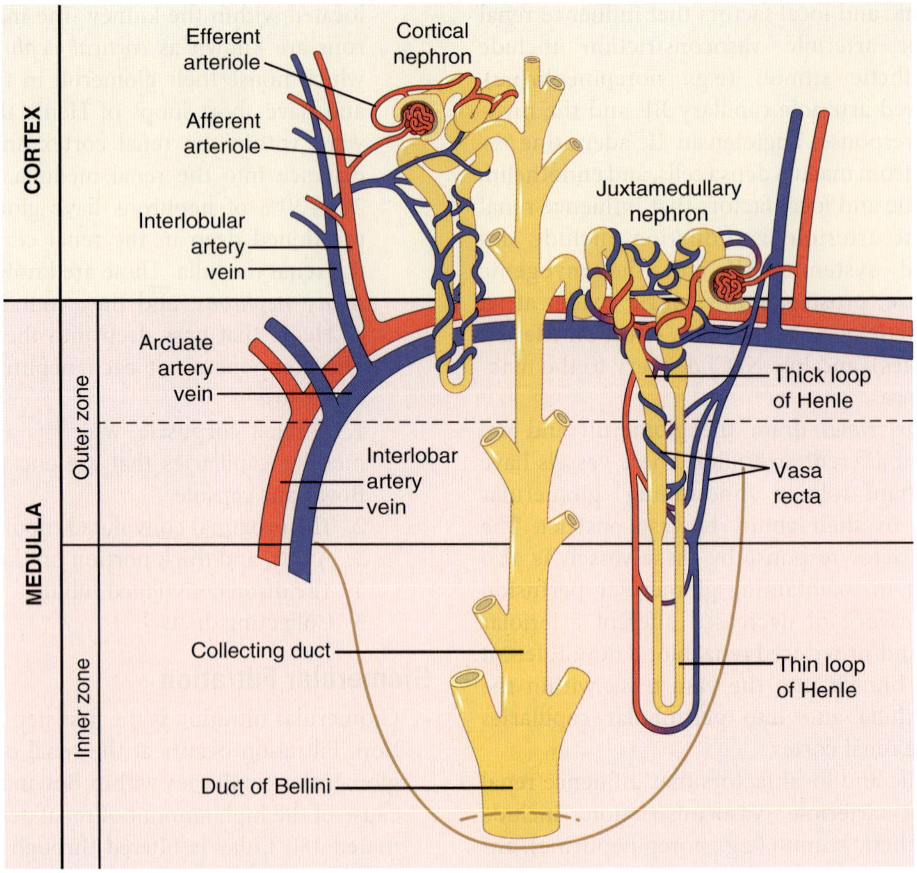

Fig. 3.47 Schematic of relationships between blood vessels and tubular structures and differences between cortical and juxtamedullary nephrons. (From Hall JE, Hall ME. *Guyton and Hall Textbook of Medical Physiology*. 15th ed. Elsevier; 2026.)

TABLE 3.45 **Substances Filtered at the Glomerular Capillaries**

Substance	Molecular Weight (Da)	Filtered at Glomerulus
Water	18	Yes
Electrolytes (e.g., sodium, potassium, magnesium, calcium, chloride)	23–40	Yes
Urea	60	Yes
Creatinine	113	Yes
Glucose	180	Yes
Amino acids	110–200	Yes
Small peptides	500–1,000	Yes
Insulin	5200	Yes
Myoglobin	17,000	Yes (in small amounts)
Albumin	66,500	No (<0.5% filtered)
Hemoglobin	64,000	No
Immunoglobulins (IgG, IgA, etc.)	150,000	No

  - The second middle layer is a *basement membrane* composed of collagen and heparan sulfate, which acts as a strainer to further restrict the passage of molecules based on size and charge.
  - The third outer layer consists of *podocytes*, which are specialized cells that have "foot-like" projections that interlock, creating small filtration openings (known as *slit pores*), creating a final barrier against protein leakage.
  - It is important to note that there is a small number of proteins (such as albumin at <0.5%) that normally filter through the glomerular barrier. These are primarily reabsorbed, with only very small amounts excreted in the urine.
  - In disease states (e.g., diabetic nephropathy), the glomerular filtration barrier is degraded, allowing large amounts of protein to leak into the glomerular filtrate, which are then excreted in the urine.
- The quantity of glomerular filtrate formed within the nephrons of the kidney each minute is the GFR. A normal GFR is approximately 125 mL/min. Most of the filtrate is reabsorbed back into the bloodstream as it moves through the renal nephron, resulting in about 1% (1–2 L) of urine produced for excretion. The primary determinants of GFR include the following:
  - Hydrostatic and oncotic pressures, creating a net filtration pressure. A primary determinant of GFR is the glomerular filtration pressure. The glomerular capillary hydrostatic pressure (60 mm Hg) is the main driving force that pushes fluid out of the capillaries and into Bowman's capsule, promoting filtration. Bowman's capsule hydrostatic pressure (18 mm Hg) opposes filtration by pushing fluid back into capillaries. Glomerular capillary oncotic pressure (32 mm Hg) is created from the amount of plasma proteins within the glomerular capillaries, which pulls water back into the capillaries, causing a reduced filtration. Bowman's capsule oncotic pressure (0 mm Hg) is normally low; however, if proteins enter the capsule (e.g., in disease states like diabetic nephropathy), there will be an increase in filtration. The sum of the "pushing" hydrostatic forces against the "pulling" oncotic forces is the net filtration pressure (10 mm Hg).
  - Blood flow that reaches the kidney is known as *renal plasma flow*. Approximately 625 mL/min of blood flows through the afferent arterioles of the nephrons of each kidney. There is a direct relationship between renal plasma flow and glomerular filtration. When renal plasma flow decreases, glomerular filtration decreases. A normal GFR is approximately 20% of the renal plasma flow, which is equal to 125 mL/min.
  - *Afferent and efferent arteriole resistance:* Glomeruli function is influenced by the balance of afferent and efferent arteriole tone. Reductions in glomerular filtration signal the afferent arterioles to dilate and improve glomerular blood flow and signal efferent arterioles to constrict, returning glomerular filtration to normal.
  - *Hormonal and neural regulation:* The majority of renal vascular resistance is located within the interlobular arteries, as well as the afferent and efferent arterioles. In general, an increase in vascular resistance before the glomerulus will reduce renal blood flow and GFR, such as sympathetic stimulation of the interlobular arteries and afferent arterioles. Angiotensin II primarily acts on the efferent arterioles to cause vasoconstriction, resulting in an increase in GFR. A decrease in vascular resistance will generally increase renal blood flow and GFR as long as autoregulatory (80- to 180-mm Hg) mechanisms remain intact.
- Several other factors influence the GFR:
  - Plasma protein concentration
    - Increased plasma proteins (e.g., dehydration states) raise oncotic pressure and decrease GFR.
    - Decreased plasma proteins (e.g., liver disease) lower oncotic pressure and increase GFR.
  - Urinary tract obstruction
    - A urinary tract obstruction (e.g., large kidney stone, tumor, or enlarged prostate) prevents urine excretion through the ureters, causing a buildup within the renal pelvis.
    - As urine accumulates, pressure increases within the renal tubules and eventually in Bowman's capsule.
    - When Bowman's capsule hydrostatic pressure rises, it reduces the pressure gradient driving filtration and leads to a decrease in GFR.
  - Pathological conditions affect GFR, such as the following:
    - Chronic kidney disease (CKD) leads to a progressive decline in GFR.

- Glomerulonephritis, as a result of inflammation of glomeruli, can impair glomerular filtration.
- Diabetes and hypertension both cause structural damage to glomeruli and affect GFR.
- Age
  - GFR declines with age as a result of loss of nephrons and decreased renal blood flow.
- The most common method for assessing kidney function in clinical practice is by measuring serum creatinine levels. However, assessment of glomerular filtration is most effective by calculating the rate at which a substance is cleared from the blood plasma. This requires that the substance be freely filtered by the glomerulus and not be reabsorbed or secreted. Insulin clearance, creatinine clearance, and cystatin C clearance are methods that can be used to assess GFR more accurately than serum creatinine values.
  - Serum creatinine is the preferred method for evaluating kidney function because it is noninvasive, cost effective, and widely available. Creatinine is a byproduct of muscle metabolism and is constantly produced and released into the bloodstream. The kidneys primarily remove creatinine through glomerular filtration with minimal tubular secretion. Serum creatinine is inversely related to GFR. As kidney function declines, less creatinine is filtered, leading to a rise in serum creatinine levels.
  - Inulin is freely filtered at the glomerulus, is not reabsorbed, and is not a secreted substance. The insulin clearance method requires an IV infusion of inulin followed by measurements of both urine and plasma inulin concentrations. This method is time-consuming and costly, which limits its clinical use. It is primarily used in research or for high-precision assessment of the GFR.
  - Urine creatinine clearance (CrCl) is currently the most accurate test used to estimate GFR in clinical practice. It is most accurate after a 24-hour urine collection in combination with a serum creatinine measurement. One limitation is that it can slightly overestimate GFR because renal tubules secrete some creatinine.
  - Cystatin C clearance can be used to assess GFR. Cystatin C is a small protein produced by nearly all cells within the body, is freely filtered by glomeruli, is not secreted, and is catabolized in the proximal tubule before being reabsorbed. It is less affected by muscle mass than creatinine and can be used as an alternative to the creatinine clearance method.

KNOWLEDGE CHECK

1. What is the primary function of the kidneys?
   a. Production and release of hormones that regulate BP
   b. Filtration of blood and concentration of urine
   c. Regulation of body temperature
   d. Production of RBCs
2. Which structure within the kidney is responsible for the initial filtration of blood?
   a. Renal pelvis
   b. Glomerulus
   c. Ureter
   d. Renal artery
3. The RAAS affects kidney function by
   a. decreasing BP and increasing urine output.
   b. increasing BP through the regulation of blood volume and vessel constriction.
   c. preventing calcium reabsorption in the kidneys and promoting calcium excretion.
   d. triggering urine storage in the bladder for later elimination.
4. What is the primary function of the renal medulla?
   a. Concentration of urine
   b. Filtration of blood
   c. Production of RBCs
   d. Detoxification of harmful substances
5. The renal medulla contains which structures that help concentrate urine?
   a. Renal corpuscles and proximal tubules
   b. Minor and major calyces
   c. Loops of Henle and collecting ducts
   d. Renal arteries and veins
6. What is the function of the juxtaglomerular apparatus in the kidney?
   a. Regulation of GFR and BP
   b. Filtration of blood and removal of toxic substances
   c. Synthesis of erythropoietin and similar hematologic stimulating hormones
   d. Conversion of vitamin D into its active form

Answers can be found in Appendix A.

Renal Tubular Reabsorption and Secretion

- The regulation of reabsorbed and secreted substances varies along the renal tubule (Fig. 3.48).
- Two additional capillary systems play essential roles in kidney function, particularly with tubular reabsorption and secretion. The peritubular capillaries are more involved with general reabsorption, whereas the vasa recta specialize in maintaining the concentration gradient within the medulla necessary for water conservation (Table 3.46).
- The formation and location of the peritubular capillaries and vasa recta depend on the type of nephron.
  - Cortical nephrons (85% of nephrons): Peritubular capillaries arise from the efferent arteriole and surround the proximal and distal convoluted tubules of cortical nephrons within the renal cortex.
    - Their primary role is to reabsorb water, nutrients, and ions from the filtrate back into circulation.
    - They also participate in secretion, where substances like drugs and waste products are moved from the blood into the tubular fluid.
  - Juxtamedullary nephrons (15% of nephrons): The efferent arterioles in this area give rise to the vasa recta, a specialized capillary network that follows the loop of Henle and extends deep into the medulla.
    - Their primary role is to help maintain the osmotic gradient in the medulla, which is an essential kidney function allowing for the concentration of urine.
    - The vasa recta is part of the countercurrent exchanger (in combination with the loop of Henle), which allows water and solutes to be exchanged in a way that avoids dissipation of the medullary concentration gradient.

Renal Tubular Reabsorption

- Renal tubular reabsorption is the process by which the kidneys selectively reclaim water, electrolytes, and other essential substances filtered from Bowman's capsule into the renal tubules and return them into the bloodstream (Table 3.47).
  - In order for a substance to be reabsorbed, it must (1) be transported across the renal tubular epithelial cell membrane and into the renal interstitial fluid and (2) move through the peritubular capillary membrane and into the blood.
  - Tubular reabsorption primarily occurs in the proximal convoluted tubule, loop of Henle, distal convoluted tubule, and collecting duct.
  - The majority of substances are reabsorbed within the proximal convoluted tubules, which include water, electrolytes (sodium, chloride, potassium), glucose, bicarbonate, and urea.
  - Tubular reabsorption helps maintain fluid and electrolyte balance; regulates BP; and prevents excessive loss of important substances such as glucose, amino acids, and bicarbonate.
- Peritubular hydrostatic and osmotic pressures help regulate tubular reabsorption.
  - Increases in peritubular hydrostatic pressure (e.g., high ABP) reduce tubular reabsorption. Renal autoregulation helps to diminish this effect.
  - Constriction of the afferent and efferent arterioles decreases the peritubular hydrostatic pressure and allows for an increase in reabsorption.
  - Increases in peritubular oncotic pressure increase tubular reabsorption. Raising the systemic plasma protein concentration increases peritubular oncotic pressure and promotes reabsorption of substances from the renal tubules.
- Reabsorption occurs through passive and active mechanisms:
  - *Active reabsorption* requires ATP to move substances against their electrochemical and concentration gradients. It requires either primary or secondary active transport mechanisms.
    - Primary active transport uses ATP. A prime example is the sodium–potassium–adenosine triphosphate (Na^+-K^+ ATPase) pump in the basolateral membrane of tubular cells throughout the renal tubule. The Na^+-K^+ ATPase pump uses the hydrolysis of ATP to actively transport sodium out of the cell and into the interstitial fluid and potassium from the interstitium back into the cell. The action of this pump maintains a low intracellular sodium concentration and a high intracellular potassium concentration.
    - Secondary active transport does not require ATP and instead uses the energy coupled from an energy source (e.g., sodium movement down its electrochemical gradient) to transport substances. This is known as *cotransport* or *countertransport*. A major example would

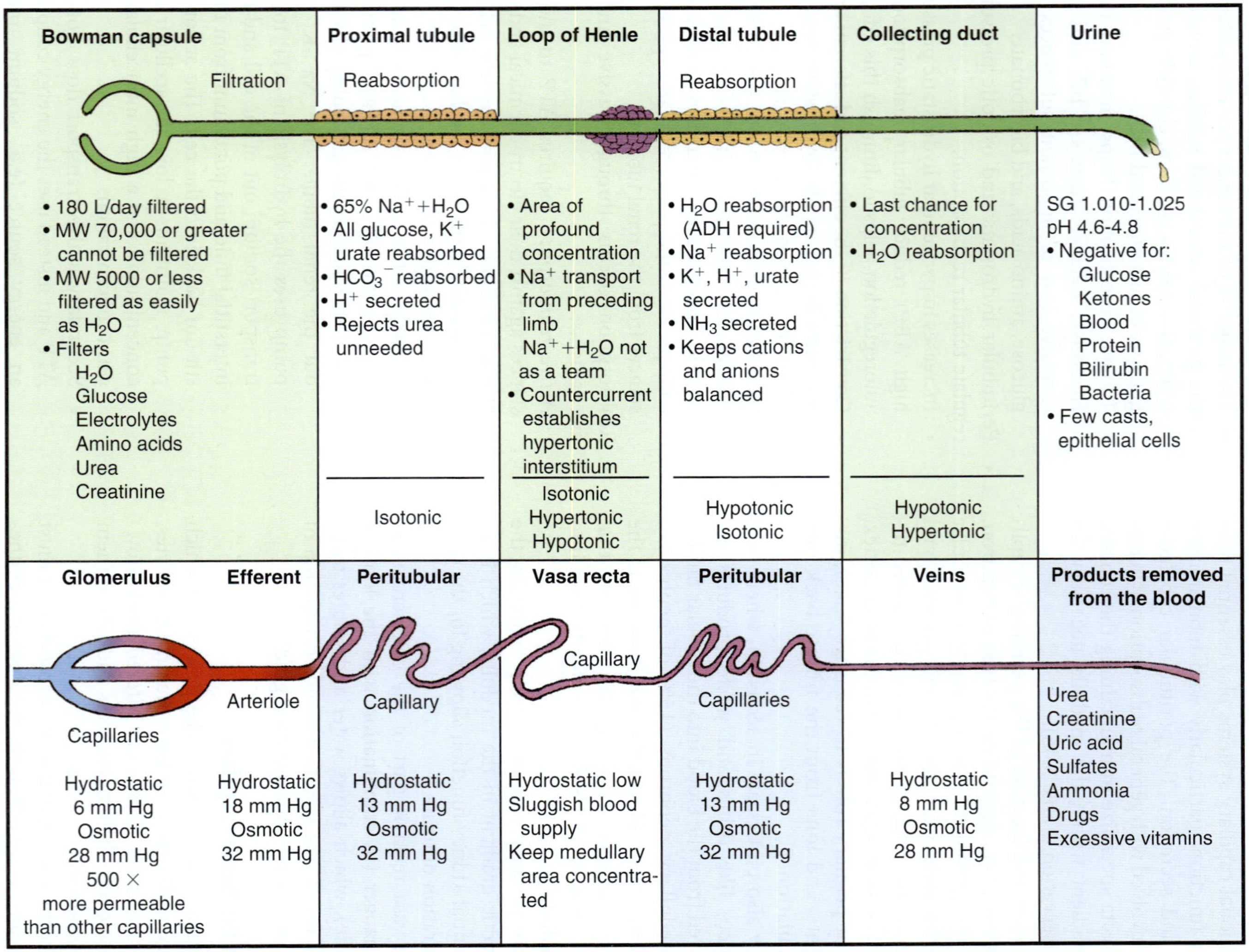

Fig. 3.48 Renal blood flow, filtration, reabsorption, and secretion. *ADH,* Antidiuretic hormone; *MW,* molecular weight; *SG,* specific gravity. (From Elisha S, Heiner JS, Nagelhout JJ. *Nurse Anesthesia.* 7th ed. Elsevier; 2023.)

TABLE 3.46 Differences Between the Peritubular Capillaries and the Vasa Recta

	Peritubular Capillaries	Vasa Recta
Location	Surround proximal and distal tubules in the cortex	Follows the loop of Henle in the medulla
Associated nephron type	Cortical nephrons	Juxtamedullary nephrons
Function	Reabsorption and secretion	Countercurrent exchange for urine concentration
Structure	Highly branched capillary network	Long, straight capillaries

TABLE 3.47 Reabsorption and Secretion of Various Substances by the Kidney Under Normal Conditions

Substance	Reabsorbed (%)	Site of Reabsorption	Secreted (%)	Site of Secretion
Water (H_2O)	99%	Proximal tubule (65%) Descending loop of Henle (15%) Distal tubule and collecting duct (19%)	None	N/A
Sodium (Na^+)	99%	Proximal tubule (65%) Ascending loop of Henle (25%) Distal tubule/collecting tubule and duct (9%)	Minimal	Distal tubule and collecting tubule and duct
Potassium (K^+)	90%	Proximal tubule (65%), loop of Henle (25%)	Variable (depends on needs)	Distal tubule and collecting duct
Glucose	100%	Proximal tubule	None	N/A
Amino acids	100%	Proximal tubule	None	N/A
Bicarbonate (HCO_3^-)	80–90%	Proximal tubule (80%) Distal tubule/collecting tubule (10%)	Minimal	Distal tubule Collecting tubule
Hydrogen ions (H^+)	None	N/A	Variable (regulates pH)	Proximal tubule, distal tubule, and collecting tubule and duct
Urea	50%	Proximal tubule and collecting duct	50%	Proximal tubule and loop of Henle
Creatinine	None	N/A	100%	Proximal tubule
Drugs and toxins	None	N/A	Variable	Proximal tubule

N/A, Not applicable.

be the active transport of sodium in the proximal tubule that pulls glucose and amino acids in a cotransport manner, which are then reabsorbed. The system is termed *sodium-glucose cotransporter* (SGLT).

- *Passive reabsorption* moves substances along their concentration gradients through diffusion or osmosis (e.g., water via osmosis, urea via diffusion).
  - *Simple diffusion:* Small solutes, like urea and lipid-soluble molecules, diffuse freely across the tubular epithelium because of their higher concentration gradients within the renal tubule.
  - *Osmosis*: Water moves in response to osmotic gradients. Water will passively follow the active transport of sodium, especially in the *proximal tubule* and descending loop of Henle via aquaporin channels and through the tight junctions between the epithelial cells of the renal tubule and into the interstitium. Water will passively move through *aquaporin* channels via osmosis

in the distal tubule, collecting tubule, and collecting ducts in the presence of ADH, which causes an increase in membrane permeability in these late tubule locations.
  - Another example is when chloride ions passively diffuse through paracellular pathways following the cation sodium (which is actively transported) in an effort to maintain electroneutrality.
- Several hormonal systems help regulate tubular reabsorption, body fluid volumes, and solute concentrations (Table 3.48).
  - *Aldosterone* is the primary mineralocorticoid released from zona glomerulosa cells within the adrenal cortex.
    - It causes (1) the reabsorption of sodium and subsequently water and (2) the secretion of potassium. It is an important hormone essential for the regulation of both serum sodium and potassium.
    - Aldosterone exerts its action on principal cells located in the late distal tubule and in the cortical areas of the collecting tubule and duct.
    - The two most important stimuli that cause the release of aldosterone are (1) an increased extracellular potassium level and (2) increased angiotensin II levels (as part of the RAAS), which result from a decreased serum sodium concentration, low intravascular volume, and/or hypotension.
    - Aldosterone deficiencies can lead to conditions such as Addison disease and result in plasma sodium loss and an accumulation of plasma potassium.
    - Excess aldosterone from adrenal tumors (e.g., Conn syndrome) results in sodium retention and decreased plasma concentrations of potassium.
  - *Angiotensin II* is formed after the release of renin causes the conversion of angiotensinogen (made and released from the liver into the blood) to angiotensin I, which then travels to the lung (and the kidney), where ACE converts it to angiotensin II.
    - The release of renin and ultimately angiotensin is caused by (1) hypotension resulting in a decreased afferent arteriole pressure, (2) low sodium concentration within the distal tubule, and (3) β-adrenergic stimulation.
    - The overall function of angiotensin II is to increase BP and extracellular volume. Angiotensin II does this by three specific mechanisms:
    - First, it stimulates aldosterone release from the adrenal cortex, which increases sodium and water reabsorption from the renal tubules.
    - Second, it causes efferent arteriole constriction (and afferent arteriole constriction to a lesser extent). Efferent arteriole constriction results in a reduced peritubular capillary hydrostatic pressure, allowing for a greater net reabsorption of tubular filtrate, especially in the proximal tubule, where sodium is primarily reabsorbed.
    - Third, it directly stimulates sodium reabsorption in the proximal tubule, loops of Henle, distal tubule, and collecting tubule. Angiotensin II directly stimulates the Na^+-K^+ ATPase pump on tubular epithelial cells, causing the reabsorption of sodium. It also stimulates other cotransport systems within the renal nephron to augment the reabsorption of sodium.

TABLE 3.48 Hormonal Regulation of Tubular Reabsorption

Hormone	Action	Site of Action
Aldosterone	Increases reabsorption of Na^+, Cl^-, and H_2O Increases secretion of K^+, H^+	Principal cells of late distal tubule, collecting tubule, and duct
Angiotensin II	Increases reabsorption of Na^+, Cl^- Increases secretion of H^+	Proximal tubule, thick ascending loop of Henle, distal tubule, collecting tubule
Antidiuretic hormone	Increases reabsorption of H_2O	Late distal tubule, collecting tubule, and duct
Atrial natriuretic peptide	Decreases reabsorption of Na^+ and Cl^-	Distal tubule, collecting tubule, and duct
Parathyroid hormone	Increases reabsorption of Ca^{2+} Decreases reabsorption of PO_4^-	Proximal tubule, thick ascending loop of Henle, distal tubule

Ca^{2+}, calcium; *Cl^-*, chloride; *H^+*, hydrogen ions; *H_2O*, water; *K^+*, potassium; *Na^+*, sodium; *PO_4^-* , phosphate.

- *ADH, or vasopressin,* is synthesized in the hypothalamus and released from the posterior pituitary gland, known as the *neurohypophysis.*
  - ADH is released in response to low blood volume, hypotension, or a high blood serum osmolarity.
  - Several osmoreceptors are located near the hypothalamus that sense the osmotic concentration of extracellular fluid. When the concentration is high (e.g., in dehydration), ADH is released.
  - Increases in extracellular volume signal atrial stretch receptors to inhibit ADH release.
  - The primary renal function of ADH is to increase the water permeability in the late distal tubule, collecting tubule, and collecting duct. This allows the body to conserve water in situations such as dehydration. In the absence of ADH, the distal tubule and collecting ducts are mostly impermeable to water, and it is excreted in the urine.
  - ADH binds to vasopressin (V_2) receptors on epithelial cells in the late distal tubule and collecting tubules and ducts, which then stimulates cyclic adenosine monophosphate (cAMP) to activate protein kinases that result in the stimulation of aquaporin-2 (AQP-2) channels that permit the rapid diffusion of water through the cells.
- *Atrial natriuretic peptide* is synthesized and released from specific cells in the cardiac atria in response to stretching of the atrium because of an increased blood volume and higher ABP.
  - ANP is a potent endogenous diuretic that has both direct and indirect mechanisms for reducing plasma volume and increasing urine flow.
  - ANP directly reduces the reabsorption of sodium and water. It acts on the collecting ducts of the renal tubule within the medulla to decrease sodium and water reabsorption, effectively promoting the excretion of sodium and water in the urine.
  - ANP indirectly reduces the reabsorption of sodium and water. It inhibits the release of renin, which then stops the formation of angiotensin II, effectively reducing the reabsorption of sodium and water from this mechanism.
- *PTH* is secreted by the parathyroid glands in response to low blood calcium (Ca^{2+}) levels.
  - Chief cells within the parathyroid gland sense low blood calcium levels (hypocalcemia), which then results in the release of PTH into the bloodstream.
  - PTH binds to receptors on the thick ascending loop of Henle and distal tubule cells of the nephron, activating cAMP and leading to an increased reabsorption of calcium from tubular filtrate.
  - PTH blocks phosphate reabsorption in the proximal tubule when serum calcium levels are low, preventing additional calcium-phosphate binding in the blood.
  - UV radiation from sunlight converts 7-dehydrocholesterol in the skin into vitamin D_3 (cholecalciferol). The liver metabolizes vitamin D_3 into 25-hydroxyvitamin D_3. PTH stimulates the kidneys to convert 25-hydroxyvitamin D_3 to 1,25-dihydroxyvitamin D_3 (calcitriol), which is activated vitamin D. Activated vitamin D helps the intestines absorb calcium.
- *SNS* stimulation increases the reabsorption of sodium.
  - Intense SNS stimulation causes renal arteriole constriction and reduced GFR, leading to a decrease in sodium and water excretion.
  - Low levels of SNS stimulation cause activation of α-adrenergic receptors on epithelial cells of the proximal tubule, thick ascending loop of Henle, and distal tubule, promoting the reabsorption of sodium and water.
  - SNS stimulation increases the release of renin and the formation of angiotensin II, which results in an increase in sodium reabsorption and a decrease in excretion.

Renal Tubular Secretion

Renal tubular secretion helps to regulate fluid balance and is the method used by the kidneys to transport substances from the peritubular capillaries into the tubular filtrate for excretion in the urine (see Table 3.47).

- Tubular secretion occurs via passive diffusion or by active transport similar to reabsorption, using ion channels or transport proteins to facilitate movement.
- Substances move from the blood and into the renal tubular cells. Once inside the tubular cells, transport

occurs into the tubule lumen by active transport, facilitated diffusion, or ion exchange mechanisms such as the sodium–hydrogen ion exchanger.

- Tubular secretion plays a crucial role in maintaining acid–base balance; regulating electrolyte levels; and clearing drugs, toxins, and metabolic waste from the bloodstream.
- Renal tubular secretion primarily occurs in the proximal and distal convoluted tubules, with some secretion activity in the cortical collecting tubule and medullary collecting ducts.
- Fluid balance, and subsequently BP, is mediated by aldosterone, causing the tubular secretion of potassium and reabsorption of sodium in the distal tubule and collecting tubule.
- Tubular secretion regulates electrolyte levels such as potassium. Hyperkalemia is managed via tubular secretion of potassium into the renal tubule.
- Creatinine is filtered at the glomerulus and is actively secreted and almost entirely excreted in urine.
- Secretion of waste and excess ions:
  - Active transport facilitates the secretion of substances like hydrogen ions (H^+), ammonium ions ($NH4^+$), potassium (K^+), creatinine, and drugs into the tubules for excretion in urine.
  - Some hydrogen ions are actively secreted into the renal tubule from the energy released from the Na^+-K^+ ATPase pump by secondary active secretion. This is termed *countertransport*, where sodium ions are reabsorbed into the blood while hydrogen ions are secreted into the renal tubule lumen.
  - Both active and passive secretory mechanisms help maintain acid–base balance and electrolyte levels.
  - Transport proteins use active transport to secrete waste products and medications into the renal tubules for elimination.

KNOWLEDGE CHECK

1. What is the primary role of the peritubular capillaries?
   a. Maintenance of the osmotic gradient within the medulla
   b. Surrounding the loop of Henle to facilitate countercurrent exchange
   c. Reabsorption of sodium, water, and other ions from the filtrate into circulation
   d. Transportation of urine from the renal pelvis to the bladder for excretion
2. Which section of the nephron is primarily associated with the vasa recta?
   a. Proximal tubule
   b. Loop of Henle
   c. Distal tubule
   d. Collecting tubule
3. How does aldosterone affect renal tubular reabsorption and secretion?
   a. Inhibits sodium and water reabsorption while promoting potassium secretion
   b. Stimulates sodium and water reabsorption while promoting potassium secretion
   c. Directly increases calcium reabsorption in the proximal tubule
   d. Prevents angiotensin II formation, reducing sodium reabsorption
4. Which process is primarily responsible for the movement of water during renal tubular reabsorption?
   a. Primary active transport
   b. Secondary active transport
   c. Simple diffusion
   d. Osmosis
5. What is the primary function of the Na^+-K^+ ATPase pump in renal tubular cells?
   a. Actively transport sodium out of the cell and potassium into the cell
   b. Passively diffuse sodium into the renal tubule while excreting potassium
   c. Facilitate water reabsorption by opening aquaporin channels
   d. Regulate creatinine excretion in the collecting duct
6. Which hormone increases water permeability in the collecting ducts by stimulating AQP-2 channels?
   a. Aldosterone
   b. Angiotensin II
   c. ADH
   d. Atrial natriuretic peptide (ANP)
7. How does the SNS influence the renal tubular reabsorption of sodium?
   a. SNS activation increases sodium reabsorption by stimulating the RAAS.
   b. SNS activation decreases renin release, leading to reduced sodium reabsorption.
   c. SNS stimulation causes vasodilation of renal arterioles, increasing the GFR of sodium
   d. SNS activity has no effect on renal function

Answers can be found in Appendix A.

Sites of Renal Tubular Reabsorption and Secretion

- The reabsorption and secretion of substances along the renal tubule vary depending on the characteristics of the individual tubular segments (see Fig. 3.48).
- Proximal tubule reabsorption:
  - The epithelial cells within the proximal tubule contain large amounts of mitochondria, allowing for significant active transport of substances into and out of proximal tubule cells.
  - Under normal circumstances, approximately 65% of sodium, water, chloride, potassium, and bicarbonate are reabsorbed within the proximal tubule.
  - Proximal tubule epithelial cells also have an extensive surface area that is loaded with protein transport molecules that facilitate the cotransport of sodium with glucose or amino acids.
  - Under normal circumstances, 100% of glucose and amino acids are reabsorbed in the proximal tubule.
- Proximal tubule secretion:
  - The proximal tubule is a site for secretion of substances such as hydrogen, organic acids, and bases into the tubular lumen.
  - Countertransport mechanisms reabsorb sodium while hydrogen and other substances are secreted into the tubular filtrate.
    - In addition to initial bicarbonate (HCO_3^-) reabsorption, it is further removed from the tubular filtrate by combining with secreted hydrogen ions (H^+) to form carbonic acid (H_2CO_3), which then dissociates into water (H_2O) and carbon dioxide (CO_2).
  - A significant amount of creatinine is filtered from the glomeruli through Bowman's capsule into the tubule filtrate. The concentration of creatinine increases as creatinine is also secreted into the proximal tubule.
  - The proximal tubule is the site of secretion for metabolic wastes (e.g., bile salts, oxalate, urate, catecholamines), drugs and toxins (e.g., penicillin, salicylates), and para-aminohippuric acid (PAH).
- Loop of Henle reabsorption:
  - There are three important functional segments within the loop of Henle: (1) thin descending segment, (2) thin ascending segment, and (3) thick ascending segment.
  - The loop of Henle is located within the renal medulla, which contains a high-solute hypertonic environment.
- The thin descending and ascending segments contain thin epithelial membranes with few mitochondria and reduced levels of metabolic activity.
  - The thin descending segment is highly permeable to water, allowing for an estimated 15% of the total water reabsorption into the hypertonic medullary interstitium.
  - This area is mostly impermeable to solutes such as sodium and chloride.
  - As tubular filtrate moves down the loop of Henle, water is reabsorbed, causing a concentrated filtrate.
- The thick ascending segment begins halfway up the ascending pathway and contains thick epithelial cells with several mitochondria that produce significant metabolic activity.
  - The thin ascending and thick ascending segments are impermeable to water.
  - Active reabsorption accounts for an estimated 25% of the filtered sodium, chloride, and potassium.
  - Other ions, such as calcium, magnesium, and bicarbonate, are actively reabsorbed, but to a lesser extent.
  - The primary method by which sodium is reabsorbed from the tubular fluid is by the 1-sodium, 2-chloride, 1-potassium cotransporter (NKCC2) mechanism.
  - Loop diuretics (e.g., furosemide, ethacrynic acid, bumetanide) inhibit the NKCC2 cotransporter, impeding sodium and potassium reabsorption and promoting diuresis. Excretion of potassium occurs concurrently.
- *Countercurrent multiplier mechanism:* Fluid flows in opposite directions within the loop of Henle, with water reabsorption occurring in the thin descending loop and sodium reabsorption (and other ions) occurring in the thick ascending loop. This, along with other factors, contributes to the increased osmolarity within the medullary interstitial fluid, affecting the countercurrent multiplier. Major factors include the following:
  - Active sodium ion transport, along with potassium, chloride, magnesium, and calcium ion cotransport, out of the thick ascending loop of Henle
  - Active transport of ions from the collecting ducts into the interstitial medullary areas of the kidney

        - Urea-facilitated diffusion from the collecting ducts into the medullary interstitium
        - The vasa recta capillary system surrounds the loop of Henle and augments the countercurrent mechanism by maintaining the osmotic gradient without washing out the solutes that are being reabsorbed.
- Loop of Henle secretion
    - Minimal amounts of hydrogen are secreted in the thick ascending loop of Henle via the sodium-hydrogen countertransport mechanism, which facilitates sodium reabsorption and hydrogen secretion.
- Distal tubule reabsorption
    - The initial segment of the distal tubule forms the macula densa, which is a specialized group of cells that help regulate kidney function.
        - They function by sensing sodium-chloride (NaCl) concentration in the tubular fluid and influence both GFR and renin release from the juxtaglomerular cells.
        - When NaCl levels are low, the macula densa signals the juxtaglomerular cells to release renin, initiating the RAAS to increase BP and sodium reabsorption.
        - Macula densa cells of the distal tubule are located next to the glomeruli and afferent arterioles, forming the juxtaglomerular apparatus. These cells help modulate afferent arteriole dilation or constriction, allowing adjustments of GFR.
    - After the macula densa is a convoluted portion of the distal tubule that functions similarly to the thick ascending portion of the loop of Henle, allowing the reabsorption of ions (e.g., sodium, chloride, potassium, calcium, magnesium) but not water, causing dilution of renal filtrate.
    - Sodium-chloride cotransporters reabsorb sodium and chloride out of the distal tubular lumen and into the tubular cell. These are the sites where *thiazide diuretics* function to inhibit sodium reabsorption and promote diuresis.
    - The late distal tubule contains two primary cell types known as *principal cells* and *intercalated cells*.
    - Principal cells function to reabsorb sodium and water from the tubular lumen.
        - Reabsorption of sodium and secretion of potassium are dependent on the function of the Na^+-K^+ ATPase pump on the basolateral (interstitial fluid side) of the principal cell's membrane. It pumps sodium out of the cell into the interstitial fluid and potassium into the cell from the interstitial fluid (potassium is then secreted into the tubular lumen).
        - *Aldosterone* exerts its action on principal cell mineralocorticoid receptors to increase the reabsorption of sodium (and water) and the secretion/excretion of potassium.
        - Potassium-sparing diuretics such as sodium channel blockers and aldosterone antagonists (e.g., amiloride, triamterene, spironolactone, eplerenone) act on principal cells to inhibit sodium reabsorption and potassium secretion, effectively decreasing excreted potassium.
        - ADH (also known as *vasopressin*) acts on the distal tubule (and collecting tubule/duct) by binding to V2 receptors on the basolateral (interstitial fluid side) membrane of principal cells. This activates a cAMP-mediated signaling pathway that leads to the insertion of AQP2 channels into the apical membrane. AQP2 channels increase water reabsorption, concentrating urine and reducing water excretion.
    - Intercalated cells within the later segments of the distal tubule and collecting tubule/duct play a major role in the regulation of acid–base balance.
        - Type A intercalated cells are very effective at reabsorbing potassium and bicarbonate from the tubular lumen in acidotic states. Potassium is reabsorbed via the hydrogen-potassium-ATPase transporter, and bicarbonate is reabsorbed via a chloride-bicarbonate countertransporter on the renal interstitial fluid side of the cell.
        - Type B intercalated cells function opposite to type A intercalated cells and reabsorb hydrogen ions from the tubular lumen in alkalotic states.
- Distal tubule secretion
    - Principal cells secrete potassium into the tubular lumen.
    - Type A intercalated cells secrete hydrogen ions (in acidosis) into the tubular lumen through two transport systems: (1) hydrogen-ATPase transporter and (2) hydrogen-potassium-ATPase transporter.
    - Type B intercalated cells secrete bicarbonate into the tubular lumen during alkalosis via a

chloride-bicarbonate countertransporter called *pendrin*; this is different from the countertransport system on type A cells.

- Cortical collecting tubule and medullary collecting duct reabsorption
  - The initial portions of the collecting segments of the nephron exist within the cortical segments of the kidney and are referred to as the *cortical collecting tubules*.
  - The cortical collecting tubule has the same receptors as the later segments of the distal tubule and has similar functions.
  - Aldosterone exerts significant action on principal cells within the cortical collecting tubules, causing the reabsorption of sodium and secretion of potassium.
  - Intercalated cells make up 30%–40% of the cells in the collecting tubules and ducts.
    - Type A intercalated cells are very effective at reabsorbing potassium and bicarbonate from the tubular lumen during acidosis. The transport of these ions is the same as in the distal tubule.
    - Type B intercalated cells reabsorb hydrogen ions from the tubular lumen during alkalosis.
  - The concentration of urine is majorly influenced by the amount of ADH present within the collecting tubule/duct.
    - Vasopressin (ADH) acts on the collecting tubule/duct (and distal tubule) by binding to V2 receptors, which ultimately opens AQP2 channels to increase water reabsorption and improve intravascular volume while at the same time concentrating urine.
    - Lower amounts of ADH reduce the cellular membrane permeability to water, reducing its reabsorption and causing more dilute urine.
  - The medullary collecting ducts allow for the reabsorption of urea via special urea transporters that facilitate urea being reabsorbed into the medullary interstitium, which increases the osmolality and assists in the kidney's ability to concentrate urine.
- Cortical collecting tubule and medullary collecting duct secretion
  - In the collecting tubules, principal cells secrete potassium into the tubular lumen.
  - In the cortical collecting tubules, type B intercalated cells secrete bicarbonate into the tubular lumen during alkalosis.
  - In the cortical collecting tubules and medullary collecting ducts, type A intercalated cells have the ability to secrete hydrogen ions against large concentration gradients during acidosis.

Renal Excretion

- Urine excretion is the final step in urine formation and is the sum of glomerular filtration, tubular reabsorption, and tubular secretion within the nephron.
- Tubular filtrate that passes from the collecting ducts and into the renal papillae, then into the minor and major calyces, and finally into the renal pelvis is considered urine.
  - Urine then travels through the ureters to the bladder, where it is stored until excretion through the urethra during urination.

KNOWLEDGE CHECK

1. What percentage of sodium, water, chloride, potassium, and bicarbonate is reabsorbed in the proximal tubule under normal conditions?
   a. 25%
   b. 50%
   c. 65%
   d. 100%
2. Which transport system is primarily responsible for sodium reabsorption in the thick ascending limb of the loop of Henle?
   a. Sodium–potassium ATPase pump
   b. Sodium-chloride cotransporter
   c. Sodium-hydrogen countertransporter
   d. NKCC2
3. Loop diuretics, such as furosemide, inhibit which of the following transporters, leading to increased diuresis?
   a. Sodium-chloride cotransporter
   b. Sodium-glucose cotransporter
   c. NKCC2
   d. Hydrogen-potassium-ATPase transporter
4. Which distal tubule cell type and collecting tubule cell type is primarily responsible for sodium and water reabsorption?
   a. Type A intercalated cells
   b. Type B intercalated cells
   c. Principal cells
   d. Juxtaglomerular cells

Continued

KNOWLEDGE CHECK—cont'd

5. What effect does ADH have on the distal tubule and collecting tubule/duct?
   a. Inhibits sodium reabsorption, which promotes both sodium and water elimination
   b. Affects AQP2 channels, resulting in increased water reabsorption
   c. Enhances the secretion of potassium into the tubular lumen for excretion
   d. Decreases bicarbonate reabsorption via intercalated cells
6. Which nephron structure is responsible for sensing sodium-chloride (NaCl) concentration and regulating renin release?
   a. Juxtaglomerular cells
   b. Macula densa
   c. Principal cells
   d. Vasa recta
7. What is the primary function of type A intercalated cells?
   a. Reabsorption of hydrogen ions during alkalosis
   b. Secretion of potassium into the tubular lumen when hyperkalemia is present
   c. Reabsorption of bicarbonate and potassium during acidosis
   d. Facilitation of sodium reabsorption through aldosterone stimulation

Answers can be found in Appendix A.

Alternative Functions of the Kidneys

- The kidney also provides functions other than the formation of urine; regulation of fluid and electrolyte balance; and excretion of metabolic waste, drugs, and hormone metabolites. These alternative functions include the following:
  - *Gluconeogenesis*: The kidneys have the ability to synthesize glucose from amino acids during periods of prolonged fasting, similar to hepatic responses. This process is disrupted during CKD or acute kidney failure.
  - *Regulation of ABP*: The kidneys affect ABP via the reabsorption of sodium and water, as well as the secretion of hormones (e.g., renin) that lead to the formation of vasoactive substances (e.g., angiotensin II).
  - *Regulation of acid–base balance*: In combination with the lungs and body fluid buffers, the kidneys help maintain appropriate acid–base balance. Renal tubular reabsorption and secretion/excretion of hydrogen ions and bicarbonate ions are influenced by either acidosis or alkalosis. Finally, some acids (e.g., sulfuric acid, phosphoric acid) generated by the metabolism of certain proteins can be eliminated only by the kidneys.
  - *Regulation of erythrocyte production*: The kidneys normally secrete all of the erythropoietin needed for RBC production. Erythropoietin acts on hematopoietic stem cells in the bone marrow to stimulate the production of RBCs. Hypoxia stimulates an increased release of erythropoietin. CKD reduces the amount of erythropoietin produced by the kidney, resulting in anemia.
  - *Regulation of 1,25-dihydroxyvitamin D_3 (calcitriol) production*: Calcitriol is the active form of vitamin D (also known as *1,25-dihydroxyvitamin D_3*). It plays an important role in regulating calcium and phosphate metabolism. Calcitriol also influences calcium deposition within bones and calcium reabsorption by the gastrointestinal tract.

KNOWLEDGE CHECK

1. Which process is similar to hepatic functions during periods of prolonged fasting?
   a. Regulation of ABP
   b. Regulation of erythrocyte production
   c. Gluconeogenesis
   d. Regulation of acid–base balance
2. What is the most effective way the kidneys contribute to the regulation of ABP?
   a. Secretion of erythropoietin to stimulate RBC production
   b. Secretion of renin to form vasoactive substances like angiotensin II
   c. Synthesis of glucose from amino acids during fasting
   d. Elimination of sulfuric acid and phosphoric acid from protein metabolism
3. What is the primary role of erythropoietin secreted by the kidneys?
   a. Regulation of calcium and phosphate metabolism
   b. Stimulation of hematopoietic stem cells to produce RBCs
   c. Regulation of acid–base balance by excreting hydrogen ions
   d. Enhancement of sodium and water reabsorption to regulate BP

Answers can be found in Appendix A.

Renal Pathophysiologic Concepts

Acute Kidney Injury

- *AKI* is a sudden decline in kidney function that results in impaired filtration and excretion of waste products. It can develop over hours to days and is typically reversible if treated quickly. It most commonly occurs in hospitalized patients in the ICU.
  - *Acute renal failure* was a term previously used to describe AKI, but this term is now reserved for the most severe cases of AKI in which the kidneys abruptly cease to function, necessitating dialysis.
  - Causes of AKI are classified into prerenal AKI, intrarenal AKI, and postrenal AKI (Table 3.49).
    - *Prerenal AKI* is caused by a decreased amount of blood flow to the kidney, resulting in activation of the RAAS and causing sodium and water retention. Prolonged hypoperfusion producing ischemia results in renal tubular cellular hypoxia that can progress to intrarenal AKI if not promptly corrected.
    - Potential causes could include hypovolemia, hypotension, renal artery disease, or some medications that decrease renal blood flow.
    - *Intrarenal (or intrinsic) AKI* is caused by direct kidney damage.
    - Examples include acute tubular necrosis, glomerulonephritis, acute interstitial nephritis, and some vascular problems.
    - Acute tubular necrosis is destruction of the renal tubular epithelial cells and is the most common cause of intrarenal AKI. Common causes are the result of (1) inadequate oxygen supply to the epithelial cells, causing cellular ischemia, or (2) toxins, poisons, or medications that damage and destroy the epithelial cells.
    - *Postrenal AKI* results from an obstruction to urine flow, causing increased renal tubular pressure, dysfunction, and a decrease in GFR.
    - Possible causes include kidney stones, benign prostatic hyperplasia, prostate cancer, urethral stricture, neurogenic bladder, and tumors.
- *Signs and symptoms* of acute AKI include overall fatigue and weakness, confusion (due to uremia),

TABLE 3.49 Potential Causes of Acute Kidney Injury (AKI)

Type of AKI	Causes	Examples
Prerenal AKI (decreased blood flow to kidneys)	Hypovolemia	Dehydration, hemorrhage, excessive vomiting/diarrhea, burns
	Hypotension	Heart failure, sepsis, shock
	Renal artery disease	Renal artery stenosis, embolism
	Medications	NSAIDs, ACE inhibitors, ARBs (reduce glomerular perfusion)
Intrarenal AKI (direct kidney damage)	Acute tubular necrosis (ATN)	Hypoperfusion ischemic injury, nephrotoxic drugs or toxins (aminoglycosides, some chemotherapeutic agents such as cisplatin, contrast dye), myoglobin from rhabdomyolysis
	Glomerulonephritis	Poststreptococcal glomerulonephritis, lupus nephritis
	Acute interstitial nephritis (AIN)	Drug-induced (antibiotics, NSAIDs, PPIs, diuretics such as furosemide or thiazides, some chemotherapeutic agents), infections, autoimmune diseases, heavy metal toxic exposure (lead, mercury)
	Vascular causes	Thrombotic microangiopathy (HUS, TTP, DIC), malignant hypertension
Postrenal AKI (obstruction of urine flow)	Urinary tract obstruction	Kidney stones, ureteral strictures
	Bladder outlet obstruction	Benign prostatic hyperplasia, prostate cancer
	Neurogenic bladder	Spinal cord injury, multiple sclerosis, diabetes
	Tumors or masses	Bladder cancer, pelvic tumors, retroperitoneal fibrosis

ACE, Angiotensin-converting enzyme; *ARB*, angiotensin receptor blockers; *DIC*, disseminated intravascular coagulation; *HUS*, hemolytic uremic syndrome; *NSAIDs*, nonsteroidal antiinflammatory drugs; *PPIs*, proton pump inhibitors; *TTP*, thrombotic thrombocytopenic purpura.

urinary changes, fluid overload, electrolyte imbalances, and uremic symptoms.

- Urinary changes can result in oliguria (<400 mL/day), anuria (<100 mL/day), or polyuria (during the recovery phase).
  - Urine output of less than 0.5 mL/kg/hour for greater than 6 hours with a precipitating cause within the last 7 days is a criterion for AKI.
- Rise in serum creatinine of 0.3 mg/dL or a serum creatinine increase of 1.5 times baseline—creatinine levels may not begin to rise until GFR has decreased by half in AKI.
- Decrease in GFR by 50% or greater
- Evidence of fluid overload, including edema, hypertension, dyspnea, and/or pulmonary crackles
- Electrolyte imbalances can be lethal and may include hyperkalemia (fatigue and weakness, arrhythmias, cardiac arrest), metabolic acidosis (low serum pH, Kussmaul breathing, tachycardia, hypotension), hyponatremia (fatigue, confusion, seizures), and/or hyperphosphatemia and hypocalcemia (muscle cramps, tetany, arrhythmias, hypotension).
  - Hyperkalemia can cause peaked T waves, widened QRS complexes, and a disappearance of the P wave. These ECG changes can be an early warning of hyperkalemia and signal the potential for life-threatening arrhythmias. Arrhythmias associated with severe hyperkalemia include VF, VT, asystole, and/or complete heart block.
- Uremic symptoms include nausea, vomiting, pruritus, and pericarditis (in severe cases).

- Prevention of AKI is the most successful management strategy.
- Addressing and correcting potential prerenal, intrarenal, and postrenal risk factors; correcting electrolyte and fluid abnormalities; and maintaining adequate renal perfusion are the most effective approaches to the treatment of AKI (Table 3.50).
  - It is important to note that AKI can be reversed if the cause is identified and reversed before cellular hypoxia occurs.
  - The kidneys can briefly tolerate reductions in perfusion as long as renal blood flow does not fall below 25% of normal.
  - General management strategies include improving intravascular fluid status (e.g., correction of hypovolemia and fluid overload), restoring appropriate electrolyte (e.g., hyperkalemia, hypocalcemia, hyperphosphatemia) and acid–base balances, and avoidance of nephrotoxic medications or other substances.
  - Renal replacement therapy using dialysis may be necessary depending on the severity of AKI.
  - The mnemonic *AEIOU* identifies indications for dialysis in AKI: acidosis, electrolyte abnormalities (especially hyperkalemia), ingestion/intoxication, overload of fluid, and uremia.
    - A—Acidosis: Severe metabolic acidosis (pH <7.1) that is refractory to medical management
    - E—Electrolyte Abnormalities: Primarily hyperkalemia (potassium levels >6.5 mEq/L) that is refractory to medical treatment or rapidly rising potassium levels

TABLE 3.50 Management Strategies for Acute Kidney Injury (AKI)

Type of AKI	Management Strategy
Prerenal AKI (decreased perfusion)	• Restore fluid balance (isotonic IV fluids, blood products) • Treat underlying cause (e.g., stop bleeding, manage sepsis, optimize cardiac function) • Avoid nephrotoxic drugs (NSAIDs, ACE inhibitors, ARBs)
Intrinsic AKI (kidney damage)	Treat specific cause: • Acute tubular necrosis: Maintain perfusion, stop nephrotoxins, dialysis if needed • Acute interstitial nephritis: Stop offending drug, consider corticosteroids • Glomerulonephritis: Immunosuppressive therapy (steroids, cytotoxic drugs)
Postrenal AKI (obstruction)	• Relieve obstruction (e.g., catheterization of bladder for BPH, nephrostomy tube, or other surgical treatments for kidney stones) • Treat underlying cause (e.g., remove tumors, surgery for strictures)

ACE, Angiotensin-converting enzyme; *ARB*, angiotensin receptor blockers; *BPH*, benign prostatic hyperplasia; *IV*, intravenous; *NSAIDs*, nonsteroidal antiinflammatory drugs

- I—Ingestions/Intoxication: Ingestion of substances or toxins that can be removed with dialysis (e.g., salicylates, lithium, isopropanol, methanol, ethylene glycol)
- O—Overload: Severe fluid overload (edema) that is unresponsive to diuretics, especially with signs of heart failure or pulmonary edema
- U—Uremia: Symptomatic uremia, including encephalopathy, pericarditis, neuropathy, bleeding, and intractable nausea/vomiting

- *Anesthetic considerations* in patients with AKI should focus on (1) correction of reversible renal dysfunction, (2) volume administration to achieve euvolemia, (3) optimization of cardiac output, and (4) ongoing assessment of cardiac and renal function throughout the perioperative period.
  - *Preoperative management*: Address any laboratory anomalies such as coagulation deficiencies, acidosis, and/or electrolyte abnormalities (e.g., hyperkalemia).
    - In addition to standard monitors, consider direct arterial line monitoring for BP.
    - Consider the placement of a central venous catheter for the administration of vasopressors, inotropes, and/or rapid fluid administration as indicated.
    - A balanced salt solution such as normal saline or lactated Ringer's should be used to help prevent low serum sodium, aldosterone secretion, and oliguria.
    - A fluid challenge of 500–1000 mL may be indicated if hourly urine output goals fall below acceptable levels.
    - Avoid hydroxyethyl starches.
    - Replace blood loss with blood products if hemorrhage has occurred or anemia is present.
    - Prepare vasopressor and inotropic infusions such as norepinephrine, dopamine, vasopressin, and/or epinephrine.
    - Monitor cardiac and volume status with transesophageal echocardiography, point-of-care ultrasonography (POCUS), and/or goal-directed fluid therapy such as SV variation or pulse pressure variation as indicated.
    - Place a urinary catheter to monitor urine output.
    - Diuretic use to prevent oliguria is not indicated. However, diuretic use in the presence of confirmed volume overload can be considered.
    - Consider dialysis during any part of the perioperative period if indicated using the AEIOU mnemonic.
  - *Induction of anesthesia* should focus on avoiding (1) significant hypotension (e.g., reduced amounts of propofol or consider etomidate) and (2) medications that rely on significant renal excretion.
    - Avoid succinylcholine if potassium level is >5.5 mEq/L or if ECG changes are evident.
    - Use caution with the use of rocuronium because it relies on roughly 30%–40% of renal excretion for clearance and will likely be prolonged in AKI.
  - *Intraoperative management*: The primary focus is maintenance of adequate perfusion to the kidney, with a MAP goal of 70–80 mm Hg.
    - Avoid any nephrotoxic agents (e.g., NSAIDs, aminoglycosides, IV contrast).
    - All volatile anesthetics can be used in patients with AKI, including sevoflurane.
    - Cisatracurium may be considered for neuromuscular blockade because it relies on Hoffman elimination and non–esterase-dependent hydrolysis for cessation of action.
    - Rocuronium may be considered if using sugammadex for reversal, but this complex may have delayed elimination in AKI and may require dialysis for removal.
    - Norepinephrine is preferred over dopamine to increase MAP values when administration of a vasopressor infusion is indicated.
    - Obtain baseline electrolyte values, serum creatinine, hematologic assays, and ABG status as indicated.
    - Prevent hypothermia by providing warm fluids and forced-air warming.
  - *Postoperative management*: Key goals during the postoperative period include pain management; close renal monitoring; continuous monitoring of electrolyte, hematologic, and acid–base status; early mobilization; and nephrology consultation.
    - Pain management may consider regional anesthesia (epidural or peripheral nerve blocks or fascial plane blocks) if feasible. Opioids such as fentanyl or hydromorphone are appropriate, but prolonged duration should be considered. Morphine should be avoided because of its

metabolites and prolonged duration of action. Acetaminophen is safe. Avoid NSAIDs.
- Monitor renal function tests and ensure strict fluid balance monitoring.
- Early mobilization reduces the risks of thromboembolism and pneumonia.
- Nephrology consultation is indicated if worsening renal function or need for dialysis arises.

Chronic Kidney Disease

- *CKD* is the progressive decline in kidney function over months or years, often as a result of underlying systemic diseases or direct injury to the kidneys. It is described as kidney damage or decreased kidney function (e.g., GFR of less than 60 mL/min/1.73 m^2) persisting for 3 months or more and is characterized by the progressive and irreversible loss of nephrons and nephron function.
  - When CKD is severe enough to require dialysis or renal transplantation it is termed *end-stage renal disease (ESRD)*.
  - Causes of CKD can result from dysfunction or disorders of renal blood vessels, glomeruli, renal tubules, renal interstitium, and/or the lower urinary tract (Table 3.51).
    - DM and hypertension are the most common causes of CKD that result in ESRD.
- *Signs and symptoms* of CKD manifest in multiple body systems and include problems with (1) overall fatigue and weakness, (2) the renal system, (3) metabolic management, (4) the cardiovascular system, (5) the neurological system, (6) the gastrointestinal system, (7) the musculoskeletal system, and (8) the integumentary system (Table 3.52).
  - Several laboratory values in CKD will be altered. Those values that are elevated include potassium, magnesium, creatinine, blood urea nitrogen (BUN), phosphorus, parathyroid, cystatin C, and anion gap (acidosis). Those that are decreased include calcium, sodium (in late stages), GFR, hemoglobin, hematocrit, bicarbonate, and albumin (Table 3.53).
  - Ultrasound evaluation of the kidneys that suggests a chronic problem may demonstrate smaller-than-normal kidneys with reduced cortical thickness, increased echogenicity, scarring, and/or multiple cysts.
  - CT can also be used to evaluate kidney size, echogenicity, the collecting duct system, and any possible obstruction.
  - Renal angiography assists with the diagnosis of renal vascular problems such as systemic vasculitis or renal artery stenosis.
- *Treatment and management* of CKD initially focus on slowing the progression of the disease, followed by strategies that manage complications and prepare for advanced disease.
  - Slowing the progression of CKD can be accomplished by incorporating lifestyle modifications, as well as BP and glycemic control.

TABLE 3.51 Potential Causes of Chronic Kidney Disease With Associated Pathophysiology

Cause	Pathophysiology
Diabetes mellitus	Chronic high blood sugar damages kidney glomeruli and causes renal inflammation, resulting in glomerular sclerosis, proteinuria, and renal fibrosis.
Hypertension	High blood pressure damages renal arteries, causing nephrosclerosis, ischemia, and reduced glomerular filtration.
Glomerulonephritis	Inflammation of kidney glomeruli causes scarring and loss of nephron function.
Polycystic kidney disease	Genetic disorder results in fluid-filled cysts within the kidneys that replace normal tissue, resulting in reduced kidney function.
Obstructive uropathy	Chronic blockage (e.g., kidney stones, enlarged prostate, urethral constriction) causes pressure buildup, hydronephrosis, and nephron damage.
Chronic infections	Recurrent kidney infections (e.g., pyelonephritis, renal tuberculosis) lead to scarring and gradual loss of kidney function.
Autoimmune diseases	Conditions like lupus attack kidney tissue, triggering inflammation and chronic kidney damage.

- Antibiotics are given for cyst infections.
- Cyst decompression may help for severe pain due to large cysts.
- When ESRD develops, dialysis or kidney transplantation is required.

- Anesthesia management is similar to that for patients with advanced kidney disease and ESRD.
  - See the Renal Transplantation section for anesthesia management strategies in those patients receiving a donor kidney.

Renovascular Hypertension

- Renovascular hypertension is a form of secondary hypertension resulting from a narrowing of the renal arteries caused by fibromuscular dysplasia or, more commonly, by atherosclerotic renal artery stenosis. The exact mechanism that causes the systemic hypertension is not fully understood, but it is believed that reduced renal perfusion activates the RAAS.
- It is characterized by a sudden and severe onset of hypertension, often in patients less than 30 years of age, and is refractory to multiple antihypertensives.
- An abdominal bruit may be heard over the flanks or epigastrium.
- Headache and dizziness are common symptoms.
- Medical management may consist of ACE inhibitors or ARBs, β-receptor blockers, calcium channel blockers, diuretics, statins, and/or lifestyle modifications (e.g., cessation of smoking, weight loss).
- Revascularization therapy may be indicated and consists of percutaneous transluminal angioplasty with stent placement or renal artery endarterectomy.
- Nephrectomy may be indicated in some cases.
- Anesthesia management should primarily focus on BP optimization to avoid a hypertensive crisis.
  - An arterial line should be placed, and vascular access should support the use of both vasopressors and vasodilators to account for perioperative BP variations.
  - The overall perioperative management is similar to that for both AKI and CKD.

Benign Prostatic Hyperplasia

- Benign prostatic hyperplasia (BPH) is a nonmalignant enlargement of the prostate gland due to hyperplasia of prostatic stromal and epithelial cells. It is a common condition in aging males (>50 years) and leads to compression of the urethral canal and alterations of normal urine flow.
- Bladder outlet obstruction and irritative voiding symptoms due to an enlarged prostate can cause obstructive symptoms (e.g., weak urinary stream, intermittency, incomplete bladder emptying) and irritative symptoms (e.g., increased frequency, urgency, nocturia, incontinence).
- Pharmacologic therapy includes α_1 blockers (e.g., tamsulosin, doxazosin), 5-alpha reductase inhibitors (e.g., finasteride, dutasteride), or a combination of these to relax prostate smooth muscle and reduce prostate size.
  - Anticholinergics or β_3 agonists (e.g., mirabegron) may be prescribed for irritative symptoms.
- Surgical treatments include transurethral resection of the prostate (TURP), transurethral laser therapy, or prostatectomy.
- Anesthesia management for prostate resection or removal uses either neuraxial or general anesthesia techniques.
  - Spinal anesthesia is preferred for TURP (allows for assessment of neurologic status and signs of TURP syndrome).
  - General anesthesia with neuromuscular blockade is needed for laparoscopic or open prostatectomies.
  - TURP involves bladder irrigation, which can lead to TURP syndrome (hyponatremia due to absorption of irrigation fluid).
  - Monitor for fluid overload and electrolyte imbalances.
  - α-Blockers used for BPH can cause hypotension under anesthesia.
  - Monitor for blood loss, especially during an open prostatectomy.
  - Temporary catheterization is often needed postoperatively.

KNOWLEDGE CHECK

1. Which is a common cause of secondary glomerulonephritis?
   a. Membranous nephropathy
   b. Poststreptococcal infection
   c. Minimal change disease
   d. Focal segmental glomerulosclerosis

2. Which clinical finding is most characteristic of nephrotic syndrome?
   a. Proteinuria
   b. Hematuria
   c. Hyperlipidemia
   d. Hypoalbuminemia

Continued

KNOWLEDGE CHECK—cont'd

3. Which type of kidney stone is most commonly associated with renal nephrolithiasis?
   a. Uric acid
   b. Magnesium ammonium phosphate
   c. Calcium oxalate
   d. Cystine
4. PKD is often associated with which extrarenal manifestation?
   a. Hepatic cysts
   b. Pulmonary fibrosis
   c. Retinal detachment
   d. Hypothyroidism
5. Which clinical sign is associated with renovascular hypertension?
   a. Proteinuria
   b. Bilateral flank pain
   c. Abdominal bruit
   d. Hematuria
6. Which medication is commonly used to promote prostate smooth muscle relaxation in BPH?
   a. Finasteride
   b. Dutasteride
   c. Tamsulosin
   d. Spironolactone
7. Which anesthesia technique is preferred for TURP?
   a. General anesthesia
   b. Spinal anesthesia
   c. Epidural anesthesia
   d. Local anesthesia
8. Which complication is most commonly associated with TURP syndrome?
   a. Hyperkalemia
   b. Hypotension
   c. Metabolic acidosis
   d. Hyponatremia

Answers can be found in Appendix A.

THERMOREGULATION

Mechanism of Heat Exchange

- The rate of heat transfer is related to the temperature difference (Fig. 3.49).

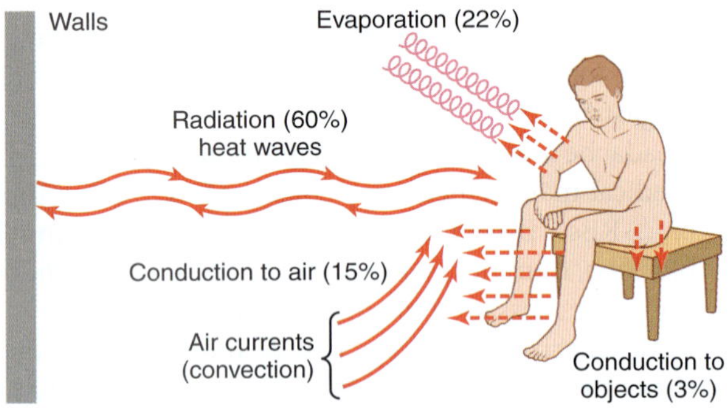

Fig. 3.49 Mechanisms of heat loss from the body. (From Hall JE. *Guyton and Hall Textbook of Medical Physiology*. 3rd ed. Elsevier; 2016.)

Conduction

- Loss/gain of heat from movement of heat from *surface to surface*
- Molecules at the surface of the skin or other exposed surfaces are transmitted to molecules of the medium adjacent to the skin.
- *Example:* Heat is lost from the patient's body when in contact with the colder operating table.

Convection

- Loss/gain of heat from movement of *air over a surface.*
- Air that is warmed by exposure to the surface of the body rises and is replaced by colder air from the environment.
- *Example:* Heat is lost from the patient's body to the colder air in the operating room.

Radiation

- All objects that have a temperature above absolute zero produce electromagnetic radiation. Therefore *if the temperature of an object is less than the temperature of the body, then there is a net loss of heat from the body to the environment through electromagnetic radiation.*
- *Example:* Most forced-air warming blankets have a metallic surface that reflects radiant heat given off by the patient back to the patient's body.
- Radiation heat loss represents the greatest mechanism of heat loss from the body, approximately 60%.

Evaporation

- Loss/gain of heat *from contact between the vapor temperature of the body and the environment*

TABLE 3.55 Methods of Monitoring Body Temperature

Temperature Site	Method of Placement	Advantages	Disadvantages
Axillary	High in axilla with arm adducted	Ease of insertion, noninvasive	Easily dislodged, trend monitor, influenced by intravenous fluid temperature
Rectal	Well lubricated past rectal sphincter	Ease of insertion	Bleeding, influenced by peritoneal/bladder cooling
Nasopharyngeal	Insert to depth between nares and auditory canal	Ease of insertion, accurate core temperature	Epistaxis
Esophageal	Insert to depth two-thirds the length of the esophagus	Ease of insertion, accurate core temperature	Esophageal perforation
Tympanic	Insert into external auditory meatus	Most accurate core temperature	Contraindicated with otitis media, damage to tympanic membrane
Skin	Place liquid crystal strip on forehead	Ease of placement	Trend monitor only

BOX 3.21 Methods to Prevent Hypothermia

- Increasing operating room temperature
- Heating blankets
- Radiant heat lights
- Heated fluids and irrigation
- Covering the patient's head
- Heated and humidified fresh gas
- Low total fresh gas flows

- Occurs through the skin and the lungs
- Accounts for 22% of total body heat loss (Table 3.55)
- Evaporation is intensified with higher-liter flows and occurs with cool, dry anesthetic gases.
- Humidified moisture exchangers provide 30% humidification, but after 1.5 hours of use, they become less effective than a heated humidified circuit.
- *Example:* Heat is lost during mechanical ventilation as fresh gas flows from the anesthesia machine into the lungs. Radiation is the mechanism by which the greatest amount of heat is lost from a patient to the environment.

Preventing Hypothermia

- The most effective method used to maintain normothermia is to warm the operating room.
- The most effective method of rewarming a patient who has become hypothermic is via forced -air rewarming (Box 3.21).

KNOWLEDGE CHECK

1. Which mechanism of heat loss is described as movement of heat between two surfaces?
   a. Conduction
   b. Convection
   c. Evaporation
   d. Radiation
2. Which mechanism accounts for the greatest amount of heat loss during surgery and anesthesia?
   a. Conduction
   b. Convection
   c. Evaporation
   d. Radiation
3. Which is the most effective method of rewarming a patient who has become hypothermic in the operating room?
   a. Warning IV fluids
   b. Warming the operating room
   c. Forced-air warming
   d. Decreasing fresh gas flow

Answers can be found in Appendix A.

Malignant Hyperthermia

Etiology

- MH is a rare metabolic disorder that is caused by *ryanodine receptor type 1* sensitization.
- MH susceptibility is caused by a genetically inherited trait (autosomal dominant gene).
- Anesthetic medications that are implicated as triggering agents for MH include inhalational agents and succinylcholine.

- Rapid physiologic deterioration can occur with MH because the patient's temperature can increase 1°C every 5 minutes.
- Each 15-minute delay in treatment increases mortality by 15%.
- Dantrolene sodium administration is the curative pharmacologic agent for MH.
- Preepisodic diagnosis can be made via an associated family history and genetic blood testing. The halothane-caffeine contracture test remains the gold standard for diagnosis.

Physiology/Pathophysiology

MH is a hypermetabolic disorder that is caused by uncontrolled and sustained full-body muscle contractions. Within a myocyte, the sarcoplasmic reticulum (SR) sequesters and then releases calcium as a part of normal muscle contraction. During normal muscular relaxation, calcium is resequestered into the SR. MH initially occurs as sensitization of ryanodine receptors present on the SR decrease the reabsorption of calcium back into the SR. The remaining calcium is available to interact with skeletal muscle fibers that cause contraction. Sustained muscle contractions dramatically increase the body's requirements for oxygen and cellular energy. Unless treatment occurs, the hypermetabolism associated with MH can result in tissue hypoxia, lactic acidosis, and cardiovascular collapse.

Pathologic conditions that predispose a patient to developing MH include muscular dystrophy. Specific muscular pathophysiologic conditions include King-Denborough syndrome and SR ATP deficiency. Duchenne muscular dystrophy is associated with anesthesia-induced rhabdomyolysis (AIR). The exact mechanism of AIR is poorly understood. Triggering agents, signs, symptoms, and treatment are identical to those for MH.

Signs/Symptoms

- *Tachycardia:* First sign present; however, nonspecific
- *Increased ETco2*: Most sensitive and specific sign
- Exhausted CO_2 absorbent
- Increased temperature
- ABG: Increased $Paco_2$, decreased Pao_2, decreased pH
- Acute hyperkalemia (dysrhythmias) and lactic acidosis
- Mottled and cyanotic skin
- Masseter muscle spasm
- Diaphoresis
- Increased creatinine kinase
- Increased myoglobin
- Myoglobinuria caused by rhabdomyolysis
- DIC
- Renal failure
- Cardiovascular collapse

Note: Although rare, the onset of MH can occur within 24 hours after an anesthetic triggering agent is administered.

Treatment

- Declare an MH emergency; call for additional assistance.
- Discontinue the administration of anesthetic triggering agents (all inhalational agents).
- Ventilate patient with 100% oxygen with "clean" anesthesia machine/circuit and charcoal filters on expiratory and inspiratory limbs.
- Consult with Malignant Hyperthermia Association of the United States (MHAUS; 1-800-MHHYPER [1-800-644-9737]).
- Dantrolene: Administer initial bolus dose of 2.5 mg/kg (total dose may exceed 10 mg/kg) based on actual body weight.
- Dantrolene sodium is the antidote used for the treatment of MH.
- The associated mechanism of action: Decreasing the release and increasing the resequestration of calcium by the SR within the myocyte
- The onset of action of dantrolene is rapid, and abatement of symptoms frequently begins to occur within 6 minutes after administration.
- The initial loading dose of dantrolene is 2.5 mg/kg, which should be based on actual body weight. This recommendation is suggested by MHAUS because dantrolene is highly lipid-soluble.
- Dantrolene can be administered up to a total dose of 30 mg/kg.
- If the continued administration of dantrolene does not produce an improvement in the patient's condition, other causes of extreme hypermetabolism (e.g., thyroid storm, pheochromocytoma) should be considered.
- The primary side effects associated with dantrolene include muscle weakness and hepatic dysfunction.
- Dantrolene sodium is present in a powder form in 20-mg vials (Revonto, Dantrium). It must be

reconstituted with 50 mL of *sterile water* to avoid precipitation.
- *Example:* Initial loading dose 2.5 mg/kg for a 70-kg patient = 175 mg; 175 mg/20 mg per vial = approximately 9 vials (180 mg).
- A newer preparation of dantrolene (Ryanodex) must be reconstituted with 5 mL of sterile water, but each vial contains 250 mg.
- Palliative treatment of hypermetabolism and muscle tissue destruction
  - Cooling measures: Forced air, cool IV fluids, intragastric lavage
  - Treat acidosis: Increase minute ventilation; administer sodium bicarbonate 1–2 mEq/kg.
  - Treat acute hyperkalemia: Calcium chloride 10% (100 mg/mL), 10 mL of regular insulin, 10 units IV combined with 50% dextrose, 50 mL
  - Obtain serial laboratory test results:
    - ABG
    - Electrolytes
    - Coagulation panel
    - Serum/urine myoglobin
- Treatment after acute MH management:
  - Transfer to ICU
  - Dantrolene 1 mg/kg q6h for 24 hours
  - Monitor for the following:
    - Muscle weakness
    - Renal failure
    - DIC
- After the initial treatment and stabilization of MH, patients must continue to be observed for an exacerbation of MH symptoms for 24 hours. To decrease the possibility of a second MH episode, dantrolene is administered 1 mg/kg every 6 hours for 24 hours.

KNOWLEDGE CHECK

1. Which sign is most reliably associated with an acute onset of MH?
   a. Sustained muscle contraction
   b. Tachycardia
   c. Elevated $Paco_2$
   d. Decreased renal function
2. Which medication can trigger an episode of MH?
   a. Sevoflurane
   b. Vecuronium
   c. Fentanyl
   d. Nitrous oxide
3. Which intervention is the curative treatment for MH?
   a. Increasing minute ventilation
   b. Administering dantrolene sodium
   c. Treating hyperkalemia
   d. Instituting cooling measures
4. How many milligrams of dantrolene should be administered for the initial dose in a patient who weighs 78 kg?
   a. 195 mg
   b. 200 mg
   c. 205 mg
   d. 210 mg

Answers can be found in Appendix A.

4

Anesthesia Equipment and Technology

INFECTION CONTROL: DISINFECTION

- The Centers for Disease Control and Prevention (CDC) estimates that over 50 million surgical and invasive procedures are performed in the United States each year. Approximately 1.7 million hospital-acquired infections (HAIs) of all types contribute to 99,000 deaths each year. Surgical site infections are the third most common type of nosocomial infection. The most frequent mode of HAI transmission is by direct contact.

Common Definitions

- *Antimicrobial:* A chemical or material capable of destroying or inhibiting the growth of microorganisms.
- *Antiseptic:* A chemical germicide that has antimicrobial activity and can be safely applied to human tissue. Antiseptics are regulated as drugs.
- *Asepsis:* A scheme or process that prevents contact with microorganisms.
- *Bactericide:* A chemical or compound that kills bacteria.
- *Bacteriostatic:* An agent that will prevent bacterial growth without necessarily killing the bacteria. Bacteriostatic action is reversible; when the agent is removed, bacteria will resume normal growth.
- *Cleaning:* The physical removal of organic and inorganic material from devices and other surfaces. Cleaning is required to prepare for sterilization. It reduces the number of microorganisms and is achieved using detergents and enzymatic products. It requires manual scrubbing to mechanically loosen contaminating material/bioburden and prepares items for safe handling.
- *Decontamination:* A process that renders contaminated inanimate items safe for handling by personnel who are not wearing protective attire. Decontamination can range from simple cleaning to sterilization.
- *Disinfectant:* A chemical germicide that is used on inanimate objects.
- *Disinfection:* A process capable of destroying most microorganisms but normally not bacterial spores. The CDC has adopted a classification that includes three levels of disinfection:
    - *Low-level disinfection:* A procedure that kills most vegetative bacteria but not *Mycobacterium tuberculosis,* as well as some fungi and viruses but not bacterial spores.
    - *Intermediate-level disinfection:* A procedure that kills vegetative bacteria, including *M. tuberculosis,* as well as most fungi and viruses but not bacterial spores.
    - *High-level disinfection:* A procedure that kills all organisms except for bacterial spores and certain species such as Creutzfeldt-Jakob prions.
- *Germicide:* An agent that destroys microorganisms.
- *Nosocomial:* An infection that is acquired in a healthcare facility.
- *Resterilization:* Sterilization of an unopened or wrapped sterile device that is past its expiration date.
- *Standard precautions:* Standards set by the CDC that include universal precautions, airborne precautions, droplet precautions, and contact precautions. Standard precautions apply to all patients, regardless of their diagnosis or infection status.
- *Sterilization:* Process capable of removing or destroying all viable forms of microbial life, including bacterial spores.
- *Universal precautions:* Recommendations by the CDC that healthcare workers use protective barriers and workplace practices to reduce the risk of exposure to blood and other bodily fluids that may contain contagious microorganisms. Universal precautions have been incorporated into standard precautions.

Infection Prevention in the Operating Room and Anesthesia Work Area

- Infection prevention and control policies specific to anesthesia care in the operating room (OR) are not universal in U.S. healthcare facilities.
- Not all anesthesia work areas are cleaned and disinfected between patients, and the anesthesia cart is an item of risk for cross-contamination.
- Certain anesthesia provider practices remain problematic, especially the use of multiple-dose vials for more than one patient, less than 100% use of gloves for airway management, lack of hand hygiene (HH) after removing gloves, and entry into anesthesia cart drawers without HH.
- Facilities should conduct regular monitoring and evaluation of infection prevention practices. To promote adherence, improvement efforts should be collaborative and should include input from frontline anesthesia personnel and local champions. Hospital and physician leadership should identify clear expectations and goals, ensure data transparency, and facilitate use of process measures to improve performance.

Hand Hygiene (HH)

Activities in anesthesia care should always result in hand hygiene. *Recommendation*: Ideally, HH should be performed according to the World Health Organization's My 5 Moments for Hand Hygiene. It is recommended that HH be performed at minimum before aseptic tasks (e.g., inserting central venous catheters [CVCs], inserting arterial catheters, drawing medications, spiking intravenous [IV] bags), after removing gloves, when hands are soiled or contaminated (e.g., oropharyngeal secretions), before touching the contents of the anesthesia cart, and when entering and exiting the OR (even after removing gloves).

Providers should wear double gloves during airway management and discard the outer glove immediately after airway manipulation. *Recommendation*: To reduce risk of contamination in the OR, providers should consider wearing double gloves during airway management and should remove the outer gloves immediately after airway manipulation. As soon as possible, providers should remove the inner gloves and perform HH. It is recommended that facilities locate alcohol-based hand-rub dispensers at the entrance to ORs and near anesthesia providers inside the OR to promote frequent HH.

Environmental Disinfection

Reusable laryngoscopes or video laryngoscopes can be replaced with single-use laryngoscopes/video laryngoscopes. *Recommendation*: Facilities should ensure that standard direct laryngoscope or video laryngoscope reusable handles and blades undergo high-level disinfection (at minimum) or sterilization before use or that reusable laryngoscopes are replaced with single-use standard direct laryngoscopes or video laryngoscopes. Clean blades and handles should be stored in packaging appropriate for semicritical items designated for "high-level" disinfection.

Cleaning and disinfection of the anesthesia machine and anesthesia work areas. *Recommendation*: To reduce the bioburden of organisms and the risk of transmitting these organisms to patients, the facility should ensure the cleaning and disinfection of high-touch surfaces on the anesthesia machine and anesthesia work area between OR uses. A hospital disinfectant approved by the Environmental Protection Agency and compatible with the equipment and surfaces based on the manufacturer's instructions should be used. Because of challenges in consistent cleaning and disinfection of the anesthesia machine and anesthesia work area between cases, priority should be given to high-touch surfaces.

Provider Clinical Practices

Injection ports used by anesthesia providers in the OR should be disinfected before use. *Recommendation*: Anesthesia providers should only use disinfected ports for IV access. Ports may be disinfected either by scrubbing the port with a sterile alcohol-based disinfectant immediately before each use or by using sterile isopropyl alcohol–containing caps that cover ports continuously. Before use, isopropyl alcohol–containing caps should cover the port for the minimum time recommended by the manufacturer. Ports should be properly disinfected before each individual drug injection or at the beginning of a rapid succession of injections, such as during induction of anesthesia. It is suggested that providers consider using isopropyl alcohol. Stopcocks should have closed injection ports installed to convert them into "closed ports," or they should be covered with sterile caps. Anesthesia providers should wipe medication vials' rubber stoppers and the necks of ampules with 70% alcohol before vial access and medication withdrawal.

General Care Principles

Intravenous and interarterial catheters should be placed with full barrier precautions. *Recommendation*: All CVCs and axillary and femoral arterial lines should be placed with full maximal sterile barrier precautions. Full maximal sterile barrier precautions include wearing a mask, cap, sterile gown, and sterile gloves and using a large sterile drape during insertion. Peripheral arterial lines (e.g., radial, brachial, or dorsalis pedis arterial lines) should be placed with a minimum of a cap, mask, sterile gloves, and a small sterile fenestrated drape.

Anesthesia providers should always recap a medication syringe after giving a portion of the syringe contents to the patient if the syringe and medication may be used again on the same patient. *Recommendation*: To reduce the risk of bacterial contamination of the syringe and syringe contents, it is recommended that anesthesia providers cap needleless syringes that will be used to administer multiple doses of a drug to the same patient after each administered dose. Needleless syringes should be capped with a sterile cap that completely covers the Luer connector on the syringe.

The anesthesia supply cart should be cleaned between cases. *Recommendation*: The anesthesia supply cart should have its accessible outer surfaces wiped clean between cases. To prevent contamination of communal supplies, anesthesia providers should always perform HH before opening the drawers or bins of the cart and handling the contents of the drawers or bins. Storing supplies on the top surface of the cart should be avoided as much as possible, and any supply items on the cart's top surface should be removed between cases to facilitate cleaning. The interior surfaces of the supply cart should be cleaned periodically.

Anesthesia providers should be aware of expiration times for sterile injectable medications and intravenous solutions. *Recommendation (sterile injectable medications):* Provider-prepared sterile injectable medications, such as a medication drawn from a vial into a syringe, are more likely to be subject to contamination than medications prepared in a pharmacy. Therefore, provider-prepared sterile injectable medications should be used as soon as practicable after preparation. Because propofol contains a preservative, the package insert typically specifies that the use of propofol should commence within 12 hours of preparation. The *United States Pharmacopeia* suggests that a medication withdrawn from a single-dose vial may be used until the end of a case.

Recommendation (intravenous solutions): Anesthesia practitioners should minimize the time between spiking intravenous solution bags and patient administration; nevertheless, certain emergent or urgent circumstances may require advance setup of IV fluids, and anesthesia providers should comply with their hospital protocols.

Syringes and medication vials should not be reused on multiple patients. *Recommendation*: Single-dose medication vials and flushes should be used whenever possible. If multiple-dose medication vials must be used, they should be used for only one patient and should only be accessed with a new sterile syringe and new sterile needle for each entry. Syringes and needles are single-patient devices, and syringes should never be reused for another patient, even if the needle is changed.

Keyboards and touchscreens in the anesthesia work area should be cleaned and protected from contamination. *Recommendation:* Facilities should require cleaning and disinfection of computer keyboards and touchscreen computer monitors after each anesthesia case using a hospital-approved disinfectant consistent with manufacturers' recommendations. Additionally, cleaning and disinfection should also occur every time there is obvious soiling or contamination of anesthesia work surfaces. Facilities should consider use of commercial plastic keyboard shields, sealed medical keyboards, or washable keyboards and touchscreens to facilitate thorough disinfection.

KNOWLEDGE CHECK

1. Which of the following levels of disinfection is the minimum required to eliminate *M. tuberculosis* from anesthesia equipment surfaces?
   a. Low-level disinfection
   b. Intermediate-level disinfection
   c. High-level disinfection
   d. Sterilization
2. What is the most frequent mode of transmission for hospital-acquired infections?
   a. Airborne particles
   b. Droplet transmission
   c. Direct contact
   d. Contaminated food or water
3. According to recommended practices, when should anesthesia providers perform hand hygiene in the OR?
   a. Only after airway manipulation
   b. Before aseptic tasks and after removing gloves
   c. Once per case, before induction
   d. Only if visible contamination is present

Answers can be found in Appendix A.

MONITORING MODALITIES

Cardiovascular System Monitoring

- Fundamental monitoring/assessment techniques include inspection (visual examination), auscultation, and palpation.
- *Inspection* of the patient can provide information regarding the adequacy of oxygen delivery and carbon dioxide elimination, fluid requirements, and positioning and alignment of body structures.
- *Auscultation* is used to verify correct placement of airway devices such as an endotracheal tube (ETT) or laryngeal mask airway, to assess arterial blood pressure (BP), and to continually monitor heart sounds and air exchange throughout the pulmonary system.
- *Palpation* can aid the anesthetist in assessing the quality of the pulse and degree of skeletal muscle relaxation, as well as locating major landmarks when placing arterial lines or performing regional anesthesia techniques.

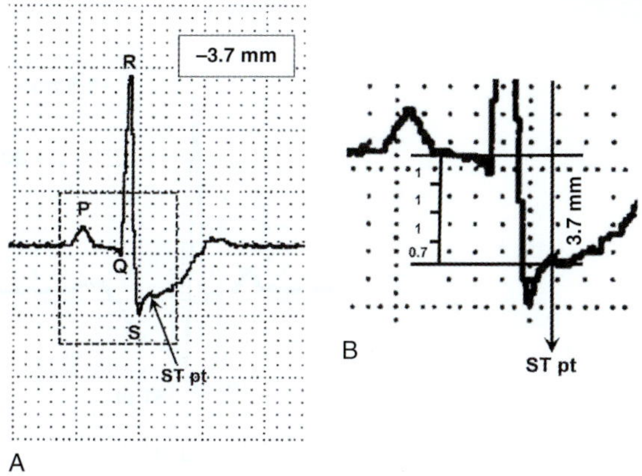

Fig. 4.1 A single cardiac cycle (ST snippet) and enlarged section of the snippet providing greater details. The PR segment is measured from the end of the P wave to the beginning of the QRS complex. (A) A depressed ST segment that is upsloping. The ST junction is synonymous with the J point, and the ST segment defines the ST point. (B) The PR segment is extended out via a horizontal line. This serves as an isoelectric reference (no deviation of the electrocardiogram stylus upward or downward) to determine the degree of ST-segment shift. The distance from the extended PR segment to the ST point demonstrates that the ST segment is depressed 3.7 mm (i.e., J-point depression of 3.7 mm). (Reprinted with permission from Kossick MA. *EKG Interpretation: Simple, Thorough, Practical.* 2nd ed. AANA Publishing; 1999.)

Electrocardiographic Monitoring

- Recommendations for ST-segment deviation thresholds account for gender, electrocardiogram (ECG) lead, age, and ethnicity on position of the ST segment.
- Leads V_2 and V_3 have been shown to exhibit the greatest shift of the ST junction (e.g., J point) and must be accounted for when applying diagnostic criteria for myocardial injury.
- The degree of ST-segment elevation (or depression) is relative to an isoelectric line that is commonly referenced as the *PR segment.* The PR segment extends from the end of the P wave to the start of ventricular depolarization (e.g., appearance of a Q wave) (Fig. 4.1).
- The ST junction is defined as the location where the QRS complex ends and the ST segment begins. It is also synonymous with the J point (Fig. 4.2).
- Recommended threshold values for ST-segment elevation are listed in Table 4.1. For ST-segment depression, the threshold values are -0.5 mm (-0.05 mV) for males and females of all ages in ECG leads V_2 and V_3 and -1.0 mm (-0.1 mV) in all other ECG leads.
- Caution should be exercised when considering numerical ST-segment deviation values. Shortened ST segments are predictably associated with tachyarrhythmias, which can result in T waves that encroach on ST segments.
- In this circumstance, the computer-derived ST-segment deviation value would reflect either (1) a falsely elevated ST segment, suggesting myocardial injury (false-positive result), or (2) the masking of a significant ST-segment depression (false-negative result) (Fig. 4.3).
- Regarding the significance of the various forms of ST-segment depression, it is important to recall that a horizontal or downward-sloping depressed ST segment has greater specificity (fewer false-positive results) than an upward-sloping depressed ST segment.
- It is more challenging to identify the regions of the myocardium affected by the appearance of ST-segment depression versus elevation.

Electrocardiographic electrode placement

- In patients with risk factors for coronary artery disease (CAD), incorrect lead placement may cause high false positives (overdiagnosis) or false negatives (underdiagnosis).

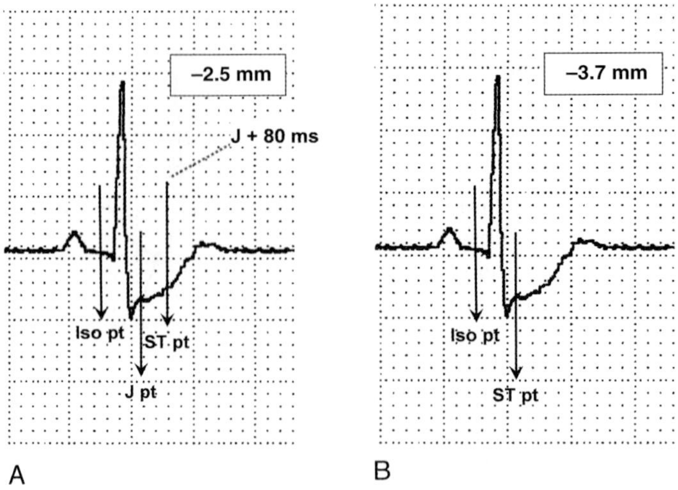

Fig. 4.2 Two ST rhythm strips illustrating two different techniques to calculate ST-segment depression values. (A) ST rhythm strip measures ST-segment deviation 80 ms (2 mm) from the J point. (B) ST rhythm strip measures ST-segment depression at the J point. The most recent American Heart Association/American College of Cardiology Foundation/Heart Rhythm Society recommendations for standardizing and interpreting the electrocardiogram advocate measuring ST-segment changes at the J point (i.e., B). (Reprinted with permission from Kossick MA. *EKG Interpretation: Simple, Thorough, Practical.* 2nd ed. AANA Publishing; 1999.)

TABLE 4.1 Threshold Values for ST-Segment Elevation

Gender and Age	ECG Leads	J-Point Elevation
Males >40 years of age	I, II, III, aVR, aVL, aVF V_1, V_4, V_5, V_6	1 mm (0.1 mV)
	V_2, V_3	2 mm (0.2 mV)
Males <40 years of age	V_2, V_3	2.5 mm (0.25 mV)
Females	I, II, III, aVR, aVL, aVF V_1, V_4, V_5, V_6	>1 mm (0.1 mV)
	V_2, V_3	1.5 mm (0.15 mV)
Males and females	V_3R, V_4R[a]	0.5 mm (0.05 mV)
Males <30 years of age	V_3R, V_4R[a]	1 mm (0.1 mV)
Males and females	V_7, V_8, V_9[b]	0.5 mm (0.05 mV)

ECG, Electrocardiogram; *mV,* millivolt.

[a]Right ventricular electrocardiogram leads.

[b]Posterior chest leads.

Data from Wagner GS, Macfarlane P, Wellens H, et al. AHA/ACCF/HRS recommendations for the standardization and interpretation of the electrocardiogram: part VI: acute ischemia/infarction: a scientific statement from the American Heart Association Electrocardiography and Arrhythmias Committee, Council on Clinical Cardiology; the American College of Cardiology Foundation; and the Heart Rhythm Society. Endorsed by the International Society for Computerized Electrocardiology. *J Am Coll Cardiol.* 2009;53:1003–1011.

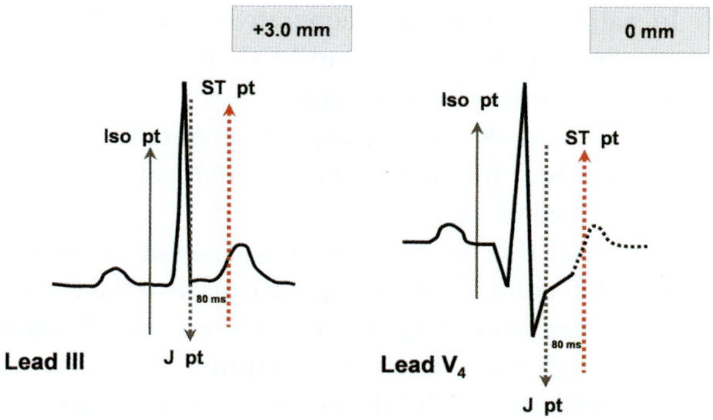

Fig. 4.3 Two cardiac cycles from leads III and V_4 illustrating a shortened ST segment. Use of a value of J + 80 ms to measure ST-segment deviation in each lead results in the ST point intersecting the T wave, thus producing inaccurate ST-segment deviation values. For lead III, the misplaced ST point produces a false-positive result, and for lead V_4, it produces a false-negative result. (Reprinted with permission from Kossick MA. *EKG Interpretation: Simple, Thorough, Practical.* 2nd ed. AANA Publishing; 1999.)

- Proper placement of the limb lead and chest lead electrodes is described in Table 4.2. For emphasis, the precordial leads should be placed via palpation of the costae, not by gross visual estimation of an intercostal space (Fig. 4.4).

Electrocardiographic lead selection

- Improper lead selection can result in unrecognized myocardial ischemia, injury, or infarction.
- The use of a single ECG lead for ischemic monitoring in patients with documented CAD is inadequate; monitoring with multiple leads enhances patient safety.
- For patients who are at risk for myocardial ischemia, it is recommended that the maximum number of ECG leads be displayed (e.g., 5, 7, 12 [derived 12-lead ECG]) during the perioperative period to enhance continuous and comprehensive assessment of ST-segment and T-wave changes (Figs. 4.5 and 4.6). The potential value of a preoperative 12-lead ECG is relative to its being correctly

TABLE 4.2 **Proper Placement of Electrocardiographic Electrodes for Monitoring Chest Leads and Limb Leads via the Mason-LikarLead Position**

RA	Over the outer right clavicle[a]
LA	Over the outer left clavicle[a]
LL	Near the left iliac crest or midway between the costal margin and left iliac crest, anterior axillary line[a]
RL	At any convenient location on the body (e.g., upper right shoulder or between right costal margin and iliac crest)
V_1	Fourth intercostal space right of the sternal border (this is the one anterior chest electrode in a five-lead ECG)
V_2	Fourth intercostal space left of the sternal border
V_3	Equidistant between V_2 and V_4
V_4	Midclavicular line at the fifth intercostal space
V_5	Horizontal to V_4 on the anterior axillary line or, if difficult to identify (anterior axillary line), midway between V_4 and V_6
V_6	Horizontal to V_5 on the midaxillary line
V_7	Horizontal to V_6 on the posterior axillary line
V_8	Horizontal to V_7 below the left scapula
V_9	Horizontal to V_8 at the left paravertebral border
V_3R	Placed right side of chest wall in mirror image to chest lead V_3
V_4R	Placed right side of chest wall in mirror image to chest lead V_4

ECG, Electrocardiographic; *LA,* left arm ECG electrode; *LL,* left leg ECG electrode; *RA,* right arm ECG electrode; *RL,* right leg ECG electrode.

[a]Mason-Likar ECG electrode placement.

Data from Kligfield P, Gettes LS, Bailey JJ, et al. Recommendations for the standardization and interpretation of the electrocardiogram: part I: the electrocardiogram and its technology a scientific statement from the American Heart Association Electrocardiography and Arrhythmias Committee, Council on Clinical Cardiology; the American College of Cardiology Foundation; and the Heart Rhythm Society endorsed by the International Society for Computerized Electrocardiology. *J Am Coll Cardiol* 2007;49:1109–1127.

recorded by the ECG technician (e.g., each ECG electrode was properly placed, the patient was in a supine position while it was recorded, and the low-frequency cutoff was set with a lower limit not exceeding 0.67 Hz).

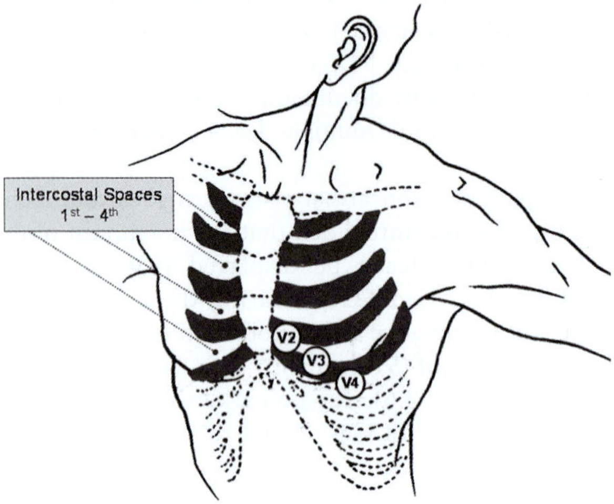

Fig. 4.4 Precordial electrodes V_2, V_3, and V_4 positioned across the ventrolateral aspect of the thorax. V_2 placement: fourth intercostal space (ICS) left of the sternum; V_3: equal distance between V_2 and V_4; V_4: left midclavicular line at the fifth ICS. (Reprinted with permission from Kossick MA. *EKG Interpretation: Simple, Thorough, Practical.* 2nd ed. AANA Publishing; 1999.)

- In patients without a preoperative 12-lead ECG or who have a baseline 12-lead ECG that is unremarkable (unknown ST fingerprint), leads V_3, V_4, V_5, limb lead III, and aVF (in this order of preference) should be selected for continuous monitoring for ST-segment elevation or depression.
- Limb lead II is recommended for assessment of narrow QRS complex rhythms, particularly if the P wave is significant for diagnostic criteria (e.g., atrial flutter, atrial fibrillation, junctional rhythms).
- The following ECG lead combinations (for ST-segment elevation or depression) are recommended in patients with documented or identified significant risk factors for ischemic heart disease:
  - For a five-cable ECG recording system, the three-lead set of V_3, MCL5, and aVF (the use of MCL5 precludes the use of limb lead III) or V_3 combined with limb lead III and aVF
  - For a three-cable ECG recording system, a two-lead set comprising MCL5 combined with limb lead aVF

Gain setting and frequency bandwidth

- Two potential problems with continuous ST-segment monitoring relate to the amplitude at which the ECG monitor has been set and whether filtering of the electrical signal is excessive.
- When accurate visual assessment of ST segments is a priority during an anesthetic, the gain of the ECG

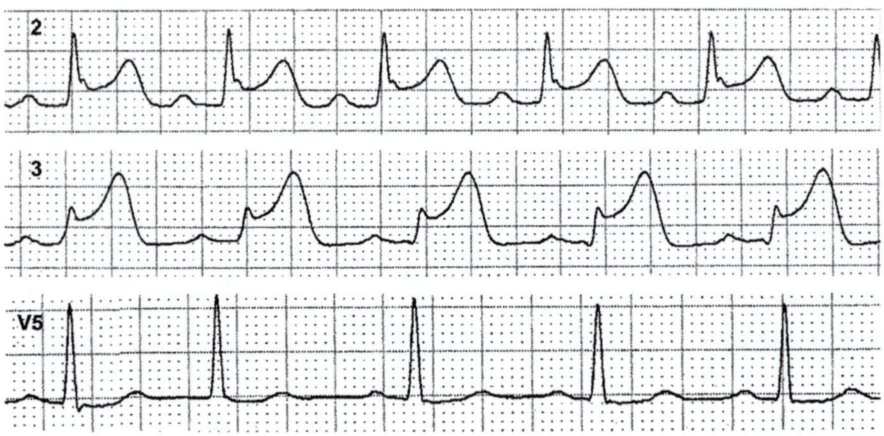

Fig. 4.5 Monitoring in three electrocardiogram leads during anesthetic administration captured significant ST-segment elevation. The greatest change in ST segments occurred in limb lead III, followed by limb lead II. Noteworthy was the failure of lead V_5 to demonstrate any appreciable change in the ST segment. Postoperatively, a cardiology consultation resulted in a diagnosis of Prinzmetal angina. (From Elisha S, Heiner JS, Nagelhout JJ. *Nurse Anesthesia.* 7th ed. Elsevier; 2023.)

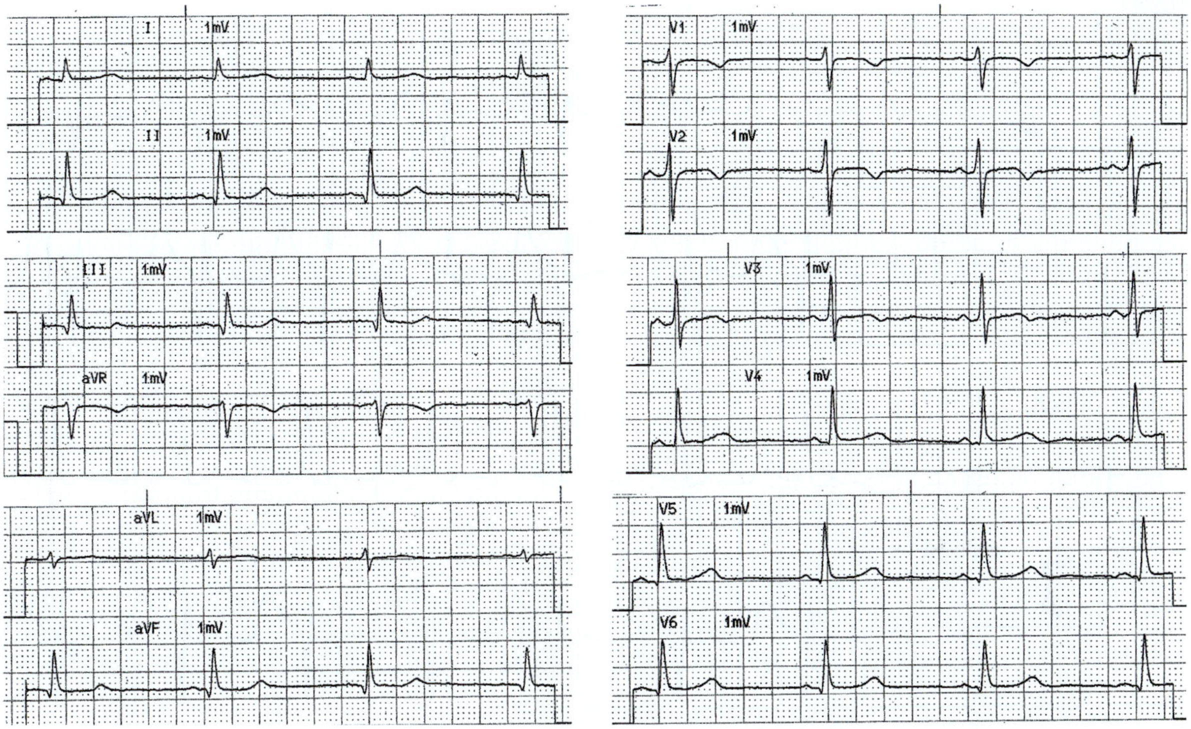

Fig. 4.6 Derived 12-lead electrocardiogram (ECG [EASI model]) recorded just before anesthetic induction in the operating room. The ECG monitor can be configured to continuously display all 12 leads for comprehensive assessment of ST segments and rhythm changes. (From Elisha S, Heiner JS, Nagelhout JJ. *Nurse Anesthesia*. 7th ed. Elsevier; 2023.)

monitor should be set at standardization (i.e., a 1-mV signal delivered by the ECG monitor produces a 10-mm calibration pulse).

- This gain setting fixes the ratio of the ST-segment and QRS-complex size so that a 1-mm ST-segment change is accurately assessed (e.g., potential myocardial injury).
- Failure to recognize the use of other gain settings can lead to overdiagnosis or underdiagnosis of myocardial injuries (ST-segment changes). Fig. 4.7 illustrates how changes in gain settings, incorrect ECG electrodes, and/or lead wire placement can confound ST-segment assessment.
- The sensitivity and specificity of computerized real-time ST-segment analysis software are dependent on the ability of the anesthetist to critically analyze the large number of factors that influence displayed ST-segment values. Attentiveness to variables such as the patient's physical status, ECG lead placement and selection, verification of proper placement of the Iso point, ST point, type of electronic filtering used by the ECG monitor, and gain setting may affect anesthetic outcome in patients at risk for myocardial ischemia or injury.

KNOWLEDGE CHECK

1. The degree of ST-segment elevation or depression is relative to the
   a. QRS complex.
   b. isoelectric line.
   c. *a* wave.
   d. QT segment.
2. Which type of dysrhythmia is associated with a short ST-segment interval?
   a. Tachyarrhythmia
   b. Bradyarrhythmia
   c. Torsade de pointes
   d. Pulseless electrical activity

Answers can be found in Appendix A.

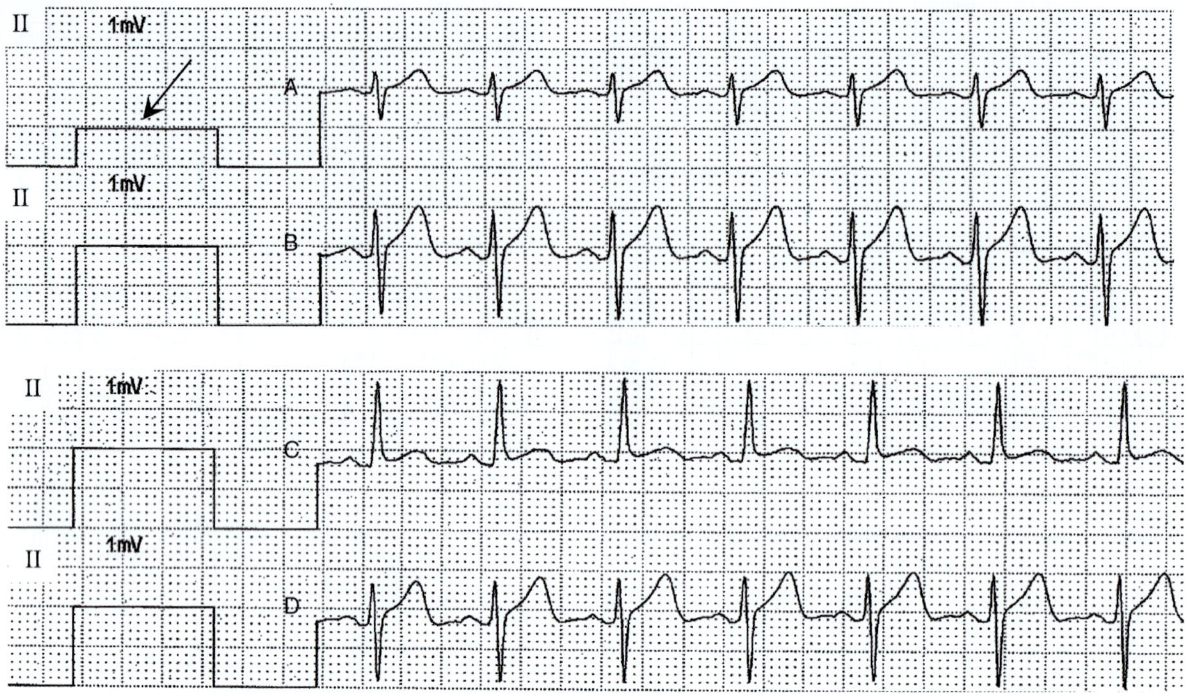

Fig. 4.7 Series of electrocardiogram (ECG) recordings illustrating how the gain setting and incorrect ECG electrode placement can lead to misinterpretation of ST-segment changes. In strip *A*, the gain setting *(arrow)* on the ECG monitor has been set at half-standardization (1 mV = 5 mm); it grossly gives the appearance of a minor ST-segment change. When concurrent strip *B* is compared with strip *A*, it becomes apparent that use of smaller gain settings can mask ST-segment deviation. Therefore, if a 0.5-mm ST-segment deviation in ECG strip *A* were to occur, it would equate to a 1-mm change. A similar error in assessment of ST-segment changes can occur secondary to misplaced ECG electrodes. ECG strip recording *C* has all limb lead electrodes properly placed and displays an ST-segment elevation of approximately 0.75 mm. In contrast, ECG rhythm strip *D* mistakenly has the left leg electrode placed in the second intercostal space, midclavicular line, and therefore is not representative of lead II. The end result is an ST segment that is falsely elevated (approximately 1.5 mm), suggesting inferior transmural myocardial injury. (Reprinted with permission from Kossick MA. *EKG Interpretation: Simple, Thorough, Practical.* 2nd ed. AANA Publishing; 1999:26–27.)

Central Venous and Arterial Hemodynamic Measurements

- Since the introduction of pulmonary artery catheterization in 1970, the frequency of its use as a monitoring tool for significant surgical procedures has diminished because of a lack of data showing improved outcomes.
- Even during cardiac or invasive vascular surgical procedures, many surgeons and anesthesia providers have opted for less invasive means to assess hemodynamic measurements (e.g., FloTrac sensor).

Physiology and morphology of hemodynamic waveforms

- Essential to accurate interpretation of hemodynamic data derived from central venous lines is a foundation in what constitutes "normal" distances, pressures, and waveform morphology for central venous pressure (CVP), right ventricular pressure (RVP), pulmonary artery pressure (PAP), and pulmonary artery occlusive pressure (PAOP) recordings. Table 4.3 illustrates the approximate distances for reaching the junction of the vena cava and the right atrium (RA) from various distal anatomic sites.

- Table 4.4 lists the anticipated distances for reaching various cardiac and pulmonary structures from the right internal jugular vein.
- Advancement of a CVP catheter 10 cm beyond these distances without the production of a characteristic waveform could indicate coiling of the central line. If this problem arises with a pulmonary artery catheter (PAC), the balloon should be deflated, and the catheter should be withdrawn.

TABLE 4.3 Distance to the Junction of the Vena Cava and Right Atrium From Various Distal Anatomic Sites

Location	Distance (cm)
Subclavian	10
Right internal jugular vein	15
Left internal jugular vein	20
Femoral vein	40
Right median basilic vein	40
Left median basilic vein	50

From Elisha S, Heiner JS, Nagelhout JJ. *Nurse Anesthesia*. 7th ed. Elsevier; 2023.

TABLE 4.4 Distance From the Right Internal Jugular Vein to Distal Cardiac and Pulmonary Structures

Location or Structure	Distance (cm)
Junction of the vena cava and right atrium	15
Right atrium	15–25
Right ventricle	25–35
Pulmonary artery	35–45
Pulmonary artery wedge position	40–50

From Elisha S, Heiner JS, Nagelhout JJ. *Nurse Anesthesia*. 7th ed. Elsevier; 2023.

- If any resistance is met during withdrawal, the provider should cease withdrawal, and a chest radiograph should be taken to rule out knotting or entanglement with the chordae tendineae or another cause.

Right atrial pressure waveform

- Familiarity with the anticipated distances of relevant hemodynamic anatomy and normal intracardiac pressures, pulmonary pressures (Table 4.5), and waveform morphology facilitates accurate interpretation of PAC data and placement of central lines.
- A normal CVP tracing will generate mean RA pressures in the range of 1–10 mm Hg.
- The fidelity of the transducing system determines whether discernible *a*, *c*, and *v* waves will be displayed once the distal tip of a central line lies just above the junction of the vena cava and the RA (Fig. 4.8).
- The *a* wave is produced by contraction of the RA.

TABLE 4.5 Normal Intracardiac and Pulmonary Artery Pressures

Location	Absolute Value (mm Hg)	Range (mm Hg)
MRAP	5	1–10
RV	25/5[a]	15–30/0–8
PA S/D	25/10[a]	15–30/5–15
MPAP	15	10–20
PAOP	10	5–15
MLAP	8	4–12
LVEDP	8	4–12

LVEDP, Left ventricular end-diastolic pressure; *MLAP,* mean left atrial pressure; *MPAP,* mean pulmonary artery pressure; *MRAP,* mean right atrial pressure; *PA,* pulmonary artery; *PAOP,* pulmonary artery occlusive pressure; *RV,* right ventricular; *S/D,* systolic/diastolic.

[a]Values are systolic pressure/diastolic pressure.

From Elisha S, Heiner JS, Nagelhout JJ. *Nurse Anesthesia*. 7th ed. Elsevier; 2023.

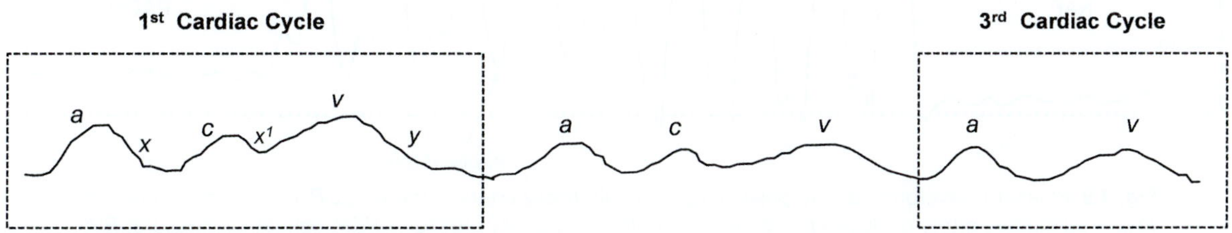

Fig. 4.8 Positive and negative waveforms of a central venous pressure tracing. The third cardiac cycle in this figure does not produce a *c* wave. (From Elisha S, Heiner JS, Nagelhout JJ. *Nurse Anesthesia*. 7th ed. Elsevier; 2023.)

- The *c* wave is produced by retrograde bulging of the closed tricuspid valve into the RA during right ventricle (RV) systole.
- The *v* wave is produced by passive filling of the RA.
- The reason the *a* wave is commonly larger than the *c* wave is based on the position of the catheter relative to the physiologic event responsible for the pressure change.
- RA systole and the subsequent increase in atrial pressure are detected by a catheter positioned just above (or inappropriately within) the RA, whereas RV systole (a more distal physiologic event relative to the position of a CVP catheter) indirectly increases RA pressure by closure of the tricuspid valve.

Right ventricular pressure waveform

- Further advancement of a PAC (approximately 10 cm) produces dramatic changes in the morphology of the hemodynamic waveform.
- As shown in Fig. 4.9, a brisk upstroke (isovolumetric contraction and rapid ejection [RV systole]) and steep downslope (reduced ejection and isovolumetric relaxation [RV systole and diastole]) are viewed on an oscilloscope when a PAC is advanced through the right intraventricular cavity.
- A PAC with the distal balloon inflated should remain in the RV for as short a time as possible to reduce the incidence of ventricular ectopy or the development of a conduction defect such as right bundle branch block.
- Pressures generated during RV systole and RV diastole are assessed indirectly via the CVP port of a PAC and the distal tip of the PAC. The former is used to estimate RV end-diastolic pressure, and the latter is used to estimate RV systolic pressure via the PA systolic recording.
- Thus right ventricular end-diastolic pressure (RVEDP) is used to estimate right ventricular end-diastolic volume (RVEDV), which approximates RV preload (and less accurately, left ventricular [LV] preload).

Pulmonary artery pressure waveform

- When a catheter enters the PA, the diastolic pressure is acutely increased, with little change in systolic pressure.
- The upstroke of the PA tracing is produced by opening of the pulmonic valve, followed by RV ejection.
- The downstroke contains the dicrotic notch, which is produced by closure of the aortic or pulmonic valve before the onset of RV diastole.

Pulmonary artery occlusive pressure waveform

- Final advancement of a PAC by 5–10 cm should produce a PAOP tracing.
- This waveform appears similar to a CVP (the *a* wave is produced by left atrial [LA] systole, the *c* wave by closure of the mitral valve, and the *v* wave by filling of the LA and upward displacement of the mitral valve during LV systole).
- It is less common to detect a *c* wave on a PAOP tracing because retrograde transmission of LA pressure (produced by closure of the mitral valve) is significantly attenuated within the pulmonary circulation.
- The characteristic waveform morphologies of a PAOP tracing are shown in Fig. 4.9.

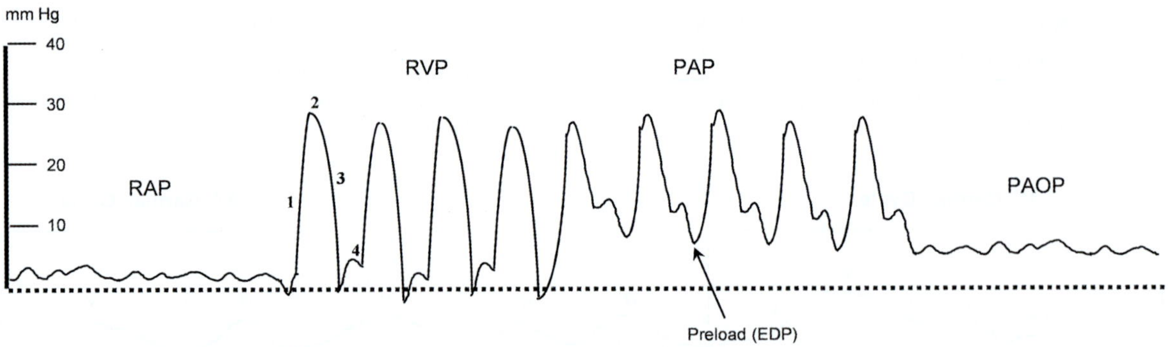

Fig. 4.9 Pressure waveforms during positioning of a pulmonary artery catheter. *EDP*, End-diastolic pressure; *PAOP*, pulmonary artery occlusive pressure; *PAP*, pulmonary artery pressure; *RAP*, right atrial pressure; *RVP*, right ventricular pressure. *1*, Isovolumetric contraction (ascent of pressure waveform); *2*, rapid ejection; *3*, isovolumetric relaxation (middescent of pressure waveform); *4*, atrial systole (slight increase in pressure). (From Elisha S, Heiner JS, Nagelhout JJ. *Nurse Anesthesia*. 7th ed. Elsevier; 2023.)

Negative deflection waveforms

- The *x* descent represents the period of RA relaxation resulting in a decrease in RA pressure. It occurs during ventricular systole as the tricuspid valve is closed.
- The x^1 descent is produced by downward pulling of the septum during ventricular systole, and the *y* descent corresponds to opening of the tricuspid valve and RV filling.
- The descents that follow the *a*, *c*, and *v* waves of a CVP or PAOP tracing are labeled as *x*, x^1, and *y* (see Fig. 4.8).

Correlation of pressure waveforms and the electrocardiogram

- The interpretation of hemodynamic waveforms can be facilitated by correlating their morphology and timeline with the ECG.
- The electrical event of the ECG precedes the physiologic effect (waveform).
- The *a* wave of a CVP tracing, which is produced by atrial contraction, will follow depolarization of the atria (P wave on the ECG).
- The *c* and *v* waves occur after the beginning of ventricular depolarization (QRS complex), or the *v* wave may not appear until shortly after the T wave (Figs. 4.10 and 4.11).

Distortion of pressure waveforms

- Arrhythmias can produce significant alterations in hemodynamic waveforms.
- Atrial fibrillation, junctional rhythms, and premature ventricular contractions (PVCs) can alter the shape of *a* waves.
- With atrial fibrillation, no synchronized atrial contraction occurs. In the CVP or PAOP tracing, this can lead to the loss of *a* waves or the appearance of small fibrillatory *a* waves.
- Complete atrioventricular (AV) block and some forms of junctional arrhythmias cause the atria to contract against a closed tricuspid valve, which can produce large cannon *a* waves (Fig. 4.12).
- Ventricular pacing can be associated with either the presence or the absence of cannon *a* waves.
- Valvular defects can also produce dramatic changes in the CVP and PAOP tracings, causing an increase in the amplitude of the *v* wave secondary to regurgitation (e.g., with mitral regurgitation [MR], a portion of the stroke volume is ejected retrograde into the pulmonary circuit, owing to an incompetent mitral valve).
- Recognition of such abnormalities is critical for accurate recording of pressure measurements and proper placement of central lines.
- Significant tricuspid regurgitation can cause a CVP recording to mimic an RV tracing, and MR can cause a PAOP recording to appear as a PA tracing. Specifically, large *v* waves become superimposed on *a* waves.

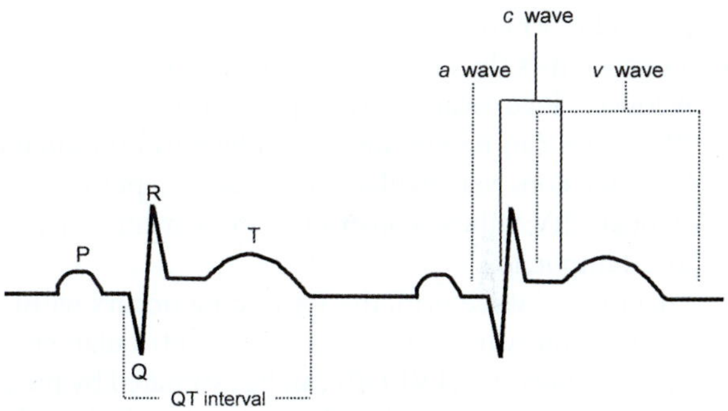

Fig. 4.10 Temporal relationship between the electrocardiogram and hemodynamic waveforms. (From Elisha S, Heiner JS, Nagelhout JJ. *Nurse Anesthesia*. 7th ed. Elsevier; 2023.)

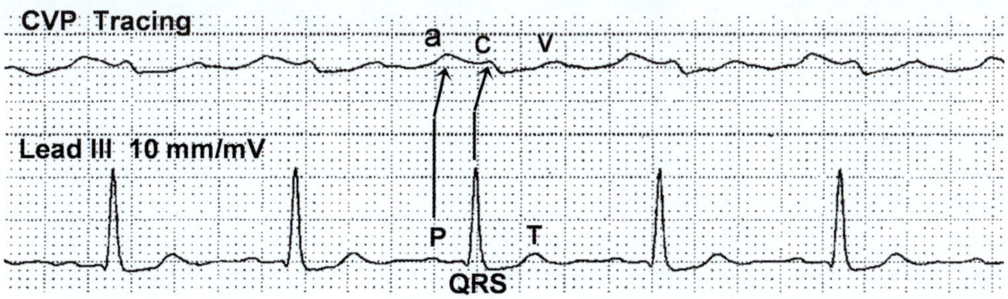

Fig. 4.11 Electrocardiographic recording with a concurrent central venous pressure tracing that demonstrates hysteresis between atrial depolarization (P wave) and the production of an *a* wave, as well as the QRS complex and the associated *c* and *v* waves. *CVP*, Central venous pressure. (From Elisha S, Heiner JS, Nagelhout JJ. *Nurse Anesthesia*. 7th ed. Elsevier; 2023.)

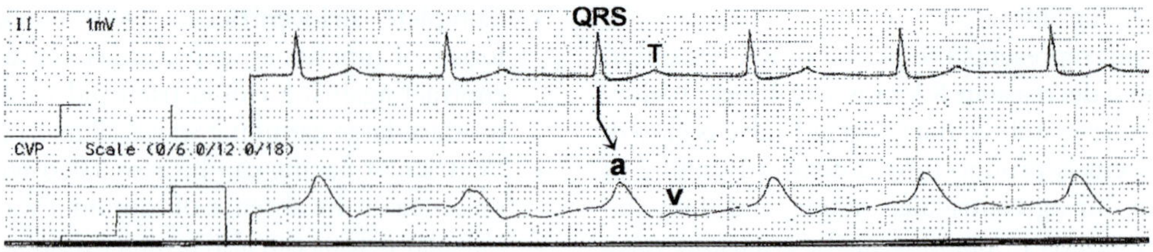

Fig. 4.12 Electrocardiographic recording of a junctional rhythm *(top)* in which there is simultaneous retrograde atrial and antegrade ventricular depolarization (as evidenced by the lack of a P wave in each cardiac cycle). This results in the right atrium contracting against a closed tricuspid valve. Therefore, the central venous pressure tracing *(bottom)* has cannon *a* waves. (From Elisha S, Heiner JS, Nagelhout JJ. *Nurse Anesthesia.* 7th ed. Elsevier; 2023.)

- Although the overall incidence of PA rupture is low (0.064%), flushing of a wedged catheter (as well as balloon overinflation) can result in vascular damage ranging from minor endobronchial hemorrhage to massive hemoptysis.
- Box 4.1 indicates how various rhythm disturbances, pacing, and valvular defects can distort the CVP tracing.

Implications of abnormal hemodynamic values

- The CVP serves as an estimate of right ventricular preload (RVEDP).
- Table 4.6 lists the causes of an elevated CVP.
- A low CVP correlates with hypovolemia.
- RV values can be elevated secondary to pulmonary hypertension, ventricular septal defect, pulmonary stenosis, RV failure, constrictive pericarditis, or cardiac tamponade.
- Like the RV waveform, the PA tracing occurs within the QT interval of the ECG. Left ventricular end-diastolic pressure (LVEDP) can be estimated by measuring the pressure value that exists just before the upstroke of the pulmonary artery (PA) waveform

BOX 4.1 Factors That Can Distort Central Venous Pressure and Pulmonary Artery Occlusive Pressure Tracings

Loss of *a* Waves or Only *v* Waves
- Atrial fibrillation
- Ventricular pacing in the setting of asystole

Giant or "Cannon" *a* Waves
- Junctional rhythms
- Complete AV block
- PVCs (simultaneous atrial and ventricular contraction)
- Ventricular pacing (asynchronous)
- Tricuspid or mitral stenosis
- Diastolic dysfunction
- Myocardial ischemia
- Ventricular hypertrophy

Large *v* Waves
- Tricuspid or mitral regurgitation
- Acute increase in intravascular volume

AV, Atrioventricular; *PVCs,* premature ventricular contractions.
From Elisha S, Heiner JS, Nagelhout JJ. *Nurse Anesthesia.* 7th ed. Elsevier; 2023.)

TABLE 4.6 Potential Causes of Elevated Central Venous Pressure, Pulmonary Artery Pressure, and Pulmonary Artery Occlusive Pressure

CVP	PAP	PAOP
RV failure	LV failure	LV failure
Tricuspid stenosis or regurgitation	Mitral stenosis or regurgitation	Mitral stenosis or regurgitation
Cardiac tamponade	L-to-R shunt	Cardiac tamponade
Constrictive pericarditis	ASD or VSD	Constrictive pericarditis
Volume overload	Volume overload	Volume overload
Pulmonary HTN	Pulmonary HTN	Ischemia
LV failure (chronic)	"Catheter whip"	

ASD, Atrial septal defect; *CVP,* central venous pressure; *HTN,* hypertension; *L,* left; *LV,* left ventricular; *PAOP,* pulmonary artery occlusive pressure; *PAP,* pulmonary artery pressure; *R,* right; *RV,* right ventricular; *VSD,* ventricular septal defect.
From Elisha S, Heiner JS, Nagelhout JJ. *Nurse Anesthesia.* 7th ed. Elsevier; 2023.

(see Fig. 4.9). See Table 4.6 for a list of causes of an increase in the PAP.

- A falsely high value can also be produced by a phenomenon called *catheter whip*, which is exaggerated oscillation of the PA tracing.
- This can occur with excessive catheter coiling if the tip of the PA catheter is near the pulmonic valve.
- To ensure that accurate pressure recordings are documented, the mean or diastolic pressure should always be determined at end expiration whether the patient is spontaneously breathing or receiving positive-pressure ventilation.
- End expiration is the time when pleural pressures are approximately equal to atmospheric pressures except when positive end-expiratory pressure (PEEP) is being used. The rationale for this timing relates to the fact that vascular pressure recordings are calibrated relative to atmospheric pressure. As stated previously, the correct area on the pressure recording to determine preload (e.g., LVEDP) is just before the upstroke of the *v* wave (or *c* wave if present).
- Causes of elevated PAOP are listed in Table 4.6.
- Table 4.7 lists clinical factors that can skew these pressure–volume relationships.
- A review of the gross interpretation of CVP and PAOP values is presented in Table 4.8.

TABLE 4.7 Factors That Alter the Relationships Among Central Cardiovascular Pressures and Volumes

CVP ≠ PADP	• Change in RV compliance (e.g., PS) • Tricuspid valve disease
PADP ≠ PAOP	• Pulmonary HTN • MR or AR • Lung zone I or II • Tachycardia • ARDS • RBBB
PAOP ≠ MLAP	• Juxtacardiac pressure (e.g., PEEP) • Lung zone I or II • Mediastinal fibrosis • RBBB
MLAP ≠ LVEDP	• Juxtacardiac pressure (e.g., PEEP) • Mitral valve disease • Change in LV compliance (e.g., AS)
LVEDP ≠ LVEDV	• Juxtacardiac pressure (PEEP) • Ventricular interdependence • Change in LV compliance (e.g., ischemia)

AR, Aortic regurgitation; *ARDS*, acute respiratory distress syndrome; *AS*, aortic stenosis; *CVP*, central venous pressure; *HTN*, hypertension; *LV*, left ventricular; *LVEDP*, left ventricular end-diastolic pressure; *LVEDV*, left ventricular end-diastolic volume; *MLAP*, mean left atrial pressure; *MR*, mitral regurgitation; *PADP*, pulmonary artery diastolic pressure; *PAOP*, pulmonary artery occlusive pressure; *PEEP*, positive end-expiratory pressure; *PS*, pulmonic stenosis; *PVR*, pulmonary artery vascular resistance; *RBBB*, right bundle branch block; *RV*, right ventricular.
From Elisha S, Heiner JS, Nagelhout JJ. *Nurse Anesthesia*. 7th ed. Elsevier; 2023.

TABLE 4.8 Potential Clinical Diagnosis via the Use of Hemodynamic Values: Interpretation of Pulmonary Artery Catheter Data

CVP	PADP	PAOP	Interpretation
Low	Low	Low	Hypovolemia, transducer not at phlebostatic axis[a]
Normal or high	High	High	LV failure
High	Normal or low	Normal or low	RV failure, TR, or TS
High	High	Normal or low	Pulmonary embolism
High	High	Normal	Pulmonary HTN
High	High	High	Cardiac tamponade, ventricular interdependence, transducer not at phlebostatic axis[a]
Normal	Normal or high	High	LV myocardial ischemia or MR
Low	High	Normal	ARDS[b]

ARDS, Acute respiratory distress syndrome; *CVP*, central venous pressure; *HTN*, hypertension; *LV*, left ventricular; *MR*, mitral regurgitation; *PADP*, pulmonary artery diastolic pressure; *PAOP*, pulmonary artery occlusive pressure; *RV*, right ventricular; *TR*, tricuspid regurgitation; *TS*, tricuspid stenosis.
[a]Phlebostatic axis is the fourth intercostal space, midanteroposterior level (not midaxillary line); for the right lateral decubitus position, fourth intercostal space midsternum; for the left lateral decubitus position, fourth intercostal space at the left parasternal border.
[b]Patients with ARDS commonly require initial fluid administration for hemodynamic stability.
From Elisha S, Heiner JS, Nagelhout JJ. *Nurse Anesthesia*. 7th ed. Elsevier; 2023.

Other hemodynamic indexes

- When pulmonary artery vascular resistance (PVR) is used clinically, it should be viewed as a gross *estimate* of RV afterload; similarly, systemic vascular resistance (SVR) is associated with LV afterload.
- In the intact heart, *afterload* is defined as systolic wall stress or the impedance the ventricle must overcome to eject its stroke volume.
- PVR, like SVR, can affect afterload, but neither formula accounts for changes in ventricular wall thickness or radius, which are components of afterload.
- The SVR index is calculated as the systemic input pressure (mean arterial pressure [MAP]) minus the output pressure (RA pressure or CVP), divided by the cardiac output (CO) multiplied by 80.
- The normal range is 800–1200 dynes-sec/cm^5.
- Determination of CO assists critical care specialists in providing rational hemodynamic therapy, evaluating the response to therapy, and along with SvO_2, determining the adequacy of tissue perfusion.
- It also permits the calculation of other hemodynamic indices (e.g., PVR and SVR).
- A "normal" CO value can be qualified by considering age differences, metabolic activity (declines with anesthesia and increases with hyperthermia), and patient size.
- This last factor may be adjusted for by converting a CO to a cardiac index (CI), which attempts to normalize CO for the large number of values found in the general population.
- However, CI adjusts only for the variables of height and weight. It does not address the lack of uniformity of predicted basal oxygen consumption and metabolic rates resulting from differences in sex and age.
- CI is calculated by dividing CO by body surface area (BSA). The plotting of height and weight on a body surface chart estimates the BSA in square meters (Fig. 4.13).
- Commonly quoted "normal" values are 4–8 L/min for CO and 2.8–3.6 L/min/m^2 for CI.
- The most commonly used technique for determining CO is thermodilution.
- Thermodilution entails the injection of a known quantity of an indicator solution (most commonly 5% dextrose in water, although 0.9% normal saline has a similar density factor) through the proximal port of a thermodilution PAC.
- The injected solution is considered a thermal indicator because it is cold relative to body temperature.
- The thermodilution injectate rapidly mixes with the incoming blood and is carried through the RV until it is detected by the thermistor near the end of the catheter in the PA.
- The computer plots a time–temperature curve, with the area under the curve being inversely proportional to the CO; therefore, larger curves are not desired.
- Variables that can influence recorded values include (1) the computation constant which varies with catheter size, injectate volume, and temperature; (2) the temperature of the injectate (desired range of 0–24°C); (3) the volume of injection; (4) the speed of injection (should be done in 4 seconds or less); and (5) the timing of injection (it should be consistent and performed at the same time during each respiratory cycle). A list of variables that can skew CO measurements is provided in Table 4.9.
- Further advancement in CO technology has been achieved via the placement of thermal filaments within the RV portion of the PAC and near the tip of the thermistor (Vigilance system, Edwards Lifesciences Corporation; OptiQue system, Abbott Labs). A computer algorithm permits analysis of a thermal signal created by small quantities of heat being emitted from the PAC—a pulsed warm thermodilution continuous cardiac output (TDCCO) technique.
- This heat signal is eventually transmitted by the blood to the distal thermistor, which permits continuous cardiac output (CCO) assessment.
- One advantage of a CCO catheter is the elimination of the time-consuming administration of a thermal injectate through the proximal port of the PAC.
- It also reduces the number of discrepancies in thermodilution CO values that can occur with inconsistent injectate administration relative to the respiratory cycle.
- A drawback to the CCO device is the hysteresis in recording hemodynamic information. Although the monitor displays updated CO figures every 30 seconds, they nonetheless do not represent real-time data.
- Other investigators have examined a variation of the TDCCO PAC, specifically a PAC (truCATH, HR HealthCare, York, PA) that measures the amount of energy required to maintain a fixed blood

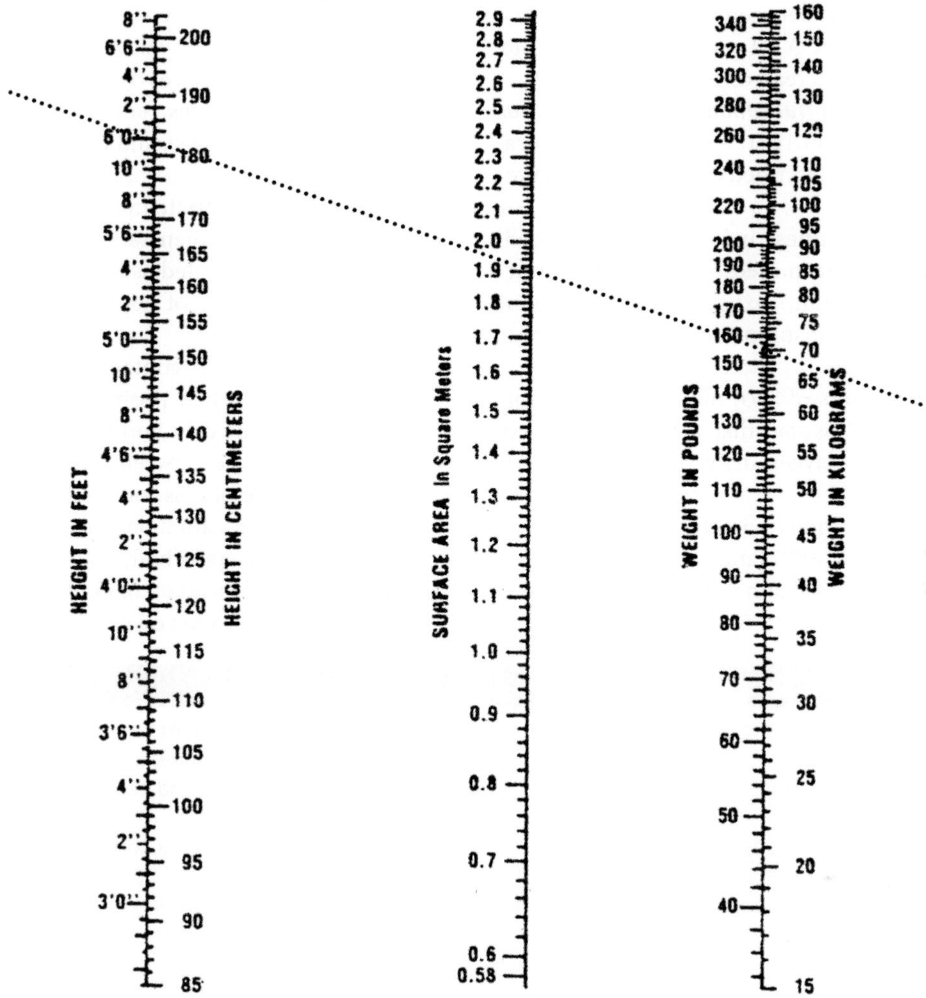

Fig. 4.13 Chart used to calculate body surface area. In this example, a height of 6 ft and a weight of 155 lb translates into a surface area of approximately 1.9 m². (From Elisha S, Heiner JS, Nagelhout JJ. *Nurse Anesthesia*. 7th ed. Elsevier; 2023.)

TABLE 4.9 **Variables That May Influence Thermodilution CO Values**

Overestimates	Underestimates	Unpredictable
• Low injectate volume	• Excessive injectate volume	• Right-to-left ventricular septal defect
• Injectate solutions that are too warm	• Injectate solutions that are too cold	• Left-to-right ventricular septal defect
• Thrombus on the thermistor of the PAC		• Tricuspid regurgitation
• Partially wedged PAC		

CO, Cardiac output; *PAC*, pulmonary artery catheter.
From Elisha S, Heiner JS, Nagelhout JJ. *Nurse Anesthesia*. 7th ed. Elsevier; 2023.

temperature gradient between two distal thermistors. Although the truCATH provides ultrafast data, it is associated with decreased reliability.

Mixed venous and central venous oxygen saturation

- Since its introduction in 1981, venous oxygen saturation (Svo_2) has been described to indirectly monitor oxygen delivery.
- This purported usefulness is based on the knowledge that Svo_2 is determined by pulmonary function, cardiac function, oxygen delivery, tissue perfusion, oxygen consumption, and hemoglobin concentration.
- Therefore, proponents of Svo_2 monitoring state that it is reasonable to assume that a decrease in Svo_2 reflects a change in oxygen delivery, presumably via a reduction in CO.
- Continuous mixed venous oximetry is measured with the use of fiberoptic reflectance spectrophotometry through two fiberoptic channels housed in the PAC.
- The normal range of Svo_2 is 65%–77%.
- Factors that increase Svo_2 values include left-to-right shunts, hypothermia, cyanide toxicity, a wedged PAC, and an increase in CO. Svo_2 decreases with hyperthermia, shivering, seizures, reduced pulmonary transport of oxygen, hemorrhage, and decreased CO.
- Sustained low values (e.g., 50%) merit investigation, followed by appropriate intervention(s).
- Central venous oxygen saturation ($Scvo_2$) monitoring has been advocated as a surrogate for Svo_2 when a less invasive form of hemodynamic monitoring is indicated.
- Modified CVCs that contain a fiberoptic lumen can measure $Scvo_2$ when positioned at the junction of the superior vena cava and RA.
- A major difference between Svo_2 and $Scvo_2$ measurements is that the latter is considered a regional indicator of venous oxygen saturation; it measures venous O_2 saturation from the upper body and head. In contrast, Svo_2 measurements depend on blood flow from the superior vena cava, inferior vena cava, and coronary sinus.

KNOWLEDGE CHECK

1. Which is the correct anatomic position for the distal tip of a central line?
   a. Between the RA and RV
   b. 2 cm within the RA
   c. At the junction of the vena cava and the RA
   d. Proximal to the tricuspid valve
2. Which portion of the ECG does the *a* wave on the CVP tracing immediately precede?
   a. P wave
   b. QRS complex
   c. T wave
   d. QT interval
3. Which physical event is represented by the *c* wave on the CVP tracing?
   a. Opening of the aortic valve
   b. Closure and bulging of the tricuspid valve
   c. Closure of the mitral valve
   d. Opening of the pulmonic valve
4. Which value is represented by CVP?
   a. LV end-systolic pressure
   b. RVEDV
   c. LV end-systolic volume
   d. Right ventricular end-diastolic pressure
5. Mean CVP values should be measured
   a. at end expiration.
   b. at the beginning of systole.
   c. at a peak pressure of 20 mm Hg.
   d. during the QRS complex.
6. Which factors can influence CO monitoring? *(Select two.)*
   a. Volume of injectate
   b. Position of patient
   c. Level of the transducer
   d. Size of the catheter
7. Which factors decrease Svo_2? *(Select two.)*
   a. Hypothermia
   b. Shivering
   c. Septic shock
   d. Cyanide toxicity

Answers can be found in Appendix A.

Blood Pressure Monitoring

- The concomitant disruption of homeostatic reflexes caused by anesthetic medications can lead to substantive changes in hemodynamics—even in relatively healthy patients.
- It is also known that the hemodynamic response to many anesthetic medications used during induction of anesthesia can cause significant variability.
- Currently, noninvasive blood pressure (NIBP) monitoring most often uses automated BP cuffs that can

be configured to measure systolic blood pressure (SBP), diastolic blood pressure, and MAP in a standard mode or stat mode and allow for varied frequencies of assessment and adjustments for patient age and habitus.

- BP cuffs should have a bladder dimension of approximately 40% of the circumference of the extremity.
- BP cuffs that are not properly sized or applied firmly to the extremity can lead to inaccurate recordings. BP cuffs that are applied loosely to the extremity, are positioned below the level of the heart, or are too small can produce arterial BP values that are falsely elevated.
- Injury and harm can occur with automatic NIBP measurements and may include damage to peripheral nerves (e.g., ulnar), development of a compartment syndrome, or interference with delivery of drugs through an IV line.
- In morbidly obese patients, it is not unusual to have to relocate a BP cuff from the upper arm because of the conical shape of the extremity.
- An alternative site for BP monitoring is the forearm. However, NIBP measurements taken in the forearm with the patient in supine or sitting position or the head of the bed elevated 45 degrees can *overestimate* the BP measured at the brachial artery site.

Arterial line assessment of blood pressure

- The most common site for direct arterial BP measurement is the radial artery.
- Other sites include the ulnar, brachial, axillary, femoral, and dorsalis pedis.
- A displaced transducer (no longer level with the phlebostatic axis) can cause a falsely elevated arterial BP if positioned substantially below the level of the heart.
- Direct arterial BP monitoring offers several distinct advantages, including beat-to-beat assessment of BP, limited hysteresis in measured values, and easy access for arterial sampling of blood for any number of laboratory tests (e.g., arterial blood gases, serum electrolytes, glucose, hemoglobin levels).
- Indications for direct arterial BP monitoring include surgical procedures in which there is potential for acute and/or gross changes in hemodynamics, such as complex vascular procedures.
- Even with lower-risk surgical procedures, direct arterial BP monitoring may be indicated, particularly if preoperative BP is poorly controlled (labile) or when intraoperative monitoring of somatosensory evoked potentials (SSEPs) produces frequent gross movement of the upper extremities, which can mitigate the effectiveness of NIBP measurements.
- Patients with comorbidities may be at substantial risk for a stroke or heart attack during periods of acute stress (e.g., laryngoscopy or emergence from an anesthetic) if BP is not directly monitored.
- Risks associated with placement of an intraarterial catheter include infection (i.e., localized and systemic infections), thrombus formation, hematoma, vasospasm, embolization, injury to adjacent nerves and veins, ischemia to extremities or digits, loss of a limb secondary to poor collateral circulation, iatrogenic injuries (e.g., air embolization, intraarterial injection of drugs meant to be administered intravenously), and acute blood loss due to an unexpected disruption of the transducing system (e.g., cracked or disconnected stopcock). Interventions used to minimize complications include positioning of the hand and wrist on an arm board.

Arterial line insertion

- Initial positioning for arterial line insertion consists of a roll that is placed beneath the wrist, with the fingers and thumb taped securely across the board. This position keeps the hand from interfering with manipulation and placement of the needle–catheter system; it also facilitates palpation of the radial artery (which is the most common artery used for arterial BP monitoring).
- A 20-gauge nontapered catheter is used (a 22-gauge catheter is optional) to penetrate an area of skin that has been prepared with antiseptic solution and infiltrated with local anesthetic.
- The needle, with bevel pointing upward, is directed at a 45-degree angle toward the palpated pulse. If bone is encountered with the tip of the needle during advancement, the complete catheter system (catheter and needle) is slowly withdrawn while observing for the free flow of arterial blood; sometimes the artery can be pierced without a "flash back" (i.e., unintentional transfixation-withdrawal method). If no blood is seen during catheter withdrawal, the needle system is redirected laterally or medially and advanced.
- Once arterial blood is seen in the lumen of the catheter, the angle of the needle is reduced to approximately 30 degrees, then advanced slightly a few millimeters.
- It is common for the Seldinger technique and a guidewire to be used when inserting an arterial catheter.

- Once the needle accesses the artery, a wire is threaded into the inner arterial lumen, and the catheter is subsequently threaded off the needle, over the wire, and into the artery.
- Ultrasound-guided placement of an arterial catheter is also common practice. A translinear probe is used to visualize the needle, either in-plane or out-of-plane, as it penetrates the artery, with confirmation of blood flow back through the needle chamber.
- After verifying correct placement of the catheter within the lumen of the artery (i.e., free flow of blood through the rigid tubing when vented to air), it is important to securely fasten the arterial catheter to the skin and apply a sterile dressing on top of the puncture site.
- The transducing system should be zeroed to atmospheric pressure with the stopcock vented to air, and referenced at the level of the LA.
- In patients with poor vascular compliance, the arterial tracing can produce an "overshoot" or "ringing" phenomenon. If not recognized, BP recordings will overestimate SBP and MAP values.
- In contrast, a dampened waveform, which can develop with a flexed wrist or low pressure in the continuous flush device, can lead to an underestimation of BP recordings (Fig. 4.14).
- Direct arterial BP measurements, although very accurate in many clinical circumstances, can still produce BP recordings that are significantly skewed and can lead to inappropriate interventions (e.g., preload augmentation, indiscriminate use of vasoactive drugs). Thus, correlation with NIBP cuff data is recommended.

KNOWLEDGE CHECK

1. The bladder dimension of a BP cuff should be approximately ___% of the circumference of the extremity.
   a. 30
   b. 40
   c. 50
   d. 60
2. Which pathologic state is associated with falsely increased arterial line SBP?
   a. Portal hypertension
   b. Diabetes
   c. Arteriosclerosis
   d. Chronic renal failure
3. Which artery is most often used for arterial blood pressure monitoring?
   a. Ulnar
   b. Branchial
   c. Radial
   d. Femoral

Answers can be found in Appendix A.

Transesophageal Echocardiographic Monitoring

- Transesophageal echocardiography (TEE) has been established as a safe diagnostic tool for monitoring numerous cardiac parameters to guide medical, surgical, and nursing care.
- Detection of systolic wall motion abnormalities (SWMAs) and vascular aneurysms, calculation of ejection fraction and ventricular preload, and measurement of blood flow within heart chambers and across valves are a few of the uses of ultrasound imaging during TEE.

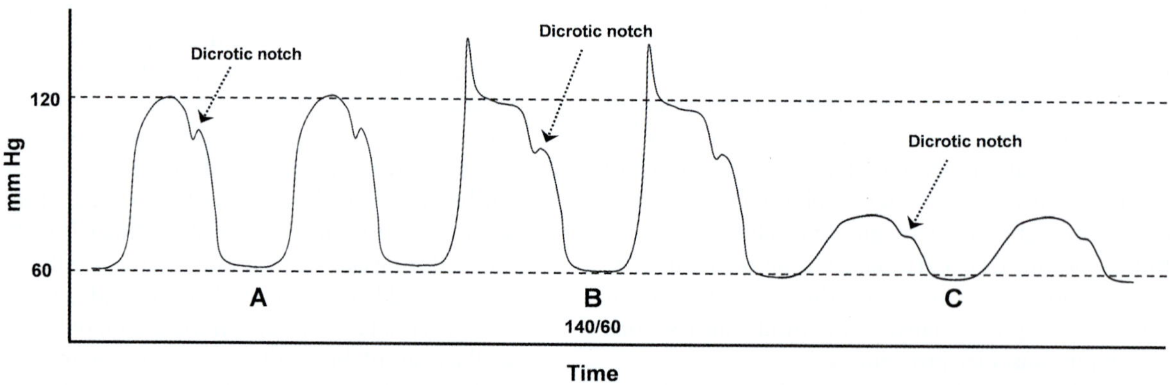

Fig. 4.14 Radial arterial pressure waveforms. (A) Normal morphology. (B) Overshoot. (C) Dampened. With waveform B, the overshoot should be ignored regarding the displayed systolic blood pressure. (From Elisha S, Heiner JS, Nagelhout JJ. *Nurse Anesthesia*. 7th ed. Elsevier; 2023.)

- The TEE probe consists of a controller, a flexible endoscopic shaft, and a probe head. The probe head is at the distal end of the endoscopic shaft and contains piezoelectric crystals that create an ultrasound beam.
- Ultrasound waves are inaudible to the human ear, having a frequency greater than 20,000 Hz.
- Piezoelectric crystals are known to produce ultrasound by vibrating when exposed to an electric current. The opposite also occurs in that they produce voltage in response to an ultrasound echo or when pressed (mechanical stress) or released. The electric current produced has been shown to be of sufficient magnitude to temporarily illuminate a small bulb. Thus, these crystals function as both generators and receivers of ultrasound waves and electric currents.
- Within the esophagus, ultrasound waves emitted by piezoelectric elements are absorbed, reflected, or scattered. When reflected by an organ (e.g., heart), the ultrasound echo produced is received by the piezoelectric elements housed within the TEE probe. These elements then generate an electrical impulse that is processed, amplified, and subsequently displayed as an image on the echograph machine.
- The frequency of the piezoelectric crystals in TEE probes ranges from 3.7 to 7 MHz. This frequency range allows greater detail in displayed images. Unfortunately, the trade-off for clearer images is lower tissue penetration. Smaller-frequency values (e.g., 2.5 MHz) are required in transthoracic echocardiographic probes because of greater distances between elements and distal anatomic structures.
- Clinically, three primary ultrasound imaging techniques are used: the M-mode, two-dimensional (2-D) imaging, and the Doppler examination.
- The M-mode provides high picture resolution with 1000 images per second. It is commonly referenced as being unidimensional and produces a well-focused, narrow ultrasound beam. It is sometimes referred to as an *ice-pick view*.
- With the 2-D scan, the ultrasound beam is electronically steered across a target field. The intermittent pulses of ultrasound are produced by varying the firing sequence (phasing) of individual piezoelectric crystals. The monitor subsequently displays an image that is triangular or appears as a "slice of pie." This produces excellent spatial orientation; however, at 30 images per second, the pictures are less well defined.
- The Doppler examination incorporates the concept of frequency shift. The clinical application of this concept involves viewing red blood cells (RBCs) as moving reflectors of ultrasound. As ultrasound reflects off the moving RBCs, echoes are produced, which are then recorded by the TEE transducer.
- With the flow of RBCs toward the TEE probe, the distance between the sound source and its reception changes. This phenomenon is referred to as a *frequency shift*. It is analogous to the change in pitch of a train whistle as the locomotive approaches the station; sound waves are compressed, and the pitch increases (frequency shift). In contrast to RBCs, body fluids (plasma) only minimally reflect ultrasound.
- Spectral and color flow Doppler examinations performed with echographs incorporate this concept by assigning different colors to RBCs that move toward and away from the source of ultrasound. This permits easy visualization of retrograde flow of blood across incompetent heart valves, as may occur with MR.
- Doppler examinations are recognized as being beneficial in determining the etiology of regurgitation and the adequacy of valve repair, as well as influencing surgical management, such as the use or nonuse of cardiopulmonary bypass.

Fundamental elements: TEE examination

- When performing a TEE, the probe is inserted into the esophagus. Positioning the TEE probe in the esophagus can be done either under sedation or after induction of the anesthetic (Fig. 4.15).

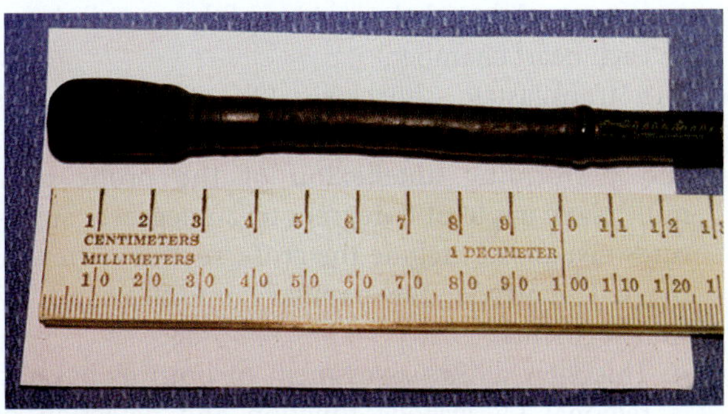

Fig. 4.15 Transesophageal echocardiography probe. Distal tip contains thermistor and piezoelectric elements. (From Elisha S, Heiner JS, Nagelhout JJ. *Nurse Anesthesia.* 7th ed. Elsevier; 2023.)

- Cardiac anatomy can be assessed, myocardial ischemia can be diagnosed via the presence of SWMA, and blood flow through heart chambers and across valves can be seen.
- The posterior structures are displayed at the top of the screen (apex of the sector), with anterior structures at the bottom.
- There are many standard views, but four primary or foundational TEE views are commonly emphasized for basic and comprehensive exams. These views provide key perspectives for evaluating cardiac function and pathology.
- The first view is the midesophageal four-chamber (ME 4C) view. The probe is placed in the midesophagus (30–40 cm from the incisors), with the multiplane angle at 0 degrees to 20 degrees. Structures visualized include the left and right atria, left and right ventricles, and mitral and tricuspid valves.
  - This view is used to assess ventricular function and chamber size, evaluate mitral/tricuspid valve anatomy and regurgitation, and look for septal defects.
- Rotation and angulation of the probe can allow for the midesophageal long-axis (ME LAX) view. The probe is also in the midesophagal position, and in this view, a multiplane angle (typically ~120°–140°) allows for the following structures to be visualized: LV and LA, aortic valve (AV) and root, and mitral valve (MV).
  - This view is useful for assessing stenosis or regurgitation of both the aortic and mitral valves, as well as overall valvular function. It all allows for assessment of the left ventricular outflow tract (LVOT), identification of masses within the atria or ventricles, and observation of the overall size of each heart chamber.
- The transgastric short-axis (TG SAX) view is achieved by advancing the probe into the stomach and performing anteflexion of the probe at a multiplane angle of 0 degrees to 20 degrees. Structures visualized include the cross-sectional view of the left ventricle, the papillary muscles, and LV wall segments.
  - This view allows assessment of both global and regional LV systolic function and detection of wall motion abnormalities (e.g., ischemia).
- The fourth view is the midesophageal bicaval, which is obtained with the probe in the midesophagal position with a multiplane angle of 90 degrees to 110 degrees. Structures visualized include the superior vena cava (SVC) and inferior vena cava (IVC), RA, and interatrial septum.
  - This view allows for evaluation of venous return and right atrial anatomy and detection of atrial septal defects (ASDs) or patent foramen ovale (PFO), and it also helps to guide central line or pulmonary catheter placement.
- Normal ventricular wall motion thickens during systole, and the endocardial surface moves inward. Approximately 87% of the normal stroke volume is derived from shortening in the short axis of the ventricle, with little contribution from the long axis.
- Abnormal wall motion can be described by three terms: hypokinesia, akinesia, and dyskinesia.
  - *Hypokinesia* represents contraction that is less vigorous than normal; wall thickening is decreased.
  - *Akinesia* depicts the absence of wall motion and can be associated with myocardial infarction.
  - *Dyskinesia* correlates with paradoxical movement (i.e., outward motion during systole) and is a hallmark of myocardial infarction and ventricular aneurysm (Fig. 4.16).
- Not all wall motion abnormalities are diagnostic of an imbalance between myocardial oxygen supply and demand. Abnormal loading conditions, asynchronous ventricular depolarization (e.g., left bundle branch block), echo dropout due to haphazard reflection of ultrasound off myocardial walls in lateral fields of the sector arc, or improper use of the gain controls of the TEE probe can lead to an erroneous diagnosis of SWMA. Also, the duration of SWMA can persist well after coronary reperfusion has been restored (e.g., 6 hours), indicating a stunned myocardium.
- The best single view for routine monitoring for SWMA (myocardial ischemia) is the short axis at the midpapillary muscle level (see Fig. 4.16), followed by the apical segment in the same axis. The midpapillary muscle level includes segments of the myocardium perfused by all three coronary arteries. This level is created by dividing the long axis of the left ventricle into three parts that include basal, mid-, and apical regions.

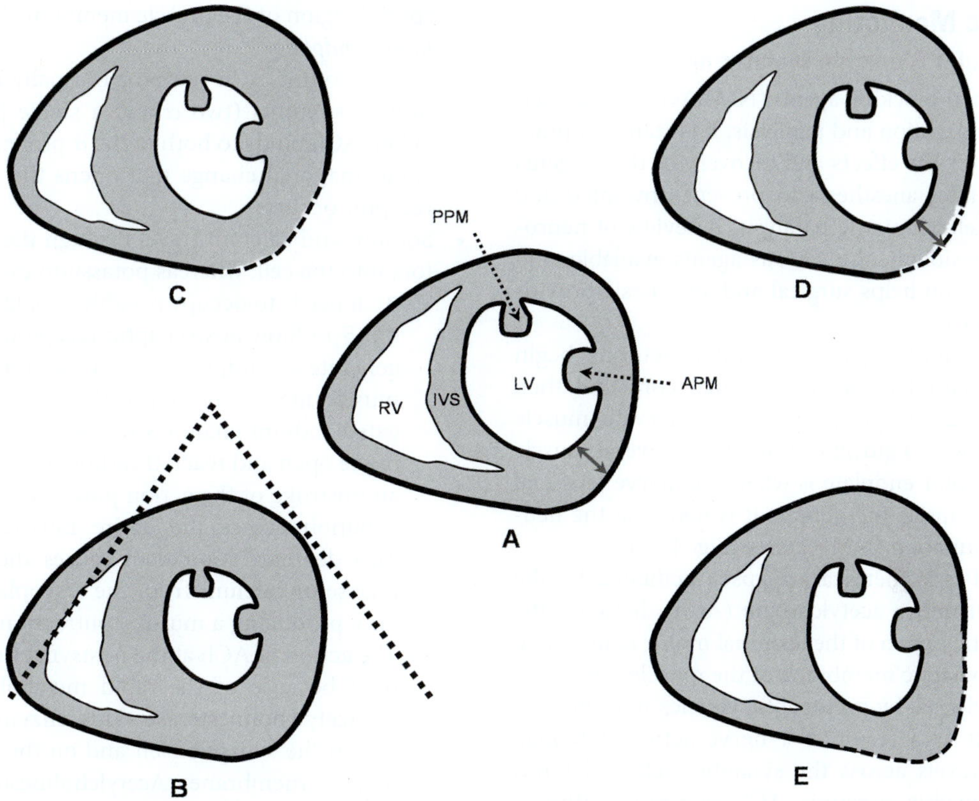

Fig. 4.16 Midpapillary muscle level short-axis view of the heart (A) during diastole, (B) during systole with normal wall thickening and inward movement of endocardial surface, (C) during systole with area of hypokinesia (decreased wall thickening), (D) during systole with an area of akinesia (no change in wall thickness), and (E) during systole with an area of dyskinesia (paradoxical movement). *APM*, Anterior papillary muscle; *IVS*, interventricular septum; *LV*, left ventricle; *PPM*, posterior papillary muscle; *RV*, right ventricle. (From Elisha S, Heiner JS, Nagelhout JJ. *Nurse Anesthesia*. 7th ed. Elsevier; 2023.)

KNOWLEDGE CHECK

1. Which ultrasound mode is associated with a triangular or "pie slice" image?
   a. M-mode
   b. 2-D imaging
   c. Doppler examination
   d. C mode
2. Which view is most efficacious to assess SWMAs?
   a. Short axis
   b. Long axis
   c. Midaxillary line
   d. M-mode
3. Which cardiac wall motion abnormality is associated with paradoxical movement during systole?
   a. Akinesia
   b. Dyskinesia
   c. Hypokinesia
   d. Tardive dyskinesia
4. Which position is the most common for placement of the TEE?
   a. Upper esophagus
   b. Midesophagus
   c. Lower esophagus
   d. Stomach
5. Which primary TEE view allows for assessment of the AV?
   a. ME 4C
   b. TG SAX
   c. ME LAX
   d. Midesophageal bicaval

Answers can be found in Appendix A.

Neurologic Monitoring

Neuromuscular Blockade Monitoring

Neuromuscular blocking agents (NMBAs) provide skeletal muscle relaxation and paralysis. It is standard practice to monitor the effects and recovery of these agents during and after anesthesia to prevent unwanted and persistent skeletal muscle paralysis. A review of neuromuscular physiology, the various agents available, and neurostimulation helps surgical and anesthesia providers offer safe care.

Neuromuscular physiology. Motor neurons begin within the ventral horn of the spinal cord and then extend their axons peripherally to innervate muscle fibers. One motor neuron can innervate several muscle fibers. The motor endplate is where the nerve terminal contacts the muscle membrane. It is here that the neuromuscular junction (NMJ) exists (Fig. 4.17).

- The NMJ is a chemical synapse, facilitated by the neurotransmitter acetylcholine (ACh), between the presynaptic region of the terminal motor neuron and the postsynaptic membrane of the muscle fiber.
- ACh is released by presynaptic vesicles into the synaptic cleft as a result of a nerve action potential. It then travels across the synaptic cleft and binds to postsynaptic nicotinic ACh receptors within a special region of the muscle membrane known as the *motor endplate*.
- Each nicotinic ACh receptor normally contains five protein subunits (two α and a single β, δ, and ε). When ACh binds to both of the α protein subunits, a conformational change that opens the postsynaptic receptor occurs.
- Sodium and calcium travel through the open receptors into the cell, whereas potassium exits the cell.
  - ACh needs to occupy roughly 250,000–500,000 of the 5 million postsynaptic receptors in order to generate an endplate potential and depolarize the muscle membrane. Once this happens, voltage-gated sodium channels within the muscle membrane open and reach threshold potential, causing an upstroke of the action potential and a full distribution across the entire muscle membrane. This depolarization then causes the subsequent release of calcium from the sarcoplasmic reticulum, producing a muscle contraction.
  - The action of ACh at the postsynaptic receptors is brief because of the rapid metabolism of ACh by acetylcholinesterase. This enzyme is present within the synaptic cleft and on the postsynaptic muscle membrane. Acetylcholinesterase causes ACh to unbind from the postsynaptic receptors

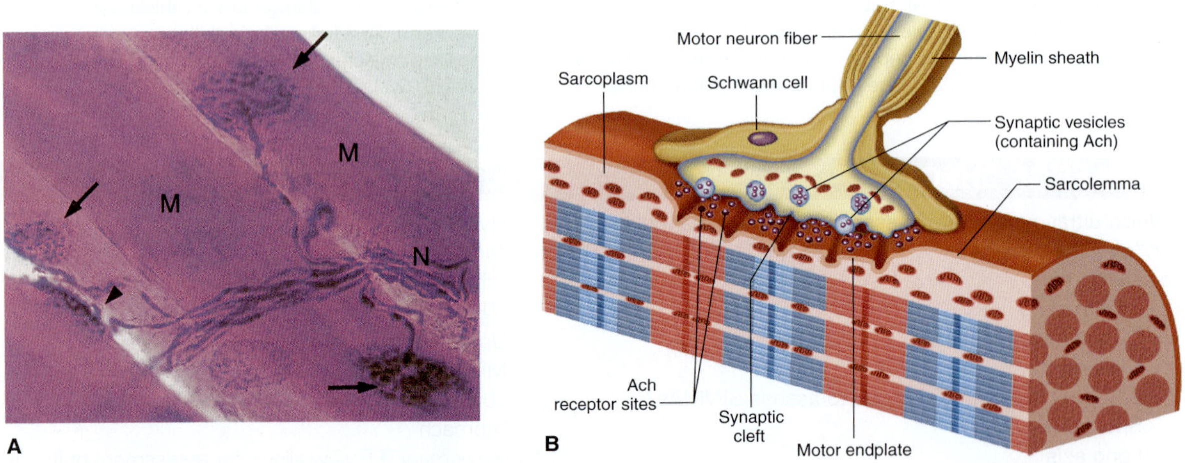

Fig. 4.17 Neuromuscular junction (NMJ). (A) Micrograph showing four NMJs. Three are surface views (*arrows*), and one is a side view (*arrowhead*). (B) This sketch shows a side view of the NMJ. Note how the distal end of a motor neuron fiber forms a synapse, or "chemical junction," with an adjacent muscle fiber. Neurotransmitter molecules (specifically, acetylcholine) are released from the neuron's synaptic vesicles and diffuse across the synaptic cleft. There, they stimulate receptors in the motor endplate region of the sarcolemma. *Ach*, Acetylcholine; *M*, muscle fibers; *N*, nerve fibers. (From Patton KT, Thibodeau GA. *Anatomy & Physiology*. 9th ed. Elsevier Mosby; 2016:367.)

and rapidly hydrolyzes it into acetate and choline. The unbinding of ACh closes postsynaptic receptors, causing closure of voltage-gated sodium channels and repolarization of the muscle membrane. Finally, the muscle relaxes when calcium is reintroduced into the sarcoplasmic reticulum.

- The amount of ACh released and the number of postsynaptic receptors stimulated are usually more than the minimum needed to generate a muscle action potential. However, problems with muscle contraction can occur with (1) decreased release of ACh at the presynaptic region (Eaton-Lambert myasthenic syndrome) or (2) a decreased amount of postsynaptic receptors (myasthenia gravis).

Neuromuscular blocking agents and other mechanisms of neuromuscular blockade. These are discussed in greater detail in Chapter 2. There are two classes of NMBAs: depolarizing and nondepolarizing.

Depolarizing muscle relaxant. A depolarizing muscle relaxant (e.g., succinylcholine) is an ACh agonist that similarly binds to the α protein subunits on postsynaptic receptors to stimulate an endplate depolarization. Succinylcholine is not metabolized by acetylcholinesterase but rather by plasma cholinesterase, allowing greater concentrations within the synaptic cleft and resulting in prolonged depolarization of the muscle membrane.

- Succinylcholine causes muscle relaxation and a phase I block because voltage-gated sodium channels initially open but then inactivate with prolonged depolarization. They cannot reopen until the endplate repolarizes; however, the endplate cannot repolarize as long as the depolarizing muscle relaxant is bound to the ACh receptor.
- Increased doses of succinylcholine can cause an extended depolarization of the muscle membrane that may result in a phase II block that is similar to that of nondepolarizing muscle relaxants. The mechanisms associated with depolarizing phase II block are poorly understood.

Nondepolarizing muscle relaxants. Nondepolarizing muscle relaxants act as competitive ACh antagonists. They prohibit postsynaptic ion channel opening and endplate depolarization by binding to one or both of the α protein subunits. Thus, they cause neuromuscular blockade by effectively preventing ACh from binding to postsynaptic ACh receptors.

Other mechanisms of neuromuscular blockade. Several diseases and other mechanisms can create neuromuscular blockade by decreasing the release of ACh at the presynaptic membrane, by altering the transmission of ACh within the synaptic cleft, or by altering the postsynaptic receptors.

- Disease states that affect the release of ACh at the presynaptic region can result from injury or autoimmunity or can be congenital in nature. Examples include muscle denervation injuries, Eaton-Lambert myasthenic syndrome, neuromyotonia, congenital myasthenia, and botulism.
- The postsynaptic muscle membrane adapts to the decrease in ACh release by generating an increase (upregulation) in postsynaptic receptors. Therefore, if succinylcholine is administered, an exaggerated response occurs because of the depolarization of many more receptors. Consequences can include hyperkalemia.
- The most common disease at the postsynaptic membrane is any form of myasthenia gravis. This disease causes a degradation of ACh receptors. The reduced number of ACh receptors results in resistance to depolarizing muscle relaxants and a sensitivity toward nondepolarizing muscle relaxants.
- Inhaled anesthetics, local anesthetics, aminoglycoside antibiotics (e.g., gentamycin), and ketamine can interfere with ACh transport and binding, leading to muscle relaxation and paralysis.

Neurostimulation. The primary method for clinically monitoring neurostimulation is with a direct current stimulator that uses subcutaneous needles or surface electrodes. These neurostimulators are monophasic and have the ability to vary both the pulse duration and intensity. This type of monitoring is recommended with the use of any NMBA. The same stimulus should be applied to the same muscle fibers over a period of time in order to assess the effectiveness of the NMBA. Upper extremity muscles or facial muscles are routinely used to assess neuromuscular function. Multiple patterns of stimulation are available, such as single twitch, train of four (TOF), tetanic stimulation (TET), and double-burst stimulation (DBS) (Table 4.10).

Single twitch. Single twitch assesses neuromuscular response to a single stimulus. The stimulus can vary from 0.1 Hz (one stimulus every 10 seconds) –1.0 Hz (one stimulus every 1 second). This is the least sensitive method for monitoring neuromuscular function because it requires a baseline stimulus response, and the response

TABLE 4.10 Common Neuromuscular Monitoring Tests

Monitoring Test	Definition	Comments	Stimulation Characteristics
Single twitch	A single supramaximal electrical stimulus ranging from 0.1 to 1.0 Hz	Requires baseline before drug administration; generally used as a qualitative rather than quantitative assessment	
Train of four (TOF)	A series of four twitches at 2 Hz every ½ second for 2 seconds	Reflects blockade from 70%–100%; useful during onset, maintenance, and emergence; TOF ratio is determined by comparing T_1–T_4	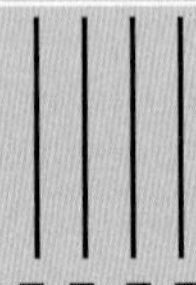
Double-burst simulation	Two short bursts of 50-Hz tetanus separated by 0.75 seconds	Similar to TOF; useful during onset, maintenance, and emergence; may be easier to detect fade than with TOF; tactile evaluation	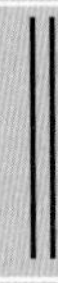
Tetanus	Generally consists of rapid delivery of a 30-, 50-, or 100-Hz stimulus for 5 seconds	Should be used sparingly for deep block assessment; painful	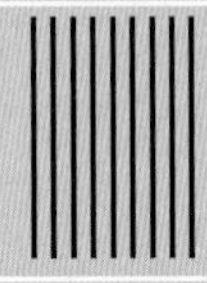
Posttetanic count	50-Hz tetanus for 5 seconds, a 3-second pause, then single twitches of 1 Hz	Used only when TOF and double-burst stimulation are absent; count of less than 8 indicates deep block, and prolonged recovery is likely	

From Elisha S, Heiner JS, Nagelhout JJ. *Nurse Anesthesia*. 7th ed. Elsevier; 2023.

to a single stimulus will not decrease until 75%–80% of the receptors are blocked. In addition, a single-twitch response can vary depending on the temperature, skin resistance, and electrode conductance.

Train of four. TOF assesses neuromuscular function by providing four repetitive stimuli at a frequency of 2 Hz. This is the most common method for monitoring neuromuscular response to NMBA. When using nondepolarizing NMBAs, the response to TOF will manifest as fade unless more than 90% of the receptors are blocked. Fade can first be detected with 70%–75% receptor blockade. Loss of the first twitch represents 75% receptor blockade. Loss of the second twitch correlates to approximately 80% receptor blockade. The third twitch is lost at 90% receptor blockade. The height of the first twitch decreases with an increase in receptor blockade. The fourth twitch disappears when 90%–100% of receptors are blocked (Fig. 4.18).

- A depolarizing block will affect all four twitches to the same degree. The four twitch heights will be similar, although they will decrease in height and then disappear as the depolarizing block progresses. This changes in a phase II block because the depolarizing relaxant assumes the qualities of a nondepolarizing relaxant and is manifested as fade on the TOF.

Tetanic stimulation. TET assesses neuromuscular function in response to high-frequency stimulation. The most common TET stimulus is 50 Hz for 5 seconds. In an unblocked individual, this will result in sustained muscle contraction. However, when nondepolarizing NMBAs are used, the muscle response will fatigue and fade over time, meaning these agents are still bound to ACh receptors. It is also possible to get fade with the use of TET when using only potent inhalational agents.

- *Posttetanic count* is useful with 100% postsynaptic receptor blockade and when there is no response to TOF or TET. The degree of neuromuscular blockade is assessed after a TET stimulus and a subsequent response to single-twitch stimulations. The method

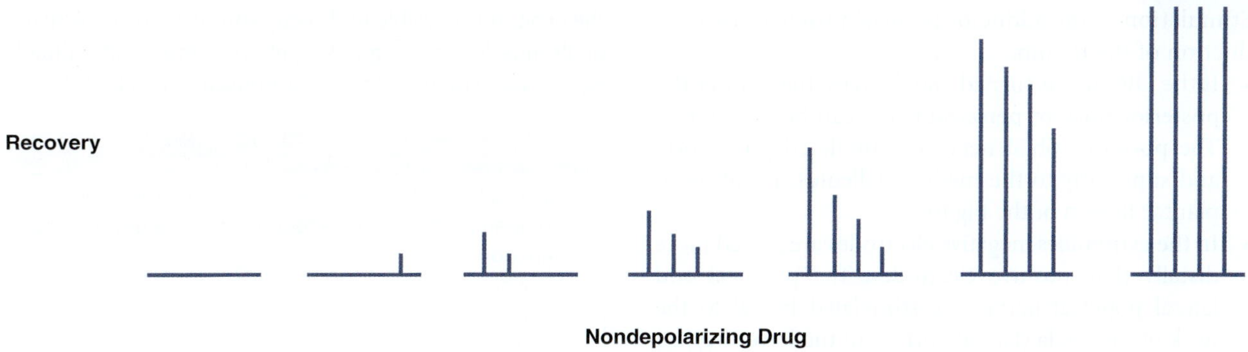

Fig. 4.18 Characteristic train-of-four response during recovery from a nondepolarizing muscle relaxant. (From Elisha S, Heiner JS, Nagelhout JJ. *Nurse Anesthesia*. 7th ed. Elsevier; 2023.)

consists of providing a 5-second stimulation at 50 Hz, then waiting 3 seconds to apply a sequence (usually 10 twitches) of single-twitch stimulations at 1 Hz. The greater the number of posttetanic responses (single twitches), the less the degree of neuromuscular blockade and the sooner the recovery.

Double-burst stimulation. DBS is an alternative method to evaluate fade during neuromuscular blockade. It consists of three 0.2-millisecond impulses at a frequency of 50 Hz, followed by an identical burst 750 milliseconds later. The second response height is compared with the first to detect any difference or fade. The intensity of DBS is of greater magnitude than TOF (but not as great as a tetanic stimulus) to evaluate neuromuscular fade.

Sites of stimulation. Relaxation of upper airway muscles, laryngeal muscles, and the diaphragm is helpful when placing tracheal tubes. Monitoring of neuromuscular blockade helps determine when these optimal intubating conditions occur.

Airway muscles. Airway muscles are rarely monitored clinically unless there is a surgical indication to do so. The airway muscle groups have a faster onset of neuromuscular blockade but are more resistant to blockade over time and thus recover sooner. Increased blood flow to the respiratory muscles may explain why they have a faster onset of blockade.

- Bilateral recurrent laryngeal nerve stimulation can be monitored externally by placing the negative electrode over the thyroid notch and the positive electrode on the chest or forehead. The negative electrode (black) should be placed distally from the nerve being assessed. The positive electrode (red) should be placed along the nerve being assessed. The current moves from the positive (hot) to the negative (ground). Therefore, the positive electrode should be placed over the thyroid notch and the recurrent laryngeal nerve (RLN), and the negative should be placed distally.
- The diaphragm can be stimulated by placing a needle electrode near the phrenic nerve at the inferior posterior border of the sternocleidomastoid muscle.

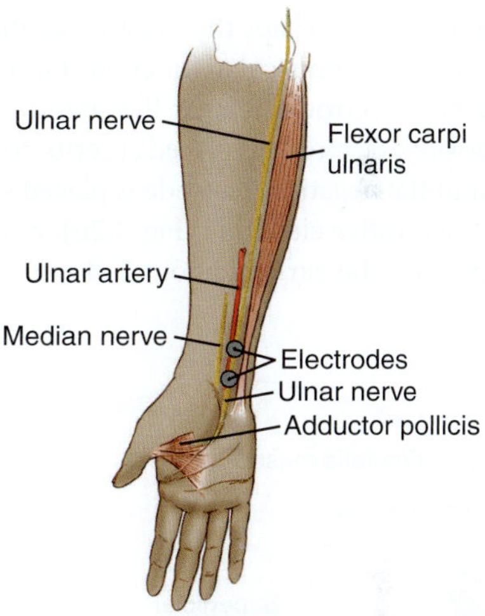

Fig. 4.19 Ulnar neuromuscular blockade testing. (From Elisha S, Heiner JS, Nagelhout JJ. *Nurse Anesthesia*. 7th ed. Elsevier; 2023.)

Upper extremity muscles. The adductor pollicis, abductor digiti quinti, and first dorsal interosseous muscles are innervated by the ulnar nerve. For optimal neuromuscular monitoring of these muscles (primarily the adductor pollicis), the negative electrode is placed distally on the radial side of the flexor carpi ulnaris (closer to center wrist) and 1 cm proximal to the wrist, and the positive electrode is placed proximally either on the volar forearm (inside flat part of the forearm) or over the olecranon groove (Fig. 4.19).

Stimulation of the adductor pollicis muscle causes adduction of the thumb.

- If the OR table is turned 180 degrees, then either the posterior tibial or peroneal nerve can be monitored. The posterior tibial nerve is stimulated posteriorly and superiorly to the medial malleolus, resulting in plantar flexion of the big toe.
- In the extremities, negative electrodes are placed more distally than positive electrodes. The peroneal and lateral popliteal nerves are stimulated lateral to the neck of the fibula (lateral portion of the lower leg just below the knee), resulting in dorsiflexion of the foot.

Facial muscles. Assessment of the orbicularis oculi muscle (surrounding the eye) in response to stimulation of the facial nerve is perhaps the most accessible method for monitoring neuromuscular function. Optimal placement of surface electrodes is near the stylomastoid foramen. The positive electrode is placed anterior to the tragus of the ear, and the negative electrode is placed superior or inferior to the positive electrode (Fig. 4.20). Both are relatively in line with the ear and about 2–3 cm posterior to the orbit. It is possible to directly stimulate the orbicularis oculi muscle, resulting in varying responses and an inadequate assessment of true neuromuscular blockade.

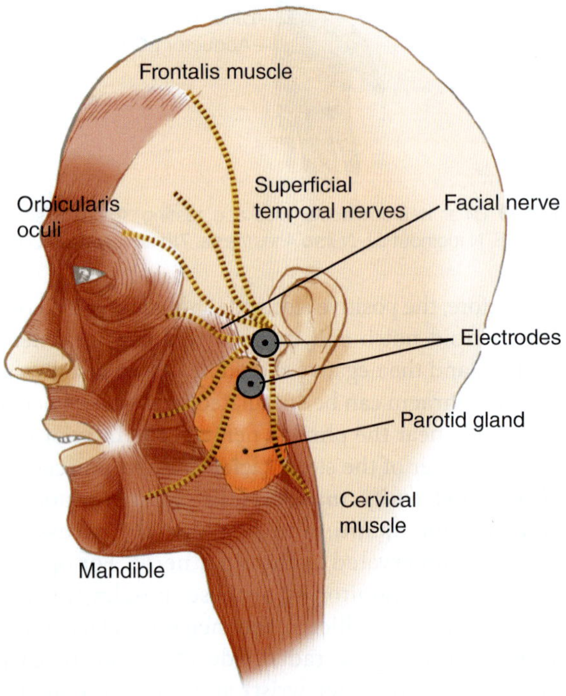

Fig. 4.20 Facial neuromuscular blockade testing. (From Elisha S, Heiner JS, Nagelhout JJ. *Nurse Anesthesia*. 7th ed. Elsevier; 2023.)

KNOWLEDGE CHECK

1. Acetylcholine binds to two _______ receptor subunits to open postsynaptic receptors at the neuromuscular junction.
   a. α
   b. β
   c. δ
   d. ϵ
2. Which ion, released from the sarcoplasmic reticulum, is primarily responsible for muscle contraction?
   a. Sodium
   b. Potassium
   c. Calcium
   d. Magnesium
3. At what percentage of neuromuscular receptor blockade is fade first detected with a TOF stimulus?
   a. 50%
   b. 60%
   c. 70%
   d. 80%
4. Which nerve is best evaluated in the upper extremity during neuromuscular monitoring?
   a. Radial
   b. Ulnar
   c. Median
   d. Axillary
5. A 45-year-old patient undergoing general anesthesia is administered a nondepolarizing NMBA. TOF monitoring shows a loss of the third and fourth twitches. Approximately what percentage of postsynaptic acetylcholine receptors are blocked?
   a. 25%
   b. 50%
   c. 75%
   d. 90%
6. Which of the following best explains why succinylcholine can cause hyperkalemia in patients with denervation injuries?
   a. Decreased acetylcholine release at the presynaptic terminal
   b. Decreased metabolism of succinylcholine by acetylcholinesterase
   c. Upregulation of postsynaptic acetylcholine receptors
   d. Resistance to nondepolarizing muscle relaxants

Answers can be found in Appendix A.

Electroencephalography

Electroencephalography (EEG) is used during cerebrovascular surgery to assess the adequacy of cerebral oxygenation. It records electrical potentials generated by cerebral cortex cells and reports the signals as a waveform with both frequency and amplitude.

- EEG can be used to assess depth of anesthesia because its signals are sensitive to both inhalational and IV anesthetics. EEG monitoring during neurosurgery detects global neurologic changes such as decreased cortical responses, symmetry between the left and right hemispheres, and brain ischemia.
- EEG waveforms include α waves (frequency 7.5–14 Hz) that indicate a resting or relaxing individual whose eyes are closed. Beta waves (frequency 14–40 Hz) are found in persons who are conscious, concentrating, and alert. These waves are more frequently seen during lighter states of anesthesia. Delta waves (frequency 0.5–4 Hz) are present during general anesthesia, deep sleep, or a brain injury. Theta waves (frequency 4–7.5 Hz) are found in persons who are lightly sleeping. Gamma waves (frequency >40 Hz) are present during awake states with high-level information processing (Table 4.11).
- Burst suppression is detected by the EEG and is characterized by periods of high electrical activity followed by no brain activity. Burst suppression is seen during inactivated brain states such as deep general anesthesia, significant hypothermia, or coma.

TABLE 4.11 Comparison of EEG Waveforms

Waveform and Frequency (Hz)	Characteristics
Alpha (7.5–14)	Occurs with eyes closed during deep relaxation
Beta (14–40)	Normal awake consciousness, alertness, logic, and critical thinking
Theta (4–7.5)	Light sleep
Gamma (> 40)	High-level information processing
Delta (0.5–4)	High amplitude, associated with deep sleep

EEG, Electroencephalogram.
From Elisha S, Heiner JS, Nagelhout JJ. *Nurse Anesthesia*. 7th ed. Elsevier; 2023.

- Isoelectricity is a flat EEG signal and signifies deep coma or brain death.
- An easier method for monitoring EEG signals is through power spectral analysis. This method processes the raw EEG signals and frequencies into a series of sine waves that are more easily reported.

Bispectral Index Monitoring

The bispectral index (BIS) monitor is a neurologic monitor developed to detect cognitive awareness during anesthesia. The exact algorithm used to process the EEG data is proprietary.

- The BIS monitor measurement allows the anesthetist to assesses four components within the EEG related to the anesthetized state: (1) processing of low frequencies that are found during deep anesthesia, (2) evaluation of high-frequency β activity that is found during lighter anesthesia, (3) assessment of suppressed and isoelectric EEG, and (4) measurement of the occurrences of burst suppression.
- BIS monitoring also accounts for electromyographic signals when calculating its algorithm. The result of the BIS algorithm is a single number that correlates with anesthesia depth.
- BIS values of 85–100 correlate with a resting or awake individual. Values between 60 and 85 are consistent with varying degrees of sedation. Values between 40 and 60 are recommended for general anesthesia. BIS values less than 40 are associated with burst suppression and isoelectricity (Fig. 4.21). These values indicate very deep anesthesia and are not recommended for prolonged periods of time.

Evoked Potentials

Noninvasive monitors use electrical potentials to assess neural function and detect spinal cord or cerebral ischemia and/or damage. Evoked potentials (EPs) measure electrophysiological responses to both sensory and motor pathways. They can be used as monitoring devices to prevent postoperative deficits and irreversible damage to these pathways. Surgical procedures that use specific EP monitoring and the anesthetic recommendations are listed in Table 4.12. Numerous factors can negatively affect EPs, including anesthetic medications, anemia, hypotension, hypoxia, surgical damage to the brain and/or spinal cord, electrocautery, and monitoring equipment failure.

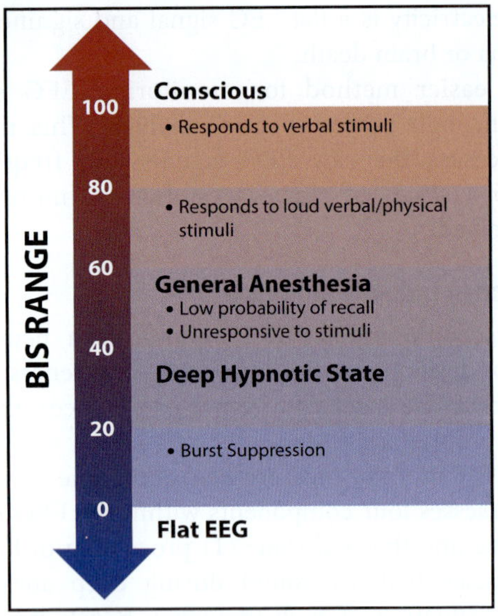

Fig. 4.21 Methods for assessing central nervous system integrity. *BIS*, Bispectral index; *EEG*, electroencephalogram. (From Elisha S, Heiner JS, Nagelhout JJ. *Nurse Anesthesia*. 7th ed. Elsevier; 2023.)

- Neurologic pathway compromise is apparent with an increase in the latency and/or a decrease in the amplitude of EP waveforms.
- Most anesthetics affect EPs to some degree. An important consideration is to maintain constant anesthetic drug levels during EP monitoring because bolus doses or changes in minimum alveolar concentration (MAC) values can distort EP readings.

Somatosensory evoked potentials. SSEPs evaluate the dorsal column (fasciculus cuneatus and gracilis) and lateral ascending sensory pathways of the spinal cord for any damage or ischemia to peripheral nerves. An SSEP consists of an electrical stimulus, via needle electrodes, applied to peripheral sensory nerves.

- The posterior tibial nerve is frequently monitored in the lower extremities, and the median nerve is monitored in the upper extremities. If these sites are not accessible, secondary sites include the common peroneal nerve and the ulnar nerve. As long as the intervening pathways are intact, the electrical impulses will ascend the spinal cord through the posterior columns.

TABLE 4.12 Recommended Monitoring Modalities and Anesthetic Regimens for Surgical Procedures

	MONITORING MODALITIES					ANESTHETIC RECOMMENDATION	
			ELECTROMYOGRAPHY				
Type of Procedure	Somatosensory Evoked Potentials	Transcranial Motor Evoked Potentials	Free Run	Stimulated	Auditory Brainstem Responses	Volatile Inhalational Anesthetics	Total Intravenous Anesthesia
Spine Skeleton							
Cervical	*	*	*				*
Thoracic	*	*	*	*			*
Lumbar instrumentation	*		*	*		*	
Lumbar disc			*	*		*	
Head and Neck							
Parotid			*	*		*	
Radical neck			*	*		*	
Thyroid			*	*		*	
Cochlear implant			*	*		*	
Mastoid			*	*		*	
Neurosurgery							
Spine							
Vascular	*	*					

TABLE 4.12 Recommended Monitoring Modalities and Anesthetic Regimens for Surgical Procedures—cont'd

	MONITORING MODALITIES					ANESTHETIC RECOMMENDATION	
			ELECTROMYOGRAPHY				
Type of Procedure	Somatosensory Evoked Potentials	Transcranial Motor Evoked Potentials	Free Run	Stimulated	Auditory Brainstem Responses	Volatile Inhalational Anesthetics	Total Intravenous Anesthesia
Tumor	*	*					
Posterior fossa							
Acoustic neuroma			*	*	*	*	
Cerebellopontine	*	±	*	*	±		*
Vascular	*	*	*		±		*
Supratentorial							
Middle cerebral artery aneurysm		*					
Tumor in motor cortex	*	*					*

*Recommended for most surgeries; ± recommended for some procedures (depending on specific location of pathology).
Adapted from Jameson LC, Sloan TB. Monitoring of the brain and spinal cord. *Anesthesiol Clin.* 2006;24(4):777–791.

- The impulses are recorded over the dorsal columns (posterior cervical spine). As the electrical volley ascends, it has a primary synapse with several nuclei (e.g., dorsal column nuclei) near the cervicomedullary junction. It then crosses the midline, ascends within the contralateral medial lemniscal pathways, and has a second synapse within the thalamus. The stimulus ends within the contralateral sensory cortex, where it is then measured (Fig. 4.22).
- SSEPs waveforms are affected by volatile inhalational anesthetics. Nitrous oxide potentiates the depressant effects of volatile agents; therefore, it should be minimized or avoided. Small doses of an inhalation agent (<0.5 MAC) can be used in combination with a propofol infusion. Etomidate and ketamine have been shown to cause changes in SSEP latency and amplitude readings and should be avoided. NMBAs, propofol, dexmedetomidine, and opioids cause minimal changes when given within standard dosage ranges. A total intravenous anesthetic (TIVA) using propofol or dexmedetomidine and an opioid is frequently administered via infusion.
- Muscle relaxants do not affect the SSEP waveform monitoring. However, if paralysis is achieved, motor evoked responses cannot be measured.

Visual evoked potentials. Visual evoked potentials (VEPs) are a type of sensory EP that is produced by light stimulation to the eyes. This measures visual pathways that include the retina, optic nerve, optic chiasm, and pathways into the occipital cortex.

- Stimulus during anesthesia is done by stroboscopic flash (luminescence) in front of closed eyelids with goggles. The retinal response is assessed with electrodes that are placed near the eye. These types of EPs can be used to monitor the anterior visual pathways during craniofacial procedures, pituitary surgery, or surgeries that involve the occipital cortex and retrochiasmatic visual tracts.
- Practically, VEPs are less useful than other types of EP monitoring because the bulky goggles used for stimulation are cumbersome, flash stimulation may not provide adequate stimulation, and VEPs are extremely sensitive to anesthetics.

Brainstem auditory evoked potential. Brainstem auditory evoked potential (BAEP) is another type of sensory EP. BAEPs use various sound frequencies to activate the auditory pathways.

- Sound is transmitted through the external and middle ear, the vibrations activate the hair cells of the cochlea, and the stimulus is then transmitted by the distal auditory nerve (cranial nerve VIII) to

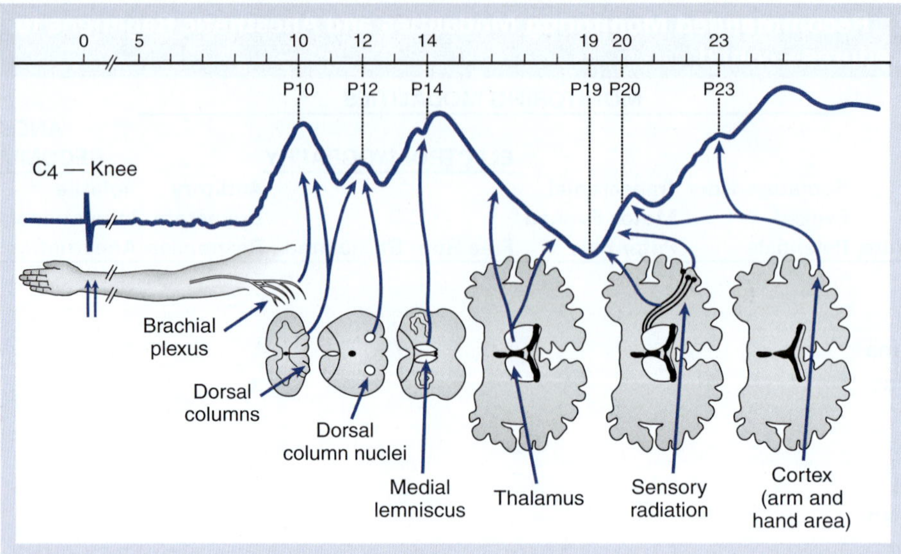

Fig. 4.22 Example of somatosensory-evoked-potential peaks. (From Wiederholt WC, Meyer-Hardting E, Budnick B, et al. Stimulating and recording methods used in obtaining short-latency somatosensory evoked potentials [SEPs] in patients with central and peripheral neurologic disorders. *Ann N Y Acad Sci.* 1982;388:349.)

the midbrain, allowing monitoring of brainstem function.

- The stimulus travels via the brainstem acoustic nuclei and lemniscal pathways to neurons in the auditory cortex. Measurements are taken here, at the brainstem, and over the sensory cortex.
- BAEPs are used during tumor resections of the posterior fossa because this is an area important for hearing, as well as during surgeries involving the brainstem.
- BAEPs are very resistant to interference; therefore most anesthetic regimens are acceptable. Opioids, benzodiazepines, ketamine, nitrous oxide, propofol, and muscle relaxants do not significantly affect BAEPs when administered within standard dosage ranges. Lidocaine infusions and high-dose volatile agents affect BAEP monitoring.
- Hypothermia and hypocapnia should be avoided because they can cause increased latency and prolonged interpeak intervals during BAEP readings.

Motor evoked potentials. Motor evoked potentials (MEPs) monitor the descending motor pathways of the anterior spinal cord for functionality, ischemia, or damage. These can be used to indicate which patients may develop a postoperative motor deficit.

- An MEP is initiated by electrical stimulation of the motor cortex or at the spinal cord itself. The MEP then sends an electrical impulse of stimuli that descends through the anterior horn of the spinal cord via the corticospinal tract. It then synapses with peripheral motor nerves and elicits a motor response to targeted muscles. Monitoring methods for cranial nerves are shown in Table 4.13, and methods for spinal nerves are shown in Table 4.14.
- The stimulus can be recorded from the spinal cord, peripheral nerves, and muscles.
- MEPs are thought to be a more sensitive indicator of spinal cord ischemia than SSEPs. Frequently, both monitoring modalities are used together, especially in spinal surgery.
- NMBAs should be avoided while MEPs are being monitored.
- IV anesthetic techniques using propofol and opioids are frequently used as primary anesthetics for patients undergoing MEP monitoring.

Cerebral Oximetry

Cerebral oximetry involves continuous noninvasive cerebral oxygen saturation using near-infrared spectroscopy (NIRS). The NIRS monitor is ideal because it can penetrate thick brain tissue and evaluate the transmission and absorption of infrared light by hemoglobin.

TABLE 4.13 Monitoring of Cranial Nerves

Cranial Nerve		Monitoring Site or Method[a]
I	Olfactory	No monitoring technique
II	Optic	Visual evoked potentials
III	Oculomotor	Inferior rectus muscle
IV	Trochlear	Superior oblique muscle
V	Trigeminal	Masseter muscle and/or temporalis muscle (sensory responses can also be monitored)
VI	Abducens	Lateral rectus muscle
VII	Facial	Orbicularis oculi and/or orbicularis oris muscles
VIII	Auditory	Auditory brainstem responses
IX	Glossopharyngeal	Stylopharyngeus muscle (posterior soft palate)
X	Vagus Superior laryngeal branch (motor) Recurrent laryngeal branch (motor)	Cricothyroid muscle Posterior cricoarytenoid Lateral cricoarytenoid Thyroarytenoid Transverse arytenoid Oblique arytenoid Thyroepiglottic Aryepiglottic
XI	Spinal accessory	Sternocleidomastoid and/or trapezius muscles
XII	Hypoglossal	Genioglossus muscle (tongue)

[a]Unless otherwise specified, monitoring is performed via electromyographic activity of the muscle(s) listed.
Adapted from Cottrell JE, Patel P. *Cottrell and Patel's Neuroanesthesia*. 6th ed. Elsevier; 2017.

TABLE 4.14 Spinal Nerve Roots and Muscles Most Commonly Monitored

Spinal Cord Nerve(s)		Muscle(s)
Cervical	C2–C4	Trapezius, sternocleidomastoid
	C5, C6	Biceps, deltoids
	C6, C7	Flexor carpi radialis
Thoracic	C8–T1	Adductor pollicis brevis, abductor digiti minimi
	T5–T6	Upper rectus abdominis
	T7–T8	Middle rectus abdominis
	T9–T11	Lower rectus abdominis
	T12	Inferior rectus abdominis
Lumbar	L2	Adductor longus
	L2–L4	Vastus medialis
Lumbosacral	L4–S1	Tibialis anterior
	L5–S1	Peroneus longus
Sacral	S1–S2	Gastrocnemius
	S2–S4	Anal sphincter

From Cottrell JE, Patel P. *Cottrell and Patel's Neuroanesthesia*. 6th ed. Elsevier; 2017.

- Cerebral oximetry and NIRS can help correctly identify decreased oxygenation in the brain areas most vulnerable to changes in oxygen supply and demand (those with high cerebral metabolic rate of oxygen), such as the frontal cortex.
- A probe is placed on the scalp that emits near-infrared light to superficial and deep tissues. Two photodetectors within the probe detect the reflected light from both deep and superficial sources. This technique is similar to pulse oximetry (as described by the Beer-Lambert law) in that oxygenated and deoxygenated hemoglobin absorb light at different frequencies, which can then be reported as a saturated amount. Unlike pulse oximetry, cerebral oximetry and NIRS use two photodetectors with each light source, absorb the light from venous hemoglobin better, and penetrate deep into thick brain tissue, but they do not have the capability to detect arterial pulsatile flow.
- Changes of greater than 25% of the baseline measurement or saturations less than 40% are consistent with decreased cerebral oxygenation. When decreased cerebral oxygenation is identified, management strategies to increase cerebral oxygenation can be promptly initiated. These include increasing the fraction of inspired oxygen (Fio_2), correcting patient position or intravascular cannula position, improving BP and CO, increasing hemoglobin concentration, and/or decreasing cerebral oxygen demand.
- Certain conditions, such as decreased BP, changes in partial pressure of carbon dioxide ($Paco_2$), administration of vasopressors, variations in regional blood flow and volume, hemoglobin concentration, and anatomic tissue variabilities, can affect the accuracy of the NIRS reading. This technology is most often used during neonatal cardiac surgery and during carotid endarterectomy. If cerebral oximetry is employed, a baseline reading should be taken before induction of anesthesia and then used to evaluate for trends. A reading that is maintained within 75% of baseline is considered normal.

Transcranial Doppler Ultrasonography

Transcranial Doppler ultrasonography (TCD) monitors hyperperfusion and hypoperfusion within large arteries of the brain, frequently via the middle cerebral artery, by assessing blood flow velocity and the intensity of pulsatile blood flow.

- Continuous pulsed Doppler ultrasound waves are transmitted and received by an ultrasound probe placed on the temporal bone. These ultrasound waves can detect shifts in frequency that demonstrate the velocity of flowing blood within vessels at the base of the brain.
- Specific parameters measured by TCD include flow direction, peak systolic and end-diastolic flow velocity, flow acceleration time, and the intensity of pulsatile flow.
- This type of monitoring is useful during cerebral aneurysm surgery, carotid endarterectomy, and cardiac surgery to assess for cerebrovascular integrity and the presence of microemboli. TCD is also used to assess for cerebral vasospasm in patients with subarachnoid hemorrhage, can evaluate for hyperperfusion after arteriovenous malformation resections, and has shown value as part of a multimodal monitoring strategy in the assessment of poor cerebral perfusion as a result of increased intracranial pressure (ICP).
- Thick temporal bones, large intracranial lesions, increases in ICP, and cerebral vasospasm can decrease the accuracy of TCD. Factors that affect blood vessel diameter, such as changes in $Paco_2$, alterations in BP, vasoactive drugs, and anesthetic agents, have less influence on TCD.

Jugular Bulb Oxygen Venous Saturation

Jugular bulb oxygen venous saturation monitors mixed venous blood as it exits the brain to provide an estimation of oxygen extraction by the brain.

- Near the inner ear at the base of the skull and within the jugular foramen exists the origin of the interior jugular vein. This is an expanded venous area known as the *jugular bulb*. The jugular bulb is not present at birth but develops in early childhood.
- Each jugular bulb receives blood from both the left and right cerebral hemispheres. The interior jugular vein can be accessed inferior to the mastoid process, and a small jugular venous catheter can be advanced into the jugular bulb under fluoroscopic guidance.
- Mixed venous hemoglobin saturations can be taken from the jugular bulb and provide information regarding cerebral oxygen consumption. This monitoring technique is useful in patients with elevated ICP.

Intracranial Pressure Monitoring

ICP monitors assess for high ICP (i.e., above 15 mm Hg). Invasive monitors are more accurate and include intraventricular catheters, intraparenchymal probes, subdural screws, or epidural sensors placed by a neurosurgeon. Noninvasive monitors are less specific and can be accomplished by evaluating the optic nerve sheath diameter using an ultrasound probe and TCD, by evaluating tympanic membrane displacement, or by computed tomography or magnetic resonance imaging.

- An *intraventricular catheter* (also known as a *ventriculostomy catheter*) is the most precise method for assessing ICP because it measures both direct and global ICP within the ventricles of the brain.
  - These can be difficult to place in patients with existing high ICP levels that cause ventricular compression or displacement. These catheters are placed through a burr hole drilled into the skull and then maneuvered via a ventriculostomy into the lateral ventricle. Cerebrospinal fluid (CSF) can be drained out through the catheter in a process called *external ventricular drainage* in order to help reduce ICP.
  - These catheters are frequently used in patients with hydrocephalus or intraventricular hemorrhage or after a traumatic brain injury with elevated ICP.
  - When ICP values are being monitored, transducers are routinely zeroed at the level of the external auditory meatus. Complications of these monitors include infection, CSF leak or blockage, craniotomy, subdural hematoma, direct cerebral damage from the catheter, and intraventricular hemorrhage.
- *Intraparenchymal probes* are placed through a burr hole and include either a microsensor or fiberoptic transducer that is placed directly into brain tissue (usually the right frontal region). This is another monitor that allows accurate assessment of global ICP. Complications are similar to those with intraventricular catheters.
- *Subdural screws (bolts)* are useful when ICP needs immediate assessment, such as in the emergency department after an acute head injury or if placement of an intraventricular catheter is difficult.
  - These are less accurate techniques for monitoring global ICP. A hollow screw is inserted into the subarachnoid or subdural space through a burr hole. Once in place, these monitors can measure ICP within either the subarachnoid or subdural space and can also drain CSF as needed.
- *Epidural sensors* are the least invasive and least accurate of the four invasive monitors. These sensors are also placed through a burr hole. They are used when placement of an intraventricular catheter is difficult or impossible. The sensor is positioned between the skull and the dural tissue. Unlike the other ICP monitors, this monitoring modality is unable to remove CSF from within the cranial vault.
- *Optic nerve sheath diameter assessment* using ultrasound is a noninvasive method for assessing the presence of increased ICP. This monitoring method can determine the difference between normal and increased (>20 mm Hg) levels.
  - The dural sheath envelops the optic nerve, thus capturing it as part of the central nervous system (CNS). Between the dura and the white matter is the subarachnoid space that communicates with the subarachnoid space surrounding the brain.
  - A normal optic nerve sheath diameter is 5 mm. An increase in ICP causes the dural sheath surrounding the optic nerve to expand to greater than 5 mm. This expansion can be evaluated using transocular ultrasound.
  - Other conditions can affect the diameter of the optic nerve sheath and include tumors, inflammation, Graves disease, and sarcoidosis. Patients with glaucoma or cataracts or those who have experienced facial and orbital trauma should not undergo a transocular ultrasound assessment of the optic nerve.

KNOWLEDGE CHECK

1. Which of the following EEG waveforms is most consistent with a patient under general anesthesia or in deep sleep?
   a. Alpha waves
   b. Beta waves
   c. Delta waves
   d. Gamma waves
2. Which of the following BIS values would most likely indicate a level of anesthesia too deep for prolonged surgical procedures?
   a. 85
   b. 70
   c. 55
   d. 30

Continued

KNOWLEDGE CHECK—cont'd

3. When monitoring SSEPs during spine surgery, which of the following anesthetic techniques is most appropriate?
   a. High-dose volatile agents with nitrous oxide
   b. Etomidate and ketamine boluses
   c. TIVA with propofol and opioid infusion
   d. Large boluses of dexmedetomidine
4. Which of the following statements regarding MEP monitoring is true?
   a. Muscle relaxants enhance the quality of MEP signals.
   b. MEPs monitor the posterior (sensory) spinal pathways.
   c. Volatile anesthetics have no effect on MEPs.
   d. MEPs are more sensitive to spinal cord ischemia than SSEPs.
5. Which EEG waveform is associated with deep sleep and general anesthesia?
   a. α (alpha)
   b. β (beta)
   c. θ (theta)
   d. δ (delta)
6. Which BIS value is within the range for general anesthesia?
   a. 76
   b. 65
   c. 52
   d. 38
7. Which MAC value is recommended if inhalation agents are used during SSEP monitoring?
   a. 0.5
   b. 1.0
   c. 1.3
   d. 1.5
8. Which medication should be avoided when measuring MEPs?
   a. Sevoflurane
   b. Ketamine
   c. Vecuronium
   d. Sufentanil
9. Which factor can cause disruption of evoked potential monitoring? *(Select all that apply.)*
   a. Hypertension
   b. Electrocautery
   c. Sevoflurane
   d. Normothermia
   e. Anemia
10. Which is the most precise method for monitoring increases in ICP?
    a. Intraventricular catheter
    b. Intraparenchymal probe
    c. Subdural screws
    d. Ultrasound of the optic nerve sheath diameter

Answers can be found in Appendix A.

Respiratory Monitoring

Respiratory Gas Monitoring

The most common technologies used to measure anesthetic gases, oxygen, and carbon dioxide include infrared absorption analysis, Raman scattering analysis, and mass spectrometry.

- *Infrared absorption analysis*, also known as *infrared spectroscopy*, is a technique for monitoring how gases absorb specific radiation frequencies on the infrared spectrum. Individual gases can be identified by the specific infrared frequencies each gas absorbs. For example, polar molecules such as carbon dioxide, nitrous oxide, and all of the volatile anesthetic gases absorb infrared radiation at unique points and have unique signatures on the infrared spectrum, allowing them to be recognized individually. Nonpolar molecules such as argon, helium, nitrogen, xenon, and oxygen do not absorb infrared radiation. The concentration of a gas is calculated by the infrared radiation energy it absorbs.
- *Raman scattering analysis*, also known as *Raman spectroscopy*, evaluates the interaction of electromagnetic radiation with matter. This method of gas analysis can be identified either individually or as mixtures of oxygen, carbon dioxide, nitrogen, nitrous oxide, and all volatile anesthetics. Raman scattering analysis uses an intense, coherent, monochromatic laser beam (light) to penetrate a gas mixture. The laser is a high-intensity beam with a known specific electromagnetic radiation frequency. As the laser beam passes through the gas mixture, the gas molecules become excited and scatter while also absorbing light. Each anesthetic gas absorbs specific laser beam frequencies while also scattering at unique laser frequencies. Both scatter frequencies and the amount of laser beam frequency absorption can be measured to identify the concentration of an anesthetic gas. Raman scattering analysis

does not analyze helium and is less accurate when higher gas flow rates or lower tidal volumes (VTs) are used. Therefore, this type of gas analysis is less effective in pediatric patients.

- *Mass spectrometry* was the primary method of gas analysis before newer infrared absorption and scattering technologies. Mass spectrometry essentially identifies and analyzes gases on the basis of their level of deflection by a magnetic field. Gases are collected and passed through a gas ionizer. After the gas molecules are ionized, they are then directed past a magnetic field, which causes them to be deflected. Smaller gas molecules deflect more, and larger gas molecules deflect less. An ion detector collects all of the deflected ionized gases for analysis and can identify them on the basis of their level of deflection by the magnetic field.
- *Oxygen analysis* is of primary importance when delivering an anesthetic. Frequently, more than one technology is used to measure oxygen concentrations during anesthesia. Oxygen has a unique physicochemical property and interaction with electromagnetic radiation, allowing its evaluation by several different technologies.
  - These technologies include electrogalvanic cell (fuel cell) electrochemical oxygen analysis, polarographic electrode (Clark electrode) analysis, paramagnetic oxygen sensor analysis using the magnetomechanical dumbbell principle, paramagnetic transduction, and fluorescence quenching.
  - When a fluorescent molecule is excited to a high-energy state, it releases a proton. If oxygen is present, it will absorb this proton, effectively "quenching" or suppressing the molecules from fluorescing. Therefore, the amount of quenched fluorescence is directly proportional to the concentration of oxygen.
- *Carbon dioxide analysis* can also be performed using several technologies apart from those already discussed.
  - Fluorescence quenching can be used to analyze the concentration of carbon dioxide, although carbon dioxide does not directly "quench" a fluorescent molecule such as oxygen. Instead, carbon dioxide causes a change in pH, which in turn releases hydrogen ions that react with a quenching agent or a fluorescent dye in the sensor. The amount of fluorescent quenching is directly proportional to the concentration of carbon dioxide.
  - Colorimetric carbon dioxide sensor analysis uses a dry-state sensor that undergoes a color change (yellow) in the presence of carbon dioxide. These are sensors that are placed on the end of an ETT and indicate only the presence of carbon dioxide and not the concentration amount. They are helpful immediately after an intubation to verify correct ETT placement. A recommended minimum of six breaths is given to avoid misinterpretation.
  - The Severinghaus carbon dioxide pressure electrode is immersed in bicarbonate solution with a gas-permeable membrane. Carbon dioxide diffuses through this membrane and into the sensor. It then converts to hydrogen ions, creating an electrical charge. This electrical current is proportionate to the concentration of carbon dioxide.

Monitoring Respiration and Ventilation

Monitoring the adequacy of respiration and ventilation is among the most important responsibilities during anesthesia. It is considered one of the primary standard monitoring techniques. In addition to clinically observed patient assessments (i.e., chest rise, lung auscultation, depth and rate of respirations, skin color [cyanosis], capillary refill at nail beds, and upper airway patency), there are several devices that allow the monitoring of both adequate and inadequate respiration.

- *Pulse oximetry* measures the percentage of oxygen bound to hemoglobin. In other words, it calculates the amount of oxygen that saturates hemoglobin. The principles that govern the functions of pulse oximetry primarily focus on the Beer-Lambert law and the fact that oxygenated hemoglobin and deoxygenated hemoglobin are uniquely different molecules and absorb different types of light.
  - The Beer-Lambert law describes how light is absorbed through a medium (e.g., body tissue, blood, and hemoglobin). The Beer portion of this law describes how the amount of light absorbed is proportional to the *concentration* of the light-absorbing substance (e.g., hemoglobin concentration). The Lambert portion of the law describes how the amount of light absorbed is proportional to the *length of the path* that the light travels within the absorbing substance (e.g., vasodilation causing more hemoglobin molecules to be present and absorb light). The application of the Beer-Lambert law in pulse oximetry explains the absorption of

the two light frequencies (infrared and red) by hemoglobin.

- The pulse oximetry probe emits two electromagnetic light sources on one side of the probe, one infrared (not seen by the human eye) and one red (seen by the human eye). The other side contains a light detector that reads how much of each light is absorbed. Oxyhemoglobin and deoxyhemoglobin absorb infrared and red light differently. Oxyhemoglobin absorbs infrared light (at 950 nm) better than deoxyhemoglobin, whereas deoxyhemoglobin absorbs red light (at 650 nm) better than oxyhemoglobin. An alternative way of explaining this concept is that oxyhemoglobin absorbs infrared light better than red light, whereas deoxyhemoglobin absorbs red light better than infrared light. The pulse oximeter calculates the ratio of infrared light to red light absorbed and presents it as an oxygen saturation number.
- The advantages of pulse oximetry include the ability to verify a hemoglobin saturation by viewing a digital display and hearing its corresponding auditory tone. In addition, these devices are inexpensive and portable; readings can be taken from a digit, ear, nose, or the forehead; and these monitors allow the detection of hemoglobin desaturation and hypoxemia.
- Disadvantages of pulse oximetry include (1) reading distortions and errors from artifact and ambient light sources, (2) the inability to detect respiratory rates (RRs), (3) a lag time of several seconds between the real oxygen saturation and pulse oximeter reading, and (4) poor peripheral perfusion (i.e., vasoconstriction, hypothermia, and hypotension) causing difficulty with pulse oximetry readings.
- Other practical applications of the pulse oximeter include the following:
  1. Nondisposable pulse oximeters are a likely source of contamination; therefore, disposable probes should be used whenever possible.
  2. Nail polish has a minimal impact on pulse oximetry readings. If readings are unreliable, rotate the probe 90 degrees so that it is measuring from the sides of the fingertip.
  3. The photoplethysmogram waveform indicates a true mechanical (perfusing) heart rate.
  4. If a probe has been repositioned and continues to remain unreliable, consider poor peripheral perfusion or hypoxemia as causes of the low reading.
  5. Fingertips, earlobes, the nose, and the forehead are the best locations for pulse oximetry readings because they contain many capillaries and arterioles.
- *End-tidal carbon dioxide (ETco2) capnography* is a standard respiratory monitor that allows continuous CO_2 waveform analysis throughout the respiratory cycle. Continuous $ETco_2$ measurements are performed using infrared analysis with primarily a diverting monitor (extracts gas from sample tubing attached to the patient and pumps it to a monitor for evaluation). This type of monitoring can assess RR and the quality of ventilation. The capnometry value that is expressed on the monitor is routinely 4–7 mm Hg lower than the actual blood $Paco_2$ in patients with zero pulmonary shunt. This is due to dilution of CO_2 within the anatomical dead space of the airway before it reaches the sampling line.
  - There are four phases of a normal capnogram waveform that are present in an intubated patient who is mechanically ventilated: (1) baseline (inspiration and inspiratory pause), which approximates zero because it is measuring the anatomic dead space where no CO_2 is present; (2) expiratory upstroke is a combination of dead-space gases and alveolar gases with some CO_2; (3) expiratory plateau represents the exhalation of CO_2 from the alveoli; and (4) the descent to original baseline signals a rapid decrease in CO_2 as a result of the inspiration of air and O_2. At the end of the expiratory plateau, just before the descent to baseline, is the point where the $ETco_2$ concentration is measured.
  - The capnogram can discriminate between normal and abnormal patterns of ventilation (Figs. 4.23 and 4.24), discriminate between spontaneous and

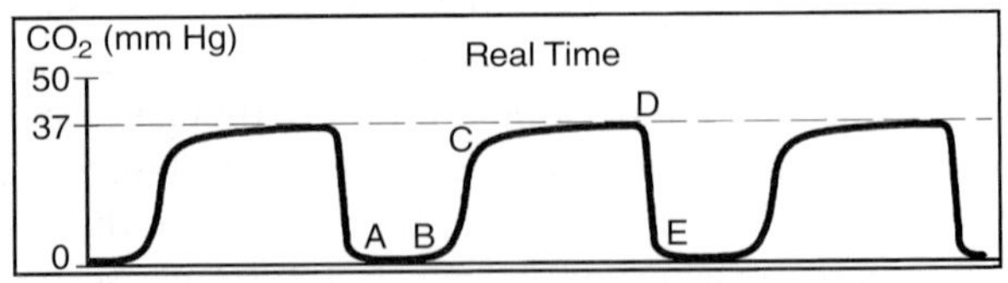

Fig. 4.23 The four phases of a normal capnogram. *A–B* represents baseline, *B–C* represents expiratory upstroke, *C–D* represents expiratory plateau, *D* represents end-tidal concentration, and *D–E* represents inspiration and descent to original baseline. (Courtesy Respironics, Inc., Murrysville, PA.)

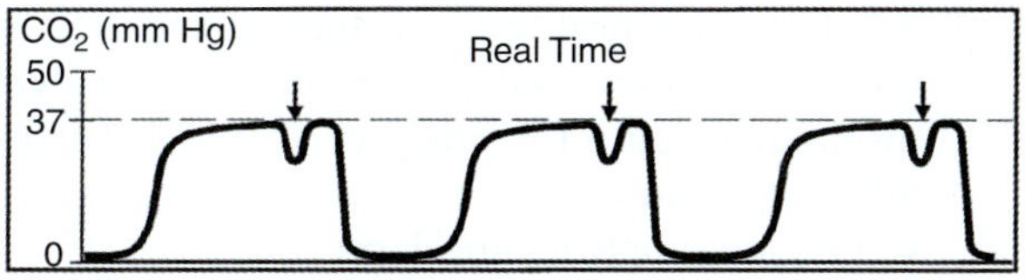

Fig. 4.24 Clefts displayed as an asynchronous spontaneous respiration with controlled ventilation. (Courtesy Respironics, Inc., Murrysville, PA.)

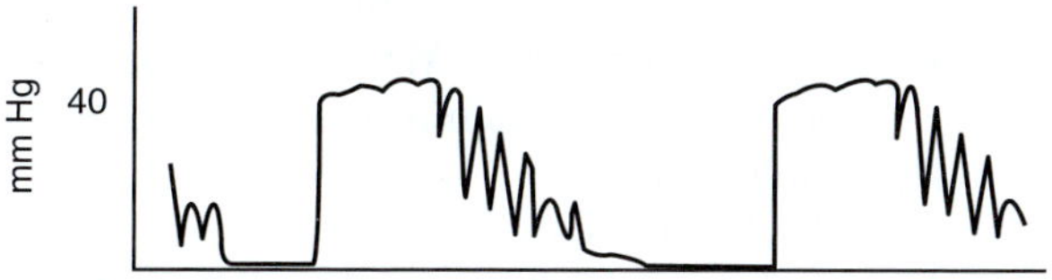

Fig. 4.25 Cardiac oscillations occur as a result of contractions of the heart and great vessels. (From Miller RD. *Miller's Anesthesia.* 8th ed. Elsevier; 2015.)

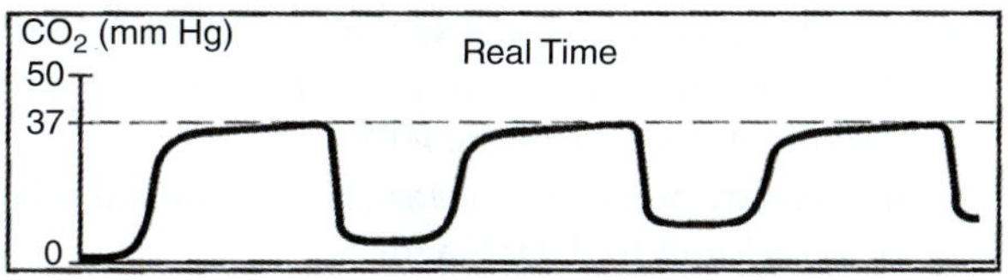

Fig. 4.26 Elevation of the baseline indicates rebreathing of CO_2. (Courtesy Respironics, Inc., Murrysville, PA.)

mechanical ventilation, indicate anesthesia system problems, and indicate patient responses during anesthesia (i.e., initiation of spontaneous breathing during positive-pressure ventilation). Altered capnographic values are possible when the patient has significant ventilation and perfusion mismatching, when values are obtained from the stomach after an esophageal intubation, from cardiac oscillations that occur as a result of heart and great vessel contractions (Fig. 4.25), or if the patient shows any type of expiratory airflow obstruction (i.e., bronchospasm). The capnogram waveform may not return to baseline if there is an inadequate fresh gas flow or an exhausted carbon dioxide absorber (Fig. 4.26). Several conditions cause an increase or decrease in $ETco_2$ (Box 4.2).

- The *precordial* or *esophageal stethoscope* is a respiratory monitoring device that provides information on both respiration and ventilation. A precordial stethoscope is placed on the patient's left chest and allows the operator to hear the quality of breath sounds as well as the RR. It is placed on the left chest in order to identify a right mainstem intubation because this side is more common. Additionally, heart sounds may also be auscultated. The stethoscope uses a bell-type device connected distally to a monophonic tube that tracks up to the operator's ear and proximally connects to a customized single-side earpiece. Some

BOX 4.2 Causes of High and Low End-Tidal Carbon Dioxide

Increased $ETco_2$

Increased CO_2 Delivery/Production

Malignant hyperthermia, fever, sepsis, seizures, increased metabolic rate or skeletal muscle activity, bicarbonate administration/medication side effect, laparoscopic surgery, clamp/tourniquet release

Hypoventilation

COPD, neuromuscular paralysis or dysfunction, CNS depression, metabolic alkalosis (if spontaneously breathing), medication side effect, inadequate minute ventilation

Equipment Problems

CO_2 absorbent exhaustion, ventilator leak, rebreathing, malfunctioning inspiratory or expiratory valve

Decreased $ETco_2$

Decreased CO_2 Delivery/Production

Hypothermia, hypometabolism, pulmonary hypoperfusion, low cardiac output or arrest, pulmonary artery embolism, hemorrhage, hypotension, hypovolemia, V/Q mismatch or shunt, auto-PEEP, medication side effect

Hyperventilation

Pain/anxiety, awareness/"light" anesthesia, metabolic acidosis (if spontaneously breathing), medication side effect

Equipment Problems

Ventilator disconnection, esophageal intubation, bronchial intubation, complete airway obstruction or apnea, sample line problems (kinks), endotracheal tube or laryngeal mask airway leaks

CNS, Central nervous system; *CO_2,* carbon dioxide; *COPD,* chronic obstructive pulmonary disease; *$ETco_2$,* end-tidal carbon dioxide; *PEEP,* positive end-expiratory pressure; *V/Q,* ventilation–perfusion.

Adapted from Sandberg WS, Urman RD, Ehrenfeld JM. *The MGH Textbook of Anesthetic Equipment.* Elsevier; 2011.

precordial devices now have Bluetooth wireless capabilities and do not require a monophonic tube. Placement is recommended after the patient is in the OR and before the induction of anesthesia in order to assess for left-sided breath sounds immediately after intubation or supralaryngeal device placement. These devices are also helpful when monitoring the quality of a patient's respiration during sedation only.

- *Acoustic monitoring transducers* are devices that can be placed on the chest of pediatric patients or on the upper neck of adult patients in order to sense turbulent airflow within the upper airway. Signal-processing algorithms convert the acoustic patterns detected by the sensors into breath cycles in order to calculate an RR. The primary purpose of these respiratory monitors is to alert to the presence of apnea. They are useful in obese patients with large amounts of chest tissue or with loud room noises, both of which are limitations of the precordial stethoscope. Acoustic monitoring devices have been used successfully in the postanesthesia care unit to identify postoperative apnea.
- *Oxygen analyzers and apnea (disconnect) alarms* are required components of the anesthesia workstation and are based on standard ASTM F1850 regulated by the American Society for Testing and Materials (ASTM). All anesthesia workstations must include the following:
  - An inspired oxygen analyzer with a high-priority alarm sounding within 30 seconds of oxygen falling below 18%. The paramagnetic analyzer is the most widely used inspired oxygen analyzer. An electrochemical (galvanic fuel cell) analyzer is the other sensor that may be used to analyze inspired oxygen. The analyzer should have the following features:
  - Oxygen supply failure alarm
  - A nitrous oxide–oxygen proportioning system (hypoxic guard or fail-safe) that prohibits inspired oxygen from falling to less than 23%–25%
  - High-priority alarms that are unable to be silenced for more than 2 minutes
  - Apnea (disconnect) alarms that are enabled as soon as the first breath is sensed and assess for the following:
    - Lack of $ETco_2$
    - Failure to reach a normal peak inspiratory pressure (PIP)
    - Failure to sense an exhaled volume
    - Low-pressure leak
    - Failure of the bellows to fill during exhalation
- The most common site for an anesthesia circuit disconnection is between the breathing circuit and the connector to the ETT.
- The electrical supply cord is either nondetachable or is resistant to detachment.
- Alarm fatigue resulting in missed alarm recognition is considered a serious health technology hazard. Hence, safety recommendations include avoiding permanently silencing alarms.
- If a machine failure occurs, immediately proceed to manual ventilation with a bag-mask device connected to high-flow oxygen.

KNOWLEDGE CHECK

1. Which type of gas analysis uses the deflection of ionized gas molecules to determine their total concentrations?
   a. Infrared absorption
   b. Photoacoustic gas
   c. Raman scattering
   d. Mass spectrometry
2. A pulse oximeter uses which type of light on the electromagnetic spectrum to assess for oxygenated hemoglobin?
   a. Infrared
   b. Red
   c. Ultraviolet
   d. Visible
3. Safety regulations prohibit high-priority alarms from being silenced for more than
   a. 30 seconds.
   b. 60 seconds.
   c. 90 seconds.
   d. 120 seconds.
4. Which phase of the capnography waveform measures the concentration of exhaled CO_2?
   a. 1
   b. 2
   c. 3
   d. 4

KNOWLEDGE CHECK—cont'd

5. Which of the following respiratory gas monitoring technologies is *ineffective* at measuring oxygen concentrations because of the gas's nonpolar nature?
   a. Infrared absorption analysis
   b. Raman scattering analysis
   c. Mass spectrometry
   d. Paramagnetic oxygen analysis
6. Which monitoring technique is most appropriate for verifying ETT placement immediately after intubation?
   a. Severinghaus CO_2 electrode
   b. Stethoscope auscultation
   c. Capnography with waveform analysis
   d. Pulse oximetry
7. Which of the following causes of decreased $ETCO_2$ is *not* related to ventilation–perfusion mismatch?
   a. Esophageal intubation
   b. Pulmonary embolism
   c. Hypovolemia
   d. Bronchospasm
8. Which of the following is a limitation of Raman scattering analysis for gas monitoring?
   a. Inability to detect volatile anesthetic agents
   b. Inability to analyze mixtures of gases
   c. Reduced accuracy at low tidal volumes and high flow rates
   d. Interference by ambient light sources

Answers can be found in Appendix A.

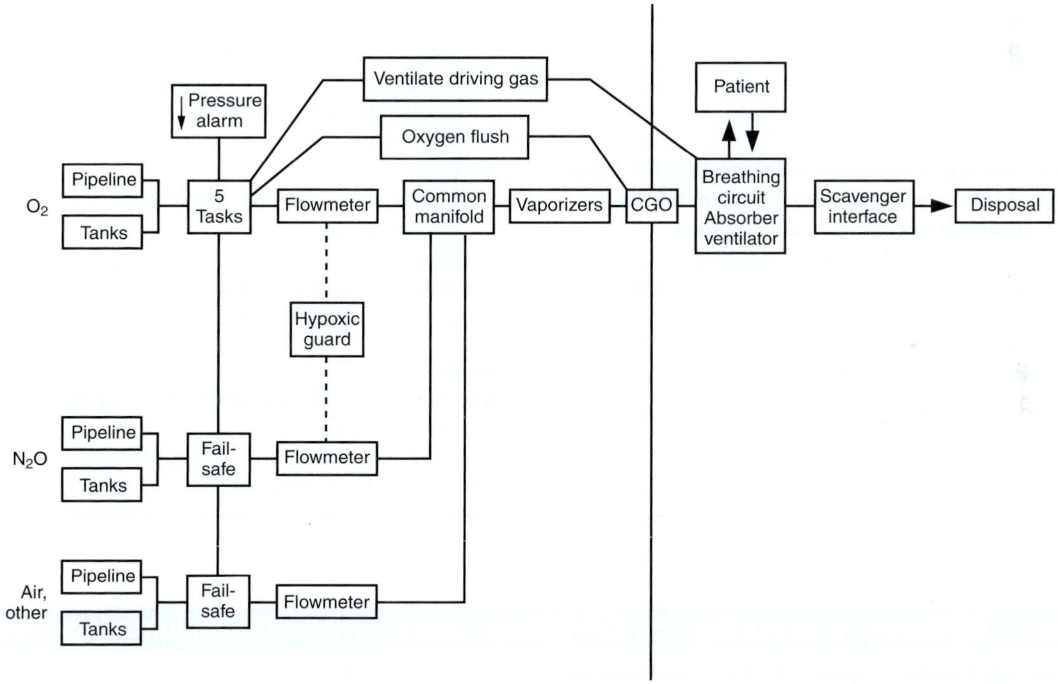

Fig. 4.27 Supply, processing, delivery, and disposal (SPDD) model. *CGO*, Common gas outlet. (Courtesy Michael P. Dosch.)

ANESTHESIA GAS MACHINE

Organization of an Anesthesia Gas Machine

- The model in Fig. 4.27 depicts the path of gas flow from entering the OR to disposal.
- Gas flows in the diagram generally proceed from left to right.
- The vertical bar separates components within the machine and proximal to the common gas outlet (left side) from external components downstream from the common gas outlet (right).
- Oxygen is central to the figure because it is the most essential gas delivered.

- The model organizes the information on the basis of how components are used rather than the pressures to which they are exposed.
- From the viewpoint of pressure to which components are exposed, components are classified as part of the high-, intermediate-, or low-pressure systems within (proximal to the common gas outlet) the gas machine (see Boxes 4.3 and 4.4; see Fig. 4.27).

BOX 4.3 Components in Supply, Processing, Delivery, and Disposal (Spdd) Model

Supply

How Do Gases Come to the Anesthesia Gas Machine? (Site: Back of the Machine)

- Pipeline
  - Wall outlets
  - Connecting valves and hoses
  - Filters and check valves
  - Pressure gauges
- Cylinders
  - Hanger yokes (yoke block)
  - Filters and check valves
  - Pressure gauge
  - Pressure regulators

Processing

How Does the Anesthesia Gas Machine Prepare Gases Before Their Delivery to the Patient? (Site: Within the Machine, Proximal to Common Gas Outlet)

- Fail-safe (oxygen pressure-failure devices)
- Flowmeters (main, auxiliary, common gas outlet, scavenging)
- Oxygen flush
- Low-oxygen-pressure alarms
- Ventilator-driving gas
- Proportioning systems (hypoxic guard)
- Oxygen second-stage regulator (if present)
- Vaporizers
- Check valves distal to vaporizers (if present)
- Common gas outlet

Delivery

How Is the Interaction of Gases With the Patient Controlled and Monitored? (Site: Breathing Circuit)

- Gas delivery hose connecting common gas outlet and breathing circuit
- Breathing circuits
  - Nonrebreathing
  - Circle
- Carbon dioxide absorption
- Ventilators
- Integral monitors
  - Oxygen analysis
  - Disconnect
  - Spirometry (volumes and flows), capnography, airway pressure
- Ventilator alarms
- Addition of positive end-expiratory pressure
- Means of humidification

Disposal

How Are Gases Disposed of? (Site: Scavenger)

- Scavenger systems
  - Interface: closed (active and passive) or open
  - Scavenger flowmeter

From Elisha S, Heiner JS, Nagelhout JJ. *Nurse Anesthesia*. 7th ed. Elsevier; 2023.

BOX 4.4 Components in the High-, Intermediate-, and Low-Pressure Pneumatic Systems

High-Pressure System (Exposed to Cylinder Pressure)

- Hanger yoke
- Yoke block with check valves
- Cylinder pressure gauge
- Cylinder pressure regulators

Intermediate-Pressure System (Exposed to Pipeline Pressure of Approximately 50 psi)

- Pipeline inlets, check valves, and pressure gauges
- Ventilator power inlet
- Oxygen pressure-failure devices
- Flowmeter valve
- Oxygen second-stage regulator (if present)
- Flush valve

Low-Pressure System (Distal to Flowmeter Needle-Valve)

- Flowmeter tubes
- Vaporizers
- Check valves (if present)
- Common gas outlet

From Elisha S, Heiner JS, Nagelhout JJ. *Nurse Anesthesia*. 7th ed. Elsevier; 2023.

Pipeline Supply

Configuration

- Oxygen is delivered to facilities and stored as a liquid at a temperature of −160°C.
- The liquid oxygen is converted to a gas and supplied to hospital pipelines at a pressure of 50 psi.
- In the OR, main and partial area shutoff valves are present to isolate sections with leaks, interrupt supply in case of fire, and allow repair work on subsections.
  - Wall outlets or hoses dropped from the OR ceiling are finished with quick-connect couplers. These couplers are used so that the connection of gas machine supply hoses to wall outlets does not require tools.
  - Nitrous oxide is delivered to the hospital in large (size H) cylinders, which are connected to a manifold. Regulators reduce the pressure so that nitrous oxide, like oxygen, is supplied to the pipelines at 50 psi.
  - 50 psi is the normal working pressure of the anesthesia gas machine.
  - Delivery piping for both nitrous oxide and oxygen uses the *Diameter Index Safety System* to prevent misconnections.
- Supply hoses connect the pipeline inlets on the back of the machine to the wall outlets.
- At the pipeline inlet, a filter, check valve, and pressure gauge are present, ensuring unidirectional forward flow so that a machine running on cylinder supplies, with the hoses disconnected at the wall outlet, does not leak.

Loss of oxygen pipeline pressure

- Loss of oxygen pipeline pressure is indicated by the pipeline pressure gauge.
- If pressure loss is profound, the oxygen low-pressure alarm sounds, and the fail-safe valves halt the delivery of all other gases.
  - Newer machines are designed to switch to air to drive the ventilator bellows when oxygen pipeline pressure is lost.
  - A "whistle" or audio alarm will sound if oxygen pipeline pressure becomes low.
  - With complete loss of oxygen pipeline pressure, the anesthetist should fully open the E cylinder of oxygen, disconnect the pipeline, and consider the use of low fresh gas flows and manual ventilation (using the circle system) to conserve the emergency cylinder supply of oxygen (Box 4.5).

Cylinder Supply

- Cylinders are present on the anesthesia gas machine as reserves for emergency use.

BOX 4.5 Management of Oxygen Pipeline Supply Failure or Crossover

Always check for the presence of a full E cylinder and an alternative means of ventilation (bag-valve-mask [Ambu] device) before using an anesthesia machine. If pipeline pressure fails or fraction of inspired oxygen drops, follow these steps:

1. Do not attempt to fix the oxygen analyzer—it must be trusted until it can be proved that the measurement is incorrect.
2. Turn on backup oxygen cylinder on back of anesthesia gas machine, and disconnect pipeline hose. Ensure that the measured fraction of inspired oxygen (FiO_2) begins to rise.
3. If the FiO_2 does not increase (with fresh gas flow adequate to wash in the O_2 quickly), ventilate the patient by using Ambu bag with room air.
4. Use low flows of oxygen. Maintain anesthesia with a volatile agent. Ensure that FiO_2 and agent concentration are appropriate.
5. Turn off the ventilator and ventilate manually through the circle system.
6. Call for help if needed; calculate the time remaining for the current cylinder; call for additional oxygen cylinders and install them on the machine if needed.
7. Find out how long the problem is expected to last; participate in the hospital disaster plan, which may require prioritizing oxygen for those patients who need it most.
8. Do not reconnect patient to pipeline gas until the gas supply is tested.
9. If unable to use the circle, ventilate with an oxygen source (freestanding cylinder) or with room air via a bag-valve-mask device, and institute total IV anesthesia.

From Elisha S, Heiner JS, Nagelhout JJ. *Nurse Anesthesia*. 7th ed. Elsevier; 2023.

- Cylinders should be opened only when they are checked or when the pipeline supply is unavailable.
- An oxygen cylinder must be checked daily and changed if the PSI (pounds per square inch) is inadequate.
  - Cylinders are labeled, marked, and color-coded.
  - Each cylinder valve has a unique arrangement of holes that correspond to its intended contents. The *Pin Index Safety System (PISS)* decreases the potential for the incorrect cylinder contents to be administered. The holes mate with pins in the yoke, which is the point where cylinders are attached to the anesthesia machine. The PISS is also another means of preventing misconnections (Table 4.15).

Electrical Power Supply

- New gas machines must be equipped with battery backup sufficient for at least 30 minutes of limited operation.
- Patient monitors (e.g., ECG, NIBP, gas analysis, pulse oximetry), fresh gas flowmeters, vaporizers, and ventilators may or may not continue to function during the period that battery backup is used. Electrical receptacles are usually found on the back of the machine so that monitors or other equipment can be plugged in.
- It is not advised to plug devices that convert electrical power into heat into plugs on the back of the anesthesia machine (air or water warming blankets, IV fluid warmers); they are likely to cause a circuit breaker to open, resulting in a power failure.
- Devices that typically require wall outlet electrical power include mechanical ventilators, physiologic monitors, room and surgical field illumination, digital flowmeter displays for electronic flowmeters, cardiopulmonary bypass pump/oxygenators, air warming blankets, gas/vapor blenders (Tec 6, GE HealthCare, Chicago, IL), and vaporizers with electronic controls (Aladin cassettes in the Aisys, GE HealthCare).

Loss of main electrical power

- With power failure in older anesthesia gas machines, the principal problems are loss of room illumination and failure of mechanical ventilators and electronic patient monitoring.
- New anesthesia gas machines have battery backup sufficient for 30 minutes of operation; however, they are typically without patient monitors (e.g., ECG, pulse oximetry, gas analysis).
- Mechanical ventilation may or may not be powered by the backup battery (depending on the model).
- New flowmeters that are entirely electronic (Aisys and Avance, GE HealthCare) require a backup pneumatic/mechanical (needle-valve and flow tube) flowmeter.
- Mechanical flowmeters with digital display of flows have a backup glass flow tube that indicates total fresh gas flow (ADU65 and Fabius GS66, GE HealthCare; Apollo, Dräger Medical, Lübeck, Germany).
- New gas machines with mechanical needle-valve flowmeters and variable bypass vaporizers (e.g., Fabius GS, Apollo, Aespire, and Aestiva, GE HealthCare) have an advantage in that delivery of gases and agents can continue indefinitely during electrical power failure.
- It is essential to have a self-inflating manual ventilation device (i.e., Ambu bag) always available during use of the anesthesia gas machine as a backup bag-mask ventilation strategy.

TABLE 4.15 E-Cylinder Characteristics[a]

Gas	Color, US (International)	Service Pressure psi ($kPa \times 10^{-2}$)	Capacity (L)	Pin Position
Oxygen	Green (white)	1900 (131)	660	2–5
Nitrous oxide	Blue (blue)	745 (51)	1590	3–5
Air	Yellow (black and white)	1900 (131)	625	1–5

[a]Note that slightly different values may be found in different sources.

Data from Dorsch JA, Dorsch SE. *A Practical Approach to Anesthesia Equipment.* Lippincott Williams & Wilkins; 2011; American Society for Testing and Materials. *Standard Specification for Particular Requirements for Anesthesia Workstations and Their Components* (F1850-00). American Society for Testing and Materials; 2005; National Fire Protection Association, *NFPA 99. Health Care Facilities.* National Fire Protection Association; 2012: Table 5.1.11.

Oxygen Pathway Through the Anesthesia Gas Machine

Oxygen flows from the oxygen inlet to the (1) fresh gas flowmeter and (2) oxygen flush valve.

Oxygen Analysis and Hypoxic Guard

- All current anesthesia gas machines incorporate nitrous oxide–oxygen proportioning (hypoxic guard) systems designed to prevent the delivery of hypoxic breathing mixtures.
- All link oxygen and nitrous oxide flows so that final breathing mixtures at the common gas outlet are at least 23%–25% oxygen.
- The ratio of nitrous oxide to oxygen is thus kept at no more than 3 to 1.
- The proper use of a calibrated oxygen analyzer in each general anesthetic is vital.
- Systems that warn of trouble with oxygen supply (low-pressure alarms) or lessen the chances of hypoxemia (hypoxic guard system, fail-safe system) are based on pressure within the oxygen circuitry of the gas machine.
- Monitoring inspired oxygen is mandatory with every general anesthetic, and the function of the oxygen monitor must be checked before providing anesthesia care.
- Two types of sensors are in current use: the electrochemical or galvanic fuel cell (Aestiva, Aespire) and the paramagnetic analyzer (in most other models).

Carbon Dioxide Absorption

- Carbon dioxide absorption makes rebreathing of exhaled gas possible while preventing rebreathing of CO_2.
- Fresh gas flow determines the amount of rebreathing in the circle system.
- Exhausted CO_2 granules cause an increase in expired and inspired CO_2.
- The correct response to hypercarbia associated with exhausted absorbent is increasing fresh gas flow (and then changing the absorbent at the end of the case), whereas this can be accomplished during the delivery of anesthesia and other gases with the newer absorbent canister designs.
- The two most common reasons for an increase in inspired CO_2 are that the absorbent granules have been exhausted or the unidirectional valves are faulty (Boxes 4.6 and 4.7).

BOX 4.6 Recommendations on the Safe Use of Carbon Dioxide Absorbents

1. Use carbon dioxide absorbents with lower (or no) amounts of strong bases (particularly potassium hydroxide [KOH]).
2. Create institutional, hospital, and/or departmental policies regarding steps to prevent desiccation of the carbon dioxide absorbent.
3. Turn off all gas flow when the machine is not in use.
4. Change the absorbent regularly (e.g., every Monday morning).
5. Change absorbent whenever the color change indicates exhaustion.
6. Change all absorbent, not just one canister in a two-canister system.
7. Change absorbent when uncertain of the state of hydration, such as when the fresh gas flow has been left on for an extensive or indeterminate time period.
8. If compact canisters are used, consider changing them more frequently.
9. Low flows also have a role in preserving humidity in absorbent granules. Using relatively low fresh gas flows for most procedures and changing flows from high to low as soon as practical is desirable.

From Elisha S, Heiner JS, Nagelhout JJ. *Nurse Anesthesia*. 7th ed. Elsevier; 2023.

BOX 4.7 Clinical Signs of Carbon Dioxide–Absorbent Exhaustion

Early

- Increase in partial pressure of end-tidal carbon dioxide; an increase in inspired (a specific sign) and expired (a nonspecific sign) carbon dioxide
- Respiratory acidosis
- Hyperventilation
- Signs of sympathetic nervous system activation (flushed appearance, cardiac irregularities, sweating)
- Increased bleeding at surgical site
- Color of indicator

Late

- Increase (and later a decrease) in heart rate and blood pressure
- Dysrhythmias

From Elisha S, Heiner JS, Nagelhout JJ. *Nurse Anesthesia*. 7th ed. Elsevier; 2023.

Use of Vaporizers

- Contemporary vaporizers are secured to the anesthesia machine in manifolds that hold two or three units.
- The operator is prevented from delivering more than one agent simultaneously by an interlock system.
- The interlock mechanism ensures that only one vaporizer is on, that gas enters only the one that is on, that all vaporizers are locked in so that leaks are decreased, and that trace vapor output is minimal when a vaporizer is off.
- Keyed-filler types are preferred because they lessen the chance that filling with the incorrect agent will occur.
- Overfilling may result in discharge of liquid anesthetic from the vaporizer outlet, which can cause injury to the patient.

Modes of Ventilation

Volume-Controlled Ventilation

- During volume-controlled ventilation (VCV), the desired tidal volume (VT) is delivered at a constant flow.
- The ventilator is volume limited and time cycled, and a constant flow is used.
- Inspiration is terminated when the desired VT is delivered or if an excessive inspiratory pressure is reached (most anesthesia ventilator systems have default PIP alarms set at 35 cm H_2O).
- Patients under general anesthesia often have decreased functional residual capacity and pulmonary compliance.
- Because the volume is controlled, alveolar ventilation and arterial carbon dioxide can be maintained despite changes in pulmonary function.
- However, with VCV, the peak inspiratory pressure (PIP) is uncontrolled and rises as the patient's compliance decreases or airway resistance increases.
- VT is adjusted to prevent atelectasis, and respiratory rate (RR) is adjusted to keep $ETCO_2$ at the desired value.
- VTs in the range of 5–7 mL/kg ideal (predicted) body weight, with PEEP (5–10 cm H_2O) and alveolar recruitment maneuvers, are currently advocated to avoid the dangers of atelectasis and ventilator-induced lung injury.
- PIP is monitored but not controlled.

Pressure-Controlled Ventilation

- PIP (Pmax) is limited, and the cycle is controlled by time, with a decelerating flow pattern.
- In a decelerating flow pattern, inspiratory flow is strongest early in inspiration (to reach the set pressure quickly) and declines to flow just sufficient to maintain the set pressure later in inspiration.
- This flow pattern increases lung inflation and oxygenation at the lowest PIP.
- However, the increase in mean airway pressure may decrease venous return and CO. Inspiratory pressure is controlled rather than volume (as with VCV).
- VT is uncontrolled and increases if compliance increases or airway resistance falls.
- If the desired VT is not obtained, either Pmax or inspiratory rise (the rate of inspiratory flow) can be increased.
- Target pressure is adjusted for the desired VT; RR is adjusted to maintain a reasonable $ETCO_2$.
- In patients with low pulmonary compliance (e.g., morbidly obese), pressure control ventilation (PCV) may result in an increased VT at a lower PIP than with VCV, especially if PIP had been high when employing VCV (e.g., in laparoscopic abdominal or pelvic surgery).
- VT must be monitored closely in PCV. During PCV, if pulmonary compliance drops (e.g., application of pneumoperitoneum) or airway resistance increases (e.g., bronchospasm, kinked or obstructed ETT), delivered VT may drop substantially.
- Conversely, if pulmonary compliance improves (e.g., release of pneumoperitoneum, return to supine from steep Trendelenburg position) or airway resistance decreases, VT may increase substantially.
- Typical initial settings for PCV in an adult include pressure limit 12–20 cm H_2O, RR 6–12 breaths per minute, and inspiratory/expiratory ratio 1:2. PEEP 5–10 cm H_2O may be added to help prevent atelectasis.

Synchronized Intermittent Mandatory Ventilation

- With the advent of supraglottic airways, such as the laryngeal mask airway (LMA), and the prevalence of ambulatory or office-based surgical procedures, spontaneous unassisted breathing during general anesthesia has become much more common.
- Ventilation modes that support a spontaneously breathing patient (i.e., provide normocapnia without bucking) include synchronized intermittent mandatory ventilation (SIMV), pressure support ventilation (PSV), continuous positive airway pressure, and airway pressure release ventilation.

- On newer anesthesia machines, SIMV may be selected based on either pressure- or volume-controlled breaths.
- Typical settings for SIMV mirror those used for VCV (or PCV if a pressure-controlled mode is chosen).
- In SIMV, the intermittent mandatory breaths are delivered in synchrony with the patient's spontaneous efforts.
- Trigger window (percentage) and sensitivity may need to be adjusted. Any spontaneous breaths occurring outside the trigger window for the next large mandatory breath may also be pressure supported.

Pressure-Controlled Ventilation With Volume Guarantee

- Like PCV, the basic controls are maximum pressure and rate, but in PCV with volume guarantee (PCV-VG), a target VT is also set.
- The ventilator delivers breaths using a decelerating flow pattern at a pressure that is less than Pmax.
- In PCV-VG, the inspiratory pressure is adjusted to deliver the target VT, using the lowest possible pressure and staying within the maximum pressure limit.
- PCV-VG begins by delivering a volume breath at the set VT.
- The patient's compliance is determined from this volume breath, and the inspiratory pressure level is then adjusted for the next breath.
- PCV-VG combines the advantages of pressure-controlled ventilation and dynamically compensates for changes in the patient's lung characteristics.

Pressure Support Ventilation

- PSV is analogous to PCV in that it is a pressure-controlled ventilation mode, but the RR is zero.
- It is similar to SIMV in that it is responsive to the patient's efforts, delivering pressure to the airway (which causes inspiratory flow), provided the effort occurs within a trigger window and enough negative inspiratory pressure is generated by the patient.
- This mode of ventilation is primarily useful for patients who are breathing spontaneously and helps to overcome the airflow resistance of the airway device.
- There is no minimum minute ventilation, although some ventilators allow setting an apnea backup rate or delay (PSVPro on Aisys).
- PSV is useful to augment the VT of a spontaneously ventilating patient during maintenance or emergence.
- The primary setting is the pressure support level, which, for adults, may be started at 10 cm H_2O and adjusted on the basis of VT and $ETCO_2$.
- Trigger window, sensitivity, maximum inspiratory flow, and apnea backup rate may also be set, depending on the ventilator (Box 4.8).

Critical Incidents Related to Ventilation

- Clinical experience with anesthesia ventilators and breathing circuits has identified several situations that have led to critical incidents.
- Vigilance directed toward situations that have the potential to cause patient injury may contribute to the prevention of future occurrences.
- The variety of faults leading to low-pressure accidents emphasizes proper performance of preanesthesia equipment checklists.

BOX 4.8 Typical Ventilator Alarms

Pressure Alarms

- High (isolated or continuing)
- Subatmospheric
  - Volume—low VT or minute volume
  - Rate—high RR
  - Reverse flow (may indicate incompetence of expiratory unidirectional valve in the breathing circuit, inadvertent placement of nasogastric tube with suction through the glottic opening)

Apnea/Disconnect Alarms[a]

These may be based on the following:

- Chemical monitoring (lack of $ETco_2$)
- Mechanical monitoring:
  - Failure to reach normal inspiratory peak pressure or failure to sense return of VT
  - Spirometry
  - Failure of standing bellows to fill during exhalation
  - Failure of manual breathing bag to move and fill during mechanical ventilation (machines with fresh gas decoupling—Apollo, Fabius, Narkomed 6000 [Dräger])
  - Other—lack of breath sounds or visible chest movement.

$ETco_2$, end-tidal carbon dioxide; *RR*, respiratory rate; *VT*, tidal volume.

[a]Note that low readings on the pulse oximeter are less valuable because these are a late sign of hypoventilation.

From Elisha S, Heiner JS, Nagelhout JJ. *Nurse Anesthesia.* 7th ed. Elsevier; 2023.

- Failure to ventilate caused by disconnection has been called the most common preventable equipment-related cause of mishaps.
- The most common site for disconnection is between the breathing circuit and the ETT (at the Y-piece).
- Other associated areas that cause a disconnection within the circle system include the following:
  - Absorbent granules changed between cases by ancillary personnel but improperly reassembled or even left open
  - Defective absorber canister
  - Failure of the bag/vent switch
  - Leaks in corrugated hoses
  - Incompetent ventilator relief valve
  - Gas sampling line preventing manual ventilation by preventing closure of an adjustable pressure-limiting valve
  - Ventilator failure due to moisture in flow sensors
- A primary monitor for disconnection is continuous auscultation of breath sounds with a precordial or esophageal stethoscope, as well as direct visual observation of chest movement.
- Electronic monitors that alert the anesthetist to disconnection include capnography and pressure- and volume-based alarms.
- To manage inability to ventilate due to low pressure in the breathing circuit, the following may be tried:
  - Ensure ventilation is occurring by checking breath sounds.
  - Check for disconnects quickly.
  - Try to ventilate manually using the anesthesia breathing circuit.
  - Check settings of fresh gas flow, scavenger, and ventilator, as well as monitor artifact.
  - If necessary, initiate rapid manual ventilation with backup ventilation equipment (Ambu bag).

Barotrauma and High Pressure in the Breathing Circuit

- The causes of sustained high pressure in the breathing circuit may include the following:
  - Obstruction to exhalation
  - Endobronchial intubation
  - Kinking of the ETT or anesthesia circuit
  - Improper scavenger assembly
  - Improper use of the adjustable pressure-limiting valve
  - Failure to remove plastic wrap around a soda lime canister before installation
  - Malfunctioning ventilator relief valve
  - Occlusion of the lumen of a breathing circuit extender adaptor by plastic debris, disposable PEEP valve, and/or faulty expiratory unidirectional valve
  - Patient factors (e.g., bronchospasm, anterior mediastinal mass)
- Consequences of obstructed breathing circuits include high PEEP, decreased venous return, cardiovascular collapse, pneumothorax, massive subcutaneous emphysema, and death.
- Treatment of sustained high ventilatory pressure:
  1. Assess patient-related causes such as bronchospasm.
  2. Manually ventilate with the breathing circuit (in "bag" mode).
  3. Disconnect the patient from the breathing circuit and continue ventilation by bag-valve-mask (e.g., Ambu bag) (Box 4.9).

BOX 4.9 Causes of Critical Incidents

Underlying Causes of Critical Incidents

- Improper or infrequent maintenance
- Inadequate in-service education
- Substandard equipment monitoring
- Failure to check equipment before use
- Lack of familiarity with equipment standards

Mechanisms of Critical Incidents

Failure to Ventilate

- Disconnection
- Failure to initiate ventilation or resume it after an interruption
- Misconnections of breathing circuit
- Occlusion or obstruction of breathing circuit
  - Kinking or plugging of endotracheal tube
  - Kinking of fresh gas delivery hose
  - Mold flash or plastic emboli from wrapping material
- Leaks
- Failure or improper reassembly of bellows after cleaning
- Damage to or disconnection of pressure monitoring or other hoses
- Failure of pipeline and tank oxygen supply
- Driving a vent with cylinders (when pipeline is unavailable), causing rapid tank depletion

BOX 4.9 Causes of Critical Incidents—cont'd

- Inadvertent application of suction to the breathing circuit
- Failure of scavenger interface negative-pressure relief valve
- Intubation of trachea with nasogastric tube, which is then connected to suction

Barotrauma

- Excess inflow to breathing circuit (flushing during ventilator inspiration)
- Ventilator relief valve that is stuck closed
- Control assembly problems

From Elisha S, Heiner JS, Nagelhout JJ. *Nurse Anesthesia*. 7th ed. Elsevier; 2023.

BOX 4.10 Means of Limiting Exposure of Personnel to Waste Anesthetic Gases

- Check the scavenger (for correct level of suction) before use.
- Perform regular preventive maintenance of room ventilation systems.
- Perform regular preventive maintenance of all anesthesia equipment.
- Conduct personnel monitoring and ambient trace gas monitoring.
- Seek the source of the smell of anesthetics noted during a case.
- Maintain an effective mask fit and seal.
- Avoid unscavengeable techniques (mask induction, insufflation).
- Prevent flow from breathing system into room air (e.g., pause fresh gas flow during intubation of the trachea).
- Turn on anesthetic gases only after the mask is on the patient.
- Turn off anesthetic gases before suctioning.
- Wash out anesthetics into the scavenger at the end of the case.
- Do not spill liquid agent.
- Use cuffed endotracheal tubes.
- Use low fresh gas flows.
- Check the machine regularly for leaks.
- Disconnect nitrous oxide at the wall outlet at the end of the day.
- Use total intravenous anesthesia.
- Avoid use of nitrous oxide.

From Elisha S, Heiner JS, Nagelhout JJ. *Nurse Anesthesia*. 7th ed. Elsevier; 2023.

Scavenging Systems and Disposal of Waste Anesthetic Gases

- Scavenging is the collection of waste anesthetic gases from the breathing circuit and ventilator and their removal from the OR.
- An amount equal to the fresh gas flow must be scavenged each minute. Otherwise, the breathing circuit and the patient's lungs will either gain or lose pressure, resulting in barotrauma or failure to ventilate.
- The most important component of the scavenger system is the interface (between the breathing circuit and wall suction) because it protects the patient's airway from excessive buildup of positive pressure and from exposure to suction.
- Advisory recommendations for exposure to waste anesthetic gases are published by the Occupational Safety and Health Administration (OSHA).
- OSHA advises that no worker should be exposed to more than 2 ppm halogenated agents (0.5 ppm if used with nitrous oxide) and no more than 25 ppm nitrous oxide, based on a time-weighted 8-hour average concentration.
  - The highest levels are found in the anesthetist's workstation; between the anesthetic gas machine and the wall; and in OR personnel working in ear, nose, and throat procedures.
  - Several variables determine the attainable reduction in waste anesthetic gases in the OR, including the degree of room ventilation, the condition of anesthesia equipment, the effectiveness of the scavenger, and the airway device that is used (Box 4.10).

Anesthesia Gas Machine Checklist

- Although equipment failures are rare, they are often the result of human error in the use of the equipment.
- Failure to check anesthesia equipment adequately has been reported as a factor in up to 30% of critical incidents.
- The anesthetist should be familiar with the checkout procedure for all models of anesthesia gas machine(s) that are in use at their facility (Box 4.11).

BOX 4.11 Summary of Checkout Recommendations by Frequency and Responsible Party

#	Items to be Completed	Frequency	Responsible Parties
1	Verify auxiliary oxygen cylinder and self-inflating manual ventilation device are available and functioning.	Daily	Anesthesiologist or other qualified anesthesia professional AND technician or technologist
2	Verify patient suction is adequate to clear the airway.	Prior to each use	Anesthesiologist or other qualified anesthesia professional AND technician or technologist
3	Confirm that alternating-current (AC) power is available and turn anesthesia delivery system on.	Daily	Anesthesiologist or other qualified anesthesia professional OR technician or technologist
4	Verify availability of required monitors and check alarms.	Prior to each use	Anesthesiologist or other qualified anesthesia professional OR technician or technologist
5	Verify that pressure is adequate in the spare oxygen cylinder mounted on the anesthesia machine.	Daily	Anesthesiologist or other qualified anesthesia professional AND technician or technologist
6	Verify that piped gas pressures are greater than the minimum required by the anesthesia machine in use, typically greater than or equal to 40 or 50 pounds per square inch gauge (psig).	Daily	Anesthesiologist or other qualified anesthesia professional AND technician or technologist
7	Verify that vaporizers are adequately filled and, if applicable, that the filler ports are securely closed.	Prior to each use	Anesthesiologist or other qualified anesthesia professional
8	Detect whether leaks exist in the gas supply lines between the flowmeters and the common gas outlet.	Daily and whenever a vaporizer is changed	Anesthesiologist or other qualified anesthesia professional OR technician or technologist
9	Test scavenging system function.	Daily	Anesthesiologist or other qualified anesthesia professional OR technician or technologist
10	Calibrate, or verify calibration of, the oxygen monitor and check the low oxygen alarm.	Daily	Anesthesiologist or other qualified anesthesia professional OR technician or technologist
11	Verify carbon dioxide absorbent is not exhausted.	Prior to each use	Anesthesiologist or other qualified anesthesia professional OR technician or technologist
12	Perform breathing system pressure and leak testing.	Prior to each use	Anesthesiologist or other qualified anesthesia professional OR technician or technologist
13	Verify that gas flows properly through the breathing circuit during both inspiration and exhalation.	Prior to each use	Anesthesiologist or other qualified anesthesia professional AND technician or technologist
14	Document completion of checkout procedures.	Prior to each use	Anesthesiologist or other qualified anesthesia professional AND technician or technologist
15	Confirm proposed patient-specific ventilator settings and evaluate readiness to deliver anesthesia care.	Immediately prior to initiating the anesthetic	Anesthesiologist or other qualified anesthesia professional

psi, Pounds per square inch.

Excerpted from (Recommendations for Pre-Anesthesia Checkout Procedures (2025), ASA Committee on Equipment and Facilities, American Society of Anesthesiologists, 2025. Available at: https://www.asahq.org/standards-and-practice-parameters/-/media/8794c27e69684dc596761c9e56d263f7.ashx) of the American Society of Anesthesiologists.

KNOWLEDGE CHECK

1. Which system minimizes the chance of the hospital supply oxygen being switched to the inlet for nitrous oxide on the anesthesia machine?
   a. Diameter Index Safety System
   b. Scavenging system
   c. First-stage regulator
   d. Pin Index Safety System
2. In the event of complete loss of oxygen pipeline pressure, the anesthetist should
   a. ventilate with bag-valve-mask and turn off inhalation agent.
   b. open the E cylinder of oxygen, disconnect the pipeline, and consider manual ventilation.
   c. manually ventilate and prepare for TIVA.
   d. increase fresh gas flows and consider changing carbon dioxide absorbent.
3. Which system decreases the potential for administering a critically low fraction of inspired oxygen?
   a. Diameter Index Safety System
   b. Free scavenging system
   c. Hypoxic guard fail-safe system
   d. Pin Index Safety System
4. Which are common reasons for increased inspired carbon dioxide? *(Select two.)*
   a. Malignant hyperthermia
   b. Exhausted CO_2 granules
   c. Increased fresh gas flow
   d. Faulty unidirectional valves
5. In which ventilator setting is the inspiratory pressure adjusted to deliver the target tidal volume while using the lowest possible pressure and staying within the maximum pressure limit?
   a. VCV
   b. PSV-VG
   c. PCV
   d. SIMV
6. Which actions would be necessary in the event of inability to ventilate due to low pressure in the breathing circuit? *(Select three.)*
   a. Verify breath sounds.
   b. Reduce inspiratory alarm value.
   c. Check connections of the breathing circuit.
   d. Open E cylinder and prepare for bag-mask ventilation.
   e. Disconnect scavenging system from anesthesia circuit.
   f. If ventilation remains inadequate with anesthesia circuit, ventilate with bag-valve-mask.
7. Which of the following components is part of the *intermediate-pressure system* of the anesthesia gas machine?
   a. Common gas outlet
   b. Cylinder pressure gauge
   c. Oxygen pressure-failure device
   d. Anesthesia gas vaporizer
8. In the event of a complete oxygen pipeline supply failure, what is the first action the anesthesia provider should take?
   a. Switch to manual ventilation using the Ambu bag with room air.
   b. Trust the oxygen analyzer and open the backup oxygen cylinder.
   c. Attempt to recalibrate the oxygen analyzer.
   d. Increase fresh gas flows to flush the system.
9. Which of the following statements is true regarding the use of oxygen cylinders on the anesthesia gas machine?
   a. Oxygen cylinders should remain open at all times to ensure a backup source is immediately available.
   b. The PISS prevents connection of the wrong cylinder by controlling cylinder pressure.
   c. Oxygen cylinders are used as the primary source of oxygen during routine anesthesia.
   d. Oxygen cylinders should be opened only during machine checks or pipeline failure.
10. What is the most appropriate immediate action if there is a total electrical power failure while using a newer anesthesia machine?
    a. Recalibrate all digital monitors.
    b. Switch to a self-inflating manual ventilation device (e.g., Ambu bag).
    c. Wait for the battery backup to activate before intervening.
    d. Increase fresh gas flow to compensate for monitor loss.
11. Which of the following is the most common preventable equipment-related cause of failure to ventilate during anesthesia?
    a. Malfunctioning ventilator relief valve.
    b. Incorrect scavenger suction level.
    c. Disconnection at the Y-piece between the breathing circuit and ETT.
    d. Inadequate carbon dioxide absorbent replacement.
12. Which of the following is most likely to result in barotrauma as a result of sustained high pressure in the anesthesia breathing circuit?
    a. Use of low fresh gas flow during maintenance.
    b. Disconnection of the gas sampling line.
    c. Improper removal of plastic wrap from a new soda lime canister.
    d. Switching to manual ventilation with a bag-valve-mask.

Answers can be found in Appendix A.

STANDARDS FOR PREANESTHESIA EVALUATION AND INFORMED CONSENT

- The code of ethics for certified registered nurse anesthetists can be accessed at the American Association of Nurse Anesthetists website: https://www.aana.com/practice/clinical-practice/clinical-practice-resources/code-of-ethics-for-crnas/.
- Essential goals of the preanesthetic and preoperative assessment and preparation of the patient include the following:
  - Optimize patient care, satisfaction, comfort, and convenience.
  - Minimize perioperative morbidity and mortality by correctly assessing issues that influence anesthesia management and risk.
  - Minimize cancellations and delays on the day of surgery.
  - Evaluate the patient's overall health status to determine need for further tests and/or specialty consultations.
  - Optimize preexisting medical conditions (e.g., medication compliance, smoking cessation, reduced alcohol ingestion).
  - Communicate specific instruction (e.g., fasting and nil per os [NPO] guidelines, blood glucose management, and home medication administration).
  - Educate patient regarding surgery, anesthesia, and expected intra- and postoperative care.
  - Formulate a plan for postoperative care.
  - Communicate patient management issues among healthcare providers.
- Standards for anesthesia practice are intended to support the delivery of patient-centered, high-quality, and safe anesthesia care.
  - These standards apply anywhere anesthesia is provided and for all types of patient populations.
- There may be various circumstances or patient issues where specific standards require modification. It is the duty of the anesthesia provider to document any modification or alteration of an anesthetic standard, as well as the reason, in the patient's medical record.
- There are 14 specific standards for nurse anesthesia practice listed on the American Association of Nurse Anesthetists website: (1) patient rights, (2) preanesthesia patient assessment and evaluation, (3) plan for anesthesia care, (4) informed consent for anesthesia care and related services, (5) documentation, (6) equipment, (7) anesthesia plan implementation and management, (8) patient positioning, (9) monitoring and alarms, (10) infection control and prevention, (11) transfer of care, (12) quality improvement process, (13) wellness, and (14) a culture of safety.

1. *Patient rights* focus on respect for the patient's autonomy, dignity, and privacy, as well as providing support for the patient's needs and safety.
2. *Preanesthesia patient assessment and evaluation* are performed and documented on every patient. Assessment, evaluation, and documentation include a patient's general health, allergies, medication history, preexisting conditions, anesthesia history, and any relevant diagnostic tests.
3. A *plan for anesthesia care* is developed after assessment and evaluation of the patient. Anesthesia care plans are discussed with the patient. Formulation of an anesthesia plan may include other members of the healthcare team (additional anesthesia providers, physicians, nurses, technologists, etc.) and may include the patient's legal representative (e.g., healthcare proxy, surrogate) if the patient is incapable of understanding. After discussion of the anesthesia care options, the patient's concerns and questions should be addressed, with the anesthesia plan modified accordingly.
4. *Informed consent for anesthesia care and related services* is required before the administration of an anesthetic. This is documented and signed by the patient or the patient's legal representative (e.g., healthcare proxy, surrogate).
5. *Documentation* of anesthesia care data and activities should occur in the patient's healthcare record and be legible, timely, accurate, and complete.
6. *Equipment* is any device, machine, or product used during the administration of anesthesia. Adherence to the manufacturer's operating instructions and other safety precautions is mandatory. A daily anesthesia equipment check, before anesthetic administration, is required to verify functionality and/or problems. Operation of equipment should be done in a manner that minimizes or eliminates the risk of fire, explosion, electrical shock, and equipment malfunction.
7. *Anesthesia plan implementation and management* is the standard that encompasses the operationalization of an anesthetic. Modifications to the anesthesia plan are made on the basis of continu-

ous assessment and patient response to the anesthetic and surgical or procedural intervention. Anesthesia care is provided until the responsibility has been accepted by another anesthesia professional or until the anesthetic is terminated and care is accepted by another trained and licensed professional.

8. *Patient positioning* focuses on the assessment and monitoring of proper bodily alignment during an anesthetic procedure. Collaboration with the surgical or procedural team is necessary during the initial positioning and throughout the case. Protective measures that pad pressure points, allow the maintenance of adequate perfusion, and protect nerves should be employed.
9. *Monitoring and alarms* encompass the evaluation of oxygenation, ventilation, the cardiovascular system, thermoregulation, and neuromuscular function. Each of these areas is continuously monitored and documented from the start of an anesthetic until termination and transfer of care.
   - *Oxygenation* requires continuous monitoring using pulse oximetry and clinical observation. The risk of fire should be communicated by the surgical or procedural team, and risk factors should be mitigated.
   - *Ventilation* requires continuous monitoring using expired carbon dioxide capnography and clinical observation. Verification of ventilation after airway manipulation and device placement should always include auscultation, chest excursion, and confirmation of continuous expired carbon dioxide on the capnogram.
   - The *cardiovascular* system is continuously monitored using the ECG waveform and a noninvasive BP cuff. Invasive monitoring should be used on a case-by-case basis as appropriate.
   - *Temperature* monitoring is required when using malignant hyperthermia–triggering agents. In other instances, body temperature should be monitored when significant changes are anticipated, intended, or suspected. Active warming devices are recommended to facilitate normothermia.
   - *Neuromuscular* monitoring is required when administering NMBAs to assess neuromuscular response, depth of blockade, and degree of recovery.

   When a physiological monitoring device is used, variable pitch and threshold alarms are turned on and audible at all times. Documentation of BP, heart rate, and respiration is done at a minimum of every 5 minutes for all anesthetics. Documentation of thermoregulation, ventilation parameters, and neuromuscular function (when muscle paralysis is used) should be completed at a minimum of every 15 minutes when indicated.
10. *Infection control and prevention* standards focus on following policies and procedures established within the practice setting to minimize the risk of infection to patients, the anesthesia provider, and other healthcare providers.
11. *Transfer of care* standards require the evaluation of the patient's hemodynamic stability, neurologic function, reporting of nausea or pain, and overall condition. These factors determine when it is appropriate to transfer the responsibility of care to another qualified and licensed healthcare provider. The patient's current status, history, anesthetic course, surgical or procedural intervention, and any other essential information should be communicated during the transfer of care.
12. *Quality improvement process* allows for ongoing review and evaluation of anesthesia care to assess the quality of care provided and identify areas of improvement.
13. *Wellness* is an important standard that focuses on anesthesia providers' ability to physically and mentally perform their duties.
14. *A culture of safety* is created for both the patient and anesthesia provider through interdisciplinary engagement, open communication, and supportive leadership.

Informed Consent

Informed consent is based on the ethical and legal concept that patients have the right to understand what is being done to them (personal autonomy) and that they agree to (and have the ability to agree to) the potential consequences of anesthetic, surgical, and/or procedural interventions.

- Elements of informed consent include the following: (1) the ability of the patient to competently make decisions of their own accord or, if unable, to designate a patient representative as proxy; (2) disclosure of information regarding the purpose, risks and benefits, side effects, alternatives, and risks of not receiving anesthesia care for the operation or procedure; (3) patient acknowledgment of disclosed information; (4) voluntary consent with questions answered by anesthesia professional; and (5) signed documentation, including date and time and relationship (as applicable), indicating informed consent by the patient.

- The timing of informed consent should follow institutional policies and procedures and be based on the patient's current health status.
- Anesthesia providers have a duty to not withhold relevant healthcare information from a patient, although there may be times a patient wants certain information to be withheld. A patient also has the right to waive their right to receive this information, or they may involve family members or caregivers in the decision-making process or even appoint a family member or caregiver as a proxy.
- In emergencies, implied consent is obtained by the medical team if immediate treatment or intervention is warranted because (1) the patient is unconscious or incapable of consenting, and (2) the harm from failing to perform the procedure is imminent and outweighs the potential harm from performing the procedure.
- Failure to obtain informed consent from a patient or patient representative as a result of incomplete communication may constitute negligence, battery, breach of contract, or other legal claims and may lead to professional discipline.

KNOWLEDGE CHECK

1. Which situation requires the use of temperature monitoring?
   a. During a sedation case lasting 30 minutes.
   b. While providing TIVA.
   c. When administering a volatile inhalational agent.
   d. For every anesthetic.
2. Which is one of the 14 anesthesia practice standards?
   a. Wellness
   b. Establish a culture of care
   c. Provider rights
   d. Excellence in anesthesia
3. Which is *not* included as an element of informed consent?
   a. Designation of a patient representative as a proxy.
   b. Disclosure of risks of not receiving anesthesia care for an operation.
   c. Patient acknowledgment of disclosed information.
   d. Patient verbal agreement without signature.
4. Which of the following is a primary goal of the preoperative assessment?
   a. Ensure patients are fully sedated before transport to the OR.
   b. Avoid the need for further diagnostic tests or specialty consultation.
   c. Optimize patient care and minimize perioperative morbidity and mortality.
   d. Confirm that preprocedural antibiotics are available in the OR.

Answers can be found in Appendix A.

APPENDIX A

Knowledge Check Answers

CHAPTER 1: AIRWAY MANAGEMENT

KNOWLEDGE CHECK, 4

1. a
2. d

KNOWLEDGE CHECK, 6

1. b
2. b

KNOWLEDGE CHECK, 8

1. d
2. b
3. c

KNOWLEDGE CHECK, 13

1. c
2. c
3. b
4. a

KNOWLEDGE CHECK, 17

1. b
2. b
3. c
4. a

KNOWLEDGE CHECK, 24–25

1. c
2. c, d, e
3. c
4. b
5. a

KNOWLEDGE CHECK, 38

1. d
2. a, b, e
3. d
4. a
5. c
6. d
7. a, b, f

KNOWLEDGE CHECK, 42

1. a
2. d
3. c

KNOWLEDGE CHECK, 47

1. b
2. c
3. b
4. b

KNOWLEDGE CHECK, 62

1. d
2. d
3. a
4. c
5. d
6. b
7. a
8. d
9. b

KNOWLEDGE CHECK, 67

1. c, d, f
2. c
3. a
4. b

KNOWLEDGE CHECK, 78–79

1. a
2. c
3. a
4. a
5. d
6. d
7. c
8. c
9. c

CHAPTER 2: PHARMACOLOGY

KNOWLEDGE CHECK, 86

1. a
2. a
3. d
4. b
5. b
6. a

KNOWLEDGE CHECK, 93–94

1. b
2. c
3. c
4. a, c
5. a
6. c
7. d
8. a
9. c
10. a
11. c
12. c

KNOWLEDGE CHECK, 97

1. b, d
2. c
3. b

KNOWLEDGE CHECK, 99

1. a
2. a
3. b
4. d
5. c, d
6. c, e
7. d

KNOWLEDGE CHECK, 105–106

1. c
2. a
3. d
4. d
5. a
6. b, c, e
7. a
8. b, c, d
9. a
10. b

KNOWLEDGE CHECK, 112

1. b, d
2. a
3. b
4. c
5. b
6. c
7. a

KNOWLEDGE CHECK, 117

1. a, b
2. b
3. c
4. b, d
5. b
6. a, d, e

KNOWLEDGE CHECK, 120

1. b
2. c
3. a, c, d
4. d

KNOWLEDGE CHECK, 124

1. c
2. d
3. b
4. b
5. b

KNOWLEDGE CHECK, 128

1. a
2. c

KNOWLEDGE CHECK, 130

1. c
2. a, b, c
3. b, d
4. d

KNOWLEDGE CHECK, 130

1. a
2. b

KNOWLEDGE CHECK, 132

1. a, d
2. b
3. c, d
4. a, b

KNOWLEDGE CHECK, 136–137

1. a
2. b
3. d
4. b
5. a, b, e
6. b, c, e
7. c
8. d
9. b
10. a
11. d

KNOWLEDGE CHECK, 139

1. a, d
2. a, c
3. d

KNOWLEDGE CHECK, 141

1. a, d
2. b, c

KNOWLEDGE CHECK, 144

1. a, d
2. b
3. a, b, c

KNOWLEDGE CHECK, 147

1. a, c, d
2. d
3. c, d
4. d

KNOWLEDGE CHECK, 153

1. c
2. b
3. c
4. a, c, d
5. a
6. c
7. b
8. a
9. b
10. b

KNOWLEDGE CHECK, 155

1. a, c
2. b

KNOWLEDGE CHECK, 155

1. a
2. c
3. a, b, d

KNOWLEDGE CHECK, 163

1. a
2. b
3. a
4. a, d

KNOWLEDGE CHECK, 168
1. c
2. a, c

KNOWLEDGE CHECK, 173
1. a
2. d
3. b
4. a
5. c, d

KNOWLEDGE CHECK, 176
1. a
2. b
3. a, b, e

KNOWLEDGE CHECK, 177
1. a, d
2. a

KNOWLEDGE CHECK, 178
1. c
2. d
3. b, d

KNOWLEDGE CHECK, 181
1. b
2. b
3. a, b, d

KNOWLEDGE CHECK, 183
1. b
2. d

KNOWLEDGE CHECK, 184
1. c
2. b

KNOWLEDGE CHECK, 187
1. b
2. c, d

KNOWLEDGE CHECK, 188
1. a
2. c

KNOWLEDGE CHECK, 189
1. b, c
2. c, d
3. c

KNOWLEDGE CHECK, 193
1. a, d
2. a

KNOWLEDGE CHECK, 194
1. d
2. b
3. a, c
4. a, c, d

KNOWLEDGE CHECK, 195
1. a
2. c

CHAPTER 3: HUMAN PHYSIOLOGY, PATHOPHYSIOLOGY, AND ANESTHESIA CASE MANAGEMENT

KNOWLEDGE CHECK, 199
1. a
2. a, c
3. b
4. c, d
5. a, d

KNOWLEDGE CHECK, 202
1. c
2. b
3. a, b, c, d

KNOWLEDGE CHECK, 208
1. c
2. b
3. b
4. a, c, e
5. c

KNOWLEDGE CHECK, 211
1. b, c, f
2. a
3. c
4. d
5. b

KNOWLEDGE CHECK, 215
1. d
2. a
3. d

KNOWLEDGE CHECK, 221
1. d
2. b
3. a
4. d

KNOWLEDGE CHECK, 225
1. b, d
2. a

KNOWLEDGE CHECK, 228
1. b
2. systolic heart failure: a, c; diastolic heart failure: b, d

KNOWLEDGE CHECK, 232
1. d
2. a
3. b, c, d, f
4. c

KNOWLEDGE CHECK, 236
1. a, c
2. c, d
3. b, d

KNOWLEDGE CHECK, 239
1. c
2. d
3. b
4. c
5. b

KNOWLEDGE CHECK, 242
1. b
2. a
3. a
4. c
5. c
6. a
7. b

KNOWLEDGE CHECK, 246
1. b
2. c
3. c
4. d

KNOWLEDGE CHECK, 252–253
1. d
2. b
3. a
4. b
5. c
6. c
7. d
8. c
9. b
10. d
11. b
12. a

KNOWLEDGE CHECK, 257
1. a
2. c
3. d
4. b
5. b

KNOWLEDGE CHECK, 260
1. b
2. d
3. a
4. b
5. b

KNOWLEDGE CHECK, 264
1. c
2. c

KNOWLEDGE CHECK, 269–270
1. a
2. a
3. a, c, d
4. b
5. b

KNOWLEDGE CHECK, 275
1. a, c
2. d
3. b, c
4. c

KNOWLEDGE CHECK, 277
1. a, c, d
2. d
3. a, e
4. c

KNOWLEDGE CHECK, 281
1. a, d
2. c
3. c

KNOWLEDGE CHECK, 283
1. a, c, e
2. d
3. a
4. c

KNOWLEDGE CHECK, 285
1. a
2. c
3. b
4. c

KNOWLEDGE CHECK, 285
1. b
2. c
3. b
4. a

KNOWLEDGE CHECK, 287
1. a, b, c, d, e, f
2. a, c, e

KNOWLEDGE CHECK, 289
1. c
2. b
3. a

KNOWLEDGE CHECK, 292
1. b
2. Match the following characteristic to MG or LEMS

   LEMS __ Most often associated with small or oat cell carcinoma

LEMS __ Exercise improves strength
MG __ Occurs more often in females than in males
MG __ May be resistant to succinylcholine, increased sensitivity to nondepolarizing muscle relaxants
LEMS __ Proximal limb weakness (legs > arms)
MG __ Ptosis and diplopia

3. d

KNOWLEDGE CHECK, 300

1. b, c
2. b, d

KNOWLEDGE CHECK, 301

1. c

KNOWLEDGE CHECK, 304

1. b, d
2. d
3. a, d

KNOWLEDGE CHECK, 309

1. b
2. d
3. a
4. b
5. b

KNOWLEDGE CHECK, 312

1. a, d
2. d
3. a
4. b
5. d

KNOWLEDGE CHECK, 313–314

1. d
2. c
3. b, d
4. c
5. a, c

KNOWLEDGE CHECK, 318

1. b
2. c
3. c
4. b
5. c

KNOWLEDGE CHECK, 321

1. c
2. c
3. b
4. b
5. c

KNOWLEDGE CHECK, 325–326

1. b
2. b
3. c
4. a
5. c
6. c
7. d

KNOWLEDGE CHECK, 329

1. d
2. c
3. b
4. c

KNOWLEDGE CHECK, 333

1. b
2. d
3. c
4. b
5. c

KNOWLEDGE CHECK, 336

1. b
2. c
3. c
4. b
5. c

KNOWLEDGE CHECK, 338–339

1. b
2. b
3. c
4. c
5. c
6. b
7. b

KNOWLEDGE CHECK, 346

1. b
2. b
3. b
4. a
5. c
6. a

KNOWLEDGE CHECK, 352

1. c
2. b
3. b
4. d
5. a
6. c
7. a

KNOWLEDGE CHECK, 355–356

1. c
2. d
3. c
4. c
5. b
6. b
7. c

KNOWLEDGE CHECK, 356

1. c
2. b
3. b

KNOWLEDGE CHECK, 365

1. b
2. d
3. c
4. b
5. b
6. d
7. d
8. c
9. c
10. b

KNOWLEDGE CHECK, 367–368

1. b
2. a
3. c
4. a
5. c
6. c
7. b
8. d

KNOWLEDGE CHECK, 369

1. a
2. d
3. c

KNOWLEDGE CHECK, 371

1. c
2. a
3. b
4. a

CHAPTER 4: ANESTHESIA EQUIPMENT AND TECHNOLOGY

KNOWLEDGE CHECK, 374

1. b
2. c
3. b

KNOWLEDGE CHECK, 379

1. b
2. a

KNOWLEDGE CHECK, 388

1. c
2. a
3. b
4. d
5. a
6. a, d
7. b, c

KNOWLEDGE CHECK, 390

1. b
2. c
3. c

KNOWLEDGE CHECK, 393

1. b
2. a
3. b
4. b
5. c

KNOWLEDGE CHECK, 398

1. a
2. c
3. c
4. b
5. d
6. c

KNOWLEDGE CHECK, 405–406

1. c
2. d
3. c
4. d
5. d
6. c
7. a
8. c
9. b, c, e
10. a

KNOWLEDGE CHECK, 410–411

1. d
2. a
3. d
4. c
5. a
6. c
7. a
8. c

KNOWLEDGE CHECK, 421

1. a
2. b
3. c
4. b, d
5. b
6. a, c, e
7. c
8. b
9. d
10. b
11. c
12. c

KNOWLEDGE CHECK, 424

1. c
2. a
3. d
4. c

INDEX

Note: Page numbers followed by "f" indicate figures, "t" indicate tables, and "b" indicate boxes.

A

Abciximab, 164t
Abdominal aortic aneurysm, 233–236, 236b
  anesthetic technique for, 235–236
  endovascular aortic repair for, 234–236, 235b, 236f
  intraoperative management for, 233–234, 234t, 235t
  postoperative period for, 234, 235b
  preoperative period for, 233, 233b
Abdominal muscles, 244
Abnormal hemodynamic values, implications of, 382f, 384–385, 384t, 385t
Absolute refractory period, 215
Absorption atelectasis, 16
Acarbose, for type 2 diabetes mellitus, 185t
Acebutolol (Sectral), 129t
Acetylcholine (ACh), 394
Acetylsalicylic acid (ASA), 164t
  on cancer, 103t
Aclidinium, 131t
Acoustic monitoring transducers, 410
Acquired conditions, and associated features, in airway management, 29t, 30–34
  acute epiglottitis, 31
  ankylosing spondylitis, 33
  atlantoaxial instability, 33–34
  cervical spine instability, 33
  laryngeal edema, 31
  laryngeal papillomas, 32
  obstructive sleep apnea, 31, 32b
  oral abscesses, 32
  retropharyngeal abscesses, 32
  rheumatoid arthritis, 33
  subglottic edema, 31
  subluxation, 33–34
  submandibular space infections, 31–32
  TMJ ankylosis, 33
  tracheal/subglottic stenosis, 31
  trismus, 32–33
Acrivastine, 175–176t
Active reabsorption, 347–349
Acute adrenal crises, treatment of, 194b
Acute adrenal crisis, 304
  treatment for, 305b
Acute coronary syndrome, 221–225, 224f, 225b
  anesthetic considerations for, 225
  signs and symptoms of, 224–225
Acute coronary syndrome *(Continued)*
  sustained ischemia causing injury/infarction, 224
  transient ischemia in, 224
  treatment of, 225
    intraoperative myocardial ischemia and, 225, 226t
Acute epiglottitis, 31
Acute kidney injury, 357–360, 357t, 358t
Acute pulmonary edema, 71–72
Acute renal failure, 357
Acute respiratory distress syndrome, 257–260
  anesthetic considerations in, 260
  etiology of, 257
  signs and symptoms of, 257–260
  treatment and management of, 260
Acute tubular necrosis, 357
Adam's apple, 10
Addison disease, 303, 304b, 304t, 305t
Addition, in drug interaction terminology, 85t
Adenoid tonsil, 7
Adenosine, for arrhythmias, 138t
Adrenal gland dysfunction, 301–302, 302f
Adrenal medulla, 304–314
Adrenal supplementation therapy, 193t, 194t
β-adrenergic blocking agents, 128–130, 130b
  clinical use of, 128, 129t
  esmolol, 129
  implications of, 128b
  labetalol, 129–130
  metoprolol, 129
Adrenocortical insufficiency, 303–304
  primary, 303, 304b, 304t, 305t
Adrenocorticotropic hormone, 293–294t
Afferent arteriole resistance, 345
Afferent arterioles, 342–343
Affinity, 80
Afterload
  definition of, 386
  myocardial oxygen demand and, 198, 198t
Agonist, 80
Agonist-antagonist, 80
Airway exchange catheters (AECs), 50–51
Airway management, 1–16
  anatomy of, 1–17
    lower airway, 13–17
    upper airway, 1–13
Airway management *(Continued)*
  assessment of, 43–47, 43t
    atlanto-occipital joint mobility, 44
    Cormack and Lehane grading, 45, 46f
    external, 43
    interincisor gap (mouth opening), 44–45
    lingual tonsillar hypertrophy, 47
    Mallampati classification, 44, 45f
    mandibular protrusion test, 45, 46f
    neck circumference, 43
    percentage of glottic opening, 45–46
    previous difficult airway, 46
    thyromental distance, 43–44, 44f
    ultrasonography, 46–47
  blocks for, 39–42, 39f
    glossopharyngeal, 41, 41f
    medications that facilitate airway anesthesia, 39–40
    methemoglobinemia, 40
    superior laryngeal nerve, 41–42, 42f
    topical anesthesia, 40–41, 41f
    transtracheal, 42, 42f
  cardiovascular response to, 24–25
  complications of, 68–79
    acute pulmonary edema, 71–72
    airway fire, 74–75, 76b
    angioedema, 75–76
    bronchoconstriction, 68–69
    bronchospasm, 68–69, 69b
    endobronchial intubation, 73
    esophageal intubation, 72–73
    hemorrhage, 69–70
    laryngospasm, 68, 68b
    lingual tonsillar hyperplasia, 78–79
    mucus plug, 72
    pneumothorax, 74, 75b
    postoperative stridor, 77, 77b
    pulmonary embolism, 73–74
    recurrent laryngeal nerve damage, 76–77
    trauma, 70
    upper airway edema, 75–76
    vocal cord granulomas/lesions/tumors, 77–78
    vomiting and aspiration, 70–71
  concepts of, 62–79
    apneic oxygenation, 63–64
    cricoid pressure/rapid-sequence intubation, 62–63, 63b

Airway management *(Continued)*
denitrogenation, 63–64
expected and unexpected difficult airway and algorithms, 64–65, 64b, 66f, 67f
operating room, 65
preoxygenation, 63–64
tracheal extubation techniques, 65–67
conditions associated with, 28–34
acquired, 30–34
congenital, 28–30
double gloves during, 373
equipment for, 47–62
anesthesia circuits, 47–50
fiberoptic stylets, 51–52
flexible intubating bronchoscopes, 51–52, 52f
intubation stylets, 50–51
oxygen delivery devices, 47–62
tracheostomy tubes, 60–62
management of devices for, 47–62
pathophysiologic concepts of, 25–38
anaphylaxis, 25
asthma, 25–26
carbon dioxide abnormalities, 26–27
hypoxia, 36–37
pulmonary edema, 37–38
physiologic concepts of, 17–25
airway pressures, 18–19
closing capacity, 20–21
creation and management of secretions, 23–24
functional residual capacity, 19–21
irritant receptors, 23–24
lung volumes, 19–20, 19f, 20t
oxygen and carbon dioxide transport, 21–23
pulmonary compliance, 18–19
resistance to breathing, 17–18
procedures for
awake intubation, 55–56
direct laryngoscopy, 52–54, 53f
emergency front-of-neck access, 57–62
needle cricothyrotomy with transtracheal jet ventilation, 57, 57f
subglottic interventions, 57–62
surgical cricothyrotomy, 57–58, 59f, 60f, 61f
tracheal intubation, 52–54, 53f
video laryngoscopy, 54–55, 55f
Airway manipulation, discard outer glove after, 373
Airway muscles, 397
Airway obstruction, 36
Airway trauma, 35
Akinesia, 392
Albiglutide (Tanzeum), for type 2 diabetes mellitus, 185t
Albuterol/ipratropium, 131t
Aldosterone, 293–294t, 350, 350t
Aldosterone antagonists, 141t
Alfuzosin (Uroxatral), 125–128
Alkylamine, 175–176t
Allergic alveolitis, 258t
Allergic reactions, in local anesthetics, 150
Alogliptin (Nesina), for type 2 diabetes mellitus, 185t
Alpha-glucosidase inhibitor, for type 2 diabetes mellitus, 185t
Aluminum hydroxide, 154
Alveolar dead space, 21
Alveolar ducts, 15–16
Alveolar obstructions, 35–36
Alveolar pressure, 247
Alveolar ventilation, 237
Alveolar-capillary membrane, 16
Alveoli, 16–17
obstructions of, 35–36
Amantadine, for Parkinson disease, 156–157t
American Society for Testing and Materials (ASTM), 410–411
Amiloride (Midamor), 141t
Amino alkyl ether (ethanolamine), 175–176t
Aminoglycosides, 161t
Amiodarone, for arrhythmias, 138t
Analgesics, miscellaneous, 145–147, 147b
anesthetic implications of, 145, 145t
anticonvulsants, 145
antidepressants, 146, 146t
corticosteroids, 146–147, 147b
Anaphylactic shock, 209, 211–213t
Anaphylaxis, 25
treatment of, 162b
Anemia, chronic kidney disease and, 362
Anemic hypoxia, 37
Anesthesia cart, protect clean supplies in, 374
Anesthesia circle system, 48
Anesthesia circuits, 47–50
Anesthesia equipment and technology, 372–12
common definitions, 372
gas machines, 411–421
infection control, 372–374
monitoring modalities, 375–411
blood pressure monitoring, 388–390
cardiovascular system, 375–393
central venous and arterial hemodynamic measurements, 380–388, 388b
electrocardiographic, 375–379, 375f, 376f, 376t, 377f, 379b
transesophageal echocardiographic, 390–393
neurologic monitoring, 394–406, 398b, 405–406b
bispectral index monitoring, 399, 400f
cerebral oximetry, 402–404
electroencephalography, 399, 399t
Anesthesia equipment and technology *(Continued)*
evoked potentials, 399–402, 400–401t
intracranial pressure, 405–406
jugular bulb oxygen venous saturation, 404
neuromuscular blockade, 394–398
transcranial Doppler ultrasonography, 404
respiratory monitoring, 406–411, 410–411b
gas, 406–407
respiration and ventilation, 407–411, 408f, 409b, 409f
work area, operating room and, infection prevention in, 373–374
environmental disinfection, 373
general care principles, 374, 374b
hand hygiene, 373
keyboards and touchscreens in, 374
provider clinical practices, 373
Anesthesia facemasks, 48
Anesthesia gas machine, 411–421
checklist, 419–421, 420b, 421b
informed consent, standards for, 423–424
organization of, 411–414, 411f, 412b
oxygen pathway through, 415–416
preanesthesia evaluation, standards for, 422–424, 424b
ventilation modes of, 416–419
Anesthesia induction medications, 94–97
benzodiazepines, 94–97, 96t, 97b
flumazenil (Romazicon), 97
implications of, 94, 95t, 96t
midazolam (Versed), 96–97
Angina ludovici, 34
Angioedema, 34, 75–76
Angiotensin II, 134, 350, 350t
Ankylosing spondylitis, 33
Antacids, oral, 154–155, 155b
Antagonism, in drug interaction terminology, 85t
Antagonists, 80
Anterior ethmoidal nerves, 4
Anterior mediastinal mass, 264–268
anesthetic considerations in, 268
etiology of, 264
signs and symptoms of, 264–268
treatment and management of, 268
Anterior pituitary hormones, 296f, 297t
Antiarrhythmics, 137–138, 138t
Antibiotics, 155–163, 163b
administration of, 161
anesthetic implications of, 155
antibiotic allergy, 162, 162b
antibiotic-anesthetic drug interactions, 162–163
clinical uses of, 157–161, 158–160t, 158b, 161t, 162t

Anticholinergics, 118–120, 119t, 120b
for nausea and vomiting, 174t
Anticholinesterase agents, 26, 112–114
Anticipated difficult airway, flexible intubating bronchoscopes for, 51
Anticoagulants, 163–168, 164t, 165–166t, 165b, 166b, 168b
anesthetic implications of, 163
antifibrinolytics, 166–168
antiplatelet drugs and noncardiac surgery, 163, 167b
thromboembolism, 166, 168b, 169t, 170t, 171t
Anticonvulsants, 145, 176–177
Antidepressants, 146, 146t, 189, 190t
Antidiuretic hormone, 293–294t, 350t, 351
Antiemetics, 168–173, 173b
anesthetic implications of, 168
clinical use of, 173, 174t
glucocorticoids, 169
5-HT_3 receptor antagonists, 169–172, 172b, 174t
metoclopramide, 173
multimodal antiemetic therapy, 168, 172b
neurokinin 1 receptor antagonists, 172, 174t
risk factors for, 168, 172b
transdermal scopolamine, 172
Antiepileptic drugs, 176–177, 177b, 177t
Antifibrinolytics, 166–168
Antifolates, 161t
Antihistamines, 174t
Antihypertensive agents, 132–135
anesthesia management of patients taking angiotensin axis blockers, 135
anesthetic implications of, 132, 133t
angiotensin 2 receptor antagonists, 134
angiotensin-converting enzyme inhibitors, 133–134
centrally acting α_2-agonists, 133
hypertension, 132–133, 133t
Antimicrobial
definition of, 372
prophylaxis, for surgery, 157, 158–160t
Antiparkinsonian drugs, 155, 155b, 156–157t
Antiplatelet drugs
classification of, 165b
in patients receiving antithrombotic therapy, 165–166t
Antipsychotics, 192–193
Antiseptic, definition of, 372
Aortic regurgitation, 207–208, 207f, 208b
anesthetic considerations for, 208
diagnostic testing/intraoperative monitoring for, 207–208
intraoperative hemodynamic considerations for, 208
medical treatment for, 207
pathophysiology of, 207
Aortic stenosis, 205–206
anesthetic considerations for, 206
diagnostic testing/intraoperative monitoring for, 205
intraoperative hemodynamic considerations for, 205–206
medical/surgical therapy for, 205
pathophysiology of, 205
Apixaban, 164t
in patients receiving antithrombotic therapy, 165–166t
for VTE, 170t
Apnea (disconnect) alarms, 410–411
Apneic mass-movement oxygenation, 63–64
Apneic oxygenation, 63–64
Apneustic center, pontine respiratory control and, 241
Apomorphine, for Parkinson disease, 156–157t
Aprepitant (Emend), 174t
Arcapta Neohaler (Novartis), 131t
Arformoterol, 131t
Arnold nerve, 8
Arrhythmia, identification and treatment for, 215–217
Arterial line
assessment, 389
insertion, 389–390, 390f
Arterial supply, of larynx, 3f, 12–13
Aryepiglottic folds, 8
Aryepiglottic muscle, 11, 12t
Arytenoid cartilages, 10
ASA. *See* Acetylsalicylic acid
Ascites, 331
Asepsis, definition of, 372
Aspart (Novolog), 183t
Astemizole (Hismanal), 175–176t
Asthma, 25–26, 238, 253–254, 255b
anesthetic considerations in, 254
etiology of, 253–254
signs and symptoms of, 254
treatment and management of, 254
ASTM. *See* American Society for Testing and Materials
Atelectasis, 16
Atenolol (Tenormin), 129t
Atherosclerosis, 221, 223f
Atlantoaxial instability, 33–34
Atlanto-occipital joint mobility, 44
Atorvastatin (Lipitor), 187t
Atrial fibrillation, 217, 218f
identification of, 217
treatment of, 217
Atrial flutter, 217, 218f
identification of, 217
treatment of, 217
Atrial natriuretic peptide, 293–294t, 350t, 351
Atrial tachyarrhythmias, 217–218
Atrioventricular block, first-degree, 218
identification of, 218
treatment of, 218
Atrioventricular bundle (bundle of his), 213
Atrioventricular node, 213
Atropine, 119
for arrhythmias, 138t
Atrovent HFA (Boehringer Ingelheim), 131t
Atypical antidepressants, 190t
Auscultation, in cardiovascular system monitoring, 375
Autoimmune diseases, chronic kidney disease and, 360t
Autonomic hyperreflexia, 284–285, 285b
Autonomic nervous system, 270–272, 271f
Awake intubation, 55–56
Azatadine, 175–176t

B

Bactericide, definition of, 372
Bacteriostatic, definition of, 372
BAEP. *See* Brainstem auditory evoked potential
Barotrauma, 418
Basement membrane, 345
Beer-Lambert law, 407–408
Benign prostatic hyperplasia, 367–368
Benzocaine, 39, 150
Benzodiazepines, 94–97, 96t, 97b
for seizure, 279
Betaxolol generic, 129t
Betrixaban, for VTE, 170t
Biguanide, for type 2 diabetes mellitus, 185t
Bilateral positive airway pressure (BiPAP), 14
Biliary tract diseases, 335–337
anesthesia management for, 337–339, 337t, 338–339b
Biliary tract malignancies, 337
BiPAP. *See* Bilateral positive airway pressure
Bisoprolol (Zebeta), 129t
Bispectral index monitoring, 399, 400f
Blood/gas solubility coefficient, 92–93t
Blood pressure monitoring, 388–390, 390b
arterial line assessment of, 389
arterial line insertion in, 389–390, 390f
Body plethysmography, 245
Bohr effect, 23
on oxyhemoglobin dissociation curve, 250
Boyle's law, 250
Bradyarrhythmias, 218–219
Brainstem, regulation of respiration and, 239–241
Brainstem auditory evoked potential (BAEP), 401–402

Breathing, physiology of, 237–242, 239b, 242b
  gas diffusion, 237–238
  gas transport, 238–239
  lung volumes and, 244–246, 244f, 245t
  muscle of respiration, 242–244, 243f
  regulation of respiration and, 239–242, 240f
Breathing circuit, high pressure in, 418
Brompheniramine (Dimetapp), 175–176t
Bronchi
  anatomy of, 14–15, 14f, 15b
  obstructions of, 35
Bronchiectasis, 16, 256
Bronchiolar obstructions, 35–36
Bronchioles
  obstructions of, 35–36
  to terminal bronchioles, 15
Bronchiolitis, 15
Bronchiolitis obliterans, 16
Bronchodilation, 17
Bronchodilators, 130, 130b, 131t
Brovana (Sunovion), 131t
Buccal artery, 6
Buccal cavity, 5
Buccal nerves, 6
Buccinator muscles, 5
Bumetanide generic, 141t
Bundle of His, 213
BURP maneuver, 10, 54f

C
Calcitonin, 293–294t
Calcium carbonate, 154
Calcium channel blockers, 130–132, 132b, 132t
Calcium chloride ($CaCl_2$), doses of, 127t
Canagliflozin (Invokana), for type 2 diabetes mellitus, 185t
Carbidopa, for Parkinson disease, 156–157t
Carbidopa/levodopa, for Parkinson disease, 156–157t
Carbidopa/levodopa/entacapone, for Parkinson disease, 156–157t
Carbon dioxide
  abnormal exchange of, 27
  abnormalities of, 26–27
  absorption, 415, 415b
  analysis, 407
  diffusion of, 238
  excess production/absorption of, 27
  transport and removal of, 22–23, 22f, 239
Carboprost (Hemabate), 195
Cardiac conduction pathway, 213
Cardiac conduction system, 210–217, 215b
  ECG wave morphology and, 213–215, 216f
  pathway, 213, 214f, 215t
  refractory period, 215, 217f, 217t
Cardiac output (CO), 386
  effect, 92–93t
Cardiogenic shock, 209, 211–213t
Cardiovascular system, 196–236
  myocardial oxygen
    demand, 197–199, 198t
    supply, 196–197, 197f, 199b
  physiologic principles in, 196, 197t
Carotid artery, external
  of oral cavity, 5
  of pharynx, 7
Carotid endarterectomy, 228–232, 229b, 232b
  anesthetic management for, 232
  indications for, 229
  intraoperative period for, 230–231
  postoperative period for, 231–232, 232t
  preoperative period for, 229–230, 230t
Carvedilol (Coreg), 129t
Catheter whip, 385
Cauda equina syndrome (CES), local anesthetics and, 150, 151b
CCO. *See* Continuous cardiac output
Ceiling effect, 81
Central chemoreceptors, regulation of respiration and, 241
Central nervous system (CNS), 270
Central venous and arterial hemodynamic measurements, 380–388, 388b
  abnormal hemodynamic values, implications of, 382f, 384–385, 384t, 385t
  hemodynamic waveforms, physiology and morphology of, 380–381, 381t
  mixed venous and central venous oxygen saturation, 388
  negative deflection waveforms, 381f, 383
  other hemodynamic indexes, 386–388, 387f, 387t
  pressure waveforms
    correlation of, 383, 383f
    distortion of, 383–384, 384b, 384f
    pulmonary artery, 382
    pulmonary artery occlusive, 382, 382f
    right atrial, 381–382, 381f, 381t
    right ventricular, 382, 382f
Central venous oxygen saturation, 388
Central venous pressure (CVP), 380
Cerebral blood flow, 272, 275b
Cerebral circulation, cerebral blood flow, 272, 275f
Cerebral cortex, regulation of respiration and, 239–241
Cerebral oximetry, 402–404
Cerebral perfusion pressure, 272
Cerebral steal phenomena, 231
Cerebrospinal fluid (CSF), 405
Cerebrovascular accident, 281–283, 283b
  anesthetic considerations for, 282–283
  etiology of, 281
  risk factors associated with, 281
  signs and symptoms of, 281
  treatment of, 281–282
Cerebrovascular autoregulation, 272–275
Cervical spine abnormalities, 28–30
Cervical spine immobilization, 51
Cervical spine instability, 33
CES. *See* Cauda equina syndrome
Cetirizine (Zyrtec), 175–176t
Cheeks, 5
Chloride shift, 22–23
Chlorothiazide (Diuril), 141t
Chlorpheniramine (Chlor-Trimeton), 175–176t
Chlorthalidone (Thalitone), 141t
Choanal atresia, 30
Cholangitis, 337
Cholecystitis, 336
Cholecystokinin, 293–294t
Choledocholithiasis, 337
Cholelithiasis, 336
Cholinergic crisis, 292
Chorda tympani, 6
Chronic infections, chronic kidney disease and, 360t
Chronic kidney disease, 360–364, 360t, 361t, 362t
Chronic obstructive pulmonary disease (COPD), 254–256
Chronic pain, analgesics and adjuncts for, 145–147
Cilia, 24
Cimetidine (Tagamet), 175–176t
Cirrhosis, 329–330, 330t, 333b
Clean-contaminated wound, 162t
Clean wound, 162t
Cleaning
  of anesthesia machine and anesthesia work area, 373
  definition of, 372
Cleft palate, 30
Clemastine fumarate, 175–176t
Clevidipine (Cleviprex), 132
  for hypertension, 132t
Clonidine (Catapres), as antihypertensive agent, 133
Clopidogrel, 164t
Closing capacity, 20–21, 246
Closing volume, 20–21, 246
CNS. *See* Central nervous system
CO. *See* Cardiac output
Coagulopathy, 331
Cobalamin deficiency, 92b
Combivent (Boehringer Ingelheim), 131t

Combivent Respimat (Boehringer Ingelheim), 131t
Complete atrioventricular (AV) block, 383
Compression atelectasis, 16
Concentration, of hemoglobin, 196–197
Concentration effect, 92–93t
Conduction, 368
Congenital conditions, and associated features, in airway management, 28–30
  cervical spine abnormalities, 28–30
  choanal atresia, 30
  cleft palate, 30
  craniofacial macrosomia, 30
  dental anomalies, 30
  glossoptosis, 28
  goiter, 30
  laryngomalacia, 30
  macroglossia, 28
  mandibular hypoplasia, 28
  maxillary hypoplasia, 28
  microcephaly, 28
  micrognathia, 28
  microstomia, 28
  prognathia, 28
  retrognathia, 28
  tracheal cartilaginous anomalies, 30
    sleeve, 30
    tracheal agenesis, 30
    tracheal stenosis, 30
    tracheoesophageal fistula, 30
    tracheomalacia, 30
Conn syndrome, 302
Contaminated wound, 162t
Context-sensitive decrement times, 84t
Continuous cardiac output (CCO), 386
Continuous positive airway pressure (CPAP), 14
Contractility, myocardial oxygen demand and, 197–198
Convection, 368
Cormack and Lehane grading, 45, 46f
Corniculate cartilages, 10
Coronary artery autoregulation, 196
Coronary artery patency, 196
Coronary stents, 163, 167b
Cortical collecting tubules, 355
Cortical nephrons, 343, 344f
Corticosteroids, 146–147, 147b, 193–194, 194b, 194t, 195t
Corticotropin-releasing hormone, 293–294t
Cortisol, 293–294t
Costovertebral skeletal deformities, 265t
CPAP. *See* Continuous positive airway pressure
Cranial nerve I, 4
Cranial nerve IX, 7
Cranial nerve V, 4, 7
Cranial nerve X, 8
Craniofacial macrosomia, 30
Cricoid cartilage, 10
Cricoid pressure, 62–63
Cricopharyngeus muscle, 7
Cricothyroid artery, 12
Cricothyroid muscles, 11, 12t
Cricothyrotomy, surgical, 57–58, 59f, 60f, 61f
Critical incidents, causes of, 418–419b
CSF. *See* Cerebrospinal fluid
Cuneiform cartilages, 10–11
Cushing syndrome, 303, 303b
CVP. *See* Central venous pressure
Cylinder supply, 413–414, 414t
Cyproheptadine, 175–176t
Cystatin C clearance, 346
Cystic fibrosis, 256–257

D
Dabigatran, 164t
Dabigatran etexilate, for VTE, 170t
Dalteparin, for VTE, 169t
Dalton's law, 250
Dantrium, 178
Dantrolene, 177–178, 178b
Dapagliflozin (Farxiga), for type 2 diabetes mellitus, 185t
DBS. *See* Double-burst stimulation
Dead space, 251–253
Decontamination, definition of, 372
Denitrogenation, 63–64
Dental anomalies, 30
Dental plexus, 6
Depolarizing muscle relaxant, 395
Desirudin, for VTE, 169t
Detemir (Levemir), 183t
Detrusor muscle, 340–341
Dexamethasone (Decadron), 174t
  on cancer, 103t
Dexmedetomidine (Precedex), 97
  as antihypertensive agent, 133
Diabetes insipidus, 298–299
Diabetes mellitus, 300, 300b
  chronic kidney disease and, 360t
Diabetic ketoacidosis (DKA), 300–301, 301t
Diameter Index Safety System, 413
Diaphragm, 243
Diastolic blood pressure, 388–389
Diastolic heart failure, 226, 228t
Diastolic time, 196
Dibucaine inhibition test, 111b
Diffusion hypoxia, 92–93t
Diffusion limitations, 27
Digitalis, 138–139, 139b, 139f, 140t
Diltiazem, 132t
  for arrhythmias, 138t
Diphenhydramine (Benadryl), 174t, 175–176t
Diphenylpyraline, 175–176t
2, 3-Diphosphoglycerate, in hemoglobin, 23
Direct and indirect α and β agonists, 124
Direct laryngoscopy, 52–54, 53f
Direct thrombin inhibitors
  in patients receiving antithrombotic therapy, 165–166t
  for VTE, 169t, 170t
Direct-acting α–agonist, 124
Dirty-infected wound, 162t
Disinfectant, definition of, 372
Disinfection, 372–374
  of anesthesia machine and anesthesia work area, 373
  definition of, 372
  environmental, 373
Distal tubule
  reabsorption, 354
  secretion, 354–355
Diuretics, 140–141, 141b
  anesthetic implications of, 140
  hypertension and, 140–141, 141t
  types of, 140
DKA. *See* Diabetic ketoacidosis
Dobutamine (Dobutrex), 126t
  doses of, 127t
Dopamine, 126t, 293–294t
  doses of, 127t
Dopamine agonists, for Parkinson disease, 156–157t
Dopamine antagonists, 174t
Dorsal respiratory group, medullary respiratory control and, 239–240
Double-burst stimulation (DBS), 109–110t, 109t, 396t, 397
Downregulation, 81
Doxazosin (Cardura), 125
Doxepin (Sinequan), 175–176t
DPP-4 inhibitors, for type 2 diabetes mellitus, 184, 185t
Droperidol (Inapsine), 174t
Ducts of Rivinus, 5
Dulaglutide (Trulicity), for type 2 diabetes mellitus, 185t
DuoNeb(dey) generic, 131t
Duopa (Abbvie), for Parkinson disease, 156–157t
Dynamic lung compliance, 18–19
Dyskinesia, 392, 393f
Dysrhythmias, 210–217
  causes of, 217

E
Echinacea, 179t
Eclampsia, seizures and, 277–278
Edoxaban, for VTE, 170t
Edrophonium (Tensilon), 114

EEG. *See* Electroencephalography
Efferent arteriole resistance, 345
Efferent arterioles, 343
Efficacy, 80
Electrical power supply, 414
  loss of, 414
Electrocardiographic electrode placement, 375–377, 377t, 378f
Electrocardiographic lead selection, 377–378, 378f, 379f
Electrocardiographic monitoring, 375–379, 375f, 376f, 376t, 377f, 379b
  electrode placement, 375–377, 377t, 378f
  gain setting and frequency bandwidth, 378–379, 380f
  lead selection, 377–378, 378f, 379f
Electroencephalography (EEG), 399, 399t
Empagliflozin (Jardiance), for type 2 diabetes mellitus, 185t
Emphysema, 238
Endobronchial intubation, 73
Endocrine system, 292–299
  anesthetic case management in, 299–303, 300b
  anesthetic considerations for, 299
  dysfunction, 297–298
End-organ damage, caused by hypertension, 200b
End-stage liver disease, 333
End-tidal carbon dioxide ($ETCO_2$)
  capnography, 408–409
  high and low, 409b
Enoxaparin, for VTE, 169t
Entacapone, for Parkinson disease, 156–157t
Environmental disinfection, 373
Ephedra (ma Huang), 179t, 180
Ephedrine, doses of, 127t
Epidural sensors, 405
Epiglotoscopy, 9
Epiglottic cartilage, 9–10
Epiglottis, 9
Epilepsy, seizures and, 277–278
Epinephrine, 126t, 293–294t
  doses of, 127t
Epistaxis, 2
Eplerenone (Inspra), 140–141, 141t
Eptifibatide, 164t
ERV. *See* Expiratory reserve volume
Erythropoietin, 293–294t
Eschmann stylet, 50, 50f
Esmolol, 129
  for arrhythmias, 138t
  for hypertension, 134t
Esophageal intubation, 72–73
Esophageal sphincter, upper, 7
Esophageal stethoscope, 409–410
Esophageal varices, 332
Essential hypertension, 199
Estrogens, 293–294t
Ethacrynic acid (Edecrin), 140, 141t
Ethmoidal arteries, 2
Ethmoidal nerves, 4
Ethmoidal sinuses, 2
Ethylenediamine, 175–176t
Etomidate, 97–98
Eustachian tube, 2
Evaporation, 368–369, 369t
Evoked potentials, 399–402, 400–401t
  brainstem auditory, 401–402
  motor, 402, 403t
  somatosensory, 400–401, 402f
  visual, 401
Exenatide (Byetta, Bydureon), for type 2 diabetes mellitus, 185t
Expiratory muscles, 243–244
Expiratory reserve volume (ERV), 19, 244, 245t
External intercostal muscles, 243
External laryngeal manipulation, 54, 54f
External ventricular drainage, 405
Extrapulmonary obstructions, 36
Extrinsic musculature, 11, 11b
Extrinsic restrictive pulmonary disease, 264, 264b, 265t

F
Facemasks
  nonrebreathing, 47–48
  simple, 47
Facial muscles, 398, 398f
Facial nerve, 6
Factor Xa inhibitors
  in patients receiving antithrombotic therapy, 165–166t
  for VTE, 169t, 170t
Famotidine, 175–176t
Fenestrated endothelial layer, 343
Fenoldopam (Corlopam)
  doses of, 127t
  for hypertension, 134t
Fexofenadine (Allegra), 175–176t
Fiberoptic scope, 56
Fiberoptic stylets, 51–52
Fick's law, 250
Finger-scalpel-bougie technique, 57–58, 61f
First-generation H_1-type antihistamines, 175–176t
Flail chest, 265t
Flexible intubating bronchoscopes, 51–52, 52f
Flumazenil (Romazicon), 97
Fluoroquinolones, 161t
Fluvastatin (Lescol), 187t
Focal (partial) seizures, 278, 279t
Follicle-stimulating hormone, 293–294t
Fondaparinux, 164t
  in patients receiving antithrombotic therapy, 165–166t
  for VTE, 169t
Foradil Aerolizer (Merck), 131t
Foreign bodies, 34
  aspirated, 35
Formoterol, 131t
Fosphenytoin (Cerebyx), for seizure, 280t
FRC. *See* Functional residual capacity
Frequency bandwidth, electrocardiographic monitoring, 378–379, 380f
Frequency shift, 391
Frontal sinuses, 2
Functional lung capacities, 245–246
Functional residual capacity (FRC), 20, 245–246, 245t
Furosemide (Lasix), 141t
  for hypertension, 140

G
Gabapentin, 145, 177
Gall bladder cancer, 336–337
Garlic, 179t, 180t
Gas diffusion, 237–238
Gas laws, 250–251
Gastrin, 293–294t
General anesthesia
  for hypertension, 201
  for carotid endarterectomy, 231
Generalized seizures, 278, 279t
Geniohyoid muscles, 5
Germicide, 372
Gingiva, 5
Ginkgo biloba, 179t, 180, 180t
Ginseng, 179t, 180, 180t
Glargine (Lantus, Toujeo), 183t
Glimepiride (Amaryl), for type 2 diabetes mellitus, 185t
Glipizide (Glucotrol), for type 2 diabetes mellitus, 185t
Glomerular filtration, 343–346, 344t
Glomerulonephritis, 365–366, 367–368b
  chronic kidney disease and, 360t
Glossopharyngeal block, 41, 41f
Glossopharyngeal nerve
  of oral cavity, 6
  of pharynx, 7
Glossoptosis, 28
GLP-1 receptor agonist, for type 2 diabetes mellitus, 184, 185t
Glucagon, 293–294t
Glucagon, doses of, 127t
Glucocorticoid excess, 303, 303b
Glucocorticoids, 174t
Gluconeogenesis, 318–319, 356
α–Glucosidase inhibitors, 184

Glulisine (Apidra), 183t
Glyburide (DiaBeta, Micronase), for type 2 diabetes mellitus, 185t
Glycogenolysis, 318
Glycopeptides, 161t
Glycopyrrolate, 40, 119–120
Glycylcyclines, 161t
Goblet cells, 23–24
Goiter, 30
Gonadotropin-releasing hormone, 293–294t
Granisetron (Kytril), 174t
Growth hormone, 293–294t
Growth hormone-inhibitory hormone (somatostatin), 293–294t
Growth hormone-releasing hormone, 293–294t
Gums, 5

H

H_1- and H_2-type antihistamines, 175–176t
H_2-type antihistamines, 175–176t
HABR. *See* Hepatic arterial buffer response
Haemophilus influenzae, 9–10
Haldane effect, 23
  on oxyhemoglobin dissociation curve, 249–250
Haloperidol (Haldol), 174t
Hand grip, 109–110t
Hand hygiene (HH), 373
  anesthesia care in, 373
Hard palate, 4
Head lift, 109–110t
Heart block, second-degree, 219
  identification of, 219
  treatment of, 219
Heart failure, 225–228, 227f, 227t, 228b
  anesthetic considerations for, 226–228, 229t
Heart rate, myocardial oxygen demand and, 197
Heat exchange, mechanism of, 368–369, 368f, 369b
Heliox, 18
Helium, 18
Hemodynamic indexes, 386–388, 387f, 387t
Hemodynamic waveforms, physiology and morphology of, 380–381, 381t
Hemoglobin, 196–197
Hemorrhagic cerebrovascular accident
  etiology of, 281
  treatment of, 281–282, 282t
Henry's law, 250
Heparin, 164t
Hepatic arterial buffer response (HABR), 316
Hepatic biliary system, 317–318, 318b
Hepatic blood flow, 315–317, 317f
Hepatic disease, anesthesia management for, 333–336, 334–335t, 336b
Hepatic encephalopathy, 332
Hepatic system, 314–339
  anatomy, 314–326, 315f, 316f
  biliary system in, 317–318, 318b
  blood flow, 315–317, 317f
  carbohydrate metabolism in, 318–319
  cholesterol extraction, synthesis, transport, and elimination in, 321, 321b
  fat metabolism in, 319–321
  filtration and detoxification of blood in, 322–323
  formation and function of bile, 325
  hormone, drug, and other substance metabolism in, 321–322
  pathophysiologic concepts of, 326–336, 327t
  physiology of, 318, 318b
  protein metabolism in, 319, 320t
  regeneration of, 325–326, 325–326b
  storage of vitamins, iron, and copper, 324–325
  synthesis of various proteins and coagulation factors in, 323, 323t, 324t
Hepatitis, 326–329, 329b
  acute, 326, 327t
  alcoholic, 327–328
  autoimmune, 329
  chronic, 326, 327t
  drug-induced, 328
  ischemic, 329
  viral, 326–327
Herbal supplements, 178–181, 181b
  adverse effects and drug interactions, 180–181, 180t
  anesthesia implications of, 178, 179t
  dietary supplements, 178–180
Herbal therapy, in patients receiving antithrombotic therapy, 165–166t
Hering-Breuer stretch reflex, regulation of respiration and, 242
HH. *See* Hand hygiene
HHS. *See* Hyperglycemic hyperosmolar state
High-level disinfection, 372
Histamine receptor antagonists, 174–176, 175–176t, 176b
Histotoxic hypoxia, 37
HMG-CoA reductase inhibitors, 187t
Homeostasis, 81
Hormone receptors, 295
Hormones, 293–294t, 293–299
  regulation, 345
  secretion, 296–297, 298f
  synthesis, 295
HPV. *See* Hypoxic pulmonary vasoconstriction
Human chorionic gonadotropin, 293–294t
Human physiology, 196–25
  cardiovascular system in, 196–236
  neurologic system, 270–292
  respiratory system in, 236–270
Human somatomammotropin, 293–294t
Hydrochlorothiazide (Microzide), 141t
Hydroxyzine (Atarax), 174t, 175–176t
Hyoid bone, 8–9
Hypercortisolism, 303
Hyperdynamic shock, 209
Hyperglycemic crises, 300–301
Hyperglycemic hyperosmolar state (HHS), 301, 301b, 301t
Hyperkalemia, chronic kidney disease and, 362
Hyperosmolar nonketotic coma. *See* Hyperglycemic hyperosmolar state
Hyperparathyroidism, 312–313, 313t
Hyperphosphatemia, chronic kidney disease and, 362
Hyperplasia, lingual tonsillar, 78–79
Hypersensitivity pneumonitis, 258t
Hypertension, 199–202, 202b, 308
  anesthesia case management for, 200–201, 201b
  chronic kidney disease and, 360t
  end-organ damage caused by, 200b
  intracranial, 275–277, 276f, 277b
    anesthetic considerations for, 277, 278t
    etiology of, 276
    signs and symptoms associated with increased ICP, 276
    treatment for, 276–277
  intraoperative goals for, 201
  portal, 330
  renovascular, 367
Hyperthyroidism, 309–310, 310b
Hypoalbuminemia, 330–331
Hypodynamic shock, 209
Hypoglossal nerve, 6
Hypoglycemics, oral, 183–184, 184b, 185t
Hypokinesia, 392
Hypoparathyroidism, 313, 313t
Hypopharynx, 6–7, 236
Hypotension, 308
  treatment of, 201–202
Hypothalamus, 295, 295f
Hypothermia, 369, 369b
Hypothyroidism, 310, 310b
Hypoventilation, 27, 36–37
Hypovolemic shock, 209, 211–213t
Hypoxemia, 36
Hypoxemic hypoxia, 36–37
Hypoxia, 36–37
  airway obstruction to, 36
  differential diagnosis for, 36–37
  hypoxemia and, 36
  management of, 37, 37b
  treatment for, 37

Hypoxic guard, 415
Hypoxic pulmonary vasoconstriction (HPV), 252–253

I
Ibutilide, for arrhythmias, 138t
IC. *See* Inspiratory capacity
Ice-pick view, 391
ICM. *See* Intravenous contrast medium
ICP. *See* Increased intracranial pressure
Idiopathic hypertension, 199
Increased intracranial pressure (ICP), 404
Indacaterol, 131t
Indapamide, generic, 141t
Induction, 94
Induction agents, 97–99, 98b, 99b
  dexmedetomidine, 97
  etomidate, 97–98
  ketamine, 98–99, 98b
  propofol, 97
Inert gas dilution test, 244–245
Inferior alveolar arteries, of oral cavity, 6
Inferior alveolar nerves, of oral cavity, 6
Inferior laryngeal artery, 12–13
Inferior nasal turbinates, 1
Inferior pharyngeal constrictor, 7
Inferior thyroid artery, 12–13
Inferior vallecula, 9
Infrahyoid muscles, 11, 11b
Infrared absorption analysis, 406
Infrared spectroscopy, 406
Inhalation anesthetics, 86–94, 93–94b
  advantages and disadvantages of, 91t
  agents, 87–94, 92–93t
  cardiovascular effects of, 90t
  characteristics of, 86t
  effects of, 90t
  implications, 86
  mechanisms of action of, 87b
  metabolism of, 90t
  on neurophysiologic monitoring of evoked potentials, 88t
  nitrous oxide, 86–87, 91t, 92f, 92b, 93–94b
  potencies of, in human, 90t
Inhalation route of administration, 82t
Inspection, in cardiovascular system monitoring, 375
Inspiratory capacity (IC), 20, 245, 245t
Inspiratory force, 109–110t
Inspiratory muscles, 243, 243f
Inspiratory reserve volume (IRV), 19, 244, 245t
Insulin, 181–183, 183b, 293–294t
  anesthetic implications of, 181
  effects of, 182
  intraoperative concerns in, 181
  in postoperative period, 181
Insulin *(Continued)*
  preoperative concerns in, 181
  preparations, 182, 183t
  timing of effects, 182–183
  in type 1 diabetes mellitus, 183
Interarterial catheter, placed with full barrier precautions, 374
Interarytenoid, 11, 12t
Interincisor gap (mouth opening), 44–45
Intermediate-level disinfection, 372
Internal intercostal muscle, 244
Internodal pathway, 213
Intracranial hypertension, 275–277, 276f, 277b
  anesthetic considerations for, 277, 278t
  etiology of, 276
  signs and symptoms associated with increased ICP, 276
  treatment for, 276–277
Intracranial pressure monitoring, 405–406
Intramuscular route of administration, 82t
Intranasal route of administration, 82t
Intraoperative bronchospasm, asthma and, 254, 255b
Intraoperative rhythm disturbances, 137–138
Intraosseous route of administration, 82t
Intraparenchymal probes, 405
Intrapulmonary pressure, 247
Intrathecal route of administration, 82t
Intravenous catheter, placed with full barrier precautions, 374
Intravenous contrast medium (ICM), 186
Intravenous dyes, 186–187, 186b, 187b
Intravenous route of administration, 82t
Intravenous solutions, expiration time for, 374
Intraventricular catheter, 405
Intrinsic activity, 80
Intrinsic laryngeal abductor muscles, 11
Intrinsic laryngeal adductor muscles, 11
Intrinsic laryngeal tensor muscles, 11
Intrinsic musculature, 11, 12f, 12t
Intrinsic restrictive pulmonary diseases, 257–260, 258t
Intubation stylets, 50–51
Inulin, 346
Inverse agonist, 80
Inverse steal phenomenon, 231
Ipratropium, 131t
Irritant receptors, regulation of respiration and, 241–242
IRV. *See* Inspiratory reserve volume
Ischemic cerebrovascular accident
  etiology of, 281
  treatment of, 282, 282b
Ischemic hypoxia, 36
Isopropyl alcohol-containing caps, injection ports covered with, 373
Isoproterenol (Isuprel), doses of, 127t
IV bags, spiking, 374

J
Jaundice, 331–332
Joint proprioceptors and mechanoreceptors, regulation of respiration and, 242
Jugular bulb oxygen venous saturation, 404
Juxtacapillary receptors, 23
  regulation of respiration and, 242
Juxtamedullary nephrons, 343, 344f

K
Kava, 179t
Ketamine, 98–99, 98b
Kidneys, alternative functions of, 356, 356b

L
Labetalol (Trandate, Normodyne), 129–130
  for hypertension, 134t
Labetalol generic, 129t
Lacosamide (Vimpat), for seizure, 280t
β-Lactams, 161t
Lambert-Eaton myasthenic syndrome (LEMS), 290, 291f, 292b
  anesthetic considerations for, 292
  etiology of, 290
  signs and symptoms of, 290
  treatment of, 290, 291t
Laminar flow, 17
Laryngeal cavity, obstructions of, 34–35
Laryngeal edema, 31
Laryngeal inlet, 11
Laryngeal musculature, 11
Laryngeal prominence, 10
Laryngeal topicalization, 41
Laryngomalacia, 30
Laryngopharynx, 6–7
Laryngoscopy, direct, 52–54, 53f
Laryngospasm, 34
Larynx, anatomy of, 8–13
Lateral cricoarytenoid muscles, 11, 12t
Lead selection, electrocardiographic, 377–378, 378f, 379f
Left bundle branches, in cardiac conduction pathway, 213
LEMS. *See* Lambert-Eaton myasthenic syndrome
Leptin, 293–294t
Levetiracetam (Keppra), for seizure, 280t
Lidocaine, 39
  in cauda equina syndrome (CES), 150
Ligand, 81
Linagliptin (Tradjenta), for type 2 diabetes mellitus, 185t
Lincosamides, 161t
Lingual arterial branches, of oral cavity, 6
Lingual nerve, of oral cavity, 6

Lingual tonsil, 7
Lingual tonsillar hyperplasia, 78–79
Lingual tonsillar hypertrophy, 7, 47
Lipid-lowering agents, 187–188, 187t, 188b
Liraglutide (Victoza), for type 2 diabetes mellitus, 185t
Lispro (Humalog), 183t
Liver, 314
  anatomy of, 315f, 316f
Lixisenatide (Lyxumia), for type 2 diabetes mellitus, 185t
LMWH. *See* Low-molecular-weight heparin
Local anesthetic systemic toxicity, 152–153, 153b
Local anesthetics, 147–153, 153b
  on cancer, 103t
  clinical differences between ester- and amide-type, 149t
  clinical effects associated with neuraxial anesthesia, 148, 149b
  implications of, 147–148
  local anesthetic systemic toxicity, 152–153, 153b
  local tissue toxicity, 150–151
  nerve fiber characteristics and sensitivity to, 148t
  side effects associated with, 148–150
  sustained release of, 151–152
  tumescent local anesthesia (TLA), 151
Local tissue toxicity, 150–151
Loop diuretics, 140, 141t
Loop of Henle
  reabsorption, 353–354
  secretion, 354
Loratadine (Claritin), 175–176t
Lorazepam (Ativan), for seizure, 280t
Lovastatin (Mevacor), 187t
Low-level disinfection, 372
Low-molecular-weight heparin (LMWH), 164t
  in patients receiving antithrombotic therapy, 165–166t
  for VTE, 169t
Lower airway, 13–17
  obstruction, 35–36
    causes of, 34–36
Ludwig angina, 34
Lung capacities, 20
Lung disease, obstructive *versus* restrictive, 253–264, 253f
Lung volumes, 244–246, 244f, 245t
Lung zones, 247–248, 248f
Luteinizing hormone, 293–294t

M

MAC. *See* Minimum alveolar concentration
MAC-BAR. *See* Minimum alveolar concentration-block adrenergic responses
Macroglossia, 28
Macrolides, 161t
Magnesium hydroxide (Milk of Magnesia), 154
Malignant hyperthermia, 369–371, 371b
Mallampati classification, 44, 45f
Mandibular hypoplasia, 28
Mandibular protrusion test, 45, 46f
Mannitol, 140
MAO-B inhibitors, for Parkinson disease, 156–157t
MAOIs. *See* Monoamine oxidase inhibitors
Mass spectrometry, 407
Maxillary hypoplasia, 28
Maxillary sinuses, 2
Mean effect time, 84t
Mechanical dead space, 21, 251
Median eminence, 295
Meglitinide, for type 2 diabetes mellitus, 184, 185t
MEPs. *See* Motor evoked potentials
Metabolic acidosis, chronic kidney disease and, 362
Metformin (glucophage), for type 2 diabetes mellitus, 185t
Metformin extended release, for type 2 diabetes mellitus, 185t
Methemoglobinemia, 40, 148–150, 150b, 150t, 238
Methylene blue, angiotensin axis blockers and, 135
Methylergonovine (Methergine), 195
Metoclopramide (Reglan), 174t
Metolazone (Zaroxolyn), 141t
Metoprolol (Lopressor, Toprol-XL), 129, 129t
  for arrhythmias, 138t
Microcephaly, 28
Micrognathia, 28
Microstomia, 28
Micturition, 340–341
Midazolam (Versed), 96–97
  for seizure, 280t
Middle nasal turbinate, 1
Miglitol, for type 2 diabetes mellitus, 185t
Milk-alkali syndrome, 154
Milrinone (Primacor), 126t, 188–189
  doses of, 127t
Minimum alveolar concentration (MAC), 92–93t
Minimum alveolar concentration awake (MAC awake), 92–93t
Minimum alveolar concentration-block adrenergic responses (MAC-BAR), 92–93t
Mirapex (Boehringer Ingelheim), for Parkinson disease, 156–157t
Mirapex ER, for Parkinson disease, 156–157t
Mitral regurgitation, 204–205, 204f
Mitral stenosis, 202–204
  anesthetic considerations for, 203–204
  diagnostic testing/intraoperative monitoring for, 203
  intraoperative hemodynamic considerations for, 203
  medical/surgical therapy for, 202–203
  pathophysiology of, 202, 203f
Mixed venous oxygen saturation, 388
Mobitz type I, 219
Mobitz type II, 219
Monoamine oxidase inhibitors (MAOIs), 190t, 192
Monro-Kellie hypothesis, 276
Motor endplate, 394
Motor evoked potentials (MEPs), 402, 403t
Mouth, anatomy of, 4–6
Mucus
  creation of, 23–24
  management of, 24
  plug, 72
Multiple endocrine neoplasia, manifestations of, 306t
Muscle rigidity, as opiates effects, 101
Muscles, of respiration, 242–244, 243f, 252–253b
Myasthenia gravis, 289, 291f, 291t, 292b
  anesthetic considerations for, 290–292
  etiology of, 290
  signs and symptoms of, 290
  treatment of, 290
Myasthenic crisis, 292
Mylohyoid paired muscles, 5
Myocardial ischemia, treatment of intraoperative, 225, 226t
Myogenic mechanism, 342

N

Nadolol (Corgard), 129t
Nasal arteries, posterior lateral, 2
Nasal awake intubation, 56
Nasal cannulas, 47
Nasal cavity
  anatomy of, 1–4
  obstructions of, 34
  openings, anatomy of, 2
Nasal topicalization, 40
Nasociliary nerve, 4
Nasolacrimal duct, 2
Nasopalatine nerves
  of nasal cavity, 4
  of oral cavity, 6
Nasopharynx, 6–7
Nateglinide (Starlix), for type 2 diabetes mellitus, 185t
Nausea and vomiting
  as opiates effects, 101
  risk factors for, 172b

Near-infrared spectroscopy (NIRS), 402–404
Nebivolol (Bystolic), 129t
Needle cricothyrotomy, with transtracheal jet ventilation, 57, 57f
Negative deflection waveforms, 381f, 383
Neostigmine (Prostigmin), 112–114
Nephrolithiasis, 366
Nephron, 341f
Nephrotic syndrome, 366
Nervous supply
  of larynx, 13
  of nasal cavity, 4
  of oral cavity, 6
  of pharynx, 7–8
Nesiritide (Natrecor), doses of, 127t
Neural regulation, 345
Neuraxial anesthesia
  on cancer, 103t
  for hypertension, 201
  in patients receiving antithrombotic therapy, 165–166t
Neurogenic shock, 210, 211–213t
Neurologic system, 270–292, 270f
  regulation of cerebral blood flow and, 272–275
Neuromuscular blockade monitoring, 394–398
  neurostimulation, 395–398, 396t
  other mechanisms of, 395
  physiology, 394–395, 394f
Neuromuscular blockade reversal, 112b
  strategies for, 116t
Neuromuscular blocking agents (NMBAs), 106–112, 112b, 113t, 394
  administration of, 111–112, 111b
  cardiac effects of, 112b
  characteristics of, 106, 107b, 108t
  common clinical signs of recovery from, 118b
  depolarizing muscle relaxant, 106, 107t
  guidelines for neuromuscular monitoring, 108–111, 109–110t, 109t, 110f, 111b, 111t
  histamine, 111–112, 111b
  nondepolarizing muscle relaxants, 106
Neuromuscular disorders, 265t
Neuromuscular junction (NMJ), 394, 394f
Neurophysiology, 272–275, 275b
Neurostimulation, 395–398, 396t
  sites of, 397–398
NIBP. *See* Noninvasive blood pressure
Nicardipine (Cardene IV), for hypertension, 134t
Nimodipine, 131
NIRS. *See* Near-infrared spectroscopy
Nitrogen washout test, 245
Nitroglycerin, for hypertension, 134t
Nitroimidazoles, 161t
Nitrous oxide, 86–87, 91t, 92f, 92b, 93–94b
  on cancer, 103t
Nitrovasodilators, 135–137
Nizatidine, 175–176t
NMBAs. *See* Neuromuscular blocking agents
NMJ. *See* Neuromuscular junction
Nonalcoholic steatohepatitis, 328
Noncardiac surgery, antiplatelet drugs and, 163, 167b
Nondepolarizing muscle relaxant, 395
Nondisposable pulse oximeters, 408
Noninvasive blood pressure (NIBP), 388–389
Nonrebreathing facemasks, 47–48
Nonshockable pulseless cardiac rhythms, 220–221, 221b, 222t
Nonstatin lipid-lowering agents, 187
Nonsteroidal antiinflammatory drugs (NSAIDs), 141–144, 143t, 144b
  acetaminophen (Ofirmev), 144
  anesthesia implications of, 141, 142f
  on cancer, 103t
  clinical uses of, 143
  ketorolac, 143–144
  meloxicam (Mobic), 144
  perioperative concerns associated with, 142–143b
Nonsteroidal antiinflammatory drugs (NSAIDs), as antithrombotic medications, 164t
Nonsulfonylurea secretagogues, 184
Norepinephrine (Levophed), 126t, 293–294t
  doses of, 127t
Nose, anatomy of, 1–4
Nosebleed, 2
Nosocomial, definition of, 372
NPH, 183t
NSAIDs. *See* Nonsteroidal antiinflammatory drugs
Nurse anesthesia, standards for, 422–423

O

Obesity, in inhalation anesthetic pharmacokinetic concepts, 92–93t
Oblique arytenoid muscle, 11, 12t
Obstructive diseases, of respiratory system, 253–257, 257b
  asthma, 253–254
  bronchiectasis, 256
  chronic obstructive pulmonary disease, 254–256
  cystic fibrosis, 256–257
Obstructive shock, 209, 211–213t
Obstructive sleep apnea, 31, 32b, 264, 269–270b
  anesthetic considerations in, 264
  etiology of, 264
  signs and symptoms of, 264
  treatment and management of, 264
Obstructive uropathy, chronic kidney disease and, 360t
Oil/gas solubility coefficient, 92–93t
Olfactory nerve, 4
Olfactory region, 1
Ondansetron (Zofran), 174t
1, 25-dihydroxycholecalciferol, 293–294t
Opiates, 99–106, 105–106b
  actions produced by, 100t
  anesthetic implications, 104–106
  cancer and, 102, 103t
  cardiac effects of, 101–102
  central nervous system effects of, 100–101
  clinical effects of, 101b
  endocrinologic effects of, 102
  gastrointestinal effects of, 102
  implications of, 99
  methadone, 104, 105t
  mixed agonist/antagonists, 104
  neuraxial effects of, 102–104
  opioid antagonist, 104
  partial agonist, 104
  side effects of, 100t
Opioids, on cancer, 103t
Optic nerve sheath diameter assessment, 405–406
Oral abscesses, 32
Oral awake intubation, 56, 56f
Oral cavity
  anatomy of, 4–6
  floor, 5
  obstructions of, 34
  skeletal framework of, 5
  structures, 4–5
Oral route of administration, 82t
Oral topicalization, 40–41, 41f
Oropharyngeal cavity, obstructions of, 34
Oropharynx, 6–7
Osmosis, 349–350
Osmotic diuretics, 140
Oxygen
  diffusion of, 238
  examples of decreased environmental, 37
  transport and delivery of, 21–22, 238
Oxygen analysis, 407, 415
Oxygen analyzers, 410–411
Oxygen delivery devices, 47–50
Oxygen extraction ratio, 248–249
Oxygen pipeline pressure, loss of, 413, 413b
Oxygen saturation, of hemoglobin, 196
Oxyhemoglobin dissociation curve, 23, 249–250, 249f
Oxymetazoline spray, 40
Oxytocin (Pitocin), 195, 293–294t

P

P wave, 213
PAC. *See* Pulmonary artery catheter

$PaCO_2$, in hemoglobin, 23
Paired laryngeal cartilages, 9f, 10–11
Palatine arteries
 descending, of nasal cavity, 2
 greater
  of nasal cavity, 2
  of oral cavity, 6
 lesser, of oral cavity, 6
Palatine nerve
 greater
  of nasal cavity, 4
  of oral cavity, 6
 lesser, of oral cavity, 6
Palatine tonsils, 7
Palatopharyngeus muscles, 7
Palpation, in cardiovascular system monitoring, 375
PAOP. *See* Pulmonary artery occlusive pressure
Papillae, 5
Parasympathetic nervous system, 272, 273–274t
Parathyroid gland dysfunction, 312, 313–314b
Parathyroid hormone, 293–294t, 350t, 351
Parkinson disease, treatment of, 155b, 156–157t
Parotid glands, 5
Partial agonist, 80
Partial pressure, 237–238
Passive reabsorption, 349–350
PDEs. *See* Phosphodiesterases
Peak airway pressure, 18
Pediatrics, in inhalation anesthetic pharmacokinetic concepts, 92–93t
PEEP. *See* Positive end-expiratory pressure
Penbutolol (Levatol), 129t
Pendin, 354–355
Percentage of glottic opening (POGO), 45–46
Perforomist (Dey), 131t
Peripheral chemoreceptors, regulation of respiration and, 241
Peripheral nerve injuries, 287–289, 287b, 288–289t, 289b
Peripheral nervous system, 270
pH, in hemoglobin, 23
Pharmacodynamics, 80–81
Pharmacogenomics, 85
Pharmacokinetics, 81–85
 binding of drugs to plasma proteins, 81
 drug distribution, 82–83, 83t
 drug metabolism, 83, 83b, 84t
 elimination of drugs by kidney, 85
 movement of drugs across cellular barriers, 81–82
 routes of administration, 82, 82t
Pharmacology, 80–4, 86b
 β–adrenergic blocking agents, 128–130, 130b
  clinical use of, 128, 129t
  esmolol, 129
  implications of, 128b
  labetalol, 129–130
  metoprolol, 129
 anesthesia induction medications, 94–97
  benzodiazepines, 94–97, 96t, 97b
  flumazenil (Romazicon), 97
  implications of, 94, 95t, 96t
  midazolam (Versed), 96–97
 antiarrhythmics, 137–138, 138t
 antibiotics, 155–163, 163b
  administration of, 161
  anesthetic implications of, 155
  antibiotic allergy, 162, 162b
  antibiotic-anesthetic drug interactions, 162–163
  clinical uses of, 157–161, 158–160t, 158b, 161t, 162t
 anticholinergics, 118–120, 119t, 120b
 anticholinesterase agents, 112–114
 anticoagulants, 163–168, 164t, 165–166t, 165b, 166b, 168b
  anesthetic implications of, 163
  antifibrinolytics, 166–168
  antiplatelet drugs and noncardiac surgery, 163, 167b
  thromboembolism, 166, 168b, 169t, 170t, 171t
 antiemetics, 168–173, 173b
  anesthetic implications of, 168
  clinical use of, 173, 174t
  glucocorticoids, 169
  5-HT_3 receptor antagonists, 169–172, 172b, 174t
  metoclopramide, 173
  multimodal antiemetic therapy, 168, 172b
  neurokinin 1 receptor antagonists, 172, 174t
  risk factors for, 168, 172b
  transdermal scopolamine, 172
 antiepileptic drugs, 176–177, 177b, 177t
 antihypertensive agents, 132–135
  anesthesia management of patients taking angiotensin axis blockers, 135
  anesthetic implications of, 132, 133t
  angiotensin 2 receptor antagonists, 134
  angiotensin-converting enzyme inhibitors, 133–134
  centrally acting α_2-agonists, 133
  hypertension, 132–133, 134t
 antiparkinsonian drugs, 155, 155b, 156–157t
Pharmacology *(Continued)*
 bronchodilators, 130, 130b, 131t
 calcium channel blockers, 130–132, 132b, 132t
 corticosteroids, 193–194, 194b, 194t, 195t
 dantrolene, 177–178, 178b
 digitalis, 138–139, 139b, 139f, 140t
 diuretics, 140–141, 141b
  anesthetic implications of, 140
  hypertension and, 140–141, 141t
  types of, 140
 drug interaction terminology, 85t
 herbal supplements, 178–181, 181b
  adverse effects and drug interactions, 180–181, 180t
  anesthesia implications of, 178, 179t
  dietary supplements, 178–180
 histamine receptor antagonists, 174–176, 175–176t, 176b
 induction agents, 97–99, 98b, 99b
  dexmedetomidine, 97
  etomidate, 97–98
  ketamine, 98–99, 98b
  propofol, 97
 inhalation anesthetics, 86–94, 93–94b
  advantages and disadvantages of, 91t
  agents, 87–94, 92–93t
  cardiovascular effects of, 90t
  characteristics of, 86t
  effects of, 90t
  implications, 86
  mechanisms of action of, 87b
  metabolism of, 90t
  on neurophysiologic monitoring of evoked potentials, 88t
  nitrous oxide, 86–87, 91t, 92f, 92b, 93–94b
  potencies of, in human, 90t
 insulin, 181–183, 183b
  anesthetic implications of, 181
  effects of, 182
  intraoperative concerns in, 181
  in postoperative period, 181
  preoperative concerns in, 181
  preparations, 182, 183t
  timing of effects, 182–183
  in type 1 diabetes mellitus, 183
 intravenous dyes, 186–187, 186b, 187b
 lipid-lowering agents, 187–188, 187t, 188b
 local anesthetics, 147–153, 153b
  clinical differences between ester- and amide-type, 149t
  clinical effects associated with neuraxial anesthesia, 148, 149b
  implications of, 147–148
  local anesthetic systemic toxicity, 152–153, 153b
  local tissue toxicity, 150–151

Pharmacology (Continued)
nerve fiber characteristics and sensitivity to, 148t
side effects associated with, 148–150
sustained release of, 151–152
tumescent local anesthesia (TLA), 151
miscellaneous analgesics, 145–147, 147b
anesthetic implications of, 145, 145t
anticonvulsants, 145
antidepressants, 146, 146t
corticosteroids, 146–147, 147b
neuromuscular blocking agents, 106–112, 112b, 113t
administration of, 111–112, 111b,
cardiac effects of, 112b
characteristics of, 106, 107b, 109t
depolarizing muscle relaxant, 106, 107t
guidelines for neuromuscular monitoring, 108–111, 109–110t, 109t, 110f, 111b, 111t
histamine, 111–112, 112b111b,
nondepolarizing muscle relaxants, 106
nonsteroidal antiinflammatory agents, 141–144, 143t, 144b
acetaminophen (Ofirmev), 144
anesthesia implications of, 141, 142f
clinical uses of, 143
ketorolac, 143–144
meloxicam (Mobic), 144
perioperative concerns associated with, 142–143b
opiates, 99–106, 105–106b
actions produced by, 100t
cancer and, 102, 103t
cardiac effects of, 101–102
central nervous system effects of, 100–101
clinical effects of, 101b
endocrinologic effects of, 102
gastrointestinal effects of, 102
implications of, 99
methadone, 104, 105t
mixed agonist/antagonists, 104
neuraxial effects of, 102–104
opioid antagonist, 104
partial agonist, 104
side effects of, 100t
oral antacids, 154–155, 155b
oral hypoglycemics, 183–184, 184b, 185t
pharmacodynamics, 80–81
pharmacogenomics, 85
pharmacokinetics, 81–85
binding of drugs to plasma proteins, 81
drug distribution, 82–83, 83t
drug metabolism, 83, 83b, 84t
elimination of drugs by kidney, 85
movement of drugs across cellular barriers, 81–82
routes of administration, 82, 82t
Pharmacology (Continued)
phosphodiesterase inhibitors, 188–189, 189b
psychopharmacology, 189–193, 193b
anesthesia implications of, 189–193
antidepressants, 189, 190t
antipsychotics, 192–193
monoamine oxidase inhibitors (MAOIs), 192
selective norepinephrine and serotonin reuptake inhibitors (SNRIs), 192
selective serotonin reuptake inhibitors, 189–191
tricyclic antidepressants, 191–192
α-receptor blocking agents, 125–128, 128b
selective muscle relaxant binding agent, 115–117, 115b, 116t, 117b, 118b
sympathomimetic amines, 120–124, 124b, 128b
dobutamine, 124
dopamine, 122–124
ephedrine, 124
epinephrine, 120–122
implications of, 120–124, 121–122t, 123t
norepinephrine, 122
phenylephrine, 124
vasopressin, 125–124, 126t, 127t
uterotonics, 194–195, 195b
vasodilators, 135–137, 136–137b
hydralazine, 136
nitric oxide (NO), inhaled, 136–137
nitroglycerin, 135–136
sodium nitroprusside, 135
Pharyngeal cavity, obstructions of, 34–35
Pharyngeal muscles, 7, 11, 11b
Pharyngeal plexus, 7
Pharyngeal sphincter, inferior, 7
Pharyngeal tonsil, 7
Pharynx, 236
anatomy of, 8–13
Phenobarbital (phenobarbital sodium; Luminal), for seizure, 280t
Phenothiazine, 175–176t
Phenoxybenzamine (Dibenzyline), 125
Phentolamine, 125
doses of, 127t
Phenylephrine (Neo-Synephrine), 126t
doses of, 127t
spray, 39–40
Phenytoin sodium (Dilantin), for seizure, 280t
Pheochromocytoma, 304–306, 306t, 309b
anesthesia case management of, 306
clinical manifestations of, 306b
intraoperative period of, 307–308, 308b
pharmacologic therapy of, 306–307
postoperative period of, 308–309
preoperative period of, 306, 307t
Phosphodiesterase 3 (PDE3) inhibitors, 188
Phosphodiesterase inhibitors, 188–189, 189b
Phosphodiesterases (PDEs), 188
Physiologic dead space, 21, 251
Physiologic difficult airway, flexible intubating bronchoscopes for, 51–52
Physostigmine (Antilirium), 114
Pin Index Safety System (PISS), 414
Pindolol generic, 129t
Pioglitazone (Actos), for type 2 diabetes mellitus, 185t
Pipeline supply, 413
configuration of, 413
oxygen pipeline pressure, loss of, 413, 413b
Piperazine, 175–176t
Piperidine, 175–176t
PISS. *See* Pin Index Safety System
Pitavastatin (Livalo), 187t
Pituitary gland
anterior, 295–299, 296f
posterior, dysfunction of, 298, 299b
Plasma cholinesterase, 111t
Plateau pressure, 18–19
Pleural effusion, 265t
Pleural pressure, 246–247
Pneumocytes, 16
Pneumonia, 238
Pneumotaxic center, pontine respiratory control and, 241
Pneumothorax, 74, 75b, 265t
Podocytes, 345
POGO. *See* Percentage of glottic opening
Poiseuille's law, 17
Polycystic kidney disease, 366–367
Polycystic kidney disease, chronic kidney disease and, 360t
Polymyxins, 161t
Pores of Kohn, 16
Positive end-expiratory pressure (PEEP), 17
Posterior cricoarytenoid muscles, 11, 12t
Posterior ethmoidal nerves, 4
Posterior pituitary hormones, 296, 297f
Postictal phase, of seizures, 278–279
Postoperative visual loss, 285–287, 286b, 287b
Posttetanic count test, 109t
Potassium-sparing diuretics, 140, 141t
Potency, 80
Potentiation, in drug interaction terminology, 85t
Pramipexole, for Parkinson disease, 156–157t
Pramlintide (Symlin), 184
Prasugrel, 164t
Pravastatin (Pravachol), 187t
Prazosin (Minipress), 125–128
Precordial stethoscope, 409–410

Pregabalin, 145, 177
Pregnancy, in inhalation anesthetic pharmacokinetic concepts, 92–93t
Preload, 198–199, 199t
Premature ventricular contractions (PVCs), 383
Preoxygenation, 63–64
Pressure-controlled ventilation, 416
with volume guarantee, 417
Pressure support ventilation (PSV), 417, 417b
Pressure waveforms
correlation of, 383, 383f
distortion of, 383–384, 384b, 384f
pulmonary artery, 382
pulmonary artery occlusive, 382, 382f
right atrial, 381–382, 381f, 381t
right ventricular, 382, 382f
Prilocaine, 39, 150
Primary adrenal insufficiency, clinical features of, 194t
Primary aldosteronism, 302
Primary hypertension, 199
Prochlorperazine (Compazine), 174t
Progesterone, 293–294t
Prognathia, 28
Prolactin, 293–294t
Prolactin-inhibiting factor, 293–294t
Promethazine (Phenergan), 174t, 175–176t
Propofol, 26, 97
Propranolol (Inderal), 129t
Proximal tubule reabsorption, 353
Proximal tubule secretion, 353
Pruritus, as opiates effects, 101–102
PSV. *See* Pressure support ventilation
Psychopharmacology, 189–193, 193b
anesthesia implications of, 189–193
antidepressants, 189, 190t
antipsychotics, 192–193
monoamine oxidase inhibitors (MAOIs), 192
selective norepinephrine and serotonin reuptake inhibitors (SNRIs), 192
selective serotonin reuptake inhibitors, 189–191
tricyclic antidepressants, 191–192
Pulmonary alveolar proteinosis, 258t
Pulmonary artery catheter (PAC), 381
Pulmonary artery occlusive pressure (PAOP), 380
waveform, 382, 382f
Pulmonary artery pressure (PA), 380
waveform, 382
Pulmonary artery vascular resistance (PVR), 386
Pulmonary edema, 37–38, 260, 261t
acute, 71–72
Pulmonary embolism, 73–74, 268–270
Pulmonary fibrosis, 258t
Pulmonary function, mechanisms of, 242–253, 246b
Pulmonary perfusion imbalances, 27
Pulmonary sarcoidosis, 258t
Pulmonary shunt, 251–252
Pulmonary shunting, 27
Pulmonary ventilation, 237
Pulmonary ventilation volumes, 19f
Pulse oximetry, 407–408
Purkinje fibers, 213
PVCs. *See* Premature ventricular contractions
PVR. *See* Pulmonary artery vascular resistance
Pyriform sinuses, 7
Pyrilamine (Triaminic), 175–176t

Q
QRS complex, 215
QT interval, 215
Quantal drug response, 81

R
Radiation, 368
Raman scattering analysis, 406–407
Raman spectroscopy, 406–407
Ranitidine (Zantac), 175–176t
Rapid sequence induction, 62
Rasagiline, for Parkinson disease, 156–157t
RBCs. *See* Red blood cells
Receptor adaptation, 81
α–receptor antagonists, 125–128
α–receptor blocking agents, 125–128, 128b
Rectal route of administration, 82t
Recurrent laryngeal nerve (RLN), 8, 13
damage of, 76–77
Red blood cells (RBCs), 391
Refractory period, in cardiac conduction system, 215, 217f, 217t
Refractory status epilepticus, medications for, 280
Regional anesthesia, for carotid endarterectomy, 231
Regular (Humulin R, Novolin R), 183t
Relative refractory period, 215
Renal autoregulation, 342
Renal blood flow, 342–343
Renal cortex, 340
Renal excretion, 355–356
Renal medulla, 340
Renal pelvis, 340
Renal plasma flow, 345
Renal system, 339–368, 346b
alternative functions of, 356, 356b
longitudinal section of, 340f
pathophysiologic concepts, 357–360
physiology, 341–342
position, 339f
transplantation, 364–365, 365b
Renal tubular reabsorption, 347–352, 348f, 349t, 350t, 352b
sites of, 353–356, 355–356b
Renal tubular secretion, 348f, 349t, 351–352, 352b
sites of, 353–356, 355–356b
Renin, 133, 293–294t
Renovascular hypertension, 367
Repaglinide (Prandin), for type 2 diabetes mellitus, 185t
Requip (GSK), for Parkinson disease, 156–157t
Residual neuromuscular block
adverse effects of, 117b
factors influencing the incidence of postoperative, 118b
Residual volume (RV), 19–20, 244, 245t
Resorption atelectasis, 16
Respiration
monitoring, 407–411
regulation of, 239–242
Respiratory bronchioles, 15–16
Respiratory conduction region, 1
Respiratory depression, as opiates effects, 101
Respiratory drive, decreased, 36
Respiratory system, 236–270, 237f
lung zones and, 247–248, 248f
pathophysiologic concepts with, 253–270
physiology of breathing and, 237–242
Resterilization, definition of, 372
Restrictive diseases, of respiratory system, 253, 257–264, 260b
extrinsic restrictive pulmonary disease, 264, 264b, 265t
intrinsic restrictive pulmonary diseases, 257–260, 258t
pulmonary edema, 260, 261t
Retrognathia, 28
Retrograde intubation, 58–60
Retropharyngeal abscesses, 32
Reusable laryngoscopes, 373
Revonto, 178
Rheumatoid arthritis, 33
Right atrial pressure waveform, 381–382, 381f, 381t
Right bundle branches, in cardiac conduction pathway, 213
Right ventricular end-diastolic pressure (RVEDP), 382
Right ventricular end-diastolic volume (RVEDV), 382
Right ventricular pressure (RV), 380
waveform, 382, 382f
Rima glottidis, 8
Rivaroxaban, 164t
in patients receiving antithrombotic therapy, 165–166t

Rolapitant (Varubi), 174t
Ropinirole, for Parkinson disease, 156–157t
Rosiglitazone (Avandia), for type 2 diabetes mellitus, 185t
Rosuvastatin (Crestor), 187t
Rotigotine, for Parkinson disease, 156–157t
RSI. *See* Rapid sequence induction
RVEDP. *See* Right ventricular end-diastolic pressure
RVEDV. *See* Right ventricular end-diastolic volume
Ryanodex, 178
Rytary (Impax), for Parkinson disease, 156–157t

S

Safinamide, for Parkinson disease, 156–157t
Salmeterol, 131t
Salpingopharyngeus muscle, 7
Saxagliptin (Onglyza), for type 2 diabetes mellitus, 185t
SBP. *See* Systolic blood pressure
Scavenging systems, 419
SCIP. *See* Surgical Care Improvement Project
Scopolamine, 119
Scopolamine transdermal (Transderm-Scop), 174t
Second-gas effect, 92–93t
Second-generation H_1-type antihistamines, 175–176t
Secretin, 293–294t
Sedation medications, 40
Seizures, 277–281, 279t, 281b
  anesthetic considerations for, 280–281
  etiology of, 277–278
  medications/drug misuse, 278
  treatment of, 279–280, 280t
Seldinger technique, 57–58, 59f, 60f
Selective muscle relaxant binding agent, 115–117, 115b, 116t, 117b, 118b
Selective norepinephrine and serotonin reuptake inhibitors (SNRIs), 146t, 190t, 192
Selective serotonin reuptake inhibitors (SSRIs), 146t, 189–191, 190t
Selective β_2–agonists, 130
Selegiline, for Parkinson disease, 156–157t
Sellick maneuver, 10, 62
Sepsis, 210
Septic shock, 210, 211–213t
Serevent Diskus (GSK), 131t
Seromucous glands, 23–24
Serotonin syndrome, 189–191, 191t
Serum creatinine, 346
SGLT2 inhibitor, for type 2 diabetes mellitus, 184, 185t
Shock states, 208–211, 211b
  classification of, 209–210, 210f
  physiology and pathophysiology of, 208–209, 209t
  treatment for, 210–211, 211–213t
Shockable pulseless cardiac rhythms, 220
SIADH. *See* Syndrome of inappropriate antidiuretic secretion
Sildenafil (Viagra, Revatio), 188
Silodosin (Rapaflo), 125–128
Simvastatin (Zocor), 187t
Sinemet (Merck), for Parkinson disease, 156–157t
Sinemet CR (Merck), for Parkinson disease, 156–157t
Single laryngeal cartilages, 9–10, 9f
Single twitch, 395–396, 396t
Single-twitch strength, 109–110t
Single-twitch test, 109t
Single-use laryngoscopes, 373
Sinoatrial node, 213
Sinus bradycardia, 218
Sinus ostium, 2
Sitagliptin (Januvia), for type 2 diabetes mellitus, 185t
Slit pores, 345
SNRIs. *See* Selective norepinephrine and serotonin reuptake inhibitors
Sodium citrate, 154
Sodium nitroprusside (Nitropress)
  doses of, 127t
  for hypertension, 134t
Soft palate, 4
Somatic nervous system, 270
Somatosensory evoked potentials (SSEPs), 389, 400–401, 402f
Spare receptor concept, 80
Sphenoid sinuses, 2
Sphenopalatine artery, 2
Spiriva HandiHaler (Boehringer Ingelheim), 131t
Spironolactone (Aldactone), 140, 141t
SSEPs. *See* Somatosensory evoked potentials
SSI. *See* Surgical site infection
SSRIs. *See* Selective serotonin reuptake inhibitors
St. John's wort, 179t, 180
ST junction, definition of, 375, 376f
ST segment, 215
Stalevo (Orion), for Parkinson disease, 156–157t
Standard precautions, definition of, 372
Staphylococcus aureus, 14
Static lung compliance, 18
Statins, 187, 187t
Status epilepticus, 278
Stenosis
  aortic, 205–206
    anesthetic considerations for, 206
    diagnostic testing/intraoperative monitoring for, 205
    intraoperative hemodynamic considerations for, 205–206
    medical/surgical therapy for, 205
    pathophysiology of, 205
  mitral, 202–204
    anesthetic considerations for, 203–204
    diagnostic testing/intraoperative monitoring for, 203
    intraoperative hemodynamic considerations for, 203
    medical/surgical therapy for, 202–203
    pathophysiology of, 202, 203f
Sterile injectable drugs, expiration time for, 374
Sterilization, definition of, 372
Steroids, preparation of, 195t
STOP-BANG scoring system, 31, 32b, 264
Stopping reflex, regulation of respiration and, 242
Strap muscles, 11
Streptokinase, 164t
Structural heart disease, intraoperative rhythm disturbances and, 137
Stylopharyngeus muscle, 7
Subclavian artery, 7
Subcutaneous route of administration, 82t
Subdural screws (bolts), 405
Subglottic edema, 31
Sublingual glands, 5
Sublingual route of administration, 82t
Subluxation, 33–34
Submandibular glands, 5
Submandibular space infections, 31
Submental arteries, of oral cavity, 6
Succinylcholine chloride, 106, 107b, 107t, 108b
Sugammadex (Bridion), 26, 115–117
Sulfonylurea, for type 2 diabetes mellitus, 184, 185t
Superior alveolar arteries, of oral cavity, 6
Superior alveolar nerves, of oral cavity, 6
Superior laryngeal artery, 12
Superior laryngeal nerve (SLN), 7
Superior laryngeal nerve block, 41–42, 42f
Superior nasal turbinate, 1
Superior pharyngeal constrictor, 7
Superior thyroid artery, 12
Superior vallecula, 9
Supplemental oxygen, on cancer, 103t
Supraglottic airway devices, 48–50, 49t
Suprahyoid muscles, 11, 11b
Supraventricular tachycardia, 218, 218f

Surfactant, decreased, 17
Surgical Care Improvement Project (SCIP), 160
Surgical cricothyrotomy, 57–58, 59f, 60f, 61f
Surgical site infection (SSI), 157, 158b
Surgical wound classification, 162t
Sustained bite, 109–110t
Sustained tetanus, 109–110t
SVR. *See* Systemic vascular resistance
SWMAs. *See* Systolic wall motion abnormalities
Sympathetic nervous system (SNS), 270–272, 351
Sympathomimetic amines, 120–124, 124b, 128b
  dobutamine, 124
  dopamine, 122–124
  ephedrine, 124
  epinephrine, 120–122
  implications of, 120–124, 121–122t, 123t
  norepinephrine, 122
  phenylephrine, 124
  vasopressin, 125–124, 126t, 127t
Synchronized intermittent mandatory ventilation, 416–417
Syndrome of inappropriate antidiuretic secretion (SIADH), 299, 300t
Synergism, in drug interaction terminology, 85t
Syringe
  medication, recap, 374
  reused, 374
Systemic inflammatory response syndrome (SIRS), 208
Systemic vascular resistance (SVR), 386
Systolic blood pressure (SBP), 388–389
Systolic heart failure, 226, 228t
Systolic wall motion abnormalities (SWMAs), 390

T
T wave, 215
Tachyphylaxis, 81
Tamsulosin (Flomax), 125–128
TCAs. *See* Tricyclic antidepressants
TCD. *See* Transcranial Doppler ultrasonography
TDCCO. *See* Thermodilution continuous cardiac output
TEE. *See* Transesophageal echocardiography
Teeth, skeletal framework of, 5
Temperature, in hemoglobin, 23
Tension pneumothorax, 265t
Terazosin (Hytrin), 125
Terminal half-life, 84t
Testosterone, 293–294t
TET. *See* Tetanic stimulation
Tetanic stimulation (TET), 396–397, 396t
Tetanus test, 109t
Tetracyclines, 161t
Therapeutic window, 81
Thermodilution continuous cardiac output (TDCCO), 386
Thermoregulation, 368–371, 369b
Thiazolidinedione, for type 2 diabetes mellitus, 184, 185t
Third-degree heart block, 219, 219f
Thoracic forces, 246–247
Thromboembolism, 166, 168b, 169t, 170t, 171t
Thrombolytics, in patients receiving antithrombotic therapy, 165–166t
Thyroarytenoid, 12t
Thyroarytenoid externus, 11
Thyroarytenoid internus, 11
Thyroepiglottic muscle, 11, 12f
Thyrohyoid membrane, 10
Thyroid cartilage, 10
Thyroid gland dysfunction, 308–310, 309f
  anesthesia case management of, 310
  intraoperative period of, 311
  pathophysiology of, 309–310
  pharmacologic therapy of, 310–311
  postoperative period of, 311–312
  preoperative period of, 310
  signs and symptoms of, 310b
  thyroid storm and, 311, 312b
Thyroid storm, 311
Thyroid-stimulating hormone, 293–294t
Thyromental distance (TMD), 43–44, 44f
Thyrotropin-releasing hormone, 293–294t
Thyroxine, 293–294t
Ticlopidine, 164t
Tidal volume, 109–110t
Timolol generic, 129t
Tiotropium, 131t
Tirofiban, 164t
Tissue plasminogen activator (tPA), 164t
TIVA. *See* Total intravenous anesthetic
TLA. *See* Tumescent local anesthesia
TMJ ankylosis, 33
TOF. *See* Train of Four
Tolcapone, for Parkinson disease, 156–157t
Tolerance, 81
Tongue, 5
Topical anesthesia, 40–41
Topical route of administration, 82t
Torsades de pointes, 220, 221f
Torsemide (Demadex), 141t
Total intravenous anesthetic (TIVA), 401
Total lung capacity, 20, 245t, 246
tPA. *See* Tissue plasminogen activator
Trachea
  anatomy of, 13–14
  obstructions of, 35
  pathology within, 35
  surgery of, 35
  trauma to, 35
Tracheal agenesis, 30
Tracheal cartilaginous anomalies, 30
  sleeve, 30
  tracheal agenesis, 30
  tracheal stenosis, 30
  tracheoesophageal fistula, 30
  tracheomalacia, 30
Tracheal cartilaginous sleeve, 30
Tracheal intubation, 52–54
Tracheal or subglottic stenosis, 31
Tracheal stenosis, 30
Trachealis muscle, 14
Tracheitis, 14
Tracheobronchial tree, 13
  irritant receptors in, 23
Tracheoesophageal fistula, 30
Tracheomalacia, 30
Tracheostomy, 14, 60
Tracheostomy tubes, 60–62
Tracheotomy, 14, 60–62
Trachlight, 50
Traditional open AAA repair, 233–234, 234t, 235t
Train of Four (TOF), 109–110t, 109t, 110f, 396, 396t, 397f
Tranexamic acid (Lysteda), 166–168
Transcranial Doppler ultrasonography (TCD), 404
Transesophageal echocardiography (TEE), 390–393
  fundamental elements of, 391–393, 391f, 393b, 393f
Transient imbalance, intraoperative rhythm disturbances and, 138
Transient ischemia, 224
Transient ischemic attack, etiology of, 281
Transpulmonary pressure, 247
Transtracheal block, 42, 42f
Transtracheal jet ventilation, needle cricothyrotomy with, 57, 57f
Transverse arytenoid, 11, 12t
Traumatic brain injury, 283–285, 284b, 285b
Triamterene (Dyrenium), 141t
Tricyclic antidepressants (TCAs), 146t, 190t, 191–192
Trigeminal nerve
  of nasal cavity, 4
  of oral cavity, 6
  of pharynx, 7
Triiodothyronine, 293–294t
Trimeprazine (Temaril), 175–176t

Trismus, 32–33
Tubal tonsils, 7
Tubuloglomerular feedback mechanism, 342
Tudorza Pressair (Forest), 131t
Tumescent local anesthesia (TLA), 151
Turbinates, 1–2
Turbulent airflow, 17

U

Ultrasonography, of airway, 46–47
Unanticipated difficult airway, 64–65
Unfractionated heparin
  in patients receiving antithrombotic therapy, 165–166t
  for VTE, 169t
Universal precautions, definition of, 372
Upper airway, 1–13
  anatomic abnormalities of, 51
  irritant receptors in, 23
  obstruction, 34–35
    causes of, 34–36
Upper extremity muscles, 397–398, 397f
Upper lip bite test (ULBT), 45
Upper respiratory infection, 268
Upregulation, 81
Urine creatinine clearance, 346
Uterotonics, 194–195, 195b
Uvula, 4

V

Vagus nerve
  of oral cavity, 6
  of pharynx, 8
Valerian, 179t
Valvular heart disease, 202–208
  aortic stenosis, 205–206, 206f
  mitral regurgitation, 204–205
    anesthetic considerations for, 205
    diagnostic testing/intraoperative monitoring for, 204
    intraoperative hemodynamic considerations for, 205
    medical/surgical therapy for, 204
    pathophysiology of, 204
  mitral stenosis, 202–204
Vaporizers, use of, 416
Vascular supply
  of nasal cavity, 2, 3f
  of oral cavity, 3f, 5–6
  of pharynx, 3f, 7
Vasodilators, 135–137, 136–137b
  hydralazine, 136
  nitric oxide (NO), inhaled, 136–137
  nitroglycerin, 135–136
  sodium nitroprusside, 135
Vasopressin (Pitressin), 355. *See also* Antidiuretic hormone
  angiotensin axis blockers and, 135
  doses of, 127t
VCV. *See* Volume-controlled ventilation
Venous drainage, 7
Venous plexus, pharyngeal, 7
Venous thromboembolism (VTE), 163
Ventilation
  critical incidents related to, 417–418
  effect, 92–93t
  modes of, 416–419
  monitoring, 407–411
Ventilation-perfusion abnormalities, 92–93t
Ventilation-perfusion mismatch, 36
Ventral respiratory group, medullary respiratory control and, 240–241
Ventricular fibrillation, 220, 220f
Ventricular folds, 8
Ventricular tachycardia, 220, 220f
Ventriculostomy catheter, 405
VEPs. *See* Visual evoked potentials
Verapamil, 132, 132t
Vestibular folds, 8
Vestibule, 5
Vials, medication, reused, 374
Video laryngoscopes, 373
Video laryngoscopy, 54–55, 55f
Visual evoked potentials (VEPs), 401
Vital capacity, 20, 109–110t, 245, 245t
Vitamin K antagonist, for VTE, 170t
Vocal cord granulomas, 77–78
Vocal cords
  false, 8
  true, 8
Vocal folds, 8
Vocalis, 11, 12t
Voice box, 8
Volatile anesthetic agents, on cancer, 103t
Volume-controlled ventilation (VCV), 416
VTE. *See* Venous thromboembolism

W

Waldeyer tonsillar ring, 7
Warfarin, 164t
  in patients receiving antithrombotic therapy, 165–166t
  for VTE, 170t
Waste anesthetic gases, disposal of, 419, 419b